Molecular Mechanisms Underlying Cancer Prevention and Intervention with Bioactive Food Components

Molecular Mechanisms Underlying Cancer Prevention and Intervention with Bioactive Food Components

Editor

Anupam Bishayee

MDPI • Basel • Beijing • Wuhan • Barcelona • Belgrade • Manchester • Tokyo • Cluj • Tianjin

Editor
Anupam Bishayee
Lake Erie College of
Osteopathic Medicine
Bradenton
United States

Editorial Office
MDPI
St. Alban-Anlage 66
4052 Basel, Switzerland

This is a reprint of articles from the Special Issue published online in the open access journal *Cancers* (ISSN 2072-6694) (available at: www.mdpi.com/journal/cancers/special_issues/Compound).

For citation purposes, cite each article independently as indicated on the article page online and as indicated below:

LastName, A.A.; LastName, B.B.; LastName, C.C. Article Title. *Journal Name* **Year**, *Volume Number*, Page Range.

ISBN 978-3-0365-8383-9 (Hbk)
ISBN 978-3-0365-8382-2 (PDF)

Cover image courtesy of Anupam Bishayee

Contents

About the Editor

Anupam Bishayee

Dr. Bishayee is a Professor of Pharmacology at the Lake Erie College of Osteopathic Medicine (Bradenton, Florida). He received his Ph.D. (cancer prevention) from Jadavpur University, Kolkata, India. Dr. Bishayee performed post-doctoral research at Rutgers University, Newark, New Jersey (formerly University of Medicine and Dentistry of New Jersey). Dr. Bishayee's primary research interest during last two decades encompasses natural products and dietary agents in health and disease. His laboratory is involved in investigating cancer preventive and therapeutic effects of medicinal plants, natural products, dietary and synthetic agents using various pre-clinical models of cancer and underlying mechanisms of action. Various projects of Dr. Bishayee are funded by the National Institutes of Health as well as private pharmaceutical and biotechnological companies. Dr Bishayee has been awarded a United States patent on development of a potential drug for breast cancer prevention and treatment. Dr. Bishayee has published more than 290 peer-reviewed original research papers and authoritative review articles, mostly in high-impact journals, 22 book chapters, and around 84 conference abstracts, and delivered more than 37 invited presentations at various national and international scientific meetings. Dr. Bishayee has been serving various reputed journals as Section Editor-in-Chief, Consulting Editor, Editorial Board Member, and reviewer. Dr. Bishayee edited an Elsevier book "Epigenetics of Cancer Prevention" and guest edited several special issues on natural products and cancer published by leading publishers, such as Elsevier, Springer Nature, MDPI, and Bentham. Dr. Bishayee is a "Highly Cited Researcher" in 2022 and his papers rank in the top 1% by citations for a field or fields (Clarivate, Web of Science). His Scopus h-index is 73 and scholars from all over the world have cited Dr. Bishayee's published work more than 17,000 times.

cancers

MDPI

Editorial

Molecular Mechanisms Underlying Cancer Prevention and Intervention with Bioactive Food Components

Anupam Bishayee

College of Osteopathic Medicine, Lake Erie College of Osteopathic Medicine, Bradenton, FL 34211, USA; abishayee@lecom.edu or abishayee@gmail.com

Cancer is the second-leading cause of death in the world, and it represents a major health challenge. According to the International Agency for Research on Cancer/GLOBOCAN, more than 19 million new cancer cases and almost 10 million cancer deaths occurred in the year 2020 [1]. The overwhelming evidence, which is based on preclinical and clinical studies, clearly indicates that diet can modify cancer outcome. Natural dietary bioactive compounds, present in fruits, vegetables, spices, whole grains, and herbs, have shown enormous potential for cancer prevention and treatment due to their easy availability, relatively low cost, high margin of safety, widespread acceptability, and human consumption.

During the last few decades, an extraordinary number of bioactive food components have been investigated, employing cell culture assays, animal tumor models, and human subjects to understand their potential for cancer prevention and treatment. I am pleased to introduce this Special Issue, which captures recent advances in our knowledge on cancer preventive and therapeutic efficacy of putative food-derived substances with understanding of the underlying cellular and molecular mechanisms of action. This thematic issue contains five original research papers and eight review articles.

Phannasorn and coinvestigators [2] evaluated the chemopreventive effects of riceberry bran oil, containing phytosterols, γ-oryzanol, and γ-tocotrienol, in chemically induced liver and colon carcinogenesis in rats. Oral administration of riceberry bran oil suppressed preneoplastic hepatic lesions and colorectal aberrant crypt foci, induced hepatocellular and colorectal cell apoptosis, and reduced the expression of proinflammatory cytokines. Additionally, the oil promoted the alteration of gut microbiota in both tumor models. This outcome of these experimental results indicates the potential health benefits of the consumption of rice constituents in preventing hepatic and colorectal cancers.

β-Caryophyllene is the primary sesquiterpene present in black pepper, cloves, hops, rosemary, copaiba, and cannabis. It has been recognized as the first known "dietary cannabinoid," a common component of food with a "Generally Recognized as Safe" status. It is approved by the United States Food and Drug Administration as a taste enhancer, food additive, and flavoring agent. According to a study conducted by Mannino and colleagues [3], β-caryophyllene has been found to suppress cell proliferation and to induce apoptosis by impacting the crosstalk between Akt, β-catenin, and cyclin D/cyclin-dependent kinase 4/6 signaling in a concentration-dependent manner in multiple myeloma. These results indicate that β-caryophyllene may represent an interesting alternative or additional therapeutic option to conventional chemotherapy for the treatment of multiple myeloma.

Polygodial, a natural sesquiterpene, can be extracted from water pepper (*Persicaria hydropiper*), Dorrigo pepper (*Tasmannia stipitata*), and mountain pepper (*Tasmannia lanceolata*). The results of a study conducted by Venkatesan et al. [4] showed that polygodial effectively inhibited the viability, cell cycle progression, and migration of taxane-resistant prostate cancer cells, possibly by increasing the generation of reactive oxygen species, disrupting the mitochondrial membrane, and activating the intrinsic cell death pathway.

Parupathi et al. [5] investigated the potential of gnetin C, a phytocompound found in the melinjo plant and commonly used in Indonesian foods, to block prostate cancer progres-

Citation: Bishayee, A. Molecular Mechanisms Underlying Cancer Prevention and Intervention with Bioactive Food Components. *Cancers* **2023**, *15*, 3383. https://doi.org/10.3390/cancers15133383

Received: 19 June 2023
Accepted: 25 June 2023
Published: 28 June 2023

sion. Their findings demonstrate that a gnetin C-supplemented diet effectively suppresses metastasis-associated protein 1-promoted tumor progression in high-risk premalignant prostate cancer transgenic mouse model. This study underscores the potential of gnetin C as a novel nutritional agent for prostate cancer prevention.

The study by Raina et al. [6] focused on elucidating the "stage-specific" efficacy of the bioactive food component inositol hexaphosphate (IP6, also known as phytic acid) against prostate cancer initiation, growth, and progression in a transgenic adenocarcinoma of the mouse prostate (TRAMP) model. Results indicated that IP6 feeding during the initial stages of cancer development prevents the progression of prostatic intraepithelial neoplasia lesions to adenocarcinoma, and IP6 feeding during the late stage of the disease reduces tumor growth and prevents its progression to the advanced stage of the disease. It has also been indicated that the anti-prostate cancer effects of IP6 are associated with its potential to eradicate the prostate cancer stem cell pool in the TRAMP model. Accordingly, IP6 intervention could have a therapeutic benefit during all stages of prostate tumorigenesis.

In this Special Issue, three review articles capture recent developments regarding research, elucidating the role of dietary phytochemicals on gastrointestinal tract cancers. Kang et al. [7] summarized the potential therapeutic effects of bioactive food components on the prevention and treatment of gastric cancer, with special focus on molecular mechanisms of action, bioavailability, and safety aspects. De et al. [8] reviewed the literature on phenolic phytocompounds endowed with anti-colorectal cancer activities, which are based on animal and human studies, to understand the impact of these results on the prevention and treatment of this cancer, which represents a significant cause of death worldwide. Dacrema et al. [9] presented an overview of the reciprocal interactions between spice-derived bioactive compounds and the gut microbiota to understand the role of dietary spices in the prevention of colorectal cancer.

There are two reviews dedicated to the impact of food-derived phytochemicals on hormone-related neoplasms. Prajapati and colleagues [10] dissected the concept of targeting luminal A-derived breast cancer stem cells with dietary phytocompounds by summarizing the signaling pathways implicated in therapy resistance. In their review, Kumar et al. [11] discussed the role of green tea catechins in the prevention of prostate cancer, presented evidence on the associations of microbiomes with prostate cancer, and evaluated the concept of utilizing the microbiome to identify biomarkers for the efficacy of green tea-derived constituents.

Nelumbo nucifera Gaertn., also known as the lotus, sacred lotus, Indian lotus, or Chinese water lily, is a recognized dietary and medicinal plant. Bishayee and colleagues [12] critically evaluated the potential of *N. nucifera*-derived products and phytoconstituents in cancer prevention and intervention with in-depth understanding of cellular and molecular mechanisms of action. Sulforaphane represents a metabolite of the phytochemical glucoraphanin, which is present in cruciferous vegetables, such as broccoli, Brussels sprouts, cabbage, and watercress. A review by Kaiser et al. [13] evaluated the recent state of knowledge on the efficacy of sulforaphane in preventing or reversing a variety of neoplasms based on preclinical and clinical studies. The authors also discussed the current limitations and challenges associated with sulforaphane research, and they suggested future research directions.

Finally, the work of Bouyahya et al. [14] focuses on recent advances in using dietary phenolic phytocompounds to sensitize various cancer cells towards chemotherapeutic agents and their values, in combination therapy, along with conventional anticancer drugs. Several phenolics, including caffeic acid, curcumin, gallic acid, resveratrol, rosmarinic acid, and sinapic acid, exhibit encouraging anticancer activities through sub-cellular, cellular, and molecular mechanisms, and they can increase the effectiveness of the approved cancer chemotherapeutic agents.

In conclusion, it is my hope that this Special Issue, featuring high-quality articles written by recognized leaders in the field, as well as young investigators from all over the world, would accelerate the translational impact of mechanism-based cancer prevention and intervention using multi-targeted dietary phytocompounds, identify current knowledge gaps, challenges, and pitfalls, as well as galvanize future research.

Conflicts of Interest: The authors declare no conflict of interest.

References

1. Sung, H.; Ferlay, J.; Siegel, R.L.; Laversanne, M.; Soerjomataram, I.; Jemal, A.; Bray, F. Global Cancer Statistics 2020: GLOBOCAN Estimates of Incidence and Mortality Worldwide for 36 Cancers in 185 Countries. *CA Cancer J. Clin.* **2021**, *71*, 209–249. [CrossRef] [PubMed]
2. Phannasorn, W.; Pharapirom, A.; Thiennimitr, P.; Guo, H.; Ketnawa, S.; Wongpoomchai, R. Enriched Riceberry Bran Oil Exerts Chemopreventive Properties through Anti-Inflammation and Alteration of Gut Microbiota in Carcinogen-Induced Liver and Colon Carcinogenesis in Rats. *Cancers* **2022**, *14*, 4358. [CrossRef] [PubMed]
3. Mannino, F.; Pallio, G.; Corsaro, R.; Minutoli, L.; Altavilla, D.; Vermiglio, G.; Allegra, A.; Eid, A.H.; Bitto, A.; Squadrito, F.; et al. Beta-Caryophyllene Exhibits Anti-Proliferative Effects through Apoptosis Induction and Cell Cycle Modulation in Multiple Myeloma Cells. *Cancers* **2021**, *13*, 5741. [CrossRef]
4. Venkatesan, R.; Hussein, M.A.; Moses, L.; Liu, J.S.; Khetani, S.R.; Kornienko, A.; Munirathinam, G. Polygodial, a Sesquiterpene Dialdehyde, Activates Apoptotic Signaling in Castration-Resistant Prostate Cancer Cell Lines by Inducing Oxidative Stress. *Cancers* **2022**, *14*, 5260. [CrossRef] [PubMed]
5. Parupathi, P.; Campanelli, G.; Deabel, R.A.; Puaar, A.; Devarakonda, L.S.; Kumar, A.; Levenson, A.S. Gnetin C Intercepts MTA1-Associated Neoplastic Progression in Prostate Cancer. *Cancers* **2022**, *14*, 6038. [CrossRef]
6. Raina, K.; Kandhari, K.; Jain, A.K.; Ravichandran, K.; Maroni, P.; Agarwal, C.; Agarwal, R. Stage-Specific Effect of Inositol Hexaphosphate on Cancer Stem Cell Pool during Growth and Progression of Prostate Tumorigenesis in TRAMP Model. *Cancers* **2022**, *14*, 4204. [CrossRef]
7. Kang, S.Y.; Hwang, D.; Shin, S.; Park, J.; Kim, M.; Rahman, M.D.H.; Rahman, M.A.; Ko, S.G.; Kim, B. Potential of Bioactive Food Components against Gastric Cancer: Insights into Molecular Mechanism and Therapeutic Targets. *Cancers* **2021**, *13*, 4502. [CrossRef] [PubMed]
8. De, S.; Paul, S.; Manna, A.; Majumder, C.; Pal, K.; Casarcia, N.; Mondal, A.; Banerjee, S.; Nelson, V.K.; Ghosh, S.; et al. Phenolic Phytochemicals for Prevention and Treatment of Colorectal Cancer: A Critical Evaluation of In Vivo Studies. *Cancers* **2023**, *15*, 993. [CrossRef] [PubMed]
9. Dacrema, M.; Ali, A.; Ullah, H.; Khan, A.; Di Minno, A.; Xiao, J.; Martins, A.M.C.; Daglia, M. Spice-Derived Bioactive Compounds Confer Colorectal Cancer Prevention via Modulation of Gut Microbiota. *Cancers* **2022**, *14*, 5682. [CrossRef] [PubMed]
10. Prajapati, K.S.; Gupta, S.; Kumar, S. Targeting Breast Cancer-Derived Stem Cells by Dietary Phytochemicals: A Strategy for Cancer Prevention and Treatment. *Cancers* **2022**, *14*, 2864. [CrossRef] [PubMed]
11. Kumar, N.B.; Hogue, S.; Pow-Sang, J.; Poch, M.; Manley, B.J.; Li, R.; Dhillon, J.; Yu, A.; Byrd, D.A. Effects of Green Tea Catechins on Prostate Cancer Chemoprevention: The Role of the Gut Microbiome. *Cancers* **2022**, *14*, 3988. [CrossRef] [PubMed]
12. Bishayee, A.; Patel, P.A.; Sharma, P.; Thoutireddy, S.; Das, N. Lotus (*Nelumbo nucifera* Gaertn.) and Its Bioactive Phytocompounds: A Tribute to Cancer Prevention and Intervention. *Cancers* **2022**, *14*, 529. [CrossRef] [PubMed]
13. Kaiser, A.E.; Baniasadi, M.; Giansiracusa, D.; Giansiracusa, M.; Garcia, M.; Fryda, Z.; Wong, T.L.; Bishayee, A. Sulforaphane: A Broccoli Bioactive Phytocompound with Cancer Preventive Potential. *Cancers* **2021**, *13*, 4796. [CrossRef] [PubMed]
14. Bouyahya, A.; Omari, N.E.; Bakrim, S.; Hachlafi, N.E.; Balahbib, A.; Wilairatana, P.; Mubarak, M.S. Advances in Dietary Phenolic Compounds to Improve Chemosensitivity of Anticancer Drugs. *Cancers* **2022**, *14*, 4573. [CrossRef] [PubMed]

cancers

MDPI

Review

Phenolic Phytochemicals for Prevention and Treatment of Colorectal Cancer: A Critical Evaluation of In Vivo Studies

Samhita De [1,†], Sourav Paul [2,†], Anirban Manna [1,‡], Chirantan Majumder [1,‡], Koustav Pal [3], Nicolette Casarcia [4], Arijit Mondal [5], Sabyasachi Banerjee [6], Vinod Kumar Nelson [7], Suvranil Ghosh [1], Joyita Hazra [8], Ashish Bhattacharjee [2], Subhash Chandra Mandal [9], Mahadeb Pal [1,*] and Anupam Bishayee [4,*]

1 Division of Molecular Medicine, Bose Institute, Kolkata 700 054, India
2 Department of Biotechnology, National Institute of Technology, Durgapur 713 209, India
3 Jawaharlal Institute Post Graduate Medical Education and Research, Puducherry 605 006, India
4 College of Osteopathic Medicine, Lake Erie College of Osteopathic Medicine, Bradenton, FL 34211, USA
5 Department of Pharmaceutical Chemistry, M.R. College of Pharmaceutical Sciences and Research, Balisha 743 234, India
6 Department of Pharmaceutical Chemistry, Gupta College of Technological Sciences, Asansol 713 301, India
7 Department of Pharmacology, Raghavendra Institute of Pharmaceutical Education and Research, Anantapur 515 721, India
8 Department of Biotechnology, Indian Institute of Technology, Chennai 600 036, India
9 Department of Pharmaceutical Technology, Jadavpur University, Kolkata 700 032, India
* Correspondence: mahadeb@jcbose.ac.in or palmahadeb@gmail.com (M.P.); abishayee@lecom.edu or abishayee@gmail.com (A.B.)
† These authors contributed equally to this work.
‡ These authors contributed equally to this work.

Simple Summary: Colorectal cancer (CRC) is a significant cause of death worldwide. The inefficacy of the current treatment regimens is reflected in the frequent recurrence and emergence of a drug-resistant form of CRC. Numerous published reports from independent investigators around the globe have shown the great potential of natural products as a source of anti-CRC drug-leads with novel functions. Here, we have reviewed the literature on phenolic phytochemicals carrying anti-CRC activity in various in vivo models and analyzed their molecular basis of action to understand the implications of these findings in the future treatment and prevention of CRC.

Abstract: Colorectal cancer (CRC) is the third most diagnosed and second leading cause of cancer-related death worldwide. Limitations with existing treatment regimens have demanded the search for better treatment options. Different phytochemicals with promising anti-CRC activities have been reported, with the molecular mechanism of actions still emerging. This review aims to summarize recent progress on the study of natural phenolic compounds in ameliorating CRC using in vivo models. This review followed the guidelines of the Preferred Reporting Items for Systematic Reporting and Meta-Analysis. Information on the relevant topic was gathered by searching the PubMed, Scopus, ScienceDirect, and Web of Science databases using keywords, such as "colorectal cancer" AND "phenolic compounds", "colorectal cancer" AND "polyphenol", "colorectal cancer" AND "phenolic acids", "colorectal cancer" AND "flavonoids", "colorectal cancer" AND "stilbene", and "colorectal cancer" AND "lignan" from the reputed peer-reviewed journals published over the last 20 years. Publications that incorporated in vivo experimental designs and produced statistically significant results were considered for this review. Many of these polyphenols demonstrate anti-CRC activities by inhibiting key cellular factors. This inhibition has been demonstrated by antiapoptotic effects, antiproliferative effects, or by upregulating factors responsible for cell cycle arrest or cell death in various in vivo CRC models. Numerous studies from independent laboratories have highlighted different plant phenolic compounds for their anti-CRC activities. While promising anti-CRC activity in many of these agents has created interest in this area, in-depth mechanistic and well-designed clinical studies are needed to support the therapeutic use of these compounds for the prevention and treatment of CRC.

Citation: De, S.; Paul, S.; Manna, A.; Majumder, C.; Pal, K.; Casarcia, N.; Mondal, A.; Banerjee, S.; Nelson, V.K.; Ghosh, S.; et al. Phenolic Phytochemicals for Prevention and Treatment of Colorectal Cancer: A Critical Evaluation of In Vivo Studies. *Cancers* **2023**, *15*, 993. https://doi.org/10.3390/cancers15030993

Academic Editor: Antonio V. Sterpetti

Received: 30 December 2022
Revised: 30 January 2023
Accepted: 30 January 2023
Published: 3 February 2023

Keywords: colorectal cancer; phenolic compounds; prevention; treatment; molecular mechanisms; in vivo

1. Introduction

The diagnosis of colorectal cancer (CRC) is a death sentence to many. CRC is the third most diagnosed and second leading cause of cancer mortality worldwide [1]. In the United States alone, there were 149,500 new cases and 52,980 deaths in 2021, with an estimated 151,030 new cases for 2022 [1]. Globally, there were 1.9 million new cases and 935,000 deaths in 2020 [2]. These numbers have risen since 2018, as at that time statistics were noted to be 1.8 million new cases and 861,000 deaths [3]. Analyses predicted the global CRC burden to rise by 60% to 2.2 million new cases and 1.1 million deaths by 2030 [3–6]. Rising cases are attributed to a more sedentary lifestyle and altered dietary habits, such as consuming processed foods, tobacco usage, and heavy alcohol consumption. India's incidence of colon cancer in 2016 was estimated to be 63,000, with a sizeable interstate variation [7,8].

Since the implementation of a screening program in the United States in 1990, CRC incidence has consistently decreased in the population of those older than 50 years [9,10]. In contrast, CRC incidence has shown a significant and steady increase (2% per year) in the population of those less than 50 years of age, which is called young-onset CRC (yCRC) [9,11,12]. While yCRC comprises only 10% of total CRC incidence, 75% of yCRC incidence affects the population of those between 40 and 49 years of age [9,11–15]. A study undertaken between 1975 and 2010 predicted that yCRC would double by 2030 in the U.S. population of those younger than 35, indicating racial disparity [9,11–15].

Current treatment options available for colorectal cancer include laparoscopic surgery, resection, palliative, neoadjuvant chemotherapy, and radiotherapy [15–22]. Chemotherapy causes undesirable side effects. In addition to being frequently ineffective, current treatments are expensive.

Utilizing phytochemicals for cancer treatment and prevention has been a matter of serious discussion for decades [3,23]. Plants have been used to treat many diseases in traditional medicine and have been a forefront in alternative approach. Over 3000 plant species have anticancer activities, with thirty plant-derived compounds undergoing preclinical testing [5]. Anticancer activity in citrus fruits, allium vegetables, and medicinal plants has demonstrated preclinical success [5,8]. Secondary plant metabolites have been shown to decrease inflammation and increase apoptosis in addition to possessing antioxidant, anticarcinogenic, and antimetastatic properties [8,23,24]. The attraction to phytochemicals arises from relatively safer and cost-efficient natural products, and their consumption by humans is widespread [5]. While research is being conducted, often with promising results, only a limited number of natural compounds have been approved for clinical use, while the clinical application of many is hindered due to low bioavailability [5,23].

Numerous literature reviews and studies on natural compounds in CRC were dissected and sorted thoroughly for relevant and vital information. It was noted that very few articles reviewed CRC and the therapeutic prospects with polyphenols [25,26]. There is no review literature explaining all classes of phenolic compounds and their signaling pathways in contrast with CRC. We have also noted that few previous reviews have focused on using plant extracts and fractions rich in phenols and pure phenolic compounds [25,26]. Some have examined flavonoids and their effects on CRC [27–36], yet no such reviews consider other classes of phenolic compounds and their effects on CRC. In contrast, numerous reviews were dedicated to discussing the deadly disease of CRC, but did not examine natural products for its treatment. A few reviews that included CRC studied general nutrition and dietary effects, but the literature examined dietary products, such as calcium, fiber, processed meats, or medicinal plants, rather than plant phenolic compounds [37–41]. Furthermore, a review was noted to include the effects of phytochemicals on CRC, but only mentioned specific biochemical properties and pathways of cancer development [42]. In view of the aforementioned limitations, our present review is up-to-date and offers the most recent information compared to previously published works. In this review, we first evaluated pertinent literature to present the characteristics of CRC and identify common risk factors and current treatment options. Then, we evaluated various in vivo studies on different phenolic phytochemicals to understand the potential of these natural agents for CRC prevention and treatment. We hope these phenolic phytocompounds spark interest in conducting new studies to eventually aid in decreasing the prevalence and lowering the risk of CRC.

2. Risk Factors

Familial, hereditary, and lifestyle factors are independent risk factors for developing CRC [43]. Genetic syndromes comprise 20–30% of CRC cases and can be divided into non-polyposis and polyposis types (Table 1). Lynch syndrome, an alternate term for the non-polyposis syndrome, is an autosomal dominant disease associated with a defect in DNA mismatch repair genes, such as *hMLH1*, *hMSH2*, *hMSH6*, or *hPMS2* [44,45]. This mutation results in microsatellite instability (MSI) regions, which is also associated with ~15% of sporadic CRC cases. As expected, individuals with MSI regions carry an increased risk for other cancers, such as endometrial carcinoma [44].

Table 1. Genes involved in different CRC syndromes and associated clinical symptoms.

Syndrome	Genetic Defects	Clinical Manifestations	References
	Hereditary nonpolyposis cancer syndromes		
Lynch syndrome	*MLH1*, *MSH2*, *MSH6*, *MSH3*, and *PMS2*	Increased risk for CRC, (10–47%) depending on gene mutated; asymptomatic unless altered bowel habits, GI bleeding due to tumors/polyps occurs; increased risk for endometrial cancer; extracolonic manifestations are associated as Muir-Torre, Turcot.	[44,46,47]
Muir-Torre syndrome (HNPCC + Sebaceous gland malignancies)	*MLH1*, *MSH2*, *MSH6*, and *PMS2*	Sebaceous skin tumor/keratoacanthoma and Lynch syndrome features.	[48,49]
Turcot syndrome type 1 (HNPCC with primary brain tumors)	*MMR*, *MLH1*, and *PMS2*	Features of Lynch syndrome + primary brain tumors.	[50–53]
	Hereditary polyposis colorectal cancers		
Familial adenomatous polyposis (FAP) syndrome	*APC*	More than colorectal adenomatous polyps; 100% cancer risk	[50,54]
Turcot syndrome type II (FAP with Primary Brain tumors)	*APC*	FAP syndrome + primary brain tumors, medulloblastoma, glioblastoma, astrocytoma.	[50–53]
Gardner syndrome	*APC*	FAP syndrome+ extraintestinal manifestations of desmoid tumors; sebaceous cysts; osteomas of mandible, skull, fibromatosis, congenital hypertrophy of retinal pigment epithelium (CHRPE); adrenal adenomas.	[55,56]
Adenomatous polyposis syndromes	*APC* and *MUTYH*	Increased number of colorectal adenomas (10–100 s), serrated polyposis, mixed polyps; duodenal adenomas are common; 43–33% increased risk of CRC; increased thyroid nodules, adrenal lesions, jawbone cysts.	[50,57–59]
Juvenile polyposis coli	*BMPR1A* and *SMAD4*	Multiple hamartomatous polyps in the GI tract- mainly colorectum; rectal bleeding due to polyps is a common presenting symptom; anemia due to bleeding is common; extracolonic manifestations hereditary hemorrhagic Telangiectasia (HHT) telangiectasias of buccal mucosa and skin, epistaxis, and anemia, with AV malformations; colorectal cancer risk 38.7% increased.	[60–62]
Peutz-Jeghers syndrome	*STK11*	Mucocutaneous pigmentation; hamartomatous polyps; 39% increased risk for CRC.	[63,64]
Cowden syndrome (multiple hamartomasyndrome)	*PTEN*	Mucocutaneous lesions and macrocephaly; skin manifestations; uterine leiomyomas, ovarian cysts; multiple hamartomas on any organ; increased risk of breast, thyroid, renal, endometrial, and colorectal cancer; 9–16% risk of CRC.; increased risk for malignant melanomas; specific dysplastic gangliocytoma of the cerebellum; Lhermitte-Duclos disease is specific to Cowden disease.	[65,66]

Abbreviations: MUTYH, mutY DNA glycosylase; STK11, serine/threonine kinase; 11SMAD4, mothers against decapentaplegic homolog 4; PTEN, phosphate and tensin homolog; BMPR1A, bone morphogenic protein receptor type 1A; MLH, MutL homolog; MSH, MutS homolog; MMR, mismatch repair.

Familial adenomatous polyposis syndrome (FAP), which is characterized by multiple polyp formations in the gastrointestinal tract, is caused by a germline mutation in the adenomatous polyposis coli (APC) gene [67–69]. Inheriting a polyposis syndrome can increase an individual's risk of developing colon cancer up to 100% [70]. Furthermore, these patients carry the risk of developing other gastrointestinal cancers and desmoid tumors. MUTYH-associated polyposis (MAP), Peutz-Jeughers syndrome (*STK11*), Juvenile polyposis syndrome (*SMAD4* and *BMPR1A*), hyperplastic polyposis (HPP), familial CRC (FCC) syndrome X, and Cowden syndrome (*PTEN*) are other polyposis syndromes that predispose individuals to an increased risk of developing CRC [50,71,72].

Chronic inflammatory bowel diseases, which encompass both ulcerative colitis and Crohn's disease, predispose individuals to CRC [73]. Additionally, previous abdominopelvic radiation is a potent risk factor for CRC, especially for childhood cancer survivors [74]. Furthermore, individuals receiving prostate cancer-related radiation therapy are at a higher risk of developing rectal carcinoma, supporting previous radiation therapy as a risk factor for CRC [75]. Cystic fibrosis is also implicated in CRC, as there is a 5–10 times greater risk of acquiring CRC in these patients. As a result, they have a separate management for CRC screening, especially post-transplant [76].

Lifestyle patterns, such as smoking, consumption of alcohol, obesity, sedentary lifestyles, and chronic diseases, pose a potent overall risk of developing sporadic CRC [77–79]. A westernized diet, rich in processed foods and red meat and deficient in fruits, fiber, and leafy vegetables, can contribute to CRC development [16,80]. Conversely, consuming more vegetables, fruits, and fiber is protective against CRC. A meta-analysis has elucidated the risk of CRC with food's dietary inflammatory index (DII). A higher DII correlating with a pro-inflammatory state increases CRC risk [81]. Numerous studies have explored the opposite end of the spectrum, examining anti-inflammatory foods and drugs for CRC chemoprevention and treatment. This is supported by a case-control meta-analysis where a higher intake of calcium, magnesium, and potassium lowered the occurrence of CRC [82].

The risk of CRC is low in vegetarians compared to meat eaters with an HR ratio of 0.49 [95% confidence interval (CI): 0.36 to 0.66], and 0.73 [95% CI: 0.54 to 0.99] when not adjusted and adjusted (for sociodemographic and lifestyle factors, multimorbidity, and body mass index) respectively. When CRC was subcategorized, the HR of 0.69 [95% CI: 0.48 to 0.99] for the colon and 0.43 [95% CI: 0.22 to 0.82] for the proximal colon was observed in vegetarians, which is much less compared to meat eaters [83]. Adherence to the Mediterranean diet was found to be associated with a low risk of rectal cancer with RR of 0.82 [95% CI: 0.71 to 0.95] for rectal cancer, 0.94 [95% CI: 0.87 to 1.02] for proximal colon cancer, and 0.91 [95% CI: 0.79 to 1.04] for distal colon cancer [84]. The unhealthy diet pattern is associated with CRC-specific mortality with RR/HR of 1.52 [95% CI: 1.13 to 2.06] [85]. The high intake of dietary calcium and magnesium is negatively associated with CRC risk with HR of 0.76 [95% CI: 0.72 to 0.80] and 0.80 [95% CI: 0.73 to 0.87], respectively. The higher intake of dietary heme, however, was positively correlated to colon cancer incidence with HR of 1.01 (95% CI: 0.82 to 1.19) and rectal cancer incidence with HR of 1.04 [95% CI: 0.67 to 1.42] [82]. The increase in DII score, and CRC are found to be positively associated with an overall increased risk of CRC by 40% with RR of 1.40 [95% CI: 1.26 to 1.55] [81]. Smoking and CRC shows a positive association with ever smoker versus never smoker, the pooled RR was 1.18 [95% CI: 1.11 to 1.25], and the pooled risk estimate was 1.25 [95% CI: 1.14 to 1.37] [77]. Alcohol consumption is also associated with an increased risk for CRC mortality. In comparison, the pooled RR was 1.03 [95% CI: 0.93 to 1.15] for any, 0.97 for light drinkers who consume $\leq$12.5 g of ethanol/day, 1.04 [95% CI: 0.94 to 1.16] for moderate drinkers who consume 12.6–49.9 g ethanol/day), 1.04 [95% CI: 0.94 to 1.16] for heavy drinking men (who consume $\geq$50 g ethanol/day), which is higher than heavy drinking women [pooled RR = 0.79 (95% CI: 0.40 to 1.54)] [78].

3. Pathogenesis

Overall, the pathogenesis of colon cancer involves three main pathways: the chromosomal instability (CIN)/classic adenoma-carcinoma sequence [86,87], the CpG island methylator phenotype (CIMP), and the microsatellite instability (MSI) pathway [88]. While these are separate pathways, there is potential overlap within them. Moreover, they involve the stepwise accumulation of multiple mutations, eventually leading to CRC development [89].

The classic adenoma-carcinoma sequence accounts for 65–70% of sporadic diseases commonly observed as left-sided CRCs [90]. This mechanism involves a dysfunctional/ inactivated APC gene located on chromosome 5q21. APC, a "gatekeeper" of colonic neoplasia, has been implicated in familial adenomatous polyposis (FAP) syndrome. The onset of CRC is inevitable in a population with an inactivating mutation in both copies of the APC gene [91,92]. APC controls cell growth and differentiation through the Wnt/ β-catenin signaling pathway. The Wnt pathway is an essential cellular signaling system by which several developmental events for embryological and tissue homeostasis occur, involving cellular proliferation and differentiation. Deregulation of the Wnt pathway can lead to the development of cancer. When the Wnt/β-catenin pathway is suppressed, there is a lower rate of cellular proliferation and fewer intestinal stem cells [93]. Activating mutations of Wnt/β-catenin leads to the pathogenesis of CRC. Over 90% of CRC cases carry mutations within this pathway [94]. It has been found that APC deletion/loss of function leads to CRC development, while restoring APC function can regress adenomas by reducing Wnt activity [93].

Apart from APC, there are other Wnt activating mutations, such as mutations in the CTNNB1 gene encoding β-catenin. R-spondins are another module of Wnt signal activators, which are associated with up to 10% of CRC mutations. Antagonism of RSPO3 with paclitaxel effectively targeted Wnt signaling in CRC [95]. A higher expression of ß-catenin in CRC cells is associated with a worse prognosis and advanced stage of the disease. Because of this, CRC metastasis was determined by the combined β-catenin odds ratio in the nucleus [96].

In the absence of APC function, β-catenin translocate to the nucleus. In cooperation with the DNA binding factor TCF, it promotes the growth of colonic epithelium via uncontrolled overexpression of its targets c-Myc and cyclin D1 [93]. Next, a mutation in KRAS contributes to molecular pathogenesis by promoting adenoma formation [97]. Finally, a mutation in p53 facilitates the progression of CRC [98]. Although important roles of p53 and KRAS were implied in the adenoma-carcinoma pathway, mouse knockout of APC develops carcinoma irrespective of its KRAS and p53 status, and re-introduction of APC restores cellular differentiation and normal crypt formation [43,93].

The microsatellite instability pathway occurs due to the inactivation of DNA mismatch repair genes, which includes ATPases hMSH2, hMSH6, hMSH3, hMLH1, hPMS2, hPMS1, and hMLH3, as involved in Lynch syndrome [99]. The MSI pathway is involved in roughly 15% of CRCs, 3% of which are Lynch syndrome while the rest are sporadic, mainly caused by MLH1 hypermethylation. Finally, the CpG island methylator phenotype (CIMP) is involved in silencing genes by hypermethylation of CpG islands on their promoters [100,101]. CIMP has been associated with older patients, female patients, and right-sided lesions with high MSI and BRAF mutations. CIMP is also associated with PI3K mutations but lacks KRAS and p53 mutations. A clearer insight and greater understanding of CIMP is required to better study the treatment and prevention of CRC [102].

4. Chemoprevention

Chemoprevention aims to intervene, prevent, suppress, and reverse the initiation and progression of carcinogenesis. It further attempts to decrease the recurrence of cancer through the usage of drugs, vitamins, and nutritional supplements [66]. Various agents, including nonsteroidal anti-inflammatory drugs (NSAIDs), such as aspirin, and other agents, such as metformin, statins, minerals, and vitamins, have been previously studied for their chemopreventive benefits regarding CRC (Table 2). There is little doubt that a significant stride has been made into the unventured territories for the chemoprevention of CRC.

Table 2. Various drugs alone and in combination tested for their effects on clinical CRC chemoprevention studies.

Drugs	Study Design	Mechanism	Main Findings	References
Aspirin	Meta-analysis	COX-2 inhibition	There was a dose-dependent reduction in the risk of CR by aspirin. An aspirin dose of 75–100 mg/day reduced the risk by 10%, and 325 mg/day reduced the risk by 35% (Meta-analysis of 45 studies [RR = 0.73, 95% confidence interval (CI) 0.69–0.78])	[103–106]
Non-aspirin NSAIDS	Meta-analysis	COX-2 inhibition	Data from 23 studies suggested using higher doses of non-aspirin NSAIDs in the general population aged 40 years or older reduced CRC risk, specifically for white women, for distal colon cancer. (Pooled ODDs ratio was 0.74 (0.67–0.81), I2 = 75.9%, $p < 0.001$.)	[107]
Sulindac+ DFMO	RCT	Sulindac inhibits COX-2 DFMO- irreversibly inhibits Ornithine decarboxylase (polyamine synthesis)	Significant reduction of recurrent adenomas (12 vs. 41%, risk ratio 0.30), advanced adenomas (0.7 vs. 8.5%, risk ratio 0.09), and multiple adenomas (0.7 vs. 13.2%, risk ratio 0.06)	[108,109]
DFMO + Aspirin	RCT	Aspirin inhibits COX-2 DFMO inhibits polyamine synthesis Both combined may have a synergistic action.	After one year of treatment, in the DFMO + aspirin arm vs. placebo, there was a significant reduction in rectal aberrant crypt foci (precursor of rectal carcinoma). (74% vs. 45%, $p = 0.020$). No statistically significant reduction of colorectal adenomas was observed.	[110]
Erlotinib + Sulindac	RCT	Erlotinib is an EGFR inhibitor; sulindac is a COX-2 inhibitor.	In 82 patients of familial adenomatous polyposis, Sulindac + Erlotinib was associated with a 69.4% decrease in those with an intact colorectum compared with placebo (95% CI, 28.8—109.2%; $p = 0.009$)	[111]
Celecoxib	Meta-analysis	Selective COX-2 inhibitor, more specific for inflammation, with fewer GI side effects. Celecoxib has higher cardiovascular mortality	3 RCTs (involving 4420 patients) and 3 post-trial studies (2159) showed a significant reduction in the incidence of adenoma RR (0.67 [95% CI, 0.62–0.72] compared with placebo). There was an increased risk of cardiovascular mortality with twice dosing 400 mg celecoxib (RR 3.42 [95% CI, 1.56–7.46]). Once-a-day dosing did not show an increased CV risk. (1.01 [95% CI, 0.70–1.46]).	[112]
Clopidogrel	Case-control Study	Clopidogrel inhibits platelet aggregation via irreversible inhibition of the P2Y12 receptor	Clopidogrel decreased CRC risk in patients receiving treatment >1 year. (0.65% AOR; 95% CI, 0.55–0.78). Dual antiplatelet therapy (Clopidogrel aspirin) had the same effect as either drug is taken as monotherapy.	[113]
Metformin	Meta-analysis	Activates AMPK, inhibits mTOR pathway	Metformin users had a significantly lower incidence. CRC (RR 0.76, CI 0.69–0.84, $p < 0.001$) compared with non-metformin users. Further analysis on the overall survival of metastatic CRC patients revealed significantly higher survival rates in metformin users (HR 0.77, CI 0.68–0.87, $p < 0.001$).	[114]
UCDA	Cohort Study	Has antioxidant action. Prevents NF-κB and AP1 activity. Inhibits c-Myc	Chronic liver disease patients with UCDA have a reduced risk of colorectal cancer. UDCA use was associated with a reduced risk of CRC (hazard ratio, 0.60; 95% confidence interval [CI], 0.39–0.92).	[115]
Statin	Meta-analysis	*3-HMGCOA* reductase inhibitor decreases cholesterol synthesis. Antioxidant activity; shows pro-apoptotic effects on human CRC lines. Anti-inflammatory properties	14 studies involving 130,994 patients. In terms of post-diagnosis statin uses, the pooled HR of all-cause mortality was 0.86 (95% CI, 0.76–0.98), and the pooled HR of CSM was 0.79 (95%CI, 0.70–0.89) (Cancer-Specific Mortality).	[116,117]

Table 2. *Cont.*

Drugs	Study Design	Mechanism	Main Findings	References
Menopausal hormone therapy (combined estrogen-progestin)	Nationwide Cohort Study (Norway)	Estrogens have been proposed to alter bile acid composition, modulate colonic transit. Decrease production of mitogenic insulin-like growth factor	The current use of postmenopausal hormone therapy was associated with a decreased CRC risk. RR (for combined estrogen-progestin therapy) in oral formulations was 0.86 (95% CI 0.71 to 1.05)	[118]
Bisphosphonates	Meta-analysis	Inhibits osteoclastic bone resorption, Anti-apoptotic effect	Meta-analysis of 34 studies and 4,508,261 participants. There was a significant reduction in the risk of CRC. (RR = 0.89, 95% CI: 0.81–0.98)	[119]

Abbreviations: RCT, randomized control trial; RR, relative risk; HR, hazard ratio; OR, odds ratio, AOR, adjusted odds ratio; CI, confidence interval; DFMO, difluoromethylornithine; UCDA, ursodeoxycholic acid.

In CRC involving the APC/β-catenin pathway, cyclooxygenase-2 (COX-2) is often implicated in the early and later stages of the adenoma sequence, driving the formation into a carcinoma [120–123]. Furthermore, COX-2 overexpression produces vascular endothelial growth factor (VEGF), which promotes tumor angiogenesis [124,125]. Hence, by targeting COX-2, various studies have shown that NSAIDs, ranging from aspirin and sulindac to the more selective COX-2 inhibitors, such as celecoxib, have proven benefits in reducing disease risk [126,127]. In the 1990s, the U.S. Preventive Services Task Force recommended aspirin to prevent non-high-risk CRC [128–130].

Other drugs, such as metformin, showed promising effects in reducing the risk of CRC development. Recent meta-analyses showed that metformin could reduce CRC risk by 22% [131]. In an ongoing ASAMET trial for the tertiary prevention of stage I–III CRC, patients were administered low doses of aspirin combined with metformin for a potential synergistic chemo-preventive action [132]. Statins, a specific inhibitor of HMG-CoA reductase in the mevalonate synthesis pathway, have been recommended to lower serum lipid levels [133]. Statins were shown to reduce CRC alone and in combination with NSAIDS [134,135]. Further investigations on multiple agents, such as antioxidants, minerals, such as selenium, and vitamins, including A, C, E, and β-carotene, were previously believed to have benefits in decreasing the risk of CRC, yet they have yielded mixed results [130,136,137]. Studies on folate's use to lower CRC risks also yielded mixed results [130]. Fiber, alcohol, monounsaturated fatty acids, polyunsaturated fatty acids, omega-3, omega-6, niacin, thiamine, riboflavin, vitamin B6, vitamin B12, zinc, magnesium, selenium, vitamin A, vitamin C, vitamin D, vitamin E, folic acid, β-carotene, anthocyanin, flavonoids, garlic, ginger, onions, thyme, oregano, saffron, turmeric, rosemary, eugenol, caffeine, and tea have all demonstrated anti-inflammatory benefits, and therefore reduce the risk of CRC development [138,139]. A higher intake of dietary fiber, pertaining to whole grains, was associated with a lower CRC risk in men [140].

5. Treatment

CRC incidence and mortality have been efficiently controlled by the routine screening and removal of polyps through colonoscopy [141]. Surgery, chemotherapy, and immunotherapy are mainstay treatments for CRC; the stage of CRC progression in each patient determines an appropriate combination. The treatment of CRC depends upon the diagnosis through tumor/node/metastasis (TNM) staging of the lesion. Adjuvant chemotherapy with fluorouracil (5-FU) decreases death rates in patients with high-risk stage II colon cancer by 3–5% and 10–15% in stage III disease alone [142]. MSI/MMR protein levels determined by IHC aid in deciding the adjuvant therapy [143–145]. Furthermore, after primary tumor resection, TNM or immunoscore can be considered to assess the tumor recurrence risk [146].

Single-agent therapy with 5-FU or therapy with multiple agents composed of 5-FU and oxaliplatin (FOLFOX), 5-FU and irinotecan (FOXFIRI) (IRI), or capecitabine and oxaliplatin (CAPOX), capecitabine (CAP), and irinotecan (CAPIRI) as first line chemotherapy is recommended based on the sensitivity and the stage of the disease. In many cases, single-agent chemotherapies yielded better results than combination therapy, given the associated systemic toxicity and unsatisfying responses [147–149]. A combination of 5-FU or CAP with oxaliplatin (OX) is recommended for stage III CRC for three to six months. Patients with intermediate-risk stage II CRC are recommended either 5-FU or CAP, which are added to OX, if the patients are high risk (stage II), for three months [145]. The International Duration Evaluation of Adjuvant Chemotherapy (IDEA) collaboration helped investigate whether three or six months of adjuvant chemotherapy was necessary, as cumulative toxicity develops from fluoropyrimidines/oxaliplatin in the form of peripheral sensory neuropathy. Results show that the overall disease-free survival was similar at 74.6% and 75.5% for three months and six months, respectively. After three months of treatment, the overall sensory peripheral neuropathy reduced from 34% to 11%. However, per ESMO guidelines, stage III CRC should still be treated with six months of FOLFOX or CAPOX if the patient falls within the high-risk category. For patients who do not tolerate oxaliplatin, capecitabine, or LVGFU2 can be acceptable alternatives [145].

Various forms of supplemental targeted immunotherapies are considered to aid chemotherapy. Monoclonal antibodies are used to attack various potential genes, such as ERFR, VEGF, and PDL-1/PDL-1. Cetuximab, an anti-EGFR chimeric monoclonal antibody, and bevacizumab, an anti-VEGF chimeric monoclonal antibody, both of which prolong OS, were the first line targeted drugs approved by the United States Food and Drug Administration (FDA) in 2004 [150,151]. An immune checkpoint blocker α-PD1/PDL-1 antibody, in combination with chemo- and radiation therapy, was approved by the FDA for MSI-H and dMMR classes of CRCs for sustained progression-free survival [152]. Cetuximab yielded a positive outcome for CRC that did not respond to single-agent IRI or fluoropyrimidine therapy. Combining cetuximab with IRI, fluorocytidine, or OX delivered promising results [151,153]. EGFR (epidermal growth factor receptor) is overexpressed in various cancers to different extents, including 25–75% in CRC [154]. Cetuximab, once bound, results in the internalization and degradation of EGFR [111]. However, cetuximab was inactive in CRCs carrying the RAS (KRAS) mutation. Like EGFR, the VEGF level is also elevated in CRC, predicting a poor prognosis [155]. Along with an elevated VEGF level, increased vascular endothelial growth factor receptor (VEGFR) activity is found in adenomas, as well as in the metastatic stage of CRC [147,156]. While cetuximab is not suitable as a second line agent, bevacizumab is often an excellent choice.

6. Literature Search Methodology

We have followed the Preferred Reporting Items for Systematic Reviews and Meta-Analysis (PRISMA) guidelines [157] for this work. Four scholarly databases, namely PubMed, Scopus, ScienceDirect, and Web of Science, were utilized to screen the literature for the last 20 years (2002 to 2022 November) by searching the title, abstract, and key words section with the key words "colorectal cancer" AND "phenolic compounds", "colorectal cancer" AND "polyphenol", "colorectal cancer" AND "phenolic acids", "colorectal cancer" AND "flavonoids", "colorectal cancer" AND "stilbene", and "colorectal cancer" AND "lignan." All search results were gathered, and duplicate files were removed. Next, literature was scanned based on title and abstract. Selected articles were then searched for retrieval. After reading the full articles, preclinical studies (in vivo animal models) with polyphenols were selected and incorporated. The methodology for literature search and study selection is depicted in Figure 1.

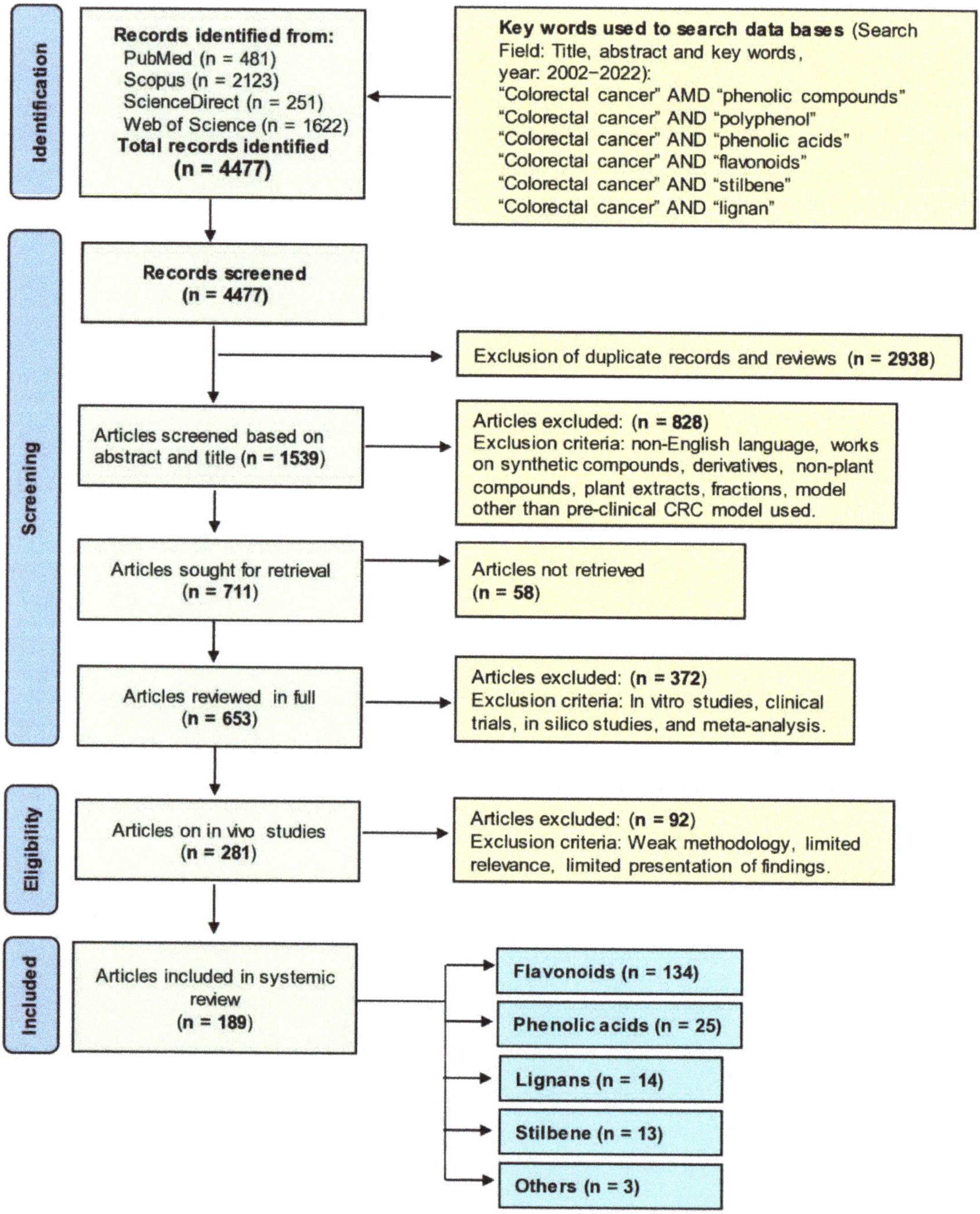

Figure 1. The PRISMA flow chart summarizing the literature search. Here "n" represents the number of articles.

7. Phenolic Compounds with In Vivo Anti-CRC Activities

Plants synthesize phenolic compounds as secondary metabolites and carry multiple aromatic rings with two or more hydroxyl groups. Phenolic compounds carry a wide (~8000 different) variety of chemical structures. Based on chemical structures, phenolic compounds are divided into different classes, such as flavonoids (e.g., anthocyanidins, flavanols, flavanones, flavones, flavonols, and isoflavoniods) and non-flavonoids, including phenolic acids (e.g., hydroxycinnamic acids and hydroxybenzoic acids), coumarins, stilbenes, lignans, and tannins [158–160]. Significant sources of phenolic compounds are fruits and vegetables. Various phenolic compounds are known for their interesting pharmacological properties, including antioxidant, anti-inflammatory, neuroprotective, and anticancer properties [161,162].

While western medicines have significant effects on CRC chemoprevention and treatment, extracts of numerous plants and plant products are still currently in use, as humanity has used plants for thousands of years as traditional or ethnic medicines for the prevention and treatment of various ailments, including cancer. The primary reasons for their popularity are fewer side effects, easy availability, and low cost compared to synthetic drugs [163–165]. Over the last several decades, steady progress has been achieved in identifying the bioactive secondary metabolites of plants, such as phenolic compounds, and understanding their mode of action to explain their health benefits [166–169]. In the following sections, we aim to summarize the anti-CRC effects of phenolic compounds based on animal studies. Table 3 describes the in vivo CRC activity of the compounds as revealed by our literature search as depicted in Figure 1. We have selected 16 relatively well-studied compounds to describe their anti-CRC activities in a greater detail in the following sections. The chemical structures of various classes of phenolic compounds with in vivo anti-CRC activities are presented in Figures 2–5.

Table 3. Anti-CRC effects and mechanisms of action of phenolic compounds based on in vivo studies.

Phytocompound	Source	Animal Model Studied	Dose and Route of Administration	Mode of Action	Reference
			Flavonoids		
2,3,5,4′-tetrahydroxystilbene-2-O-β-D-glucoside	*Polygonum multiflorum* Thunb	AOM-induced colon carcinogenesis in male F144 rats	Oral administration, 30, 150, 250 mg/kg	Decreased the number ofACF by 47–54%; suppressed tumor growth; downregulated NF-κB in nucleus and cytoplasm; downregulated CEA	[170]
4′-hydroxychalcone	Herb, teas, and spices	$APC^{Min/+}$ mice	Oral administration, 10 mg/kg	Reduced the incidences and size of adenomas; induced apoptosis; suppressed proliferation of polyps; downregulated Ki-67; downregulated *c-Myc, Axin2* and *CD44* gene expression	[171]
Aciculatin	*Chrysopogon aciculatus*	HCT116 induced tumor xenograft SCID mice	Intraperitoneal injection, 30 mg/kg	Suppressed tumor growth without losing weight; upregulated the expression of p53 and downregulated the expression of Ki-67; induced apoptosis; arrested cells in sub G_1 phase	[172]
Apigenin	Parsley, wheat, onions, apples, and tea plants	AOM-induced CF-1 mice and Min mice carrying mutant APC gene	Oral administration of 0.1% dietary apigenin	Reduced ACF formation and ODC activity	[173]
		Male BALB/c-nu mice	Intraperitoneal injection, 20 mg/kg	Induced apoptosis of CRC cells; upregulated FADD expression and its phosphorylation	[174]
		Male BALB/c-nu mice injected with SW480 cells	Route of administration not reported, 50 mg/kg	Elevated transgelin and downregulation of MMP-9 expression via reducing Akt phosphorylation at Ser473 and Thr308	[175]
		$APC^{Min/+}$ mice	Oral gavage, 25 and 50 mg/kg	Reduced the number of polyps; induced of p53 activity	[176]
		Nude BALB/c mice injected with HT-29 cells	Subcutaneous injection, 35 mg/kg	Induced apoptosis; induced autophagy through inhibition mTOR/PI3K/Akt signaling pathway	[177]
		SCID mice	Oral gavage, 25 mg/kg	Suppressed prosurvival regulators Mcl-1, Akt, and ERK	[178]
		NEDD9 knock downed DLD1 cells mediated metastasis model in female athymic nude mice	Intraperitoneal injection, 20 mg/kg	Suppressed invasion, migration, and metastasis by downregulating overexpressed Neural precursor cells expressed NEDD9	[179]

Table 3. *Cont.*

Phytocompound	Source	Animal Model Studied	Dose and Route of Administration	Mode of Action	Reference
Baicalein	*Scutellaria baicalensis* Georgi	AMO and DSS induced colon tumor in male ICR mice	Oral administration, 1,5 and 10 mg/kg	Restored colon length; reduced tissue inflammation.	[180]
		SW620 xenograft in BALB/c nude mice	Intraperitoneal injection, 50 mg/kg	Suppressed tumor growth by 55% without losing body weight	[181]
		CT-26 derived tumor in female BALB/c mice	Intraperitoneal injection, 20 and 40 mg/kg	Reduced tumor growth rate; downregulated TLR4 and p-IκBα protein expression; inhibited NF-κB	[182]
		HT-29 cell-induced tumor xenograft in male nude mice	Oral administration, 10 mg/kg	Suppressed tumor growth by 29.33% compared to the control group; induced apoptosis; upregulated p53 and p21	[183]
		DLD-1 tumor xenograft in BALB/c athymic nude mice	Intragastric administration, 20 mg/kg	Suppression of tumor growth; inhibition of ERK phosphorylation; downregulation of MMP-2 and MMP-9	[184]
		HCT116 tumor xenograft in NSG immunodeficient mice	Intraperitoneal injection, 50 mg/kg	Suppressed tumorigenesis; inhibited colon cancer growth; induced apoptosis and senescence	[185]
		HCT116 tumor xenograft in athymic BALB/c nude mice	Intraperitoneal injection, 80 mg/kg	Suppressed tumor growth; induced senescence; upregulated DEPP; activated Ras/Raf/MEK/ERK pathway	[186]
		HT-29 tumor xenograft in nude mice	Intraperitoneal injection, 50 and 100 mg/kg	Suppressed tumor growth	[187]
		HCT116 tumor xenograft in athymic BALB/c nude mice	Intraperitoneal injection, 100 and 200 mg/kg	Suppressed tumor growth; induced apoptosis; suppressed cancer stem cells; inhibited EMT and cyclin D1	[188]
		$APC^{Min/+}$ mice	Oral administration, 30 mg/kg	Reduced tumor numbers; suppressed IL-1β, IL-2, IL-6, and IL-10	[189]
		HCT116 tumor xenograft in male BALB/c nude mice	Intraperitoneal injection, 100 mg/kg	Suppressed tumor growth; decreased circMYH9, mir761 and HDGF	[190]

Table 3. *Cont.*

Phytocompound	Source	Animal Model Studied	Dose and Route of Administration	Mode of Action	Reference
Boeravinone B	*Boerhaavia diffusa*	DMH-induced CRC in Swiss albino Wistar rats	Intraperitoneal injection, 20 and 40 mg/kg	Decreased the number of tumor incidences; downregulated LPO; upregulated catalase, SOD and GSH; downregulated TNF-α, IL-1β, IL-6, COX-2, PGE2 and iNOS; upregulated levels of IL-4 and IL-10; down regulated MPO; downregulated the expression of GDI2 mRNA	[191]
Chrysin	*Passiflora caerulea, Passiflora incarnata, Oroxylum indicum*	AOM-induced ACF in male F344 rats	Dietary administration, 0.001% and 0.01%	Reduced mitotic index and increased apoptotic index; reduced the frequency of ACF	[192]
		Male albino rats injected with DMH + DSS	Oral administration, 125 and 250 mg/kg	Reduced the level of CXCL1, AREG and MMP-9	[193]
Curcumin	*Curcuma longa*	DSS-induced colitis in C57BL/6 mice	Oral consumption as dietary supplement, 0.6%	Reduced tumor incidences; inhibited nuclear translocation of β-catenin; downregulated TNF-α and interferon-γ; downregulated COX-2 and p53	[194]
		HCT116 tumor xenograft in female ICR SCID mice	Intragastric administration, 500 mg/kg	Suppressed tumor growth; inhibited proteasome; suppressed proliferation; induced apoptosis	[195]
		AOM-DSS induced CRC in male C57BL/6 mice	Oral gavage, 500 mg/kg	Reduced CRC tumor number; downregulated IL-1β, IL-6, COX-2 and β-catenin; suppressed Axin2 by inhibiting Wnt/β-catenin pathway	[196]
		AOM-induced colonic preneoplastic lesion in C57BL/KsJ-db/db obese mice	Dietary supplement, 0.2% and 2.0%	Inhibited colonic premalignant lesion	[197]
		HCT116 tumor xenograft in athymic nu/nu nude mice	Oral administration, 1 g/kg	Enhanced the efficacy of radiation therapy; suppressed NF-κB activity and expression	[198]
		Colo205 and LoVo tumor xenografts in athymic nu/nu mice	Tail vein injection, 40 mg/kg	Inhibited tumor growth; suppressed angiogenesis	[199]
		AOM-induced colon carcinogenesis in $Il10^{-/-}$ mice	Oral administration, 1%	Reduced colon tumors	[200]
		AOM/DSS-induced colitis in C5757BL/6 mice	Oral administration, 25 mg/kg	Suppressed colitis-associated colon cancer and reduced tumor number	[201]

Table 3. *Cont.*

Phytocompound	Source	Animal Model Studied	Dose and Route of Administration	Mode of Action	Reference
Cyanidin	Blackberries (*Rubus fruticosus*)	$Apc^{Min/+}$ mice	Dietary supplementation, 0.03%, 0.1% or 0.3%	Reduced adenoma counts	[202]
Daidzein	Soybeans and soy-based products, and nuts	Male albino rats injected with DMH + DSS	Oral administration, 5 and 10 mg/kg	Reduced the level of CXCL1, AREG and MMP-9	[193]
Delphinidin	Berries, pomegranates, eggplant, roselle, and wine	Male BALB/c nude mice xenograft with luciferase-transfected DLD-1 cells	Intraperitoneal injection, 100 μM	Suppressed integrin/FAK nexus; elevated miR-204–3p levels	[203]
Diosmetin	Chamomile, parsley, rosemary, rooibos tea, green tea, and other plants fof the mint and citrus family (Lamiaceae)	NCr nu/nu nude mice injected with HCT-116 cells	Oral administration, 50 and 100 mg/kg	Downregulated Bcl-2; upregulated Bax	[204]
EGCG	*Camellia sinensis* L. Ktze	SW837 xenograft in male BALB/c nude mice	Oral administration, 0.01% and 0.1%	Reduced tumor growth; inhibited phosphorylation of VEGFR-2, Akt and ERK	[205]
		AOM-induced colonic premalignant lesions C57BL/KsJ-db/db mice	Oral administration, 0.01% and 0.1%	Decreased p-IGF-IR, p-GSK-3β, β-catenin, COX-2 and cyclin D1 in colonic mucosa; reduced IGF-I, insulin, triglyceride, cholesterol and leptin in serum	[206]
		AOM-induced colonic carcinogenesis in ICR mice	Oral administration, 0.25% and 0.5%	Inhibited large ACF formation; inhibited iNOS and COX-2	[207]
		HCT116-SDCSCs tumor xenograft in athymic nude mice	Cells were pretreated, 100 μM	Suppressed tumor formation; downregulated Notch1, Bmi1, Suz12, and Ezh1; upregulated miR-34a, miR-145 and miR-200c	[208]
		DMH-induced colon carcinogenesis in Wister rats	Oral administration, 0.2%	Inhibited ACF and induced apoptosis	[209]
		DMH-induced CRC in male Wistar rats	Oral administration, 50, 100 and 200 mg/kg	Lowered ACF formation; reduced tumor volume	[210]

Table 3. *Cont.*

Phytocompound	Source	Animal Model Studied	Dose and Route of Administration	Mode of Action	Reference
Eriodictyol	*Eriodictyon californicum*	DMH-induced colon carcinogenesis in male albino Wistar rats	Intragastrical administration, 200 mg/kg	Suppressed the number of polyps, ACF and lipid peroxidation levels; upregulated catalase, SOD, GP_X, GST, GSH and GR	[211]
Euxanthone	*Polygala caudata*	HT-29 cells induced tumor in BALB/c nude mice	Intraperitoneal injection, 20 and 40 mg/kg	Suppressed tumor growth; induced apoptosis; upregulated Bax; downregulated Bcl-2; induced caspase-3 cleavage; downregulated CIP2A expression and upregulated PP2A	[212]
Fisetin	Strawberry, apple, persimmon, grapes, onion, and cucumber	AOM and DSS induced CAC in male BALB/c mice	Oral administration, 20 mg/kg	Suppressed dysplastic lesions; induced apoptosis in colonic tissue; downregulated Bcl-2 and STAT3	[213]
		FC1 mice, 3K1 mice, $Apc^{Min/+}$ males, $3K1Apc^{Min/+}$ mice, B6 congenic strain, B6 $FC13K1Apc^{Min/+}$ mice	Intraperitoneal injection, 1 mg/animal	Upregulated AMPK phosphorylation; suppressed PI3K/Akt/mTOR signaling	[214]
		Male athymic nude mice	Oral administration, 400 and 800 mg/kg	Induced apoptosis, caspase-8 and cyt.; inhibited IGF1R and Akt	[215]
		CT-26 tumor in BALB/c nude mice	Subcutaneous injection, 5 mg/kg	Suppressed oncoprotein securin in p53-independent fashion	[216]
		BALB/c mice	Tail vein injection, 50 mg/kg	Inhibited programmed cell death and angiogenesis	[217]
		HCT116 tumor xenograft in mice NOD/Shi-scid-IL2R gamma (null) (NOG)	Intraperitoneal injection, 30, 60 and 120 mg/kg	Suppressed tumor growth in a dose-dependent manner	[218]
Flavone	Fruits and vegetables	DMM-induced colon carcinogenesis in C57BL/6J mice	Subcutaneous injection, 15 and 400 mg/kg	Suppressed ACF formation and multiplicity	[219]
Formononetin	*Astragalus membranaceus*	Female BALB/c-nu/nu mice injected with HCT-116 cells	Intraperitoneal injection, 20 mg/kg	Decreased VEGF, MMP-2 and MMP-9 levels	[220]
Furowanin A	*Millettia pachycarpa* Benth	HT-29 tumor xenograft in male athymic BALB/c nude mice	Intraperitoneal injection, 20 and 40 mg/kg	Suppressed tumor growth, induced apoptosis and autophagy; upregulated cleaved caspase-3, LC3BII, Beclin and p27; downregulated Ki-67, pSTAT3, Mcl-1, p62, and cyclin D	[221]

Table 3. *Cont.*

Phytocompound	Source	Animal Model Studied	Dose and Route of Administration	Mode of Action	Reference
Genistein	*Genista tinctoria*	DMH-induced colon cancer in Wistar rats	Oral administration, 2.5 mg/kg	Regulated tumor microenvironment; upregulated SOD, CAT, GPx, GR, vitamin A, vitamin C, vitamin E and GSH; activated NRF2 and HO-1; reduced expression of CD133, CD44 and β-catenin	[222]
		AOM-induced colon cancer in Sprague-Dawley rats	Dietary supplementation, 140 mg/kg	Suppressed the expression of cyclin-D1 and c-Myc; decreased expression of Wnt5a, Sfrp1, Sfrp2, and Sfrp5; downregulated Wnt/ β-catenin pathway	[223]
		HCT116 tumor xenograft in athymic BALB/c mice	Oral administration, 75 mg/kg	Didn't inhibit tumor growth; suppress metastasis; downregulated MMP-2 and EGFR3	[224]
Genkwanin	Dried flower buds of *Daphne genkwa*	$APC^{Min/+}$ mice	Oral administration, 12.5 and 25 mg/kg	Inducted host defense; reduced proinflammatory cytokine levels	[225]
		AOM/DSS-induced C57BL/6J mice	Oral administration, 22.5 mg/kg	Suppressed colon cancer growth by triggering tumor cell death; inhibited of pro-inflammatory cytokines	[226]
Hesperidin	Citrus fruits	AOM-induced Swiss albino mice	Oral administration, 25 mg/kg	Inhibited NF-κB, iNOS and COX-2; reduced cellular oxidative indicators and improved antioxidant status	[227]
		AOM-induced male Swiss albino mice	Oral administration, 25 mg/kg	Inhibited the constitutively active Aurora-A driven PI3K/Akt/GSK-3 and mTOR; activated autophagy	[228]
		AOM-induced male F344 rats	Oral administration, 1000 ppm	Inhibited ACF formation; reduced colonic mucosal ODC activity and polyamine levels in the blood	[229]
		DMH-induced CRC in albino rats	Oral administration, 25 mg/kg	Elevated the expression of Smad4 and activin A	[230]
Hinokiflavone	*Selaginella tamariscina*, *Juniperus phoenicea*, and *Rhus succedanea*	CT-26 tumor in female BALB/c mice	Intraperitoneal injection, 25 and 50 mg/kg	Suppressed tumor growth and proliferation; induced apoptosis; downregulated Ki-67 and MMP-9	[231]
Icariside II	*Epimedi* Herba	SW620 tumor xenograft in nude BALB/c mice	Intraperitoneal injection, 25 mg/kg	Suppressed tumor growth; induced apoptosis	[232]
Icaritin	*Epimedium* sp.	HT-29 tumor xenograft in male nude mice	Oral gavage, 10 mg/kg	Suppressed tumor growth and volume	[233]

Table 3. *Cont.*

Phytocompound	Source	Animal Model Studied	Dose and Route of Administration	Mode of Action	Reference
Isoangustone A	*Glycyrrhiza* sp.	SW480 tumor xenograft in male BALB/c nu/nu mice	Intraperitoneal injection, 10 mg/kg	Suppressed tumor growth; induced autophagic cell death; upregulated phosphorylation of AMPK, ACC and LC3B-1 and II levels	[234]
Isoliquiritigenin	*Glycyrrhiza glabra*	AOM/DSS-induced colon carcinogenesis in male BALB/c mice	Intragastrical administration, 3, 15 and 75 mg/kg	Suppressed tumorigenesis; inhibited macrophage polarization; upregulated TNF-α, INF-γ and IL-12; downregulated TGF-β, IL-10 and IL-1 and COX-2	[235]
	Glycyrrhiza uralensis Fisher	AOM-treated colon carcinogenesis in 344 rats	Oral administration, 100 ppm dietary supplementation	Suppressed ACF formation; induced apoptosis	[236]
Isorhamnetin	*Opuntia ficus-indica*	HT-29 RFP xenograft in immunosuppressed mice	Oral administration, dose not reported	Elevated cleaved caspase-9, Hdac11, and Bai1 proteins	[237]
		FVB/N mice treated with AOM/DSS	Oral administration, dietary supplement, dose not reported	Inhibited nuclear translocation of β-catenin and c-Src stimulation; activated CSK	[238]
Kaempferol	Apple, tea, broccoli, and grapefruit	DMH-induced colorectal carcinogenesis in male Wistar rats	Oral administration, 200 mg/kg	Restored CAT, SOD, and GPx	[239]
		DMH-induced colon carcinoma in male Sprague Dawley rats	Oral administration, 200 mg/kg	Reduced multiple plaque lesions and preneoplastic lesions	[240]
		DMH-induced colitis in Sprague-Dawley albino rats	Oral administration, 200 mg/kg	Reduced multiplicity of the ACF; downregulated COX-2 and PCNA	[241]

Table 3. *Cont.*

Phytocompound	Source	Animal Model Studied	Dose and Route of Administration	Mode of Action	Reference
Luteolin	Celery, parsley, broccoli, onion leaves, carrots, peppers, cabbages, and tea	DMH-induced carcinogenesis in male Wistar rats	Subcutaneous injection, 0.2 mg/kg	Reduced the number of tumor polyps and colon polyploids; decreased COX-2 level in blood and colonic tissue	[242]
		AOM-induced CRC in male BALB/c mice	Oral administration, 1.2 mg/kg	Reduced the levels of alkaline phosphatase and lactate dehydrogenase; suppressed iNOS and COX-2	[243]
		AOM-induced CRC in male BALB/c mice	Oral administration, 1.2 mg/kg	Reduced cytochrome b_5, cytochrome P450 and cytochrome b_5; enhanced the expression of UDP-GT and GST in colonic tissue; upregulated Nrf2	[244]
		CT-26 mediated lung metastasis	Oral administration, 10 and 50 mg/kg	Suppressed lung nodules and nodule volume; inhibited MMP-9 expression	[245]
		AOM-induced colon carcinogenesis in BALB/c mice	Oral administration, 1.2 mg/kg	Inhibited MMP-2 and MMP-9; downregulated γ-glutamyl transferase, 5′ nucleotidase, cathepsin D, and carcinoembryonic antigen	[246]
		HT-29 tumor xenograft in BALB/c nude mice	Intragastric administration, 100 mg/kg	Suppressed CRC metastasis; upregulated miR-384; downregulated pleiotrophin expression	[247]
		HT-29 tumor xenograft in BALB/c nude mice	Intraperitoneal injection, 50 mg/kg	Inhibited tumor growth; induced apoptosis	[248]
Lysionotin	*Lysionotus pauciflorus* Maxim	HCT116 tumor xenograft in athymic nude mice	Intraperitoneal injection, 20 mg/kg	Suppressed tumor growth; induced ferroptosis	[249]
Magnolin	*Magnolia biondii*	HCT116 tumor xenograft in female BALB/c athymic nude mice	Intraperitoneal injection, 20 mg/kg	Suppressed tumor growth; downregulated LIF, STAT3 and Mcl-1	[250]

Table 3. *Cont.*

Phytocompound	Source	Animal Model Studied	Dose and Route of Administration	Mode of Action	Reference
Morin	Old fustic (*Chlorophora tinctoria*) and osage orange (*Maclura pomifera*)	Male athymic nude mice injected with HCT-116 cells	Intraperitoneal injection, 30 and 60 mg/kg	Inactivated NF-κB signaling	[251]
		Male albino Wistar rats injected with DMH	Intraperitoneal injection, 30 and 60 mg/kg	Modulated tumor metabolism via β-cateinin/c-myc signaling, glycolysis and glutaminolysis pathways	[252]
		Pirc rats (F344/NTac-Apc am1137)	Dietary supplementation, 50 mg/kg	Restored the sensitivity to apoptosis by inhibiting LMW-PTP	[253]
		Male albino Wistar rats injected with DMH	Intragastric administration, 50 mg/kg	Reduced ACF formation; suppressed fecal and mucosal biotransformation enzymes	[254]
		Male albino Wistar rats injected with DMH	Intragastric administration, 50 mg/kg	Inhibited NF-κB and inflammatory mediators; suppressed proapoptotic pathway	[255]
		DMH-induced colon carcinogenesis in a male Wistar rats	Oral administration, 50 mg/kg	Reduced lipid hydroperoxides and CD; increased superoxide SOD, CAT, GST, GPx, GR; decreased GSH	[256]
Myricetin	Tea, barriers, fruits, vegetables	DMH-induced rat colon carcinogenesis	Dietary supplementation, 50, 100 and 200 mg/kg myricetin	Restored CAT, GPx and GSH	[257]
		$APC^{Min/+}$ C57BL/6J mice	Oral gavage, 100 mg/kg	Promoted apoptosis in adenomatous polyps; lowered IL-6 and PGE2; downregulated p38 MAPK/Akt/mTOR signaling pathway	[258]
		AOM/DSS-induced in BALB/c mice	Oral gavage, 40 and 100 mg/kg	Inhibited the development of colorectal tumors and colorectal polyps; decreased the levels of TNF-, IL-1, IL-6, NF-κB, p-NF-κB, COX-2, PCNA, and cyclin D1	[259]
		AOM/DSS-induced colitis in C57BL/6 mice	Oral administration, 100 mg/kg	Decreased CSF/M-CSF, IL-6, and TNF-α in colonic mucosa; inhibited NF-κB/IL-6/STAT3 pathway	[260]

Table 3. *Cont.*

Phytocompound	Source	Animal Model Studied	Dose and Route of Administration	Mode of Action	Reference
Naringenin	Oranges, lemons, and grapefruit	AOM-induced colon carcinogenesis in rats	Dietary supplement, 0.02%	Reduce the number of HMACF by 51% and the proliferative index by 32%	[261]
		DSS-induced murine colitis model	Oral administration, 50 mg/kg	Decreased iNOS, ICAM-1, MCP-1, COX-2, TNF-α, and IL-6 transcript levels	[262]
		HT-29 tumor xenograft in athymic NIH Swiss nude mice	Oral administration, 40 mg/kg	Suppressed tumor growth; inhibited COX-1	[263]
Naringin	Oranges, lemons, and grapefruit	DMH-induced female Wistar rats	Oral gavage, 10, 100, 200 mg/kg	Reduced cell proliferation and tissue iron levels; upregulated antioxidant mineral levels	[264]
		AOM/DSS-induce Male C57BL/6 mice	Oral gavage, 50 and 100 mg/kg	Suppressed ER stress-induced autophagy in colorectal mucosal cells	[265]
		AOM-induced ACF in Sprague Dawley rats	Oral administration, 200 mg/kg	Reduced total number of ACF; suppressed proliferation; induced apoptosis; downregulated COX-2 and iNOS	[266]
Nobiletin	Peel of various *Citrus* fruits	AOM-DSS-induced colon carcinogenesis in male CD-1 mice	Oral, dietary supplement, 100 ppm	Reduced tumor incidences and multiplicity	[267]
Orientin	*Ocimum sanctum*	DMH-induced CRC in male Wister rats	Intraperitoneal injection, 10 mg/kg	Reduced NF-κB, TNF-α and IL-6; downregulated Ki-67 and PCNA; suppressed iNOS and COX-2	[268]
		DMH-induced CRC in male Wister rats	Intraperitoneal injection, 10 mg/kg	Suppressed ACF and crypt multiplicity; elevated the level of antioxidants; downregulated phase I enzymes and upregulated phase II enzymes	[269]
Oroxylin A	*Scutellaria baicalensis*	AOM-DSS induced CRC in C57BL/6 mice	Dietary supplementation, 50, 100 and 200 mg/kg	Suppressed tumor formation and colitis associated CRC; induced apoptosis; downregulated IL-6, IL-1β, p-STAT3, cyclin D, and Bcl-2; upregulated Bax	[270]
		HCT116 tumor xenograft in male athymic BALB/c nude mice and AOM-DSS induced colon carcinogenesis in male C57BL/ 6 mice	Oral administration, 150 and 300 mg/kg	Suppressed carcinogenesis and primary colon cancer progression; reduced triglyceride; downregulated HIF1α, Srebp1, FASN, ADRP and FABP7; upregulated CPT1	[271]
Pectolinarigenin	*Cirsium chanroenicum*	Murine CT26 CRC cells were introduced into BALB/C mice	Intraperitoneal injection, 25 and 50 mg/kg	Induced apoptotic death of cancer cells; suppression STAT3	[272]

Table 3. *Cont.*

Phytocompound	Source	Animal Model Studied	Dose and Route of Administration	Mode of Action	Reference
Peonidin	Sweet potato (*Ipomoea batatas*)	AOM-induced CF-1 mice	Dietary supplementation, 10 to 30%	Blocked cell cycle at the G1 phase; activated caspase-3	[273]
Petunidin	*Lycium ruthenicum*	Nude mice	Intraperitoneal injection, 25 and 50 mg/kg	Induced ferroptosis via inhibiting SLC7A11	[274]
Phloretin	*Manchurian apricot*	COLO 205 cells derived tumor in BALB/c nude mice	Route of administration not reported, 25 mg/kg	Inhibited tumor growth; upregulated p53, p21 and E-cadherin	[275]
Polyphenon E		AOM-induced colon carcinogenesis in F344 rats	Oral administration, 0.24%	Induced apoptosis; decreased eicosanoid, prostaglandin E2, and interleukin B4 in plasma; decreased nuclear β-catenin and increased expression of RXRα,β and γ in adenocarcinomas	[276]
Procyanidin	Cider apple (*Malus domestica*)	AOM-induced Wistar rats	Oral administration, 0.01%	Suppressed protein kinase; down-regulated of polyamine production; stimulated caspase-3	[277]
		Male C57/BL6 mice transfected with CT26 cells	Oral gavage, 30 mg/kg	Reduced cellular oxidative stress through modulation of Nrf2/ARE signaling	[278]
Quercetin	Apples, nuts, cauliflower, cabbage, onions, grapes, berries, broccoli, citrus fruits, cherries, green tea, and coffee	AOM-induced colon tumor in C57BL/6J male mice	Dietary supplementation, 0.5%	Induced apoptosis; upregulated CB1-R; downregulated STAT3 and p-STAT3; downregulated Bax/Bcl-2 ratio	[279]
		Subcutaneous DLD-1 human colon tumor fragment implant in male athymic nu/nu mice	Intraperitoneal injection, 30 mg/kg	Enhanced radiosensitivity by inhibiting ATM-mediated signaling pathway	[280]
		AOM-induced CRC in male weanling Sprague-Dawley rats	Dietary supplement, 4.5 g/kg	Reduced the number of crypts; inhibited proliferation; induced apoptosis; suppressed COX-1, COX-2 and iNOS	[281]
		AOM/DSS induced colon carcinogenesis in C57BL/6J mice	Dietary supplementation, 30 mg/kg	Reduced number and size of colon tumors; suppressed inflammation; downregulated LOP, NO, SOD, G6PD, and GSH	[282]
		CT-26 lung tumor metastasis in BALB/c mice	Intraperitoneal injection, 50 mg/kg	Suppressed lung metastasis; induced apoptosis	[283]
		HT-29 tumor xenograft in BALB/c nude mice	Subcutaneous injection, 10 mg/kg	Enhanced radiosensitivity; inhibited Notch-1 signaling	[284]

Table 3. *Cont.*

Phytocompound	Source	Animal Model Studied	Dose and Route of Administration	Mode of Action	Reference
Rutin	Buckwheat, Mez, Labisia pumila, *Sophora japonica* L., Schum, *Canna indica* L., and *Ruta graveolens* L.	SW480 cell-induced tumor xenograft	Intraperitoneal injection, 20 mg/kg	Suppressed tumor growth; decreased angiogenesis and VEGF levels	[285]
Scutellarin	*Scutellaria barbata*	AOM/DSS-induced male C57BL/6 mice	Intraperitoneal injection, 25, 50 and 100 mg/kg	Inhibited Wnt/β-catenin signal transduction	[286]
		RKO cells were subcutaneously implanted into female nude mice	Intraperitoneal injection, 50, 150 and 300 mg/kg	Suppressed tumor growth and metastasis	[287]
		AOM/DSS-induced mice	Intraperitoneal injection, 25, 50 and 100 mg/kg	Suppressed the Hedgehog signaling cascade	[288]
Silibinin	*Silybum marianum*	LoVo cell deposition on eight days old fertilized chicken egg	Route of administration not reported, 9.64 µg/mL	Decreased in VDI; upregulated *Flt-1* gene	[289]
		AOM-induced CRC in male Wistar rats	Intragastric intonation, 300 mg/kg	Suppressed preneoplastic lesion formation; activated apoptosis; registered sub G0/G1 cell cycle arrest; reduced MMP-7, IL-1β and TNF-α	[290]
Tangeretin	Peel of citrus fruits	HT-29 induced tumor xenograft in BALB/c nude mice	Route of administration not reported, 5 mg/kg	Suppressed tumor growth	[291]
Taxifolin	Olive oil, grapes, citrus fruits, and onion	HCT116 tumor xenograft in athymic male nude mice	Intraperitoneal injection, 15 and 25 mg/kg	Suppressed tumor growth; induced apoptosis; inhibited cyclin D; degraded β-catenin; inhibited of Akt phosphorylation	[292]
Tricin	Rice bran, oats, barley, and wheat	Colon26-Luc colon tumor and lung metastasis model in BALB/c mice	Oral gavage, 19 and 37.5 mg/kg	Suppressed tumor growth; reduced metastasis incidence	[293]
		AOM-DSS induced CRC in male Crj: CD-1 mice	Dietary supplement, 50 and 250 ppm	Restored colonic length; reduced number of incidences and multiplicity of adenomas and adenocarcinomas; downregulated PCNA and TNF-α	[294]

Table 3. *Cont.*

Phytocompound	Source	Animal Model Studied	Dose and Route of Administration	Mode of Action	Reference
Troxerutin	Tea and coffee	DMH-induced colon carcinogenesis in male albino Wistar rats	Oral administration, 12.5, 25 and 50 mg/kg	Lowered ACF formation and crypt multiplicity; reduced cytochrome P450, cytochrome b_5, cytochrome P4502E1, NADPH-cytochrome P450 reductase, and NADH-cytochrome b_5 reductase and upregulates phase GST, DTD and UDPGT	[295]
Vitexin	Passionflower, bamboo leaves, pearl, and millet	HCT116 tumor xenograft in nude BALB/c mice	Oral administration, 25, 50 and 100 mg/kg	Suppressed tumor growth; increased phosphorylation of JNK; upregulated LC3 II and ApoL1	[296]
		HCT116^{DR} tumor xenograft in female athymic BALB/c nude mice	Oral administration, 25 and 50 mg/kg	Suppressed tumor growth; induced apoptosis; downregulated HSP90, HSP70, HSP27, Atg7, Beclin-1, LC3 II and Bcl-2; upregulated Bax and PARP1; cleaved caspase-3 and caspase-9	[297]
Wogonin	*Scutellaria baicalensis*, *Scutellaria radix*	AOM/DSS-induced colitis related colon cancer in C57BL/6 mice	Gastric intubation, 60 mg/kg	Decreased cell proliferation; lowered the expression and secretion of IL-6 and IL-1β and expression of NF-κB; increased Nrf2 nuclear translocation	[298]
		AOM-DSS-induced CRC animal model in C57BL/6 mice	Route of administration not reported, 50 and 100 mg/kg	Reduced tumor multiplicity; reverted colon length to normal	[299]
		SW480 induced tumor xenograft in BALB/c nude mice	Intraperitoneal injection, 2 mM	Downregulated of YAP-1 and IRF3; upregulated p-YAP	[300]
Xanthohumol	*Humulus lupulus*	AOM-induced colorectal carcinogenesis in male Sprague-Dawley rats	Oral gavage, 5 mg/kg	Suppressed tumor growth; induced apoptosis; suppressed COX-2 and iNOS	[301]
Zapotin	Tropical fruit zapote blanco (*Casimiroa edulis*)	AOM/DSS-induced female CF-1 mice	Intragastric administration, 5 and 10 mg/kg	Induced cell cycle arrest and apoptosis	[302]

Table 3. *Cont.*

Phytocompound	Source	Animal Model Studied	Dose and Route of Administration	Mode of Action	Reference
		Phenolic acids			
Caffeic acid	Coffee, wine tea	CT-26 lung metastasis in BALB/c mice	Oral administration, 0.1 and 0.5 g/kg	Inhibited lung metastasis; suppressed MEK1, TOPK, and TAP-induced activation of AP1, NF-κB and ERK signaling; inhibited TAP, EGF and H-Ras induced neoplastic transformation	[303]
		HCT116 tumor xenograft in NSG mice	Intraperitoneal injection, 10 mg/kg	Inhibited CSC growth and self-renewal by inhibition of PI3K/Akt signaling	[304]
		HCT116 tumor xenograft in BALB/c AnN Foxn-1 nude mice	Oral administration, 50 nmol/kg	Inhibited PI3K/Akt/mTOR pathway; suppressed MMP-9, cyclin D1, Cdk4, cyclin E, PCNA, FASN c-Myc, and N-cadherin expression; upregulated p21	[305]
		HT-29 tumor xenograft in BALB/c nude mice	Intragastric administration, CAPE (10 mg/kg); CAPE-pNO2 5, (10 and 20 mg/kg)	Inhibited tumor growth and VEGF expression; upregulated p53, p27, p21, cyt. c, and cleaved caspase-3; downregulated procaspase-3, Cdk2, and c-Myc;	[306]
		HCT116 tumor xenograft in nude mice	Oral administration, 0.2 and 2 mg/kg	Suppressed tumor growth; displayed cell cycle arrest in S phase and autophagic cell death	[307]
Chlorogenic acid	Apple, betel, coffee beans, kiwi, grapes, eggplant, pear, plum, potato, and tea	MAM acetate-induced carcinogenesis hamsters	Oral administration, 0.025% dietary supplement	Reduced colon tumor incidences; registered antioxidative effect; inhibited the activity of microsomal enzyme	[308]
		AOM-induced ACF in colon of male F344 rats	Oral administration, 0.025% dietary supplement	Reduced ACF formation and growth	[309]

Table 3. *Cont.*

Phytocompound	Source	Animal Model Studied	Dose and Route of Administration	Mode of Action	Reference
Ellagic acid		AOM-induced colon tumors in rats	Oral administration, 250, 2500 and 5000 ppm	Inhibited the incidence of adenocarcinomas in the small intestine	[310]
		DMH-induced colon cancer in rats	Oral administration, 60 mg/kg	Lowered the frequency of ACF and lipid peroxidation; increased the activity of CAT, SOD, GPx, GR and GST; restored the levels of vitamin C, vitamin E and GSH	[311]
		DMH-induced colon cancer in Wistar albino rats	Oral administration, 60 mg/kg	Inhibited NF-κB, iNOS, COX-2, TNF-α and IL-6; restored the levels 5′-ND, γ-GT, CEA, AFP and LDH	[312]
		DMH-induced colon cancer in rats	Oral administration, 60 mg/kg	Inhibited PI3K-p58 activation; downregulated Akt and Bcl-2; upregulated Bax	[313]
		DMH-induced colorectal cancer in rats	Oral administration, 60 mg/kg	Inhibited ACF formation; increased the activity of CAT, SOD, GPx, and GR; inhibited ODC expression through inhibition of c-MYC	[314]
		DMH-induced colon cancer in male Laca mice	Oral administration, 10 mg/kg	Restored colon membrane alterations	[315]
Ferulic acid	Rice, wheat, pineapple, grains, and peanuts	AOM-induced colon cancer in male Fischer 344 rats	Oral administration, 250 ppm and 500 ppm	Reduced number and size of adenomas; increased the activity of GST and QR	[316]
		AOM-induced colon carcinogenesis in F344 rats	Dietary supplement of 3-(4′-geranyloxy-3-methoxyphenyl)-2propenoate (geranylated derivative of ferulic acid) 0.1% and 0.2%	Decreased the number of ACF	[317]

Table 3. *Cont.*

Phytocompound	Source	Animal Model Studied	Dose and Route of Administration	Mode of Action	Reference
Gallic acid	Barriers and pomegranates	DMH-induced colon cancer in male Wister rats	Oral administration, 50 mg/kg	Reduced lipid peroxidation, LOOH, CD, SOD, CAT, GSH, GR and GPx; reduced ascorbic acid and tocopherol levels	[318]
		SW480 induced tumor xenograft in NOD SCID gamma NSG mice	Intraperitoneal injection, 200 mg/kg	Exerted antitumor activity mediated by interaction with G-quadruplexes	[319]
		DSS-induced acute colitis in C57BL/6 mice	Oral administration, 5 and 25 mg/kg	Suppressed acute colitis; inhibited phosphorylation of STAT3	[320]
		HCT116 and HT-29 tumor xenografts in BALB/c nude mice	Intraperitoneal injection, 80 mg/kg	Suppressed p-SRC, p-EGFR, p-Akt and p-STAT3	[321]
		Ulcerative colitis in rats	Oral administration, 10 mg/kg	Suppressed colon cancer; induced ferroptosis	[322]
		DMH-induced colon cancer in male albino Wister rats	Oral administration, 50 mg/kg	Elevated the activity of cytochrome P450, cytochrome b5, GST, DT-diaphorase and γ-GT	[323]
Geraniin	*Phyllanthus amarus*	SW480 tumor xenograft in nude mice	Oral administration, 10, 20 and 40 mg/kg	Suppressed tumor growth; induced apoptosis; inhibited phosphorylation of PI3K and Akt	[324]
p-Coumaric acid	Mushrooms, apples, pears, barriers, oranges, and beans	DMH-induced colon carcinogenesis in male albino Wistar rats	Intragastric intubation, 100 mg/kg	Reduced ACF, DACF, MDF and BCAC	[325]
Syringic acid	Olives, dates, pumpkins, grapes, and palms	DSS-induced mice	Oral administration, 25 mg/kg	Decreased the level of iNOS, COX-2, TNF-α, IL-1β and IL-6; reduced activation and accumulation of p-STAT-3 by decreasing expression of p65-NF-κB	[326]
		DMH-induced colorectal cancer in male rats	Oral administration, 50 mg/kg	Reduced tumor incidences, tumor volume and average number of tumors	[327]
Lignans					
Arctigenin	*Arctium lappa*, *Forsythia suspensa.*	CT-26 cells derived lung metastasis model in BALB/c mice	Oral gavage, 50 mg/kg	Reduced the number of lung nodules; induced apoptosis in lung tissue; inhibited EMT in lung tissue; induced cleavage of caspase-3, caspase-9, and PARP; downregulated Bcl-2 and Bcl-xL; upregulated Bax	[328]

Table 3. *Cont.*

Phytocompound	Source	Animal Model Studied	Dose and Route of Administration	Mode of Action	Reference
Daurinol	*Haplophyllum dauricum*	HCT116 tumor xenograft in athymic BALB/c (*Slc/nu*) nude mice	Oral administration, 5 and 10 mg/kg	Suppressed tumor growth; upregulated p-Chk1(Ser345)/Chk1	[329]
Dehydrodiisoeugenol	*Myristica fragrans* Houtt	HCT116, zsw480, and patient-derived xenograft in female NOD/SCID mice	Intraperitoneal injection, 40 mg/kg	Suppressed tumor growth by inducing ER stress; upregulated BiP, PERK, and IRE1α	[330]
Gomisin A	*Schisandra chinesis*	CT-26 induced lung metastasis in female BALB/c mice	Intraperitoneal injection, 50 mg/kg	Suppressed lung metastasis; reduced the number of lung nodules; increased phosphorylation of AMPK and p38 in lung tissue	[331]
Honokiol	*Magnolia grandiflora*	SW620 tumor xenograft in female athymic BALB/c nude mice nu/nu	Intragastric administration, 50 mg/kg	Inhibited proliferation of CRC; upregulated TGF-β1 and p53 by upregulating BMP7	[332]
Justicidin A	*Justicia procumbens*	HT-29 tumor xenograft in NOD-SCID mice	Oral administration, 6.2 mg/kg	Suppressed tumor growth; induced autophagy in tumor tissue; induced apoptosis	[333]
Magnolol	*Magnolia officinalis*	CT-26 and HT-29 tumor in BALB/c and Cg-Foxn1^{nu}/CrlNarl nude mice respectively	Route of administration not reported, 50 and 100 mg/kg	Inhibited tumor growth; induced apoptosis; upregulation of Fas, Fas-L, cleaved caspase-3, cleaved caspase-9 and cleaved caspase-8; downregulated NF-κB, PKCδ, ERK, Akt, C-FLIP, and MCL-1; inhibition of PKCδ-NF-κB signaling	[334]
		HCT116 tumor xenograft in female BLB/c nude mice	Intraperitoneal injection, 5 mg/kg	Suppressed tumor growth without showing any toxicity	[335]
Schisandrin B	*Schisandra chinensis, Schisandra propinqua, and Schisandra rubriflora*	AOM-DSS-induced CRC in C57BL/6 mice	Oral administration, 3.7–30 mg/kg	Suppressed SIRT1	[336]
Secoisolariciresinol	*Fitzroya cupressoides* and *Crossosoma bigelovii*	HCT116 tumor xenograft in male BALB/c nude mice	Route of administration not reported, 50, 100 and 200 mg/kg	Inhibited tumor growth; induced pyroptosis; downregulated Ki-67; upregulated N-GSDMD	[337]
		DSS-induced colitis in mice	Dietary supplementation, 200 mg/kg	Suppressed tumor growth; reduced IL-1β, IL-18, TNF-α and NLRP1	[338]

Table 3. *Cont.*

Phytocompound	Source	Animal Model Studied	Dose and Route of Administration	Mode of Action	Reference
Sesaminol	*Sesamum indicum*	Ethanol-induced CRC in male C57BL/6NCr mice	Oral administration, 2.5 mg/mice	Reduced colonic lesions; downregulated iNOS and CYP2E1; lowered TNF-α, IL-6, MCP-1 and NF-κB levels; increased cell adhesion by upregulation of ZO-1, occludin and cladulin-1	[339]
Tracheloside	*Carthamus tinctorious* L. (safflower)	CT-26 lung metastasis in BALB/c mice	Oral administration, 25 and 50 mg/kg	Suppressed lung metastasis; induced apoptosis; upregulated E-cadherin RNA; downregulated N-cadherin, vimentin, snail and twist RNA	[340]
Vitexin	*Vitex negudo*	HCT116 tumor xenograft in female nu/nu mice	Intraperitoneal injection, 40 mg/kg	Inhibited tumor growth and lowered tumor volume; upregulated PUMA and p53; induced PUMA-mediated apoptosis	[341]
Stilbenes					
Piceatannol	Red and white grapes	AOM/DSS-induced colon tumor in C57BL/6J mice	Oral administration, 5 and 12.5 mg/kg	Decreased tumor number and size; decreased Ki-67- and COX-2-positive cell number; downregulated MCP1 and PD1	[342]
Polydatin	*Picea sitchensis*	Caco-2 tumor xenograft in C57BL/6 mice	Subcutaneously into the tumor, 150 mg/kg	Suppressed tumor growth; upregulated miR-382; downregulated PD-L1	[343]

Table 3. *Cont.*

Phytocompound	Source	Animal Model Studied	Dose and Route of Administration	Mode of Action	Reference
Pterostilbene	Blueberries and cranberries	AOM-induced colonic ACF preneoplastic lesions and adenomas in male ICR mice	Oral administration, 50 or 250 ppm	Reduced ACF and adenoma formation; induced apoptosis; downregulated iNOS and COX-2; inhibited Wnt/β-catenin signaling through suppressing phosphorylation of GSK3β; inhibited VEGF, cyclin D, MMPs, Ras, PI3K/Akt and EGFR	[344]
		AOM-induced colon tumors in F344 rats	Oral administration, 40 ppm	Reduced the proliferation of non-metastatic adenomas; downregulated IL-1β, IL-4, TNF-α, PCNA, β-catenin and cyclin D and p-NF-κB/p65	[345]
		AOM-induced colon tumor in male BALB/c mice	Oral administration, 50 or 250 ppm	Reduced NF-κB through inhibition of PKC-β phosphorylation; downregulated iNOS, COX-2 and aldose reductase; upregulated HO-1, GR and Nrf2 signaling	[346]
		CL187 transplantation model in BALB/c nude mice	Intraperitoneal injection, 25, 50, 100 and 200 mg/kg	Inhibited Top1-mediated DNA damage repair pathway	[347]
		AOM-induced colonic ACF preneoplastic lesions in F344 rats	Oral administration, 40 ppm	Inhibited ACF formation; blocked cell proliferation and iNOS	[348]
Resveratrol	Grapes, blueberries, raspberries, mulberries, and peanuts	LoVo cell-mediated metastasis model in mice	Intragastric administration, 50, 100 and 150 mg/kg	Inhibited metastasis; decreased tumor size; suppressed TGF-β1/Smad pathway; downregulated Snail and vimentin; upregulated E-cadherin expression	[349]
		$APC^{CKO}/Kras^{mut}$ mice	Dietary supplementation, 150 ppm and 300 ppm	Suppressed tumor formation; reduced tumor size; downregulated Kras expression	[350]
		DSS-induced colon carcinogenesis in rats	Oral administration, 60 mg/kg	Reduced ACF and MDF	[351]
		HCT116 tumor xenograft in ICR SCID mice	Oral administration, 150 mg/kg	Suppressed tumor growth; induced apoptosis; inhibited NF-κB	[352]
		COLO250-luc tumor xenograft in athymic mice	Injection in tumor, 6 μg/implant	Suppressed tumor growth	[353]

Table 3. *Cont.*

Phytocompound	Source	Animal Model Studied	Dose and Route of Administration	Mode of Action	Reference
		HT-29 tumor xenograft in BALB/c nu/nu mice	Intragastric administration, 480, 960 and 1920 mg/kg	Suppressed VEGF-mediated angiogenesis	[354]
Miscellaneous compounds					
Oleuropein	Olives (*Olea europaea*)	AOM-induced CRC in female A/J mice	Dietary supplementation, 125 mg/kg	Suppressed preneoplastic lesions; lowered tumor incidences; prevented DNA damage	[355]
Thymol	*Thymus vulgaris* L.	HCT116 tumor xenograft and lung metastasis model in BALB/c nude mice	Intraperitoneal injection, 75 and 150 mg/kg	Induced apoptosis; upregulated E-cadherin; downregulated N-cadherin; suppressed lung metastasis by inhibiting Wnt/β-catenin pathway	[356]
Verbascoside	Genus, *Cistanche*	HCT116 tumor xenograft in BALB/c nude mice	Tail vein injection, 20, 40, and 80 mg/kg	Upregulated HIPK2, p53 and Bax; downregulation Bcl-2	[357]

Abbreviation: ACC, acetyl CoA carboxylase; ACF, aberrant crypt foci; AFP, α-fetoprotein; AOM, azoxymethane; APC, adenomatous polyposis coli; BAX, B-cell lymphoma 2 associated x protein; BCAC, β-catenin accumulated crypts; BCL-2, B-cell lymphoma 2; BID, BH3 interacting-domain death agonist; CAC, colitis-associated colorectal cancer; CAT, catalase; CEA, carcinoembryonic antigen; CD, conjugated dienes; CIP2A, cancerous inhibitor of PP2A; c-MYC, cellular myelocytomatosis oncogene; COX-2, cyclooxygenase-2; CRC, colorectal cancer; CSK, C-terminal Src kinase; DACF, dysplastic aberrant crypt foci; DMH, 1,2-dimethylhydrazine; DNMT, DNA methyltransferase; EGCG, (-) epigallocatechin gallate; EGF-β, epidermal growth factor-β; EGFR, epidermal growth factor receptor; ERK, extracellular-signal-regulated kinase; FADD, Fas-associated protein with death domain; Flt-1, fms-like tyrosine kinase-1; GPx, glutathione peroxidase; GR, glutathione reductase; GSK-3β, glycogen synthase kinase-3β; GSH, glutathione; GST, glutathione S-transferase; γ-GT, γ-glutamyl transpeptidase; HMACF, high multiplicity aberrant crypt foci; IGF2, insulin like growth factor 2; IGFBP3, insulin like growth factor binding protein 3; IL-6, interleukin 6; iNOS, inducible nitric oxide synthase; KRAS, Kirsten rat sarcoma viral oncogene homolog; LC3b, light chain 3B of microtubule-associated proteins 1A/1B; LDH, lactate dehydrogenase; LMW-PTP, low molecular weight protein tyro-sine phosphatase; MAM, methyl azoxymethane; MAPK, mitogen-activated protein kinase; MDF, mucin-depleted foci; MMP, matrix metalloproteinase; mTOR, mammalian target of rapamycin; 5′-ND, 5′-nucleotidase; NEDD9, developmentally downregulated 9; NF-κβ, nuclear factor-κβ; Nrf-2, nuclear factor erythroid -2 related factor; ODC, ornithine decarboxylase; PCNA, proliferating cell nuclear antigen; PI3K, phosphoinositide 3-kinase; PP2A, protein phosphatase 2A; PTEN, phosphatase and TENsin homolog deleted on chromosome 10; QR, quinone reductase; SCID, severe combined immunodeficient; SIRT, Sirtuin 1; SOD, superoxide dismutase; STAT3, signal transducer and activator of transcription 3; TNF-α, tumor necrosis factor-α; Top1, topoisomerase 1; VDI, vascular density index; VEGF, vascular endothelial growth factor; γ-GT, γ-glutamyl transpeptidase.

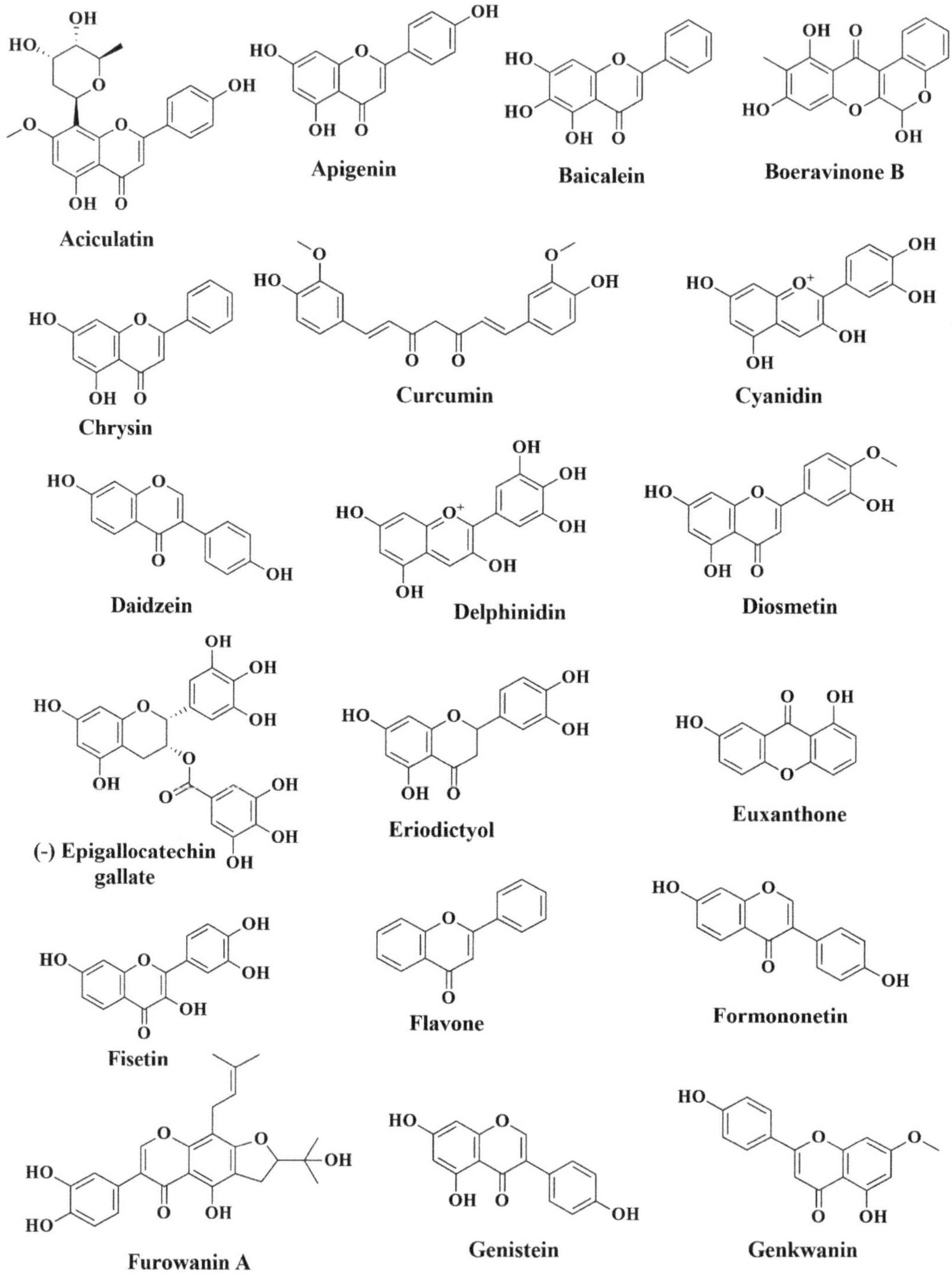

Figure 2. *Cont.*

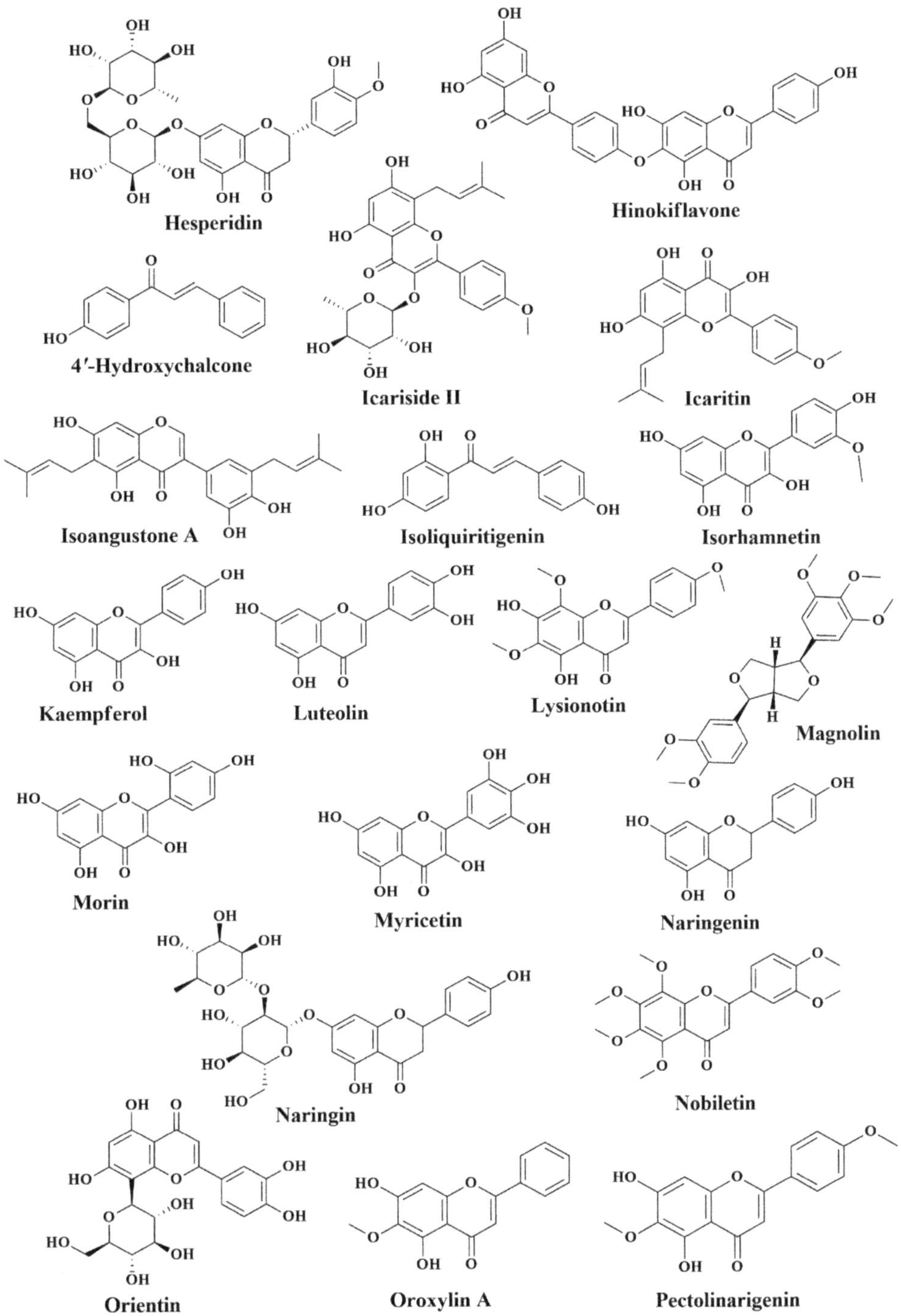

Figure 2. *Cont.*

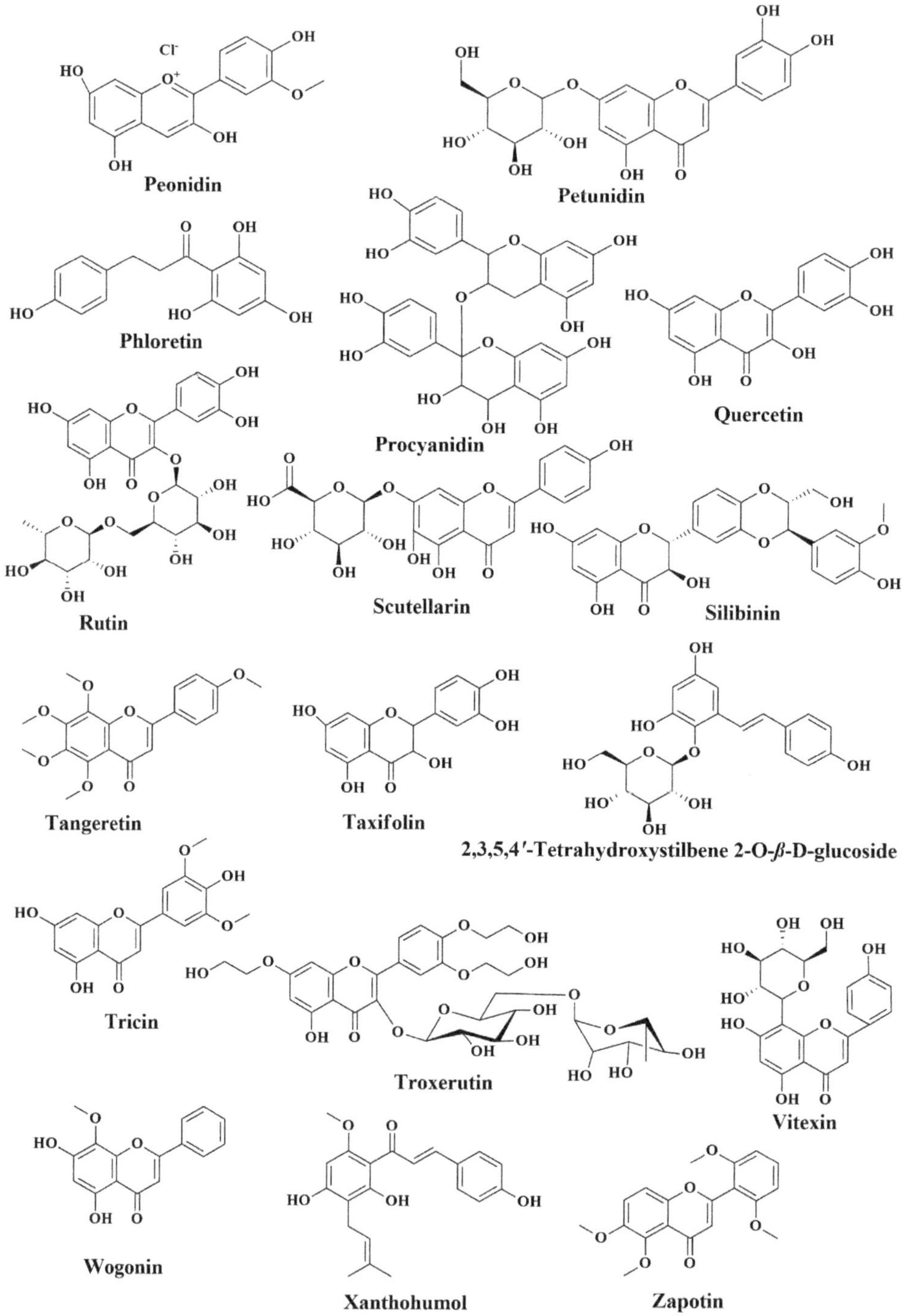

Figure 2. Chemical structures of flavonoids with in vivo anti-CRC activities.

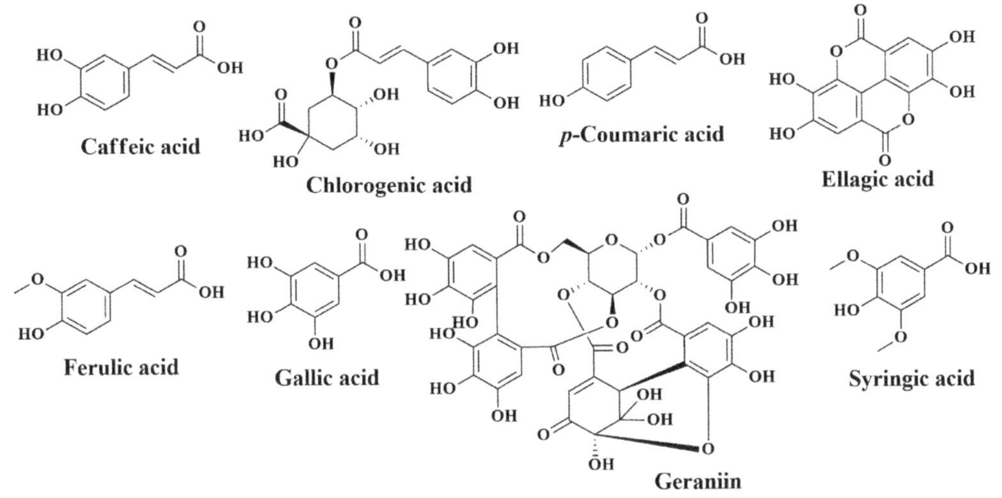

Figure 3. Chemical structures of phenolic acids with in vivo anti-CRC activities.

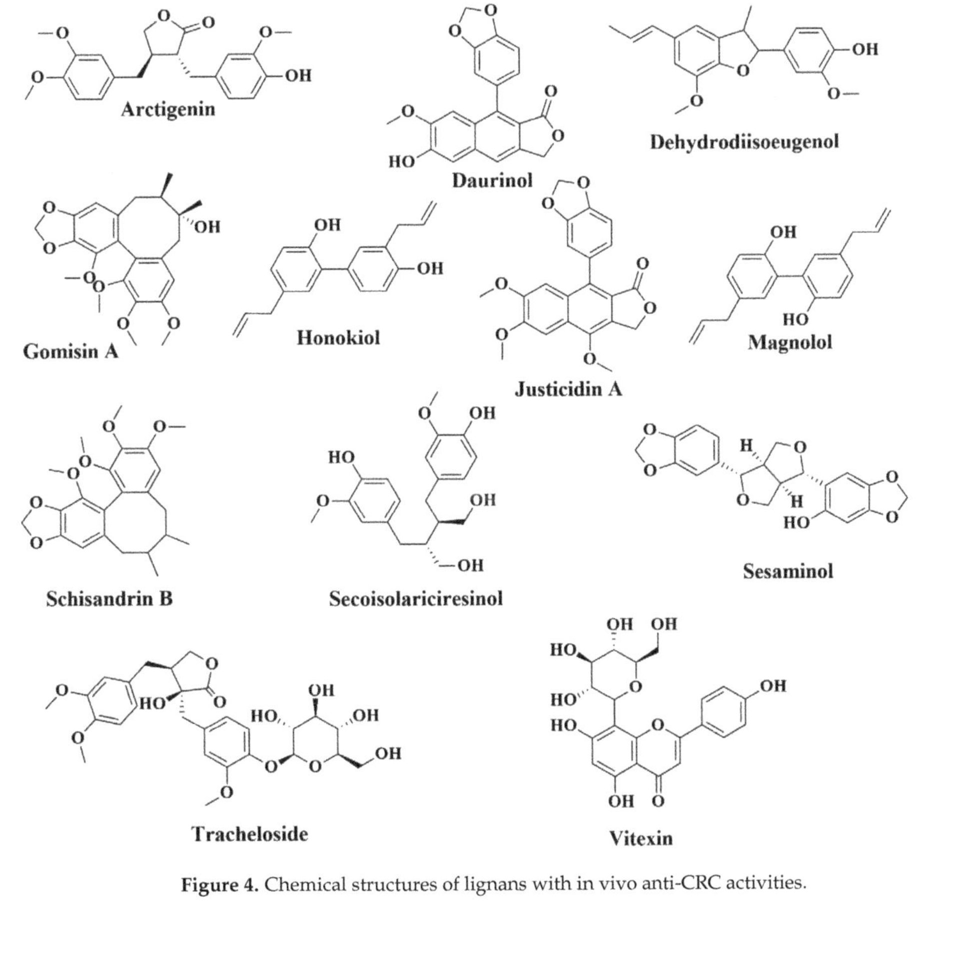

Figure 4. Chemical structures of lignans with in vivo anti-CRC activities.

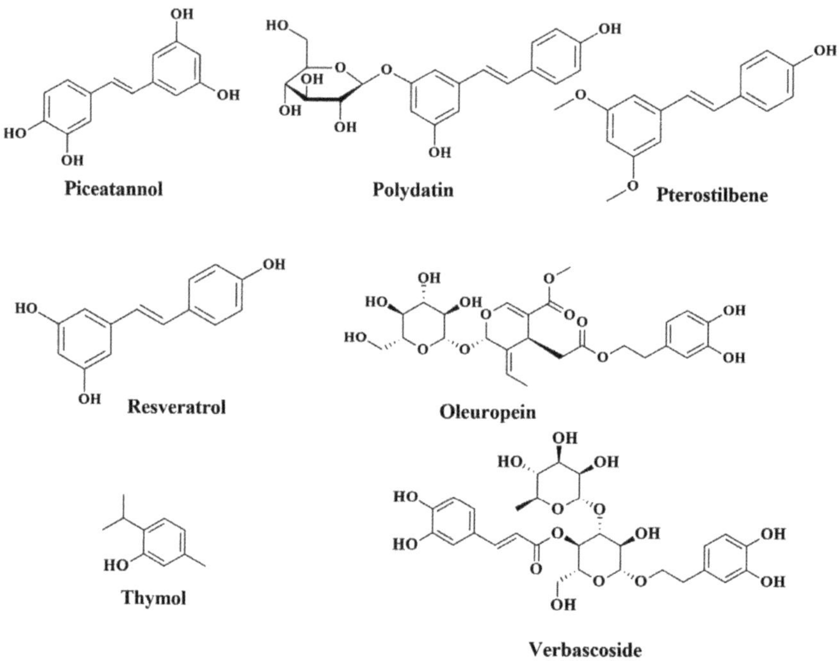

Figure 5. Chemical structures of stilbenes and miscellaneous compounds with in vivo anti-CRC activities.

7.1. Flavonoids

7.1.1. Baicalin

Baicalin (molecular weight: 446.4 g/mol), conjointly called baicalein 7-O-glucuronide and 7-D-glucuronic acid-5, 6-dihydroxyflavone or known by its chemical name, 5, 6 dihydroxy-4-oxo-2phenyl-chromen-7-yl) oxy-3, 4, 5-trihydeoxytetrahydropyran-2-carboxylic acid, is a glycosyloxyflavone. It is a key component of a variety of traditional medicine preparations, consisting of Sho-Saiko-To, Yangkun pills, Kushen decoction, and Shuanghuanglian injections. Scutellariae radix, Scutellaria planipes, Scutellaria rehderiana, and Scutellaria scandens are only a few of the Scutellaria species that contain the compound baicalin, which is extensively distributed throughout the genus [358].

Baicalein suppressed AOM/DSS-induced colon tumors in mice and induced apoptotic cell death. Baicalein suppressed inflammation by PARP1-mediated NF-κB inhibition [180]. A dose of 50 mg/kg baicalin suppressed the growth of highly metastatic SW620 tumor xenograft in BALB/c nude mice [181]. Baicalin inhibited the TLR4/NF-κB signaling and significantly suppressed CT-26 tumor growth, migration, and invasion. Anti-tumor immunity was also enhanced by an increase in $CD4^+$ and $CD8^+$ T cells in CT-26 tumors [182]. Baicalein treatment induced apoptosis in a p53-mediated Akt-dependent manner and suppressed HT-29 tumor xenograft [183]. In another study, baicalein suppressed MMP-2 and MMP-9 and inhibited DLD1 tumor growth and metastatic effects by inhibiting phosphorylation of ERK [184].

Dou et al. [185] showed that baicalein and baicalin can significantly inhibit the growth of HCT116 tumor xenograft by inducing tumor cell apoptosis and senescence through inhibiting the telomerase reverse transcriptase. It has also been hypothesized that the control of colon cancer cell apoptosis and senescence is caused by the MAPK, ERK, and p38 signaling pathways. Wang et al. [186] verified that baicalin application increased the expression of DEPP and triggered its downstream target Ras/Raf/MEK/ERK and p16INK4A/Rb pathways by serving as an antioxidant, resulting in senescence in colon carcinoma cells in HCT116 tumor model in BALB/c athymic nude mice. It was revealed that baicalin inhibited the HT-29 xenograft tumor in nude mice by suppressing c-Myc as the driver of miRNAs responsible for oncogenic development (oncomiRs). These findings demonstrated an association of c-Myc in baicalin-mediated inhibition of colon cancer growth [187]. In orthotopically transplanted tumors of CRC cells in BALB/c nude mice, baicalin administration lowered the levels of marker proteins for cell cycle, EMT, and stemness [188].

Wang et al. [189] observed that the baicalein therapy dramatically decreased tumor numbers in the small intestine and colon of $Apc^{Min/+}$ mice. Furthermore, reduced levels of inflammatory cytokines, such IL-1, IL-2, IL-6, G-CSF, and GM-CSF B, in this mouse tumor model suggested that baicalein's anti-CRC action was mediated by reducing gut inflammation. Baicalin treatment suppressed HCT116 tumor xenograft growth by downregulation of CircMYH9 and HDGF, and upregulation of miR-761 [190].

7.1.2. Curcumin

Curcumin, with the chemical name (1E, 6E)-1,7-bis(4-hydroxy-3-methoxyphenyl)-1,6-heptadiene-3,5-dione(diferuloylmethane), is a hydrophobic polyphenol derived from the roots of a well-known Indian spice, turmeric (Curcuma longa). Consumption of turmeric is believed to provide protection from numerous ailments, including CRC [359–362]. Anti-CRC activities of curcumin were demonstrated by several independent groups. Curcumin reduced putative precursor colonic lesions, e.g., aberrant crypt foci (ACF), through suppressing the levels of proinflammatory cytokines, such as TNF-α and IL-6, and proinflammatory mediators, such as COX-2, in obese and diabetic (db/db) mice [197]. Adiponectin plays an important anti-inflammatory role in the gut [363–365]. Curcumin increased the adiponectin level in both AOM-treated and untreated C57BL/KsJ-db/db (db/db) mice [197]. Leptin levels are directly proportional to body fat. High serum leptin levels can cause inflammation-mediated CRC [366,367]. Curcumin was able to reduce the body fat content along with serum leptin levels, and thus reduce the severity of CRC. This study also observed AMPK activation and COX-2 inhibition in those animals [197].

Curcumin reduced DSS-induced ACF and β-catenin accumulation. Due to its anti-inflammatory properties, curcumin suppressed pro-inflammatory cytokines and COX-2 and iNOS in DSS-induced colonic tissue [194]. Curcumin suppressed the growth of HCT116 tumor xenograft in ICR SCID mice. Curcumin treatment led to proteasome inhibition and induction of apoptosis which, in turn, suppressed the HCT116 tumor growth [195]. In another study, curcumin inhibited AOM/DSS-induced tumorigenesis in mice. Curcumin also downregulated Axin2 and exerted its anticancer activity by Axin2 mediated inhibition of the Wnt/β-catenin pathway [196].

Curcumin was found to inhibit HCT116-induced xenografts in male nude mice, along with suppressing NF-κB regulated genes, including Bcl-2, c-FLIP, IAP1, and survivin. It further cleaved procaspase-3 and procaspase-9. Curcumin pretreatment sensitized the tumor xenograft to γ-radiation and suppressed NF-κB activity by inhibiting the binding of NF-κB to its response element on its target genes, thus minimizing invasion, migration, and angiogenesis. Curcumin ameliorated the γ-radiation mediated increase of cellular proinflammatory mediator COX-2 and c-Myc in a HCT116 xenograft tumor model [198,199].

Furthermore, curcumin was found to modulate gut microbiome habitat in AOM-injected IL10-/-mice and was implicated in the function of anti-inflammation and the maintenance of gut homeostasis. The aberrant cytoplasmic and nuclear localization of β-catenin in AOM-treated wild-type and AOM/Il-10-/-mice was significantly reduced by curcumin treatment [200].

Curcumin enhanced the anti-CRC activity of capecitabine in HCT116 tumor xenografts in male athymic nu/nu mice through the induction of apoptosis and inhibition of angiogenesis, invasion, and metastatic factors, such as VEGF, ICAM-1, and MMP-9, and CXCR4. Inhibition of COX-2 and cell cycle progression mediators, cyclin D1 and c-Myc, was also observed in the curcumin-treated animals. The anti-CRC effects of liposomal curcumin alone and combined with oxaliplatin were tested on CRC xenografts induced by Colo205 and LoVo cells in athymic nu/nu mice. The combination therapy showed efficient tumor growth inhibition by apoptosis (PARP-1 cleavage). Liposomal curcumin also inhibited angiogenesis in consistence with the inhibition of VEGF, CD31, and IL-8 expression [201]. Phytosomal curcumin was tested for its ameliorative effects on an AOM/DSS model of colitis-associated CRC alone and in combination with 5-FU in in vivo. Curcumin, alone and in combination, functioned through modulating Wnt/β-catenin signaling and E-cadherin activities. Curcumin administered by oral gavage and in combination with 5-FU significantly inhibited GSK3 α/β and cyclin D1 expression. Curcumin was shown to reduce oxidative stress induced ACF and colon injuries induced by AOM/DSS by upregulating endogenous antioxidative enzymes, such as superoxide dismutase (SOD), catalase (CAT), thiolase, and inducing autophagy by upregulating beclin1 [200].

7.1.3. Catechins

Catechins are a group of polyphenols abundantly present in tea, cocoa, berries, grapes, and apples. Catechins have a myriad of health benefits, and their anticancer properties have been extensively studied [368,369]. Kim et al. [370] examined the effects of green tea polyphenol (GTP) dosage on DSS-induced acute colitis and DMH and DSS-induced colon cancer developed in male ICR mice. GTP contained 70% of total catechins, half of which were EGCG and 3% being caffeine. This study showed that a specific dosage of GTP was effective in ameliorating the carcinogenic effect of DSS/DMH. The basis of this activity was implicated in the antioxidant properties of GTP. If the dosage was higher or lower than the effective dose, GTP was ineffective. This is potentially due to a loss of, or insufficient, antioxidant properties. Depending on the treatment conditions, GTFP can exhibit antioxidant or pro-oxidant properties [371].

The anticancer effect of EGCG was also tested on azoxymethane (AOM)-induced male C57BL/KsJ-db/db (db/db) mice. EGCG caused a significant reduction in the levels of IGF-IR, phospho-IGF-IR, phospho-GSK-3β, β-catenin, COX-2, and cyclin D1. There was also an increase in serum IGFBP3 and a decrease in serum IGF-I, insulin, triglyceride, cholesterol, and leptin in the treated mice [206].

Zhong et al. [207] investigated the acetylated-EGCG activity against protumorigenic inflammatory mediators in AOM-mediated colitis-induced CRC in a male mouse model. Acetylated-EGCG inhibited the expression of pro-tumorigenic inflammatory mediators, such as inducible nitric oxide synthase (iNOS) and COX-2. iNOS is one of the enzymes that remain in ACF and causes the continuous formation of nitric oxide (NO), leading to the promotion of tumorigenesis [372–374]. Furthermore, COX-2 converts arachidonate to prostaglandin E2. A sustained overexpression of prostaglandin E2 in the tissues may lead to epithelial cell cancers, including CRC [207,375,376].

EGCG showed the antistemness and chemosensitizing effects on xenograft tumors of HCT116 spheroid-derived cancer stem cells in male nude mice. EGCG inhibited CRC stemness and sensitized 5-FU-resistant HCT116 cells. EGCG suppressed stemness markers, such as Notch-1, and upregulated the expression of tumor suppressive miRNAs, including miR34a, miR200c, and miR-145 [208].

Another study demonstrated the effects of green tea catechins alone and in combination with curcumin on DMH-induced colon cancer in male Wistar rats [209]. A 32-week-long dietary treatment with curcumin, green tea catechins, and their combination showed a significant reduction in the number of colorectal aberrant cryptic foci in these animals. Notably, the combinatorial treatment had a greater effect than that with either of the compounds acting alone. A significant decrease in the proliferation index and an increase in the apoptotic index were reported in the groups treated with a combination of the compounds, compared to the mock-treated group or those receiving only DMH [209].

The anticancer effect of polyphenol E (PPE) was tested on AOM-treated F344 rats. PPE is a standardized GTP mixture containing 65% EGCG and other catechins. After AOM treatment, the animals were given a 20% high-fat diet, with or without 0.24% PPE for 34 weeks. PPE treatment resulted in a significant reduction in tumor size and the number of tumors in these animals. PPE was shown to decrease nuclear β-catenin levels, induce apoptosis, and increase the levels of RXR-α, RXR-β and RXR-γ expression in adenocarcinomas. This was accompanied by the lowering of proinflammatory eicosanoids, prostaglandin E2, and leukotriene B4 in the plasma [276].

7.1.4. Fisetin

Fisetin is a hydroxy flavone under the subgroup of flavonoid found in various fruits and vegetables, such as strawberry, apple, persimmon, grapes, onion, and cucumber. In an AOM/DSS-induced colitis associated CRC model in BALB/c mice, fisetin suppressed dysplastic lesions through inducing apoptosis in the colonic tissue along with downregulation of Bcl-2 and STAT3, and upregulation of cleaved-caspase-3 and BAX. Fisetin treatment restored the level of enzymatic (SOD, CAT, GPx, and GR) and non-enzymatic (vitamin E, and vitamin C) antioxidants in DMH-induced colonic tissue back to normal [213].

Fisetin treatment resulted in activation of AMPKα and inhibition of PI3K/Akt/mTOR signaling pathway along with decreased expression of PI3K, reduced Akt phosphorylation in PIK3CA mutants. In $FC^1 3K^1 Apc^{Min/+}$ mice, fisetin decreased the occurrence of colonic tumor incidences. In combination with 5-FU, fisetin reduced the overall colonic tumor incidences [214].

Fisetin inhibited growth of LoVo tumor xenograft in athymic nude mouse model. Mechanistic study revealed that fisetin acted by inducing apoptosis in tumor tissue through activation of caspase-8 and increased cyt. c expression. In the tumor tissue of treated animals, inhibition of IGF1R and Akt activation was observed [215].

Although CT-26 tumor growth was suppressed upon the intratumoral injection of fisetin, HCT116 tumors were not sensitive to the similar treatment where a combination of radiation with fisetin was more effective. Fisetin suppressed the oncoprotein securin in CT-26 tumor in a p53-independent fashion, but securin null HCT116 tumors are more sensitive to fisetin treatment [216].

Fisetin suppressed HCT116 induced tumor growth in NOD/Shi-scid-IL2R gamma (null) (NOG) mice in a dose-dependent manner compared to control group [218]. Another study showed that due to poor water solubility, the fisetin micelles, composed of poly(ethylene glycol)-poly(ε-caprolactone), i.e., MPEG-PCL, are more efficient antitumor agents over free fisetin as tested in CT-26 tumor model. MPEG-PCL showed enhanced inhibition of angiogenesis through inducing apoptotic cell death [217].

7.1.5. Genistein

Genistein, a naturally occurring isoflavone, was first isolated from Genista tinctoria. Its anticancer properties have been extensively studied [377]. Sekar et al. [222] examined genistein's role in regulating the tumor microenvironment in DMH-induced colon cancer in Wistar rats. This study revealed that genistein could regulate enzymatic (SOD, CAT, GPx, and GR) and non-enzymatic (vitamin E, vitamin C, vitamin A, and GSH) antioxidants in DMH-induced colonic tissue environments. It was found that the loss of mucin secretion in DMH-induced animals was restored by genistein. There was also a reduction of mast cell population and collagen deposition in genistein-treated animals compared to mock-treated animals. Argyrophilic nuclear organizer region and proliferating cell nuclear antigen, two prognostic markers, were decreased by genistein in DMH-treated rats. Genistein activated NRF2 and its downstream target, heme oxygenase-1, and alleviated DMH-induced oxidative stress. Higher expression of colonic stem cell markers, such as CD133, CD44, and β-catenin, was found to be reduced by genistein in DMH-treated animals [222].

It was shown that oral administration of genistein to mice carrying orthotopically implanted human CRC did not inhibit tumor growth. However, it did show inhibition of distant metastasis formation at a dose non-toxic to the animals. Subsequent biochemical analyses showed genistein-mediated downregulation of matrix metalloproteinase-2 (MMP-2) and FMS-related tyrosine kinase 4, also known as vascular endothelial growth factor receptor 3, suggesting its inhibitory role against neoangiogenesis in mouse tumors [224].

Chen et al. [378] conducted a study in which clinical signatures of the anti-CRC activity of genistein were tested in clinical samples of plasma, tumor tissue samples, and standard tissue samples isolated from patients. The expression of miR-95, serum glucocorticoid kinase 1 (SGK1), Bcl-2, and Erk1 was highly elevated in samples of CRC compared to the normal samples. Furthermore, genistein could sensitize CRC SW620 cells to apoptosis with increased LDH content in a concentration-dependent manner, accompanied by downregulation of endogenous miR-95, SGK1, and Erk1 activities [378].

Zhang et al. [223] studied the effect of genistein on AOM-induced colon carcinogenesis in male Sprague Dawley rats. The animals were given a control diet, soya protein isolate (SPI), and a genistein diet orally, starting from gestation to 13 weeks of age. Pre-AOM treatment analysis was performed by taking samples at seven weeks of age, and the remaining rats were AOM-treated at this time for six weeks for analysis. Compared to the control group, AOM injections did not cause aberrant nuclear accumulation of β-catenin in SPI and genistein-treated groups. Moreover, SPI and genistein suppressed the expression of cyclin-D1 and c-Myc. In addition, the expression of Wnt signaling genes (Wnt5a, Sfrp1, Sfrp2, Sfrp5) was decreased to a level comparable to that of pre-AOM treatment by SPI and genistein. Furthermore, the rats fed SPI and genistein had lower numbers of total aberrant crypts, which correlated with the reduction in Wnt/β-catenin signaling. Genistein also lowered the number of ACF [223].

The first clinical study to assess the safety and tolerability of genistein in combination with chemotherapy for the treatment of metastatic CRC was conducted by Pivota et al. [379]. Patients diagnosed with metastatic CRC but not previously treated were administered FOLFOX or FOLFOX-bevacizumab. Genistein (60 mg/day) was given orally for seven days every two weeks. Treatment was started four days before chemotherapy and continued through days one through three of infusion chemotherapy. In this trial, thirteen patients received combinatorial treatment. Treatment with genistein alone resulted in mild side effects, such as headaches, nausea, and hot flashes, with one subject experiencing grade 3 hypertension. There was no increase in chemotherapy-related adverse events when genistein was added to FOLFLOX. The best overall response rate for the genistein supplementation of the chemotherapy regimen was 61.5%. The median progression-free survival of the same study was 11.5 months [379].

7.1.6. Kaempferol

Kaempferol, a dietary flavanol found in many plants, including apple, tea, broccoli, and grapefruit, has been demonstrated to carry antitumor effects based on preclinical studies [380]. Nirmala et al. [239] demonstrated the beneficial effects of orally administered kaempferol with intravenous irinotecan in 1,2-dimethyl hydrazine (DMH)-induced colorectal carcinoma in male Wistar rats. In the kaempferol-fed animal groups, levels of DMH-induced erythrocyte lysate levels and decreased liver thiobarbituric acid reactive substances. Levels of several antioxidant enzymes, such as catalase, superoxide dismutase, and glutathione peroxidase, were recovered, and the most successful effects were achieved at a dose of 200 mg/kg body weight of kaempferol (which is comparable to irinotecan).

The combined effect of fluoxetine, an antidepressant drug, and kaempferol in alleviation of DMH-induced colon carcinoma in male Sprague Dawley rats was also analyzed. Compared to fluoxetine and kaempferol alone, combined treatment of these two agents caused greater reduction in multiple plaque lesions and preneoplastic lesions in the colonic tissues. This combinatorial treatment also reduced tissue concentration of malondialdehyde and NO. Both serum and tissue β-catenin levels were significantly decreased by the combinatorial treatment. There was also a significant increase in serum and tissue caspase-3 levels. PCNA and COX-2 positive cells in the colon of animals receiving the combinatorial treatment were lower when compared to fluoxetine and kaempferol treatments alone [240].

Hassanein et al. [241] studied the effect of sulindac in combination with either EGCG or kaempferol in DMH-induced colon carcinogenesis in male Sprague Dawley rats. The combinations of EGCG and kaempferol with sulindac, a nonsteroidal anti-inflammatory drug, caused great enhancement of sulindac's antioxidant, anti-inflammatory, antiproliferative, and apoptotic activities. Sulindac combined with both compounds caused a decrease in thiobarbituric acid-reactive substance, tissue NO, and both serum and tissue β-catenin. Downregulation of PCNA and COX-2 and a decrease in the number of ACF caused by DMH administration were also noted [241].

7.1.7. Luteolin

Luteolin (3′,4′,5,7-tetrahydroxyflavone) was discovered in different fruits, vegetables, and medicinal herbs. Plants rich in luteolin are used for treating various ailments, such as hypertension, inflammation, and cancer in Chinese traditional medicine [381,382]. The anti-CRC activity, as well as the anti-angiogenic, anti-invasive, and antimetastatic effects of luteolin were studied using AOM-induced colitis models of male BALB/c mice. Upregulation of γ-glutamyl transferase (GGT), found in a number of human neoplasms, facilitates neoplastic progression and metastasis [246,383]. GGT and 5′-nucleotidase (5′ND) were inhibited in AOM-treated mice by luteolin. Furthermore, luteolin reduced other tumor markers in AOM-treated animals, such as cathepsin-D and carcinoembryonic antigen (CEA), which are correlated with poor prognosis [246]. Luteolin inhibited invasion and metastasis by reducing the expression of MMP-2 and MMP-9 along with enhancing expression of tissue inhibitor metalloproteinases 2 (TIMP-2) [246]. Mast cells were associated with enhanced angiogenesis and tumor malignancy [384]. It was found that luteolin also decreased giant mast cell and total mast cell populations in AOM-treated mice, compared to AOM-induced control animals [246].

Luteolin reduced the number and size polyps of DSS-treated mice. Upon luteolin treatment, DSS-induced oxidative stress, level of carcinoembryonic antigen and COX-2 were decreased in colonic tissue [242]. In another study, luteolin was shown to suppress AOM-induced CRC by downregulating iNOS and COX-2 expression level [243]. Luteolin also suppressed AOM-induced CRC by activating Nrf2/Keap1 pathway [244].

Luteolin inhibited HT29 xenograft's growth in nude mice by an activity consistent with modulation of miR-384/pleiotrophin axis [247]. miR384 expression was found to be downregulated in the majority (83%) of CRC biopsy samples, correlating with the invasiveness and migratory abilities of CRC [385]. Pleiotrophin plays a major role in angiogenesis through upregulation of VEGF in CRC [386]. Luteolin treatment of HT-29 cell-induced xenograft tumor developed in female nude BALB/c mice efficiently suppressed the migration of CRC cells from the spleen to the liver and metastasis through upregulation of miR-384/pleiotrophin axis. Luteolin upregulated the expression of miR-384, which, by targeting pleiotrophin expression, inhibited the expression of MMP-2, MMP-3, MMP-9, MMP-16, as well as invasion and metastasis of CRC [247]. Luteolin, in synergy with adenovirus CD55-TRAIL, inhibited HT-29 xenografts in female BALB/c nude mice through increasing the apoptotic activity [248].

In another study, luteolin showed antimetastatic activity against CT-26 lung metastasis by downregulating MMP-2 and MMP-9. MEK and Akt phosphorylation was suppressed by the inhibition of Raf and PI3K by luteolin [245].

7.1.8. Myricetin

Myricetin (3,3′,4′,5,5′,7-hexahydroxyflavone), a naturally occurring flavonoid pigment, is typically present in fruits, herbs, and nuts. The presence of three hydroxyl groups at 3-′, 4-′, and 5′-carbon positions makes myricetin unique from other flavanols [387]. Studies by Nirmala and Ramachandran [257] showed the efficacy of myricetin on 1,2-dimethylhydrazine-induced rat colon carcinogenesis. They demonstrated that myricetin administration reduced the incidence of tumor-bearing rats and tumors in total. Furthermore, myricetin supplementation dramatically decreased intestinal tumorigenesis developed in adenomatous polyposis coli multiple intestinal neoplasia ($APC^{Min/+}$) mice. Additionally, myricetin treatment improved the antioxidant enzymes, including catalase, glutathione peroxidase, and GSH, in a dose-dependent manner [257].

Li et al. [258] assessed the effectiveness of myricetin against intestinal tumorigenesis in adenomatous polyposis coli multiple intestinal neoplasia ($APC^{Min/+}$) mice. Promoting apoptosis in adenomatous polyps, myricetin-fed $APC^{Min/+}$ mice grew fewer, smaller polyps and did not appear to experience negative side effects. By modifying the GSK-3 and Wnt/-catenin pathways, lowering the levels of the proinflammatory cytokines IL-6 and PGE2, and downregulating the phosphorylated p38 MAPK/Akt/mTOR signaling pathway, myricetin prevents the growth of intestinal tumors [258].

AOM/DSS-induced mice were used by Zhang et al. [259] to test myricetin's effectiveness against chronic colonic inflammation and inflammation-driven carcinogenesis. Myricetin significantly decreased the levels of inflammatory factors, such as TNF-, IL-1, IL-6, NF-B, p-NF-B, COX-2, PCNA, and cyclin D1, to inhibit the development of colorectal tumors and shrink colorectal polyps [259].

M10, a new derivative of myricetin, was tested by Wang et al. [205] to show that M10 inhibits robust endoplasmic reticulum (ER) stress-induced autophagy in inflamed colonic mucosal cells of AOM/DSS-induced mice model. The decreased levels of proinflammatory mediators, such CSF/M-CSF, IL-6, and TNF-α, in colonic mucosa and the prevention of the NF-κB/IL-6/STAT3 pathway, were shown to be associated with the antitumor activity [260].

7.1.9. Naringenin

Naringenin, a flavonoid found mostly in citrus fruits and vegetables with no taste or color, carries antioxidant, anti-inflammatory, antiviral, antimicrobial, and antitumor properties [388]. In addition, naringenin was found to reduce the number of high multiplicity aberrant crypt foci (HMACF) by 51% and the proliferative index by 32% in an AOM-induced rat model. Here, naringenin was implied to prevent CRC through decreasing proliferation and increasing apoptosis of luminal surface colonocytes [261].

Naringenin inhibited a dextran sulfate sodium (DSS)-induced murine colitis model. The inhibitory action was correlated with the inhibition of iNOS, ICAM-1, MCP-1, COX-2, TNF-α, and IL-6 transcript levels. The decrease in TNF-α and IL-6 levels was consistent with the suppression of TLR4 mRNA and protein in the colon mucosa. LPS-induced nuclear translocation of p65/RelA was also inhibited by naringenin in RAW264.7 cells, suggesting its action through TLR4 inhibition [262].

6-C-(E-phenylethenyl)-naringenin (6CEPN) inhibited anchorage independent growth of CRC cells, as well as in a CRC-induced xenograft in a dose-dependent manner through the inhibition of COX-1, an underlying cause of malignant character of CRC cells [263].

Naringin was shown to reduce tumor size and growth of AMO or DSS-induced CRC model in C57BL/6 mice by suppressing ER stress-induced autophagy in colorectal mucosal cells [265]. Another study showed naringin-mediated inhibition of tumor cell proliferation and AOM-induced CRC through inducing apoptosis in an AOM-injected Sprague-Dawley rat model [266,389].

7.1.10. Quercetin

Quercetin (3,4,5,7-pentahydroxyflavone), a polyphenolic flavonoid, was isolated from vegetables, fruits, grain, seeds, and tea [282,390]. Quercetin was shown to carry various pharmacological properties, including anticancer properties. It was further found to be effective against AOM/DSS-mediated colitis induced CRC and showed a decrease in mucin-depleted foci and aberrant crypt foci development [391]. In addition, quercetin treatment was shown to efficiently reduce AOM/DSS-induced inflammation, a major cause of colon carcinogenesis [282,392,393]. In another study, quercetin was found to restore leukocyte levels lost by AOM/DSS treatment. It was also noted that quercetin efficiently downregulated various oxidative stress-related markers, such as lipid peroxide (LPO), NO, SOD, glucose-6-phosphate (G6PD), and glutathione (GSH), explaining its role in neutralizing inflammation. The metabolic profiling of sera demonstrated the effect of quercetin through the downregulation of biomarkers that are upregulated in AOM/ DSS-treated mice [282].

In a metastatic cancer model induced in BALB/c mice by CT-26 cells, quercetin was shown to be effective through inducing the intrinsic pathway of apoptosis, along with upregulating the p-38 MAPK pathway. Notably, quercetin function was correlated with modulation of the EMT markers, such as downregulation of N-cadherin, snail, MMP-2, and MMP-9, while E-cadherin, TIMP-1, and TIMP-2 were upregulated [283].

Quercetin augmented radio-sensitization of CRC cells observed in HT-29 tumor xenografts through induction of apoptosis. Combining quercetin with a low dosage of 5Gy radiation effectively suppressed CRC cell proliferation with little toxicity towards normal colonic epithelial cells, CCD-18Co. The combinational therapy was found to target cancer stem cells, as suggested by the reduction of cancer stemness factors, such as DCLK-1, CD24, Lgr5, CD29, and CD44, and the colonosphere formation. The proportion of CD133+ cells also decreased in DLD-1 and HT-29 cells under combinatorial treatments [284].

Li et al. [284] further observed that the combinational therapy of ionizing radiation and quercetin targets the notch-signaling pathway through the downregulation of γ-secretase. The combinational therapy of ionizing radiation and quercetin effectively reduced the expression of γ-secretase complex components nicastrin, PEN2, APH1, presenilin-1, and presenilin-2, which suppressed notch cleavage and thus notch signaling. The combination therapy also inhibited the expression of Jagged-1 and cleaved Notch-1 protein levels [284].

Quercetin induced antiproliferative activity and proapoptotic effects are mediated by the upregulation of cannabinoid receptor-1 (CB1-R) in AOM-treated mice. The downregulation of STAT3 and pSTAT3 was also observed [279].

When radiation therapy was used with quercetin treatment, it suppressed the tumor size of the DLD1 tumor xenograft in athymic nude mice, indicating that quercetin enhanced the radiosensitivity of DLD1 tumors [280].

7.1.11. Rutin

Rutin, a glycosidic derivative of quercetin, is also known as quercetin-3-O-rutinoside or vitamin-P. It is known to carry antimicrobial, antifungal, anti-inflammatory, anticancer, and antiallergic properties, with poor solubility in water [394]. Rutin naturally occurs in various plants, including buckwheat, Mez, Labisia pumila, *Sophora japonica* L., Schum, *Canna indica* L., and *Ruta graveolens* L. [395,396]. In a dose-dependent manner, rutin suppressed SW480 cell-induced tumor growth in a tumor xenograft model without affecting the organ or body weight. In the same model, rutin was shown to enhance mean survival time by 50 days and suppressed angiogenesis through decreasing the serum VEGF level [285].

7.1.12. Tangeretin

Fruits and vegetables contain a wide variety of flavonoids. Citrus fruit flavonoids exhibit various biological effects, such as anticancer and antitumor properties. For example, tangeretin, a polymethoxylated (5,6,7,8,4′-pentamethoxyflavone) flavone, is predominant in the peel of citrus fruits and is thought to operate as a natural resistance factor against pathogenic fungus. In addition, tangeretin has been demonstrated to have several biological properties, including the capacity to suppress cancer cell growth [397].

Bao et al. [291] sought to create a nano-system that included tangeretin (TAGE) and atorvastatin (ATST) and was embellished with RGD (cyclized arginine-glycine-aspartic acid sequences) to treat colon cancer. To assess the anticancer effects of these two drugs on colon cancer cells and in female BALB/c mice harboring cancer models, these researchers produced ATST and TAGE combination nanosystems; RGD-ATST/TAGE CNPs. Results indicated that the RGD-decorated nano-system was more hazardous to HT-29 cells than the undecorated nano-system and that the weight ratio of ATST to TAGE, at which the highest synergism was seen, was 1:1. The integrated nano-systems had a high in vivo biodistribution in the tumor site and effectively reduced in vivo tumor development without significantly harming the treated mice's primary organs and tissues [291].

7.1.13. Wogonin

The medicinal plant *Scutellaria baicalensis* and the traditional Chinese medicine of Huang-Qin (Scutellaria radix) include a significant active monoflavonoid called wogonin (5,7-dihydroxy-8-methoxyflavone). Wogonin has many therapeutic possibilities, including anti-inflammatory and anticancer effects. It has also been observed to inhibit the development of several types of cancer cells with excellent specificity between normal cells and cancer cells [398,399].

To study wogonin's role in colitis-associated colorectal cancer (CAC), Yao et al. [298] developed the AOM/DSS-induced C57BL/6 mice paradigm. They discovered that wogonin markedly reduced the prevalence of tumors and prevented the growth of colorectal adenomas by lowering the expression and secretion of IL-6 and IL-1β, as well as decreasing the cell proliferation and expression of NF-κB in adenomas and adjacent tissues. Further, it increased Nrf2 nuclear translocation in those same tissues [298].

Feng et al. [299] evaluated wogonin's anti-colon cancer effect in an AOM-DSS-induced CRC animal model. They discovered that wogonin decreased tumor abundance and kept colon length within normal range without adversely affecting other organs. In addition, wogonin administration inhibited the SW480 cell-induced xenograft growth in BALB/c mice. Another study, by You et al. [300], further examined the effects of wogonin in mice with colon cancer. Treatment with wogonin abrogated the survival and metastasis properties of colon cancer cells in vivo. A detailed analysis revealed that wogonin-mediated upregulation of p-YAP1 level was responsible for the observed anti-colon cancer effect. This suggested the involvement of the Hippo signaling pathway in the process.

7.2. Phenolic Acids

7.2.1. Caffeic Acid

Caffeic acid (3,4-dihydroxycinnamic acid) is a nonflavonoid catechol with potent antioxidant properties. It is found in almost all plants as an intermediate in the lignin biosynthesis pathway. The prime source of caffeic acid is coffee. Caffeic acid possesses various pharmacological properties, such as antioxidant, anti-inflammatory, anticancer, and neuroprotective effects [400]. Caffeic acid, by direct interaction, inhibited MEK1 and TOPK activity in an ATP non-competitive manner. Kang et al. [303] conducted experiments using caffeic acid on a mouse tumor model. It demonstrated action by inhibition of ERK and p90RSK activation. Caffeic acid suppressed the TPA-induced activation of AP1, NF-κB, and ERK signaling, and thus neoplastic transformation induced by TPA, EGF, and H-Ras. Through inhibition of ERK functions, caffeic acid inhibited lung metastasis of CT-26 cells. This study also indicated the usefulness of caffeic acid in reducing ERK activity in patient tumor samples.

Caffeic acid effectively inhibited cancer stem cells (CSC) and reduced radiation-induced sphere formation of CD133+ and CD44+ CSC in two patient-derived tumor xenograft (PDTX) models of human CRC in immune-suppressed mice. In vivo, the radiation-induced elevation of PI3K/Akt signaling pathway was also suppressed by caffeic acid. In caffeic acid-treated xenograft samples, the abundance of CD133+ and CD44+ subpopulations of CSC cells were decreased. In addition, CD44+ and CD133+ cells of CRC lost their ability for self-renewal, migration, and CSC-like properties due to caffeic acid in a PDTX xenograft model. Inhibition of PI3K/Akt signaling was described as a significant mode of action caffeic acid in inhibiting CSC proliferation [304].

Both caffeic acid phenethyl ester (CAPE) and caffeic acid phenylpropyl ester (CAPPE) could inhibit HCT116 cell-induced tumor xenograft in immune-compromised mice through inhibition of PI3K/Akt and inactivation of mTORC1 by AMPK activation. Treatment with CAPE and CAPPE reduced the MMP-9 level at a non-hepatotoxic concentration. In addition, CAPE and CAPPE suppressed expression of cyclin D1, Cdk4, cyclin E, c-Myc, and N-cadherin, and upregulated p21 in vivo. Expression of tumor biomarkers, such as PCNA and FASN, was also suppressed by CAPE and CAPPE in tumor tissue [305].

CAPE and caffeic acid p-nitro-phenethyl ester (CAPE-pNO2) upregulated the levels of p53, p27, p21, cytochrome c (cyt. C), and cleaved caspase-3, but downregulated procaspase-

3, Cdk2, and c-Myc in HT-29 tumor xenograft in mice. There was a dose-dependent inhibition of tumor growth and VEGF expression by these compounds, with no visible toxicity to normal cells [306].

Consumption of decyl caffeic acid inhibited tumor growth in mice with a HCT116-induced tumor xenograft. The mechanism of action involved the induction of cell cycle arrest at the S phase as well as autophagy [307].

7.2.2. Gallic Acid

Gallic acid (3,4,5-trihydoxy benzoic acid) is a naturally occurring polyhydroxy phenolic acid found as an active compound in various fruits, nuts, food compounds, vegetables, and numerous plants, such as green chicory, grapes, blackberries, raspberries, blueberries, and strawberries. Gallic acid is well known for its antimicrobial, antioxidant, anti-inflammatory, and anticancer potential [401,402]. In a dose-dependent manner, gallic acid was shown to inhibit DSS-induced colitis in mice through the inhibition of STAT3 phosphorylation [320]. This inhibitory mechanism includes reduced proinflammatory mediators Th1, TNF-α, and IL-6, and chemokines, such as KC and MCP-1 [320].

In another study, the inhibitory effects of gallic acid were tested in HCT116 and HT29 cells and tumor xenografts in BALB/c mice. The function of pro-oncogenic factors, such as Src, STAT3, EGFR, and Akt, along with key players in the apoptosis pathway were analyzed. The results demonstrated inhibition of STAT3 and Akt by inhibiting Src and EGFR functions. Furthermore, net enhancement of the cleaved caspase-3 and caspase-9 suggested the involvement of apoptosis as the mechanism behind cell death [321].

Gallic acid was shown to ameliorate ulcerative colitis-associated CRC induced in rats by TNBS treatment by modulating ferroptosis, an iron-dependent process of cellular necrosis [322]. Gene expression profiling interactive analysis (GEPIA) and bioinformatics analysis identified significant involvement of ferroptosis-related genes in CRC prognosis. This analysis indicated that eight ferroptosis-related genes are involved in cell survival. This docking study suggested that gallic acid could induce ferroptosis by modulating some of these genes [322].

7.3. *Stilbenes*

Resveratrol

Resveratrol (3,5,4′-trihydroxystilbene), a stilbenoid that can be found in peanuts, skin of red grapes, and blueberries, has been studied for its potential anticancer properties [403,404]. Saud et al. [350] used a mouse model with a knocked-out APC locus, and Kras activated specifically in the distant colon to study the effect of resveratrol on sporadic CRC. The mice received a diet supplemented with resveratrol (150 or 300 ppm) before the appearance of tumors. This resulted in a 60% inhibition of tumor production and loss of Kras expression in 40% of mice that developed tumors. Oral administration of resveratrol for tumor bearing mice resulted in complete tumor remission in 33% of mice and a decrease in tumor size in 97% of the remaining mice. Upregulation of miR-96, a negative regulator of Kras expression, in non-tumoral and tumoral colonic tissues suggested that resveratrol exerted its anti-CRC effects by downregulating Kras expression [350]. Alfaras et al. [351] examined the effects of oral administration of trans-resveratrol on DMH-induced precancerous colonic lesions in male Sprague-Dawley rats. This resulted in the reduction of aberrant cryptic foci by 52% and mucin depleted foci by 45% in the colon. In colonic contents, dihydroresveratrol was the most abundant compound detected, followed by trans-resveratrol and its derivatives [351]. Synergistic effects of resveratrol and curcumin on CRC were studied by Majumdar et al. [352].

One study analyzed the effects of resveratrol and its PLGA-chitosan based nanoformulation in animal models (both xenograft and orthotopic) of colon cancer. Both the compound and its nanoformulation caused an appreciable decrease in tumor growth and hemoglobin percentages of tumor mass, signifying reduced angiogenesis with nanoformulation exhibiting more bioavailability and functional efficacy than [353]. Resveratrol combined with ginkgetin, a phytochemical obtained from Ginkgo biloba, exhibited a synergistic effect in suppressing VEGF-induced endothelial cell proliferation, migration, invasion, and tube formation in HT29 cell-induced xenografts in mice. When administered together, these two compounds demonstrated a synergistic antitumor effect with 5-FU, causing a reduction in micro vessel density of the tumors. Furthermore, the combinatorial treatment relieved the 5-FU-induced inflammatory response by lowering the expression of COX-2 and inflammatory cytokines [354]. Resveratrol also suppressed TGF-β1/Smad signaling, downregulated Snail and vimentin, and upregulated E-cadherin expression, which in turn inhibited EMT [349].

8. Phenolics in Clinical Trials for CRC Treatment

Many of the compounds discussed here, such as curcumin, resveratrol, EGCG, genistein, and fisetin, entered into different phases of clinical trials. Curcumin, the most studied phytochemical in both preclinical and clinical studies, has been tested for its effectiveness as an anti-inflammatory agent as well as its potential in prevention, management and therapy of different cancer types, including CRC [405]. The anticancer potential of resveratrol has been documented through studying its efficacy, safety, and pharmacokinetics in more than 244 clinical trials, with additional clinical trials currently being carried out by independent groups [406,407]. Although the clinical utility of resveratrol is well documented, the rapid metabolism and poor bioavailability have limited its therapeutic use [406,408]. Clinical trials on green tea extract containing EGCG as the major active component were conducted, demonstrating the good tolerance of the agent with no significant advantage of its inclusion between the placebo and the treated groups [409]. The efficacy of flavonoid fisetin supplementation on the inflammatory status and MMP levels was tested in small groups of CRC patients, while several markers were measured to assess its therapeutic efficacy, treatment with this polyphenol primarily resulted in the significant changes in IL-8 concentrations compared to the placebo group [410]. The safety and tolerability of genistein in combination with a chemotherapy agent in metastatic CRC were studied in a clinical trial with a small group of patients receiving FOLFOX or FOLFOX-bevacizumab. The results demonstrated the safety and tolerability of the treatment with notable efficacy [379]. While the results of these studies are encouraging, additional studies are needed to assess the long-term use of these phytochemicals in the clinic.

9. Conclusions and Future Perspectives

CRC is the third most diagnosed and second leading cause of cancer-related death worldwide. According to recent statistics, CRC claims close to a million lives, which is about half of the population it affects globally every year. Although the CRC death rate has declined due to routine screening and early detection, CRC incidence is predicted to be doubled by the end of this decade due to various reasons, demanding an urgent need to overcome the limitations of current treatment strategies, including the development of alternative therapy regimens. This review aims to present a detailed account of the recent advances in studies on various phenolic phytochemicals with anti-CRC activities demonstrated in animal experiments with the underlying molecular basis of their actions (summarized in Table 3).

As discussed here, the phytochemicals were reported to act through inhibiting hallmarks of various CRC attributes, such as the potential of cell growth and proliferation, self-renewal, invasion, migration, and angiogenesis through inducing apoptosis, ferroptosis, and autophagy-mediated cell death pathways (Figure 6). These activities involved the modulation of various pathways, such as the levels of proinflammatory cytokines and chemokines (IL-1, IL-6, ICAM-I, TNF, COX-2, iNOS, KC, and MCP1), oxidative stress markers and pathways (SOD, catalase, thiolase, glutathione peroxidase, GSH and Keap1/NRF2/GSK-3β/HO-1), cell cycle regulators (cyclin D1, cyclin E, and CDK 4/6), apoptotic/autophagy regulators (p21, p53, caspase-3, caspase-9, Bax, Bcl-2, Bak, and Beclin1), proliferative signaling pathways regulators (PI3K/Akt/mTOR/AMPK, Wnt/β-catenin, MAPK-p38, ERK, MEK, and c-Myc), regulators of invasion, migration, metastasis, and angiogenesis (Notch1, STAT-3, VEGF, CD31, MMP-2, MMP-3, MMP-9, MMP-16, EGFR, Twist1, Vimentin, FMS-related tyrosine kinase 4, endothelial growth receptor-3, Snail, N-cadherin, E-cadherin, TIMP-1, and TIMP-2), stemness

(CD133, CD44, ALDH1, CD29, DCLK-1, and LGR5) and expression of tumor suppressive miRNAs (miR34a, miR200c, and miR145). The downregulation of COX-2 levels can be achieved upon treatment with EGCG [206], curcumin [194,197], kaempferol [239], luteolin [242,243], myricetin [259], naringenin [262], piceatannol [342], pterostilbene [344], syringic acid [326], boeravinone B [191], hesperidin [227], isoliquiritigenin [235], orientin [268], quercetin [281], and xanthohumol [301]. Caffeic acid suppressed TPA-induced activation of AP1 and NF-κB signaling [303]. Many phytophenols can induce an antioxidant response, such as EGCG, gallic acid, boeravinone B, eriodyctyol, luteolin, and morin. Caffeic acid phenethyl ester and caffeic acid phenylpropyl ester-induced mTOR inhibition through the activation of AMPK [305]. Isoangustone A upregulated AMPK phosphorylation in vivo [234]. Pterostilbene inhibited EGFR in an AOM-induced colonic adenomas in mice [344].

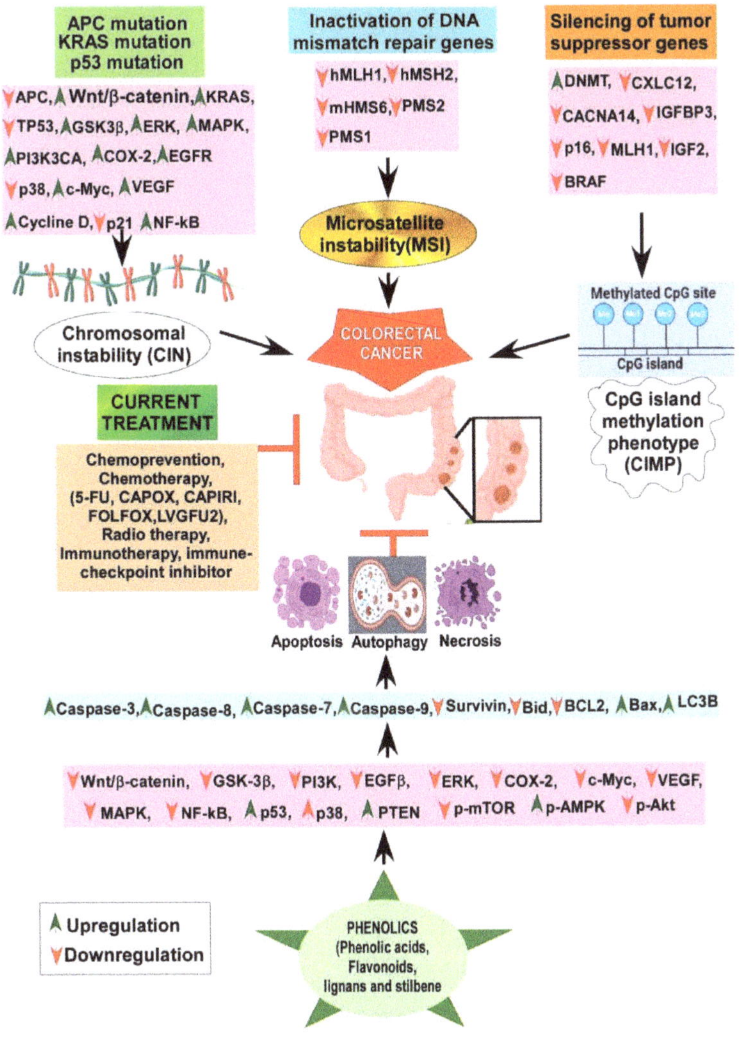

Figure 6. Genetic and molecular basis of colorectal cancer along with the current treatment strategies where potentials of phenolic compounds were indicated. CIN, MSI and CIMP are the prime factors in CRC development. Besides the currently available chemotherapeutic treatment strategies, different polyphenols are reported to induce CRC cell death by apoptosis and/or autophagy and/or necrosis.

There is increasing evidence in favor of the idea that diet can influence the intestinal microbiome and thus the risk of CRC. Diets rich in fruits and vegetables can be associated with gut microbiome rich in Prevotella compared with Bacteroides associated with good colonic health while the consumption of diet with low plant-based food rich in processed food led to the opposite effects [411,412]. Diets rich in plant-based nutraceuticals could regulate host immune and inflammatory behavior and thus gut homeostasis through modulating the composition and functionality of the gut microbiome [413]. Therefore, CRC incidence and progression can be reduced by modulating gut microbiome by careful choice of diet and phytochemicals which could be a promising and efficient way to reduce the burden of CRC [413]. Gut microbiota can digest dietary phytochemicals by their unique ability to produce short chain fatty acids, such as butyric acid, with anti-inflammatory and antineoplastic activity [414]. Phenolic phytochemicals have served us as an important source of novel drugs/leads. While the studies discussed here provided encouraging results, several issues are needed to be considered to get a step closer to the end users, such as:

1. Apparently, the functions of many phytochemicals are limited by their poor solubility, absorption, and bioavailability. Encapsulation by nano-formulation as well as chemical derivatization of the compound could resolve this issue.
2. Some cases reproducing the activity observed in preclinical animal models into the clinic/human could be challenging due to several factors. Success in this endeavor requires careful optimization in administered doses to assess functional synergy, if any, with anti-CRC regimens used in the clinic. Once positive results are obtained in the preclinical settings, testing the validity of the finding, such as safety and efficacy, in clinical trials with appropriate controls will be important to move further.
3. It is reasonable to think that a phenolic compound showing very weak and toxic activity can yield desirable effect when combined with another phytochemical. Therefore, a careful combination of selected polyphenols can yield unique anti-CRC activity. It is important to clearly determine the maximum tolerable dose of a phytochemical to better understand its therapeutic efficacy alone or in combination with another phytochemical or drug.
4. Once a phenolic compound with unique anti-CRC activity is identified, it would be important to develop strategies to synthesize the compound in the laboratory, given the very low abundance of a secondary metabolite in the plants. A detailed understanding of the pharmacophore responsible for the observed function should be helpful for chemical synthesis or semi-synthesis, and cellular target identification of the compound. Given the structural complexity of the plant secondary metabolites, it is often a major challenge for natural product chemists and medicinal chemists to solve. Ideally, the simultaneous engagement of experts from interdisciplinary areas, such as ethnopharmacology, molecular biology, biochemistry, natural product chemistry, medicinal chemistry, bioinformatics, and pharmacology, will be necessary to achieve progress in real-time in harvesting the full potential of natural products as the source of novel drug leads.

Author Contributions: Conceptualization, M.P.; methodology, S.D. and S.P.; investigation, S.D., S.P., A.B. (Ashish Bhattacharjee) and S.C.M.; data curation, S.D. and S.P.; writing—original draft preparation, S.D., S.P., K.P., A.M. (Anirban Manna), J.H., V.K.N., C.M., N.C. and A.B. (Anupam Bishayee); writing—review and editing, M.P., K.P., N.C. and A.B. (Anupam Bishayee); visualization, S.G., A.M. (Arijit Mondal) and S.B.; supervision, M.P. and A.B. (Anupam Bishayee); project administration, M.P. and A.B. (Anupam Bishayee), funding acquisition, M.P. All authors have read and agreed to the published version of the manuscript.

Funding: This research was funded by the Science and Engineering Research Board, Department of Biotechnology (DBT), and Department of Science and Technology (DST) to M.P. S.D. is a University Grant Commission (UGC) Senior Research Fellow (SRF), A.M. (Anirban Manna) is a DBT SRF, and C.M. is a DST Inspire Fellow. S.G. was an SRF of the Council of Scientific and Industrial Research.

Conflicts of Interest: The authors declare no conflict of interest. The funders had no role in the writing of the manuscript.

Abbreviations

5-FU	5-fluorouracil
5′ND	5-nucleotidase
6CEPN	6-C-(E-phenylethyl)-naringenin
ACF	aberrant crypt foci
AOM	azoxymethane
APC	adenomatous polyposis coli
ATST	atorvastatin
BAX	B-cell lymphoma 2-associated x protein
BCL-2	B-cell lymphoma 2
BID	BH3 interacting-domain death agonist
BRAF-B	rapidly accelerated fibrosarcoma/murine sarcoma viral oncogene homolog B
CAC	colitis-associated colorectal cancer
CACNA14	voltage-dependent P/Q type calcium channel subunit alpha1A
CAP	capecitabine
CAPE,	caffeic acid phenethyl ester
CAPPE	caffeic acid phenylpropyl ester
CAPE-pNO2	caffeic acid p-nitro-phenylethyl ester
CAPIRI	capecitabine and irinotecan
CAPOX	capecitabine and oxaliplatin
CEA	carcinoembryonic antigen
CIMP	CpG island methylation phenotype
CIN	chromosomal instability
CLXC12	C–X–C chemokine 12
COX-2	cyclooxygenase-2
CRC	colorectal cancer
CSC	cancer stem cell
cyt. c	cytochrome c
DII	dietary inflammatory index
Dkk	Dickkopf
DMH	dimethyl hydrazine
DNMT	DNA methyltransferase
DSS	dextran sulphate sodium
Dvl	Discevelled
EGF-β	epidermal growth factor-β
EGFR	epidermal growth factor receptor
ER	endoplasmic reticulum
ERK	extracellular signal-regulated kinase
FAP	familial adenomatous polyposis syndrome
FDA	Federal Drug Administration
FOLFOX	5-FU and oxaliplatin
FOXFIRI	5-FU and irinotecan
FZD	Frizzled receptor
G6PD	glucose-6-phosphate dehydrogenase
GEPIA	gene expression profiling interactive analysis
GGT	γ-glutamyl transferase
GSH	glutathione
GSK-3β	glycogen synthase kinase-3β
GTP	green tea polyphenol
HMACF	high multiplicity aberrant crypt foci
hMLH1	human MutL homolog 1
HPP	hyperplastic polyposis
IDEA	International Duration Evaluation of Adjuvant Chemotherapy

IGF-2	insulin like growth factor-2
IGFBP3	insulin like growth factor-binding protein 3
iNOS	inducible nitric oxide synthase
IRI	irinotecan
KRAS	Kirsten rat sarcoma viral oncogene homolog
LC3B	light chain 3B of microtubule-associated proteins 1A/1B
LPO	lipid peroxide
MAP	MUTYG- associated polyposis
MAPK	mitogen-activated protein kinase
MMP	matrix metalloproteinase
MSI	microsatellite instability
mTOR	mammalian target of rapamycin
NF-κβ	nuclear factor-κβ
NO	nitric oxide
NSAID	nonsteroidal anti-inflammatory drug
oncomiRs	oncogenic miRNAs
OPE	orange peel extract
OX	oxaliplatin
PDTX	patient-derived tumor xenograft
PI3K	phosphoinositide 3-kinase
PPE	polyphenol E
PTEN	phosphatase and tensin homolog deleted on chromosome 10
SEER	surveillance epidemiology and end results
SGK1	serum glucocorticoid kinase 1
Skip	Ski-interacting protein
SOD	superoxide dismutase
SPI	soya protein isolate
TAGE	tangeretin
TIMP	tissue inhibitor metalloproteinase
TNM	tumor/node/metastasis
TRPV1	transient receptor potential vanilloid 1
VEGF	vascular endothelial growth factor
VEGFR	vascular endothelial growth factor receptor
YAP	yes-associated protein
yCRC	young-onset colorectal cancer

References

1. Siegel, R.L.; Miller, K.D.; Fuchs, H.E.; Jemal, A. Cancer statistics, 2021. *CA Cancer J. Clin.* **2021**, *71*, 7–33. [CrossRef] [PubMed]
2. Sung, H.; Ferlay, J.; Siegel, R.L.; Laversanne, M.; Soerjomataram, I.; Jemal, A.; Bray, F. Global cancer statistics 2020: GLOBOCAN estimates of incidence and mortality worldwide for 36 cancers in 185 countries. *CA Cancer J. Clin.* **2021**, *71*, 209–249. [CrossRef] [PubMed]
3. Ferlay, J.; Colombet, M.; Soerjomataram, I.; Mathers, C.; Parkin, D.; Piñeros, M.; Znaor, A.; Bray, F. Estimating the global cancer incidence and mortality in 2018: GLOBOCAN sources and methods. *Int. J. Cancer* **2019**, *144*, 1941–1953. [CrossRef] [PubMed]
4. Arnold, M.; Sierra, M.S.; Laversanne, M.; Soerjomataram, I.; Jemal, A.; Bray, F. Global patterns and trends in colorectal cancer incidence and mortality. *Gut* **2017**, *66*, 683–691. [CrossRef] [PubMed]
5. Haque, A.; Brazeau, D.; Amin, A.R. Perspectives on natural compounds in chemoprevention and treatment of cancer: An update with new promising compounds. *Eur. J. Cancer* **2021**, *149*, 165–183. [CrossRef]
6. Swetha, M.; Keerthana, C.; Rayginia, T.P.; Anto, R.J. Cancer chemoprevention: A strategic approach using phytochemicals. *Front. Pharmacol.* **2021**, *12*, 809308.
7. Dhillon, P.K.; Mathur, P.; Nandakumar, A.; Fitzmaurice, C.; Kumar, G.A.; Mehrotra, R.; Shukla, D.; Rath, G.; Gupta, P.C.; Swaminathan, R. The burden of cancers and their variations across the states of India: The Global Burden of Disease Study 1990–2016. *Lancet Oncol.* **2018**, *19*, 1289–1306. [CrossRef]
8. Choudhari, A.S.; Mandave, P.C.; Deshpande, M.; Ranjekar, P.; Prakash, O. Phytochemicals in cancer treatment: From preclinical studies to clinical practice. *Front. Pharmacol.* **2020**, *10*, 1614. [CrossRef]
9. Siegel, R.L.; Miller, K.D.; Goding Sauer, A.; Fedewa, S.A.; Butterly, L.F.; Anderson, J.C.; Cercek, A.; Smith, R.A.; Jemal, A. Colorectal cancer statistics, 2020. *CA Cancer J. Clin.* **2020**, *70*, 145–164. [CrossRef]

10. Ranjan, A.; Ramachandran, S.; Gupta, N.; Kaushik, I.; Wright, S.; Srivastava, S.; Das, H.; Srivastava, S.; Prasad, S.; Srivastava, S.K. Role of phytochemicals in cancer prevention. *Int. J. Mol. Sci.* **2019**, *20*, 4981. [CrossRef]
11. Siegel, R.L.; Miller, K.D.; Fedewa, S.A.; Ahnen, D.J.; Meester, R.G.; Barzi, A.; Jemal, A. Colorectal cancer statistics, 2017. *CA Cancer J. Clin.* **2017**, *67*, 177–193. [CrossRef] [PubMed]
12. Mauri, G.; Sartore-Bianchi, A.; Russo, A.G.; Marsoni, S.; Bardelli, A.; Siena, S. Early-onset colorectal cancer in young individuals. *Mol. Oncol.* **2019**, *13*, 109–131. [CrossRef] [PubMed]
13. Murphy, C.C.; Lund, J.L.; Sandler, R.S. Young-onset colorectal cancer: Earlier diagnoses or increasing disease burden? *Gastroenterology* **2017**, *152*, 1809–1812.e1803. [CrossRef] [PubMed]
14. You, Y.N.; Xing, Y.; Feig, B.W.; Chang, G.J.; Cormier, J.N. Young-onset colorectal cancer: Is it time to pay attention? *Arch. Intern. Med.* **2012**, *172*, 287–289. [CrossRef] [PubMed]
15. Holowatyj, A.N.; Ruterbusch, J.J.; Rozek, L.S.; Cote, M.L.; Stoffel, E.M. Racial/ethnic disparities in survival among patients with young-onset colorectal cancer. *J. Clin. Oncol.* **2016**, *34*, 2148. [CrossRef] [PubMed]
16. Thanikachalam, K.; Khan, G. Colorectal cancer and nutrition. *Nutrients* **2019**, *11*, 164. [CrossRef]
17. Tanaka, S.; Oka, S.; Chayama, K. Colorectal endoscopic submucosal dissection: Present status and future perspective, including its differentiation from endoscopic mucosal resection. *J. Gastroenterol.* **2008**, *43*, 641–651. [CrossRef]
18. Chakedis, J.; Schmidt, C.R. Surgical treatment of metastatic colorectal cancer. *Surg. Oncol. Clin.* **2018**, *27*, 377–399. [CrossRef]
19. Mojtahedi, Z.; Koo, J.S.; Yoo, J.; Kim, P.; Kang, H.-T.; Hwang, J.; Joo, M.K.; Shen, J.J. Palliative care and life-sustaining/local procedures in colorectal Cancer in the United States hospitals: A ten-year perspective. *Cancer Manag. Res.* **2021**, *13*, 7569–7577. [CrossRef]
20. Townsend, A.; Price, T.; Karapetis, C. Selective internal radiation therapy for liver metastases from colorectal cancer. *Cochrane Database Syst. Rev.* **2009**, CD007045. [CrossRef]
21. Kanani, A.; Veen, T.; Søreide, K. Neoadjuvant immunotherapy in primary and metastatic colorectal cancer. *Br. J. Surg.* **2021**, *108*, 1417–1425. [CrossRef]
22. Loughrey, M.B. Neoadjuvant immunotherapy and colorectal cancer treatment: Implications for the primary role of surgery. *Color. Dis. Off. J. Assoc. Coloproctol. Great Br. Irel.* **2022**, *24*, 1460–1461. [CrossRef]
23. Aiello, P.; Sharghi, M.; Mansourkhani, S.M.; Ardekan, A.P.; Jouybari, L.; Daraei, N.; Peiro, K.; Mohamadian, S.; Rezaei, M.; Heidari, M. Medicinal plants in the prevention and treatment of colon cancer. *Oxidative Med. Cell. Longev.* **2019**, *2019*, 2075614. [CrossRef] [PubMed]
24. Muppala, S. Phytochemicals Targeting Colorectal Cancer Growth and Metastasis. *Crit. Rev. Oncog.* **2020**, *25*, 141–149. [CrossRef] [PubMed]
25. Sain, A.; Sahu, S.; Naskar, D. Potential of Olive oil and its phenolic compounds as therapeutic intervention against colorectal cancer: A comprehensive review. *Br. J. Nutr.* **2021**, *128*, 1257–1273. [CrossRef] [PubMed]
26. Cueva, C.; Silva, M.; Pinillos, I.; Bartolomé, B.; Moreno-Arribas, M.V. Interplay between dietary polyphenols and oral and gut microbiota in the development of colorectal cancer. *Nutrients* **2020**, *12*, 625. [CrossRef]
27. Andrews, L. Dietary flavonoids for the prevention of colorectal cancer. *Clin. J. Oncol. Nurs.* **2013**, *17*, 671–673. [CrossRef]
28. Woo, H.D.; Kim, J. Dietary flavonoid intake and risk of stomach and colorectal cancer. *World J. Gastroenterol.* **2013**, *19*, 1011. [CrossRef]
29. Kocic, B.; Kitic, D.; Brankovic, S. Dietary flavonoid intake and colorectal cancer risk: Evidence from human population studies. *J. BUON* **2013**, *18*, 34–43.
30. Jin, H.; Leng, Q.; Li, C. Dietary flavonoid for preventing colorectal neoplasms. *Cochrane Database Syst. Rev.* **2012**, CD009350. [CrossRef]
31. Han, S.; Cao, Y.; Guo, T.; Lin, Q.; Luo, F. Targeting lncRNA/Wnt axis by flavonoids: A promising therapeutic approach for colorectal cancer. *Phytother. Res.* **2022**, *36*, 4024–4040. [CrossRef] [PubMed]
32. Pereira-Wilson, C. Can dietary flavonoids be useful in the personalized treatment of colorectal cancer? *World J. Gastrointest. Oncol.* **2022**, *14*, 1115. [CrossRef] [PubMed]
33. Fernández, J.; Silván, B.; Entrialgo-Cadierno, R.; Villar, C.J.; Capasso, R.; Uranga, J.A.; Lombó, F.; Abalo, R. Antiproliferative and palliative activity of flavonoids in colorectal cancer. *Biomed. Pharmacother.* **2021**, *143*, 112241. [CrossRef] [PubMed]
34. Afshari, K.; Haddadi, N.S.; Haj-Mirzaian, A.; Farzaei, M.H.; Rohani, M.M.; Akramian, F.; Naseri, R.; Sureda, A.; Ghanaatian, N.; Abdolghaffari, A.H. Natural flavonoids for the prevention of colon cancer: A comprehensive review of preclinical and clinical studies. *J. Cell. Physiol.* **2019**, *234*, 21519–21546. [CrossRef]
35. Li, Y.; Zhang, T.; Chen, G.Y. Flavonoids and colorectal cancer prevention. *Antioxidants* **2018**, *7*, 187. [CrossRef]
36. Koosha, S.; Alshawsh, M.A.; Looi, C.Y.; Seyedan, A.; Mohamed, Z. An association map on the effect of flavonoids on the signaling pathways in colorectal cancer. *Int. J. Med. Sci.* **2016**, *13*, 374. [CrossRef]
37. Potter, J.D. Nutrition and colorectal cancer. *Cancer Causes Control* **1996**, *7*, 127–146. [CrossRef]
38. Martinez, M.E.; Willett, W.C. Calcium, vitamin D, and colorectal cancer: A review of the epidemiologic evidence. *Cancer Epidemiol. Biomark. Prev.* **1998**, *7*, 163–168.
39. Terry, P.; Giovannucci, E.; Michels, K.B.; Bergkvist, L.; Hansen, H.; Holmberg, L.; Wolk, A. Fruit, vegetables, dietary fiber, and risk of colorectal cancer. *J. Natl. Cancer Inst.* **2001**, *93*, 525–533. [CrossRef]

40. Santarelli, R.L.; Pierre, F.; Corpet, D.E. Processed meat and colorectal cancer: A review of epidemiologic and experimental evidence. *Nutr. Cancer* **2008**, *60*, 131–144.
41. Benarba, B.; Pandiella, A. Colorectal cancer and medicinal plants: Principle findings from recent studies. *Biomed. Pharmacother.* **2018**, *107*, 408–423. [CrossRef] [PubMed]
42. La Vecchia, S.; Sebastián, C. Metabolic pathways regulating colorectal cancer initiation and progression. *Semin. Cell Dev.Biol.* **2020**, *98*, 63–70. [CrossRef] [PubMed]
43. Keum, N.; Giovannucci, E. Global burden of colorectal cancer: Emerging trends, risk factors and prevention strategies. *Nat. Rev. Gastroenterol. Hepatol.* **2019**, *16*, 713–732. [CrossRef] [PubMed]
44. Lynch, H.T.; Smyrk, T.C.; Watson, P.; Lanspa, S.J.; Lynch, J.F.; Lynch, P.M.; Cavalieri, R.J.; Boland, C.R. Genetics, natural history, tumor spectrum, and pathology of hereditary nonpolyposis colorectal cancer: An updated review. *Gastroenterology* **1993**, *104*, 1535–1549. [CrossRef] [PubMed]
45. Niessen, R.C.; Berends, M.J.; Wu, Y.; Sijmons, R.H.; Hollema, H.; Ligtenberg, M.J.; de Walle, H.E.; de Vries, E.G.; Karrenbeld, A.; Buys, C.H. Identification of mismatch repair gene mutations in young patients with colorectal cancer and in patients with multiple tumours associated with hereditary non-polyposis colorectal cancer. *Gut* **2006**, *55*, 1781–1788. [CrossRef] [PubMed]
46. Seppälä, T.; Latchford, A.; Negoi, I.; Sampaio Soares, A.; Jimenez-Rodriguez, R.; Sánchez-Guillén, L.; Evans, D.; Ryan, N.; Crosbie, E.; Dominguez-Valentin, M. European guidelines from the EHTG and ESCP for Lynch syndrome: An updated third edition of the Mallorca guidelines based on gene and gender. *Br. J. Surg.* **2021**, *108*, 484–498. [CrossRef]
47. Møller, P.; Seppälä, T.T.; Bernstein, I.; Holinski-Feder, E.; Sala, P.; Evans, D.G.; Lindblom, A.; Macrae, F.; Blanco, I.; Sijmons, R.H. Cancer risk and survival in path_MMR carriers by gene and gender up to 75 years of age: A report from the Prospective Lynch Syndrome Database. *Gut* **2018**, *67*, 1306–1316. [CrossRef]
48. Ponti, G.; Manfredini, M.; Tomasi, A.; Pellacani, G. Muir–Torre Syndrome and founder mismatch repair gene mutations: A long gone historical genetic challenge. *Gene* **2016**, *589*, 127–132. [CrossRef]
49. Grzybowski, A.; Jablonska, S. Muir–Torre Syndrome—Is It Really a New Syndrome? *Am. J. Dermatopathol.* **2009**, *31*, 799–802. [CrossRef]
50. Kidambi, T.D.; Kohli, D.R.; Samadder, N.J.; Singh, A. Hereditary polyposis syndromes. *Curr. Treat. Options Gastroenterol.* **2019**, *17*, 650–665. [CrossRef]
51. Hamilton, S.R.; Liu, B.; Parsons, R.E.; Papadopoulos, N.; Jen, J.; Powell, S.M.; Krush, A.J.; Berk, T.; Cohen, Z.; Tetu, B. The molecular basis of Turcot's syndrome. *N. Engl. J. Med.* **1995**, *332*, 839–847. [CrossRef]
52. Rutz, H.P.; de Tribolet, N.; Calmes, J.M.; Chapuis, G. Long-time survival of a patient with glioblastoma and Turcot's syndrome: Case report. *J. Neurosurg.* **1991**, *74*, 813–815. [CrossRef] [PubMed]
53. Haggar, F.A.; Boushey, R.P. Colorectal cancer epidemiology: Incidence, mortality, survival, and risk factors. *Clin. Colon Rectal Surg.* **2009**, *22*, 191–197. [CrossRef] [PubMed]
54. Galiatsatos, P.; Foulkes, W.D. Familial adenomatous polyposis. *Off. J. Am. Coll. Gastroenterol. ACG* **2006**, *101*, 385–398. [CrossRef] [PubMed]
55. Coffin, C.M.; Hornick, J.L.; Zhou, H.; Fletcher, C.D. Gardner fibroma: A clinicopathologic and immunohistochemical analysis of 45 patients with 57 fibromas. *Am. J. Surg. Pathol.* **2007**, *31*, 410–416. [CrossRef]
56. Kiessling, P.; Dowling, E.; Huang, Y.; Ho, M.L.; Balakrishnan, K.; Weigel, B.J.; Highsmith, W.E.; Niu, Z.; Schimmenti, L.A. Identification of aggressive Gardner syndrome phenotype associated with a de novo APC variant, c. 4666dup. *Mol. Case Stud.* **2019**, *5*, a003640. [CrossRef] [PubMed]
57. Sutcliffe, E.G.; Thompson, A.B.; Stettner, A.R.; Marshall, M.L.; Roberts, M.E.; Susswein, L.R.; Wang, Y.; Klein, R.T.; Hruska, K.S.; Solomon, B.D. Multi-gene panel testing confirms phenotypic variability in MUTYH-Associated Polyposis. *Fam. Cancer* **2019**, *18*, 203–209. [CrossRef] [PubMed]
58. Curia, M.C.; Catalano, T.; Aceto, G.M. MUTYH: Not just polyposis. *World J. Clin. Oncol.* **2020**, *11*, 428. [CrossRef]
59. Vogt, S.; Jones, N.; Christian, D.; Engel, C.; Nielsen, M.; Kaufmann, A.; Steinke, V.; Vasen, H.F.; Propping, P.; Sampson, J.R. Expanded extracolonic tumor spectrum in MUTYH-associated polyposis. *Gastroenterology* **2009**, *137*, 1976–1985.e1910. [CrossRef]
60. Calva-Cerqueira, D.; Chinnathambi, S.; Pechman, B.; Bair, J.; Larsen-Haidle, J.; Howe, J. The rate of germline mutations and large deletions of SMAD4 and BMPR1A in juvenile polyposis. *Clin. Genet.* **2009**, *75*, 79–85. [CrossRef]
61. Gallione, C.J.; Repetto, G.M.; Legius, E.; Rustgi, A.K.; Schelley, S.L.; Tejpar, S.; Mitchell, G.; Drouin, É.; Westermann, C.J.; Marchuk, D.A. A combined syndrome of juvenile polyposis and hereditary haemorrhagic telangiectasia associated with mutations in MADH4 (SMAD4). *Lancet* **2004**, *363*, 852–859. [CrossRef] [PubMed]
62. Brosens, L.A.; Van Hattem, A.; Hylind, L.M.; Iacobuzio-Donahue, C.; Romans, K.E.; Axilbund, J.; Cruz-Correa, M.; Tersmette, A.C.; Offerhaus, G.J.A.; Giardiello, F.M. Risk of colorectal cancer in juvenile polyposis. *Gut* **2007**, *56*, 965–967. [CrossRef]
63. Kopacova, M.; Tacheci, I.; Rejchrt, S.; Bures, J. Peutz-Jeghers syndrome: Diagnostic and therapeutic approach. *World J. Gastroenterol.* **2009**, *15*, 5397. [CrossRef] [PubMed]
64. Westerman, A.M.; Entius, M.M.; De Baar, E.; Boor, P.P.; Koole, R.; Van Velthuysen, M.L.F.; Offerhaus, G.J.A.; Lindhout, D.; De Rooij, F.W.; Wilson, J.P. Peutz-Jeghers syndrome: 78-year follow-up of the original family. *Lancet* **1999**, *353*, 1211–1215. [CrossRef]
65. Smerdel, M.P.; Skytte, A.-B.; Jelsig, A.M.; Ebbehøj, E.; Stochholm, K. Revised Danish guidelines for the cancer surveillance of patients with Cowden Syndrome. *Eur. J. Med. Genet.* **2020**, *63*, 103873. [CrossRef] [PubMed]

66. Lloyd, K.M.; Dennis, M. Cowden's disease: A possible new symptom complex with multiple system involvement. *Ann. Intern. Med.* **1963**, *58*, 136–142. [CrossRef]
67. Miyaki, M.; Konishi, M.; Kikuchi-Yanoshita, R.; Enomoto, M.; Igari, T.; Tanaka, K.; Muraoka, M.; Takahashi, H.; Amada, Y.; Fukayama, M. Characteristics of somatic mutation of the adenomatous polyposis coli gene in colorectal tumors. *Cancer Res.* **1994**, *54*, 3011–3020.
68. Lamlum, H.; Ilyas, M.; Rowan, A.; Clark, S.; Johnson, V.; Bell, J.; Frayling, I.; Efstathiou, J.; Pack, K.; Payne, S. The type of somatic mutation at APC in familial adenomatous polyposis is determined by the site of the germline mutation: A new facet to Knudson's' two-hit'hypothesis. *Nat. Med.* **1999**, *5*, 1071–1075. [CrossRef]
69. Fodde, R.; Smits, R.; Clevers, H. APC, signal transduction and genetic instability in colorectal cancer. *Nat. Rev. Cancer* **2001**, *1*, 55–67. [CrossRef]
70. Kanth, P.; Grimmett, J.; Champine, M.; Burt, R.; Samadder, J.N. Hereditary colorectal polyposis and cancer syndromes: A primer on diagnosis and management. *Off. J. Am. Coll. Gastroenterol. ACG* **2017**, *112*, 1509–1525. [CrossRef]
71. Mokarram, P.; Albokashy, M.; Zarghooni, M.; Moosavi, M.A.; Sepehri, Z.; Chen, Q.M.; Hudecki, A.; Sargazi, A.; Alizadeh, J.; Moghadam, A.R. New frontiers in the treatment of colorectal cancer: Autophagy and the unfolded protein response as promising targets. *Autophagy* **2017**, *13*, 781–819. [CrossRef] [PubMed]
72. Jasperson, K.W.; Tuohy, T.M.; Neklason, D.W.; Burt, R.W. Hereditary and familial colon cancer. *Gastroenterology* **2010**, *138*, 2044–2058. [CrossRef]
73. Potack, J.; Itzkowitz, S.H. Colorectal cancer in inflammatory bowel disease. *Gut Liver* **2008**, *2*, 61. [CrossRef] [PubMed]
74. Armenian, S.H.; Robison, L.L. Childhood cancer survivorship: An update on evolving paradigms for understanding pathogenesis and screening for therapy-related late effects. *Curr. Opin. Pediatr.* **2013**, *25*, 16. [CrossRef] [PubMed]
75. Baxter, N.N.; Goldwasser, M.A.; Paszat, L.F.; Saskin, R.; Urbach, D.R.; Rabeneck, L. Association of colonoscopy and death from colorectal cancer. *Ann. Intern. Med.* **2009**, *150*, 1–8. [CrossRef]
76. Hadjiliadis, D.; Khoruts, A.; Zauber, A.G.; Hempstead, S.E.; Maisonneuve, P.; Lowenfels, A.B.; Braid, A.L.; Cullina, J.; Daggett, A.; Fink, A. Cystic fibrosis colorectal cancer screening consensus recommendations. *Gastroenterology* **2018**, *154*, 736–745.e714. [CrossRef]
77. Botteri, E.; Iodice, S.; Bagnardi, V.; Raimondi, S.; Lowenfels, A.B.; Maisonneuve, P. Smoking and colorectal cancer: A meta-analysis. *JAMA* **2008**, *300*, 2765–2778. [CrossRef]
78. Cai, S.; Li, Y.; Ding, Y.; Chen, K.; Jin, M. Alcohol drinking and the risk of colorectal cancer death: A meta-analysis. *Eur. J. Cancer Prev.* **2014**, *23*, 532–539. [CrossRef]
79. Kyrgiou, M.; Kalliala, I.; Markozannes, G.; Gunter, M.J.; Paraskevaidis, E.; Gabra, H.; Martin-Hirsch, P.; Tsilidis, K.K. Adiposity and cancer at major anatomical sites: Umbrella review of the literature. *BMJ* **2017**, *356*, j477. [CrossRef]
80. Wong, M.C.; Ding, H.; Wang, J.; Chan, P.S.; Huang, J. Prevalence and risk factors of colorectal cancer in Asia. *Intest. Res.* **2019**, *17*, 317. [CrossRef]
81. Shivappa, N.; Godos, J.; Hébert, J.R.; Wirth, M.D.; Piuri, G.; Speciani, A.F.; Grosso, G. Dietary inflammatory index and colorectal cancer risk—A meta-analysis. *Nutrients* **2017**, *9*, 1043. [CrossRef] [PubMed]
82. Meng, Y.; Sun, J.; Yu, J.; Wang, C.; Su, J. Dietary intakes of calcium, iron, magnesium, and potassium elements and the risk of colorectal cancer: A meta-analysis. *Biol. Trace Elem. Res.* **2019**, *189*, 325–335. [CrossRef] [PubMed]
83. Parra-Soto, S.; Ahumada, D.; Petermann-Rocha, F.; Boonpoor, J.; Gallegos, J.L.; Anderson, J.; Sharp, L.; Malcomson, F.C.; Livingstone, K.M.; Mathers, J.C. Association of meat, vegetarian, pescatarian and fish-poultry diets with risk of 19 cancer sites and all cancer: Findings from the UK Biobank prospective cohort study and meta-analysis. *BMC Med.* **2022**, *20*, 1–16. [CrossRef]
84. Zhong, Y.; Zhu, Y.; Li, Q.; Wang, F.; Ge, X.; Zhou, G.; Miao, L. Association between Mediterranean diet adherence and colorectal cancer: A dose-response meta-analysis. *Am. J. Clin. Nutr.* **2020**, *111*, 1214–1225. [CrossRef] [PubMed]
85. Hoang, T.; Kim, H.; Kim, J. Dietary intake in association with all-cause mortality and colorectal cancer mortality among colorectal cancer survivors: A systematic review and meta-analysis of prospective studies. *Cancers* **2020**, *12*, 3391. [CrossRef]
86. Cho, K.R.; Vogelstein, B. Genetic alterations in the adenoma–carcinoma sequence. *Cancer* **1992**, *70*, 1727–1731. [CrossRef]
87. Cho, K.R.; Vogelstein, B. Suppressor gene alterations in the colorectal adenoma-carcinoma sequence. *J. Cell. Biochem.* **1992**, *50*, 137–141. [CrossRef]
88. Tariq, K.; Ghias, K. Colorectal cancer carcinogenesis: A review of mechanisms. *Cancer Biol. Med.* **2016**, *13*, 120. [CrossRef]
89. Hermsen, M.; Postma, C.; Baak, J.; Weiss, M.; Rapallo, A.; Sciutto, A.; Roemen, G.; Arends, J.W.; Williams, R.; Giaretti, W. Colorectal adenoma to carcinoma progression follows multiple pathways of chromosomal instability. *Gastroenterology* **2002**, *123*, 1109–1119. [CrossRef]
90. Baran, B.; Ozupek, N.M.; Tetik, N.Y.; Acar, E.; Bekcioglu, O.; Baskin, Y. Difference between left-sided and right-sided colorectal cancer: A focused review of literature. *Gastroenterol. Res.* **2018**, *11*, 264. [CrossRef]
91. Gryfe, R.; Bapat, B.; Gallinger, S.; Swallow, C.; Redston, M.; Couture, J. Molecular biology of colorectal cancer. *Curr. Probl. Cancer* **1997**, *21*, 233–299. [CrossRef] [PubMed]
92. Levy, D.B.; Smith, K.J.; Beazer-Barclay, Y.; Hamilton, S.R.; Vogelstein, B.; Kinzler, K.W. Inactivation of both APC alleles in human and mouse tumors. *Cancer Res.* **1994**, *54*, 5953–5958. [PubMed]
93. Dow, L.E.; O'Rourke, K.P.; Simon, J.; Tschaharganeh, D.F.; van Es, J.H.; Clevers, H.; Lowe, S.W. Apc restoration promotes cellular differentiation and reestablishes crypt homeostasis in colorectal cancer. *Cell* **2015**, *161*, 1539–1552. [CrossRef] [PubMed]

94. Cancer Genome Atlas Network. Comprehensive molecular characterization of human colon and rectal cancer. *Nature* **2012**, *487*, 330. [CrossRef]
95. Fischer, M.M.; Yeung, V.P.; Cattaruzza, F.; Hussein, R.; Yen, W.-C.; Murriel, C.; Evans, J.W.; O'Young, G.; Brunner, A.L.; Wang, M. RSPO3 antagonism inhibits growth and tumorigenicity in colorectal tumors harboring common Wnt pathway mutations. *Sci. Rep.* **2017**, *7*, 1–9. [CrossRef]
96. Chen, Z.; He, X.; Jia, M.; Liu, Y.; Qu, D.; Wu, D.; Wu, P.; Ni, C.; Zhang, Z.; Ye, J. β-catenin overexpression in the nucleus predicts progress disease and unfavourable survival in colorectal cancer: A meta-analysis. *PLoS ONE* **2013**, *8*, e63854. [CrossRef]
97. Grady, W.M.; Markowitz, S.D. Genetic and epigenetic alterations in colon cancer. *Annu. Rev. Genom. Hum. Genet.* **2002**, *3*, 101–128. [CrossRef]
98. Armaghany, T.; Wilson, J.D.; Chu, Q.; Mills, G. Genetic alterations in colorectal cancer. *Gastrointest. Cancer Res.* **2012**, *5*, 19.
99. Lynch, H.T.; Boland, C.R.; Gong, G.; Shaw, T.G.; Lynch, P.M.; Fodde, R.; Lynch, J.F.; de la Chapelle, A. Phenotypic and genotypic heterogeneity in the Lynch syndrome: Diagnostic, surveillance and management implications. *Eur. J. Hum. Genet.* **2006**, *14*, 390–402. [CrossRef]
100. Toyota, M.; Ahuja, N.; Ohe-Toyota, M.; Herman, J.G.; Baylin, S.B.; Issa, J.-P.J. CpG island methylator phenotype in colorectal cancer. *Proc. Natl. Acad. Sci. USA* **1999**, *96*, 8681–8686. [CrossRef]
101. Weisenberger, D.J.; Siegmund, K.D.; Campan, M.; Young, J.; Long, T.I.; Faasse, M.A.; Kang, G.H.; Widschwendter, M.; Weener, D.; Buchanan, D. CpG island methylator phenotype underlies sporadic microsatellite instability and is tightly associated with BRAF mutation in colorectal cancer. *Nat. Genet.* **2006**, *38*, 787–793. [CrossRef]
102. Advani, S.M.; Advani, P.; DeSantis, S.M.; Brown, D.; VonVille, H.M.; Lam, M.; Loree, J.M.; Sarshekeh, A.M.; Bressler, J.; Lopez, D.S. Clinical, pathological, and molecular characteristics of CpG island methylator phenotype in colorectal cancer: A systematic review and meta-analysis. *Transl. Oncol.* **2018**, *11*, 1188–1201. [CrossRef]
103. Bosetti, C.; Santucci, C.; Gallus, S.; Martinetti, M.; La Vecchia, C. Aspirin and the risk of colorectal and other digestive tract cancers: An updated meta-analysis through 2019. *Ann. Oncol.* **2020**, *31*, 558–568. [CrossRef] [PubMed]
104. Cao, Y.; Nishihara, R.; Qian, Z.R.; Song, M.; Mima, K.; Inamura, K.; Nowak, J.A.; Drew, D.A.; Lochhead, P.; Nosho, K. Regular aspirin use associates with lower risk of colorectal cancers with low numbers of tumor-infiltrating lymphocytes. *Gastroenterology* **2016**, *151*, 879–892.e874. [CrossRef] [PubMed]
105. Chan, A.T.; Ogino, S.; Fuchs, C.S. Aspirin and the risk of colorectal cancer in relation to the expression of COX-2. *N. Engl. J. Med.* **2007**, *356*, 2131–2142. [CrossRef] [PubMed]
106. Rothwell, P.M.; Wilson, M.; Elwin, C.-E.; Norrving, B.; Algra, A.; Warlow, C.P.; Meade, T.W. Long-term effect of aspirin on colorectal cancer incidence and mortality: 20-year follow-up of five randomised trials. *Lancet* **2010**, *376*, 1741–1750. [CrossRef] [PubMed]
107. Tomić, T.; Domínguez-López, S.; Barrios-Rodríguez, R. Non-aspirin non-steroidal anti-inflammatory drugs in prevention of colorectal cancer in people aged 40 or older: A systematic review and meta-analysis. *Cancer Epidemiol.* **2019**, *58*, 52–62. [CrossRef]
108. Meyskens, F.L.; McLaren, C.E.; Pelot, D.; Fujikawa-Brooks, S.; Carpenter, P.M.; Hawk, E.; Kelloff, G.; Lawson, M.J.; Kidao, J.; McCracken, J. Difluoromethylornithine plus sulindac for the prevention of sporadic colorectal adenomas: A randomized placebo-controlled, double-blind trial. *Cancer Prev. Res.* **2008**, *1*, 32–38. [CrossRef]
109. Thomasset, S.; Berry, D.P.; Cai, H.; West, K.; Marczylo, T.H.; Marsden, D.; Brown, K.; Dennison, A.; Garcea, G.; Miller, A. Pilot study of oral anthocyanins for colorectal cancer chemoprevention. *Cancer Prev. Res.* **2009**, *2*, 625–633. [CrossRef]
110. Sinicrope, F.A.; Velamala, P.R.; Song, L.M.W.K.; Viggiano, T.R.; Bruining, D.H.; Rajan, E.; Gostout, C.J.; Kraichely, R.E.; Buttar, N.S.; Schroeder, K.W. Efficacy of difluoromethylornithine and aspirin for treatment of adenomas and aberrant crypt foci in patients with prior advanced colorectal neoplasms. *Cancer Prev. Res.* **2019**, *12*, 821–830. [CrossRef]
111. Samadder, N.J.; Kuwada, S.K.; Boucher, K.M.; Byrne, K.; Kanth, P.; Samowitz, W.; Jones, D.; Tavtigian, S.V.; Westover, M.; Berry, T. Association of sulindac and erlotinib vs placebo with colorectal neoplasia in familial adenomatous polyposis: Secondary analysis of a randomized clinical trial. *JAMA Oncol.* **2018**, *4*, 671–677. [CrossRef] [PubMed]
112. Veettil, S.K.; Nathisuwan, S.; Ching, S.M.; Jinatongthai, P.; Lim, K.G.; Kew, S.T.; Chaiyakunapruk, N. Efficacy and safety of celecoxib on the incidence of recurrent colorectal adenomas: A systematic review and meta-analysis. *Cancer Manag. Res.* **2019**, *11*, 561. [CrossRef] [PubMed]
113. Rodríguez-Miguel, A.; García-Rodríguez, L.A.; Gil, M.; Montoya, H.; Rodríguez-Martín, S.; de Abajo, F.J. Clopidogrel and low-dose aspirin, alone or together, reduce risk of colorectal cancer. *Clin. Gastroenterol. Hepatol.* **2019**, *17*, 2024–2033.e2022. [CrossRef] [PubMed]
114. Ng, C.-A.W.; Jiang, A.A.; Toh, E.M.S.; Ng, C.H.; Ong, Z.H.; Peng, S.; Tham, H.Y.; Sundar, R.; Chong, C.S.; Khoo, C.M. Metformin and colorectal cancer: A systematic review, meta-analysis and meta-regression. *Int. J. Color. Dis.* **2020**, *35*, 1501–1512. [CrossRef]
115. Huang, W.-K.; Hsu, H.-C.; Liu, J.-R.; Yang, T.-S.; Chen, J.-S.; Chang, J.W.-C.; Lin, Y.-C.; Yu, K.-H.; Kuo, C.-F.; See, L.-C. The association of ursodeoxycholic acid use with colorectal cancer risk: A nationwide cohort study. *Medicine* **2016**, *95*, e2980. [CrossRef]
116. Li, Y.; He, X.; Ding, Y.e.; Chen, H.; Sun, L. Statin uses and mortality in colorectal cancer patients: An updated systematic review and meta-analysis. *Cancer Med.* **2019**, *8*, 3305–3313. [CrossRef]
117. Barbalata, C.I.; Tefas, L.R.; Achim, M.; Tomuta, I.; Porfire, A.S. Statins in risk-reduction and treatment of cancer. *World J. Clin. Oncol.* **2020**, *11*, 573. [CrossRef]

118. Botteri, E.; Støer, N.C.; Sakshaug, S.; Graff-Iversen, S.; Vangen, S.; Hofvind, S.; De Lange, T.; Bagnardi, V.; Ursin, G.; Weiderpass, E. Menopausal hormone therapy and colorectal cancer: A linkage between nationwide registries in Norway. *BMJ Open* **2017**, *7*, e017639. [CrossRef]
119. Li, Y.-Y.; Gao, L.-J.; Zhang, Y.-X.; Liu, S.-J.; Cheng, S.; Liu, Y.-P.; Jia, C.-X. Bisphosphonates and risk of cancers: A systematic review and meta-analysis. *Br. J. Cancer* **2020**, *123*, 1570–1581. [CrossRef]
120. Eberhart, C.E.; Coffey, R.J.; Radhika, A.; Giardiello, F.M.; Ferrenbach, S.; Dubois, R.N. Up-regulation of cyclooxygenase 2 gene expression in human colorectal adenomas and adenocarcinomas. *Gastroenterology* **1994**, *107*, 1183–1188. [CrossRef]
121. Oshima, M.; Dinchuk, J.E.; Kargman, S.L.; Oshima, H.; Hancock, B.; Kwong, E.; Trzaskos, J.M.; Evans, J.F.; Taketo, M.M. Suppression of intestinal polyposis in ApcΔ716 knockout mice by inhibition of cyclooxygenase 2 (COX-2). *Cell* **1996**, *87*, 803–809. [CrossRef] [PubMed]
122. Castellone, M.D.; Teramoto, H.; Williams, B.O.; Druey, K.M.; Gutkind, J.S. Prostaglandin E2 promotes colon cancer cell growth through a Gs-axin-ß-catenin signaling axis. *Science* **2005**, *310*, 1504–1510. [CrossRef] [PubMed]
123. Wang, D.; DuBois, R.N. The role of COX-2 in intestinal inflammation and colorectal cancer. *Oncogene* **2010**, *29*, 781–788. [CrossRef]
124. Masferrer, J.L.; Leahy, K.M.; Koki, A.T.; Zweifel, B.S.; Settle, S.L.; Woerner, B.M.; Edwards, D.A.; Flickinger, A.G.; Moore, R.J.; Seibert, K. Antiangiogenic and antitumor activities of cyclooxygenase-2 inhibitors. *Cancer Res.* **2000**, *60*, 1306–1311. [PubMed]
125. Seno, H.; Oshima, M.; Ishikawa, T.-O.; Oshima, H.; Takaku, K.; Chiba, T.; Narumiya, S.; Taketo, M.M. Cyclooxygenase 2-and prostaglandin E2 receptor EP2-dependent angiogenesis in ApcΔ716 mouse intestinal polyps. *Cancer Res.* **2002**, *62*, 506–511. [PubMed]
126. Nan, H.; Hutter, C.M.; Lin, Y.; Jacobs, E.J.; Ulrich, C.M.; White, E.; Baron, J.A.; Berndt, S.I.; Brenner, H.; Butterbach, K. Association of aspirin and NSAID use with risk of colorectal cancer according to genetic variants. *JAMA* **2015**, *313*, 1133–1142. [CrossRef]
127. Arber, N.; Eagle, C.J.; Spicak, J.; Rácz, I.; Dite, P.; Hajer, J.; Zavoral, M.; Lechuga, M.J.; Gerletti, P.; Tang, J. Celecoxib for the prevention of colorectal adenomatous polyps. *N. Engl. J. Med.* **2006**, *355*, 885–895. [CrossRef]
128. Dehmer, S.P.; Maciosek, M.V.; Flottemesch, T.J.; LaFrance, A.B.; Whitlock, E.P. Aspirin for the primary prevention of cardiovascular disease and colorectal cancer: A decision analysis for the US Preventive Services Task Force. *Ann. Intern. Med.* **2016**, *164*, 777–786. [CrossRef]
129. Chubak, J.; Whitlock, E.P.; Williams, S.B.; Kamineni, A.; Burda, B.U.; Buist, D.S.; Anderson, M.L. Aspirin for the prevention of cancer incidence and mortality: Systematic evidence reviews for the US Preventive Services Task Force. *Ann. Intern. Med.* **2016**, *164*, 814–825. [CrossRef]
130. Katona, B.W.; Weiss, J.M. Chemoprevention of colorectal cancer. *Gastroenterology* **2020**, *158*, 368–388. [CrossRef]
131. Liu, F.; Yan, L.; Wang, Z.; Lu, Y.; Chu, Y.; Li, X.; Liu, Y.; Rui, D.; Nie, S.; Xiang, H. Metformin therapy and risk of colorectal adenomas and colorectal cancer in type 2 diabetes mellitus patients: A systematic review and meta-analysis. *Oncotarget* **2017**, *8*, 16017. [CrossRef] [PubMed]
132. Petrera, M.; Paleari, L.; Clavarezza, M.; Puntoni, M.; Caviglia, S.; Briata, I.M.; Oppezzi, M.; Mislej, E.M.; Stabuc, B.; Gnant, M. The ASAMET trial: A randomized, phase II, double-blind, placebo-controlled, multicenter, 2× 2 factorial biomarker study of tertiary prevention with low-dose aspirin and metformin in stage I-III colorectal cancer patients. *BMC Cancer* **2018**, *18*, 1–9. [CrossRef]
133. Chan, K.K.; Oza, A.M.; Siu, L.L. The statins as anticancer agents. *Clin. Cancer Res.* **2003**, *9*, 10–19. [PubMed]
134. Teraoka, N.; Mutoh, M.; Takasu, S.; Ueno, T.; Yamamoto, M.; Sugimura, T.; Wakabayashi, K. Inhibition of intestinal polyp formation by pitavastatin, a HMG-CoA reductase inhibitor. *Cancer Prev. Res.* **2011**, *4*, 445–453. [CrossRef] [PubMed]
135. Suh, N.; Reddy, B.S.; DeCastro, A.; Paul, S.; Lee, H.J.; Smolarek, A.K.; So, J.Y.; Simi, B.; Wang, C.X.; Janakiram, N.B. Combination of atorvastatin with sulindac or naproxen profoundly inhibits colonic adenocarcinomas by suppressing the p65/β-catenin/cyclin D1 signaling pathway in rats. *Cancer Prev. Res.* **2011**, *4*, 1895–1902. [CrossRef]
136. Malila, N.; Virtamo, J.; Virtanen, M.; Albanes, D.; Tangrea, J.A.; Huttunen, J.K. The effect of α-tocopherol and β-carotene supplementation on colorectal adenomas in middle-aged male smokers. *Cancer Epidemiol. Prev. Biomark.* **1999**, *8*, 489–493.
137. Papaioannou, D.; Cooper, K.; Carroll, C.; Hind, D.; Squires, H.; Tappenden, P.; Logan, R. Antioxidants in the chemoprevention of colorectal cancer and colorectal adenomas in the general population: A systematic review and meta-analysis. *Color. Dis.* **2011**, *13*, 1085–1099. [CrossRef]
138. Yusof, A.S.; Isa, Z.M.; Shah, S.A. Dietary patterns and risk of colorectal cancer: A systematic review of cohort studies (2000–2011). *Asian Pac. J. Cancer Prev.* **2012**, *13*, 4713–4717. [CrossRef]
139. Vanio, H.; Bianchini, F. Weight Control and Physical Activity. In *IARC Handbooks of Cancer Prevention*; IARC Press: Lyon, France, 2002.
140. He, X.; Wu, K.; Zhang, X.; Nishihara, R.; Cao, Y.; Fuchs, C.S.; Giovannucci, E.L.; Ogino, S.; Chan, A.T.; Song, M. Dietary intake of fiber, whole grains and risk of colorectal cancer: An updated analysis according to food sources, tumor location and molecular subtypes in two large US cohorts. *Int. J. Cancer* **2019**, *145*, 3040–3051. [CrossRef]
141. Brenner, H.; Chang-Claude, J.; Jansen, L.; Knebel, P.; Stock, C.; Hoffmeister, M. Reduced risk of colorectal cancer up to 10 years after screening, surveillance, or diagnostic colonoscopy. *Gastroenterology* **2014**, *146*, 709–717. [CrossRef]
142. Wells, K.O.; Hawkins, A.T.; Krishnamurthy, D.M.; Dharmarajan, S.; Glasgow, S.C.; Hunt, S.R.; Mutch, M.G.; Wise, P.; Silviera, M.L. Omission of adjuvant chemotherapy is associated with increased mortality in patients with T3N0 colon cancer with inadequate lymph node harvest. *Dis. Colon Rectum* **2017**, *60*, 15–21. [CrossRef] [PubMed]

143. Ribic, C.M.; Sargent, D.J.; Moore, M.J.; Thibodeau, S.N.; French, A.J.; Goldberg, R.M.; Hamilton, S.R.; Laurent-Puig, P.; Gryfe, R.; Shepherd, L.E. Tumor microsatellite-instability status as a predictor of benefit from fluorouracil-based adjuvant chemotherapy for colon cancer. *N. Engl. J. Med.* **2003**, *349*, 247–257. [CrossRef] [PubMed]
144. Sargent, D.J.; Marsoni, S.; Monges, G.; Thibodeau, S.N.; Labianca, R.; Hamilton, S.R.; French, A.J.; Kabat, B.; Foster, N.R.; Torri, V. Defective mismatch repair as a predictive marker for lack of efficacy of fluorouracil-based adjuvant therapy in colon cancer. *J. Clin. Oncol.* **2010**, *28*, 3219. [CrossRef]
145. Argilés, G.; Tabernero, J.; Labianca, R.; Hochhauser, D.; Salazar, R.; Iveson, T.; Laurent-Puig, P.; Quirke, P.; Yoshino, T.; Taieb, J. Localised colon cancer: ESMO Clinical Practice Guidelines for diagnosis, treatment and follow-up. *Ann. Oncol.* **2020**, *31*, 1291–1305. [CrossRef] [PubMed]
146. Angell, H.K.; Bruni, D.; Barrett, J.C.; Herbst, R.; Galon, J. The immunoscore: Colon cancer and beyond. *Clin. Cancer Res.* **2020**, *26*, 332–339. [CrossRef] [PubMed]
147. Xie, Y.-H.; Chen, Y.-X.; Fang, J.-Y. Comprehensive review of targeted therapy for colorectal cancer. *Signal Transduct. Target. Ther.* **2020**, *5*, 1–30.
148. Falcone, A.; Ricci, S.; Brunetti, I.; Pfanner, E.; Allegrini, G.; Barbara, C.; Crinò, L.; Benedetti, G.; Evangelista, W.; Fanchini, L. Phase III trial of infusional fluorouracil, leucovorin, oxaliplatin, and irinotecan (FOLFOXIRI) compared with infusional fluorouracil, leucovorin, and irinotecan (FOLFIRI) as first-line treatment for metastatic colorectal cancer: The Gruppo Oncologico Nord Ovest. *J. Clin. Oncol.* **2007**, *25*, 1670–1676.
149. Souglakos, J.; Androulakis, N.; Syrigos, K.; Polyzos, A.; Ziras, N.; Athanasiadis, A.; Kakolyris, S.; Tsousis, S.; Kouroussis, C.; Vamvakas, L. FOLFOXIRI (folinic acid, 5-fluorouracil, oxaliplatin and irinotecan) vs FOLFIRI (folinic acid, 5-fluorouracil and irinotecan) as first-line treatment in metastatic colorectal cancer (MCC): A multicentre randomised phase III trial from the Hellenic Oncology Research Group (HORG). *Br. J. Cancer* **2006**, *94*, 798–805.
150. Cunningham, D.; Humblet, Y.; Siena, S.; Khayat, D.; Bleiberg, H.; Santoro, A.; Bets, D.; Mueser, M.; Harstrick, A.; Verslype, C. Cetuximab monotherapy and cetuximab plus irinotecan in irinotecan-refractory metastatic colorectal cancer. *N. Engl. J. Med.* **2004**, *351*, 337–345. [CrossRef]
151. Mendelsohn, J.; Prewett, M.; Rockwell, P.; Goldstein, N.I. CCR 20th anniversary commentary: A chimeric antibody, C225, inhibits EGFR activation and tumor growth. *Clin. Cancer Res.* **2015**, *21*, 227–229. [CrossRef]
152. Oliveira, A.F.; Bretes, L.; Furtado, I. Review of PD-1/PD-L1 inhibitors in metastatic dMMR/MSI-H colorectal cancer. *Front. Oncol.* **2019**, *9*, 396. [CrossRef] [PubMed]
153. Jonker, D.J.; O'Callaghan, C.J.; Karapetis, C.S.; Zalcberg, J.R.; Tu, D.; Au, H.-J.; Berry, S.R.; Krahn, M.; Price, T.; Simes, R.J. Cetuximab for the treatment of colorectal cancer. *N. Engl. J. Med.* **2007**, *357*, 2040–2048. [CrossRef] [PubMed]
154. Roskoski, R., Jr. The ErbB/HER family of protein-tyrosine kinases and cancer. *Pharmacol. Res.* **2014**, *79*, 34–74. [CrossRef]
155. Shibuya, M. Vascular endothelial growth factor (VEGF) and its receptor (VEGFR) signaling in angiogenesis: A crucial target for anti-and pro-angiogenic therapies. *Genes Cancer* **2011**, *2*, 1097–1105. [CrossRef]
156. Guba, M.; Seeliger, H.; Kleespies, A.; Jauch, K.-W.; Bruns, C. Vascular endothelial growth factor in colorectal cancer. *Int. J. Color. Dis.* **2004**, *19*, 510–517. [CrossRef] [PubMed]
157. Page, M.J.; McKenzie, J.E.; Bossuyt, P.M.; Boutron, I.; Hoffmann, T.C.; Mulrow, C.D.; Shamseer, L.; Tetzlaff, J.M.; Akl, E.A.; Brennan, S.E. The PRISMA 2020 statement: An updated guideline for reporting systematic reviews. *Syst. Rev.* **2021**, *88*, 105906.
158. De Paulo Farias, D.; de Araujo, F.F.; Neri-Numa, I.A.; Pastore, G.M. Antidiabetic potential of dietary polyphenols: A mechanistic review. *Food Res. Int.* **2021**, *145*, 110383. [CrossRef]
159. Tsimogiannis, D.; Oreopoulou, V. Classification of phenolic compounds in plants. *Polyphen. Plants (Second Ed.)* **2019**, 263–284. [CrossRef]
160. Vuolo, M.M.; Lima, V.S.; Junior, M.R.M. Phenolic compounds: Structure, classification, and antioxidant power. *Bioact. Compd.* **2019**, 33–50. [CrossRef]
161. Kiruthiga, C.; Devi, K.P.; Nabavi, S.M.; Bishayee, A. Autophagy: A potential therapeutic target of polyphenols in hepatocellular carcinoma. *Cancers* **2020**, *12*, 562. [CrossRef]
162. Darvesh, A.S.; Carroll, R.T.; Bishayee, A.; Geldenhuys, W.J.; Van der Schyf, C.J. Oxidative stress and Alzheimer's disease: Dietary polyphenols as potential therapeutic agents. *Expert Rev. Neurother.* **2010**, *10*, 729–745. [CrossRef]
163. Karimi, A.; Majlesi, M.; Rafieian-Kopaei, M. Herbal versus synthetic drugs; beliefs and facts. *J. Nephropharmacol.* **2015**, *4*, 27. [PubMed]
164. Samec, M.; Liskova, A.; Koklesova, L.; Samuel, S.M.; Zhai, K.; Buhrmann, C.; Varghese, E.; Abotaleb, M.; Qaradakhi, T.; Zulli, A. Flavonoids against the Warburg phenotype—Concepts of predictive, preventive and personalised medicine to cut the Gordian knot of cancer cell metabolism. *Epma J.* **2020**, *11*, 377–398. [CrossRef] [PubMed]
165. Jain, A.; Madu, C.O.; Lu, Y. Phytochemicals in chemoprevention: A cost-effective complementary approach. *J. Cancer* **2021**, *12*, 3686. [CrossRef] [PubMed]
166. Rajamanickam, S.; Agarwal, R. Natural products and colon cancer: Current status and future prospects. *Drug Dev. Res.* **2008**, *69*, 460–471. [CrossRef]
167. Bishayee, A.; Sethi, G. Bioactive natural products in cancer prevention and therapy: Progress and promise. *Semin. Cancer Biol.* **2016**, *40*, 1–3. [CrossRef]

168. Huang, X.-M.; Yang, Z.-J.; Xie, Q.; Zhang, Z.-K.; Zhang, H.; Ma, J.-Y. Natural products for treating colorectal cancer: A mechanistic review. *Biomed. Pharmacother.* **2019**, *117*, 109142. [CrossRef]
169. Atanasov, A.G.; Zotchev, S.B.; Dirsch, V.M.; Supuran, C.T. Natural products in drug discovery: Advances and opportunities. *Nat. Rev. Drug Discov.* **2021**, *20*, 200–216. [CrossRef]
170. Lin, C.-L.; Jeng, J.-H.; Wu, C.-C.; Hsieh, S.-L.; Huang, G.-C.; Leung, W.; Lee, C.-T.; Chen, C.-Y.; Lee, C.-H. Chemopreventive potential of 2, 3, 5, 4′-tetrahydroxystilbene-2-O-β-D-glucoside on The formation of aberrant crypt foci in azoxymethane-induced colorectal cancer in rats. *BioMed Res. Int.* **2017**, *2017*, 3634915. [CrossRef]
171. Chen, Q.; Lei, J.; Zhou, J.; Ma, S.; Huang, Q.; Ge, B. Chemopreventive effect of 4′-hydroxychalcone on intestinal tumorigenesis in Apc Min mice Corrigendum in/10.3892/ol. 2021.12741. *Oncol. Lett.* **2021**, *21*, 213. [CrossRef]
172. Lai, C.-Y.; Tsai, A.-C.; Chen, M.-C.; Chang, L.-H.; Sun, H.-L.; Chang, Y.-L.; Chen, C.-C.; Teng, C.-M.; Pan, S.-L. Aciculatin induces p53-dependent apoptosis via MDM2 depletion in human cancer cells in vitro and in vivo. *PLoS ONE* **2012**, *7*, e42192. [CrossRef]
173. Au, A.; Li, B.; Wang, W.; Roy, H.; Koehler, K.; Birt, D. Effect of dietary apigenin on colonic ornithine decarboxylase activity, aberrant crypt foci formation, and tumorigenesis in different experimental models. *Nutr. Cancer* **2006**, *54*, 243–251. [CrossRef]
174. Wang, Q.R.; Yao, X.Q.; Wen, G.; Fan, Q.; Li, Y.-J.; Fu, X.Q.; Li, C.K.; Sun, X.G. Apigenin suppresses the growth of colorectal cancer xenografts via phosphorylation and up-regulated FADD expression. *Oncol. Lett.* **2011**, *2*, 43–47. [CrossRef] [PubMed]
175. Chunhua, L.; Donglan, L.; Xiuqiong, F.; Lihua, Z.; Qin, F.; Yawei, L.; Liang, Z.; Ge, W.; Linlin, J.; Ping, Z. Apigenin up-regulates transgelin and inhibits invasion and migration of colorectal cancer through decreased phosphorylation of AKT. *J. Nutr. Biochem.* **2013**, *24*, 1766–1775. [CrossRef]
176. Zhong, Y.; Krisanapun, C.; Lee, S.-H.; Nualsanit, T.; Sams, C.; Peungvicha, P.; Baek, S.J. Molecular targets of apigenin in colorectal cancer cells: Involvement of p21, NAG-1 and p53. *Eur. J. Cancer* **2010**, *46*, 3365–3374. [CrossRef]
177. Chen, X.; Xu, H.; Yu, X.; Wang, X.; Zhu, X.; Xu, X. Apigenin inhibits in vitro and in vivo tumorigenesis in cisplatin-resistant colon cancer cells by inducing autophagy, programmed cell death and targeting m-TOR/PI3K/Akt signalling pathway. *J. Buon* **2019**, *24*, 488–493. [PubMed]
178. Shao, H.; Jing, K.; Mahmoud, E.; Huang, H.; Fang, X.; Yu, C. Apigenin sensitizes colon cancer cells to antitumor activity of ABT-263. *Mol. Cancer Ther.* **2013**, *12*, 2640–2650. [CrossRef] [PubMed]
179. Dai, J.; Van Wie, P.G.; Fai, L.Y.; Kim, D.; Wang, L.; Poyil, P.; Luo, J.; Zhang, Z. Downregulation of NEDD9 by apigenin suppresses migration, invasion, and metastasis of colorectal cancer cells. *Toxicol. Appl. Pharmacol.* **2016**, *311*, 106–112. [CrossRef]
180. Kim, D.H.; Hossain, M.A.; Kang, Y.J.; Jang, J.Y.; Lee, Y.J.; Im, E.; Yoon, J.-H.; Kim, H.S.; Chung, H.Y.; Kim, N.D. Baicalein, an active component of Scutellaria baicalensis Georgi, induces apoptosis in human colon cancer cells and prevents AOM/DSS-induced colon cancer in mice. *Int. J. Oncol.* **2013**, *43*, 1652–1658. [CrossRef]
181. Chen, W.-C.; Kuo, T.-H.; Tzeng, Y.-S.; Tsai, Y.-C. Baicalin induces apoptosis in SW620 human colorectal carcinoma cells in vitro and suppresses tumor growth in vivo. *Molecules* **2012**, *17*, 3844–3857. [CrossRef]
182. Song, L.; Zhu, S.; Liu, C.; Zhang, Q.; Liang, X. Baicalin triggers apoptosis, inhibits migration, and enhances anti-tumor immunity in colorectal cancer via TLR4/NF-κB signaling pathway. *J. Food Biochem.* **2022**, *46*, e13703. [CrossRef]
183. Kim, S.-J.; Kim, H.-J.; Kim, H.-R.; Lee, S.-H.; Cho, S.-D.; Choi, C.-S.; Nam, J.-S.; Jung, J.-Y. Antitumor actions of baicalein and wogonin in HT-29 human colorectal cancer cells. *Mol. Med. Rep.* **2012**, *6*, 1443–1449. [CrossRef] [PubMed]
184. Chai, Y.; Xu, J.; Yan, B. The anti-metastatic effect of baicalein on colorectal cancer. *Oncol. Rep.* **2017**, *37*, 2317–2323. [CrossRef] [PubMed]
185. Dou, J.; Wang, Z.; Ma, L.; Peng, B.; Mao, K.; Li, C.; Su, M.; Zhou, C.; Peng, G. Baicalein and baicalin inhibit colon cancer using two distinct fashions of apoptosis and senescence. *Oncotarget* **2018**, *9*, 20089. [CrossRef] [PubMed]
186. Wang, Z.; Ma, L.; Su, M.; Zhou, Y.; Mao, K.; Li, C.; Peng, G.; Zhou, C.; Shen, B.; Dou, J. Baicalin induces cellular senescence in human colon cancer cells via upregulation of DEPP and the activation of Ras/Raf/MEK/ERK signaling. *Cell Death Dis.* **2018**, *9*, 217. [CrossRef] [PubMed]
187. Tao, Y.; Zhan, S.; Wang, Y.; Zhou, G.; Liang, H.; Chen, X.; Shen, H. Baicalin, the major component of traditional Chinese medicine Scutellaria baicalensis induces colon cancer cell apoptosis through inhibition of oncomiRNAs. *Sci. Rep.* **2018**, *8*, 14477. [CrossRef] [PubMed]
188. Yang, B.; Bai, H.; Sa, Y.; Zhu, P.; Liu, P. Inhibiting EMT, stemness and cell cycle involved in baicalin-induced growth inhibition and apoptosis in colorectal cancer cells. *J. Cancer* **2020**, *11*, 2303. [CrossRef]
189. Wang, C.-Z.; Zhang, C.-F.; Luo, Y.; Yao, H.; Yu, C.; Chen, L.; Yuan, J.; Huang, W.-H.; Wan, J.-Y.; Zeng, J. Baicalein, an enteric microbial metabolite, suppresses gut inflammation and cancer progression in Apc Min/+ mice. *Clin. Transl. Oncol.* **2020**, *22*, 1013–1022. [CrossRef] [PubMed]
190. Zhang, W.; Liu, Q.; Luo, L.; Song, J.; Han, K.; Liu, R.; Gong, Y.; Guo, X. Use Chou's 5-steps rule to study how Baicalin suppresses the malignant phenotypes and induces the apoptosis of colorectal cancer cells. *Arch. Biochem. Biophys.* **2021**, *705*, 108919. [CrossRef]
191. Zhou, C.; Ou, W.; Xu, Q.; Lin, L.; Xu, F.; Chen, R.; Miao, H. Chemoprotective effect of boeravinone B against 1, 2-dimethyl hydrazine induced colorectal cancer in rats via suppression of oxidative stress and inflammatory reaction. *J. Gastrointest. Oncol.* **2022**, *13*, 1832–1841. [CrossRef]
192. Miyamoto, S.; Kohno, H.; Suzuki, R.; Sugie, S.; Murakami, A.; Ohigashi, H.; Tanaka, T. Preventive effects of chrysin on the development of azoxymethane-induced colonic aberrant crypt foci in rats. *Oncol. Rep.* **2006**, *15*, 1169–1173. [CrossRef]

193. Salama, A.A.; Allam, R.M. Promising targets of chrysin and daidzein in colorectal cancer: Amphiregulin, CXCL1, and MMP-9. *Eur. J. Pharmacol.* **2021**, *892*, 173763. [CrossRef] [PubMed]
194. Villegas, I.; Sánchez-Fidalgo, S.; de la Lastra, C.A. Chemopreventive effect of dietary curcumin on inflammation-induced colorectal carcinogenesis in mice. *Mol. Nutr. Food Res.* **2011**, *55*, 259–267. [CrossRef]
195. Milacic, V.; Banerjee, S.; Landis-Piwowar, K.R.; Sarkar, F.H.; Majumdar, A.P.; Dou, Q.P. Curcumin inhibits the proteasome activity in human colon cancer cells in vitro and in vivo. *Cancer Res.* **2008**, *68*, 7283–7292. [CrossRef] [PubMed]
196. Hao, J.; Dai, X.; Gao, J.; Li, Y.; Hou, Z.; Chang, Z.; Wang, Y. Curcumin suppresses colorectal tumorigenesis via the Wnt/β-catenin signaling pathway by downregulating Axin2. *Oncol. Lett.* **2021**, *21*, 186. [CrossRef]
197. Kubota, M.; Shimizu, M.; Sakai, H.; Yasuda, Y.; Terakura, D.; Baba, A.; Ohno, T.; Tsurumi, H.; Tanaka, T.; Moriwaki, H. Preventive effects of curcumin on the development of azoxymethane-induced colonic preneoplastic lesions in male C57BL/KsJ-db/db obese mice. *Nutr. Cancer* **2012**, *64*, 72–79. [CrossRef] [PubMed]
198. Kunnumakkara, A.B.; Diagaradjane, P.; Guha, S.; Deorukhkar, A.; Shentu, S.; Aggarwal, B.B.; Krishnan, S. Curcumin sensitizes human colorectal cancer xenografts in nude mice to γ-radiation by targeting nuclear factor-κB–regulated gene products. *Clin. Cancer Res.* **2008**, *14*, 2128–2136. [CrossRef]
199. Li, L.; Ahmed, B.; Mehta, K.; Kurzrock, R. Liposomal curcumin with and without oxaliplatin: Effects on cell growth, apoptosis, and angiogenesis in colorectal cancer. *Mol. Cancer Ther.* **2007**, *6*, 1276–1282. [CrossRef]
200. McFadden, R.-M.T.; Larmonier, C.B.; Shehab, K.W.; Midura-Kiela, M.; Ramalingam, R.; Harrison, C.A.; Besselsen, D.G.; Chase, J.H.; Caporaso, J.G.; Jobin, C. The role of curcumin in modulating colonic microbiota during colitis and colon cancer prevention. *Inflamm. Bowel Dis.* **2015**, *21*, 2483–2494. [CrossRef]
201. Marjaneh, R.M.; Rahmani, F.; Hassanian, S.M.; Rezaei, N.; Hashemzehi, M.; Bahrami, A.; Ariakia, F.; Fiuji, H.; Sahebkar, A.; Avan, A. Phytosomal curcumin inhibits tumor growth in colitis-associated colorectal cancer. *J. Cell. Physiol.* **2018**, *233*, 6785–6798. [CrossRef]
202. Cooke, D.; Schwarz, M.; Boocock, D.; Winterhalter, P.; Steward, W.P.; Gescher, A.J.; Marczylo, T.H. Effect of cyanidin-3-glucoside and an anthocyanin mixture from bilberry on adenoma development in the ApcMin mouse model of intestinal carcinogenesis—Relationship with tissue anthocyanin levels. *Int. J. Cancer* **2006**, *119*, 2213–2220. [CrossRef]
203. Huang, C.-C.; Hung, C.-H.; Hung, T.-W.; Lin, Y.-C.; Wang, C.-J.; Kao, S.-H. Dietary delphinidin inhibits human colorectal cancer metastasis associating with upregulation of miR-204-3p and suppression of the integrin/FAK axis. *Sci. Rep.* **2019**, *9*, 18954. [CrossRef] [PubMed]
204. Koosha, S.; Mohamed, Z.; Sinniah, A.; Alshawsh, M.A. Evaluation of anti-tumorigenic effects of diosmetin against human colon cancer xenografts in athymic nude mice. *Molecules* **2019**, *24*, 2522. [CrossRef] [PubMed]
205. Shimizu, M.; Shirakami, Y.; Sakai, H.; Yasuda, Y.; Kubota, M.; Adachi, S.; Tsurumi, H.; Hara, Y.; Moriwaki, H. (−)-Epigallocatechin gallate inhibits growth and activation of the VEGF/VEGFR axis in human colorectal cancer cells. *Chem.-Biol. Interact.* **2010**, *185*, 247–252. [CrossRef] [PubMed]
206. Shimizu, M.; Shirakami, Y.; Sakai, H.; Adachi, S.; Hata, K.; Hirose, Y.; Tsurumi, H.; Tanaka, T.; Moriwaki, H. (−)-Epigallocatechin gallate suppresses azoxymethane-induced colonic premalignant lesions in male C57BL/KsJ-db/db mice. *Cancer Prev. Res.* **2008**, *1*, 298–304. [CrossRef]
207. Zhong, Y.; Chiou, Y.-S.; Pan, M.-H.; Ho, C.-T.; Shahidi, F. Protective effects of epigallocatechin gallate (EGCG) derivatives on azoxymethane-induced colonic carcinogenesis in mice. *J. Funct. Foods* **2012**, *4*, 323–330. [CrossRef]
208. Toden, S.; Tran, H.-M.; Tovar-Camargo, O.A.; Okugawa, Y.; Goel, A. Epigallocatechin-3-gallate targets cancer stem-like cells and enhances 5-fluorouracil chemosensitivity in colorectal cancer. *Oncotarget* **2016**, *7*, 16158. [CrossRef]
209. Xu, G.; Ren, G.; Xu, X.; Yuan, H.; Wang, Z.; Kang, L.; Yu, W.; Tian, K. Combination of curcumin and green tea catechins prevents dimethylhydrazine-induced colon carcinogenesis. *Food Chem. Toxicol.* **2010**, *48*, 390–395. [CrossRef]
210. Wang, Y.; Jin, H.-Y.; Fang, M.-Z.; Wang, X.-F.; Chen, H.; Huang, S.-L.; Kong, D.-S.; Li, M.; Zhang, X.; Sun, Y. Epigallocatechin gallate inhibits dimethylhydrazine-induced colorectal cancer in rats. *World J. Gastroenterol.* **2020**, *26*, 2064. [CrossRef]
211. Mariyappan, P.; Kalaiyarasu, T.; Manju, V. Effect of eriodictyol on preneoplastic lesions, oxidative stress and bacterial enzymes in 1, 2-dimethyl hydrazine-induced colon carcinogenesis. *Toxicol. Res.* **2017**, *6*, 678–692. [CrossRef]
212. Wang, N.; Zhou, F.; Guo, J.; Zhu, H.; Luo, S.; Cao, J. Euxanthone suppresses tumor growth and metastasis in colorectal cancer via targeting CIP2A/PP2A pathway. *Life Sci.* **2018**, *209*, 498–506. [CrossRef]
213. Kunchari Kalaimathi, S.; Sudhandiran, G. Fisetin ameolirates the azoxymethane and dextran sodium sulfate induced colitis associated colorectal cancer. *Int. J. Pharm. Clin. Res.* **2016**, *8*, 551–560.
214. Khan, N.; Jajeh, F.; Eberhardt, E.L.; Miller, D.D.; Albrecht, D.M.; Van Doorn, R.; Hruby, M.D.; Maresh, M.E.; Clipson, L.; Mukhtar, H. Fisetin and 5-fluorouracil: Effective combination for PIK3CA-mutant colorectal cancer. *Int. J. Cancer* **2019**, *145*, 3022–3032. [CrossRef]
215. Jeng, L.B.; Kumar Velmurugan, B.; Chen, M.C.; Hsu, H.H.; Ho, T.J.; Day, C.H.; Lin, Y.M.; Padma, V.V.; Tu, C.C.; Huang, C.Y. Fisetin mediated apoptotic cell death in parental and Oxaliplatin/irinotecan resistant colorectal cancer cells in vitro and in vivo. *J. Cell. Physiol.* **2018**, *233*, 7134–7142. [CrossRef] [PubMed]
216. Leu, J.D.; Wang, B.S.; Chiu, S.J.; Chan, C.Y.; Chen, C.C.; Chen, F.D.; Avirmed, S.; Lee, Y.J. Combining fisetin and ionizing radiation suppresses the growth of mammalian colorectal cancers in xenograft tumor models. *Oncol. Lett.* **2016**, *12*, 4975–4982. [CrossRef]

217. Chen, Y.; Wu, Q.; Song, L.; He, T.; Li, Y.; Li, L.; Su, W.; Liu, L.; Qian, Z.; Gong, C. Polymeric micelles encapsulating fisetin improve the therapeutic effect in colon cancer. *ACS Appl. Mater. Interfaces* **2015**, *7*, 534–542. [CrossRef]
218. Li, L.; Wang, M.; Yang, H.; Li, Y.; Huang, X.; Guo, J.; Liu, Z. Fisetin Inhibits Trypsin Activity and Suppresses the Growth of Colorectal Cancer in Vitro and in Vivo. *Nat. Prod. Commun.* **2022**, *17*, 1934578X221115511. [CrossRef]
219. Winkelmann, I.; Diehl, D.; Oesterle, D.; Daniel, H.; Wenzel, U. The suppression of aberrant crypt multiplicity in colonic tissue of 1, 2-dimethylhydrazine-treated C57BL/6J mice by dietary flavone is associated with an increased expression of Krebs cycle enzymes. *Carcinogenesis* **2007**, *28*, 1446–1454. [CrossRef]
220. Auyeung, K.K.-W.; Law, P.-C.; Ko, J.K.-S. Novel anti-angiogenic effects of formononetin in human colon cancer cells and tumor xenograft. *Oncol. Rep.* **2012**, *28*, 2188–2194. [CrossRef]
221. Ma, Z.; Bao, X.; Gu, J. Furowanin A-induced autophagy alleviates apoptosis and promotes cell cycle arrest via inactivation STAT3/Mcl-1 axis in colorectal cancer. *Life Sci.* **2019**, *218*, 47–57. [CrossRef]
222. Sekar, V.; Anandasadagopan, S.K.; Ganapasam, S. Genistein regulates tumor microenvironment and exhibits anticancer effect in dimethyl hydrazine-induced experimental colon carcinogenesis. *Biofactors* **2016**, *42*, 623–637. [CrossRef]
223. Zhang, Y.; Li, Q.; Zhou, D.; Chen, H. Genistein, a soya isoflavone, prevents azoxymethane-induced up-regulation of WNT/β-catenin signalling and reduces colon pre-neoplasia in rats. *Br. J. Nutr.* **2013**, *109*, 33–42. [CrossRef] [PubMed]
224. Xiao, X.; Liu, Z.; Wang, R.; Wang, J.; Zhang, S.; Cai, X.; Wu, K.; Bergan, R.C.; Xu, L.; Fan, D. Genistein suppresses FLT4 and inhibits human colorectal cancer metastasis. *Oncotarget* **2015**, *6*, 3225. [CrossRef] [PubMed]
225. Wang, X.; Song, Z.-J.; He, X.; Zhang, R.-Q.; Zhang, C.-F.; Li, F.; Wang, C.-Z.; Yuan, C.-S. Antitumor and immunomodulatory activity of genkwanin on colorectal cancer in the APCMin/+ mice. *Int. Immunopharmacol.* **2015**, *29*, 701–707. [CrossRef] [PubMed]
226. Yin, H.-F.; Yin, C.-M.; Ouyang, T.; Sun, S.-D.; Chen, W.-G.; Yang, X.-L.; He, X.; Zhang, C.-F. Self-Nanoemulsifying Drug Delivery System of Genkwanin: A Novel Approach for Anti-Colitis-Associated Colorectal Cancer. *Drug Des. Dev. Ther.* **2021**, *15*, 557. [CrossRef] [PubMed]
227. Saiprasad, G.; Chitra, P.; Manikandan, R.; Sudhandiran, G. Hesperidin alleviates oxidative stress and downregulates the expressions of proliferative and inflammatory markers in azoxymethane-induced experimental colon carcinogenesis in mice. *Inflamm. Res.* **2013**, *62*, 425–440. [CrossRef]
228. Saiprasad, G.; Chitra, P.; Manikandan, R.; Sudhandiran, G. Hesperidin induces apoptosis and triggers autophagic markers through inhibition of Aurora-A mediated phosphoinositide-3-kinase/Akt/mammalian target of rapamycin and glycogen synthase kinase-3 beta signalling cascades in experimental colon carcinogenesis. *Eur. J. Cancer* **2014**, *50*, 2489–2507. [CrossRef]
229. Tanaka, T.; Makita, H.; Kawabata, K.; Mori, H.; Kakumoto, M.; Satoh, K.; Hara, A.; Sumida, T.; Tanaka, T.; Ogawa, H. Chemoprevention of azoxymethane-induced rat colon carcinogenesis by the naturally occurring flavonoids, diosmin and hesperidin. *Carcinogenesis* **1997**, *18*, 957–965. [CrossRef]
230. El-Deek, S.E.; Abd-Elghaffar, S.K.; Hna, R.S.; Mohamed, H.G.; El-Deek, H.E. Effect of hesperidin against induced colon cancer in rats: Impact of Smad4 and activin a signaling pathway. *Nutr. Cancer* **2022**, *74*, 697–714. [CrossRef]
231. Zhou, J.; Zhao, R.; Ye, T.; Yang, S.; Li, Y.; Yang, F.; Wang, G.; Xie, Y.; Li, Q. Antitumor activity in colorectal cancer induced by hinokiflavone. *J. Gastroenterol. Hepatol.* **2019**, *34*, 1571–1580. [CrossRef]
232. Shi, C.-J.; Li, S.-Y.; Shen, C.-H.; Pan, F.-F.; Deng, L.-Q.; Fu, W.-M.; Wang, J.-Y.; Zhang, J.-F. Icariside II suppressed tumorigenesis by epigenetically regulating the circβ-catenin-Wnt/β-catenin axis in colorectal cancer. *Bioorganic Chem.* **2022**, *124*, 105800. [CrossRef]
233. Zhou, C.; Gu, J.; Zhang, G.; Dong, D.; Yang, Q.; Chen, M.-B.; Xu, D. AMPK-autophagy inhibition sensitizes icaritin-induced anti-colorectal cancer cell activity. *Oncotarget* **2017**, *8*, 14736. [CrossRef] [PubMed]
234. Tang, S.; Cai, S.; Ji, S.; Yan, X.; Zhang, W.; Qiao, X.; Zhang, H.; Ye, M.; Yu, S. Isoangustone A induces autophagic cell death in colorectal cancer cells by activating AMPK signaling. *Fitoterapia* **2021**, *152*, 104935. [CrossRef] [PubMed]
235. Zhao, H.; Zhang, X.; Chen, X.; Li, Y.; Ke, Z.; Tang, T.; Chai, H.; Guo, A.M.; Chen, H.; Yang, J. Isoliquiritigenin, a flavonoid from licorice, blocks M2 macrophage polarization in colitis-associated tumorigenesis through downregulating PGE2 and IL-6. *Toxicol. Appl. Pharmacol.* **2014**, *279*, 311–321. [CrossRef] [PubMed]
236. Takahashi, T.; Takasuka, N.; Iigo, M.; Baba, M.; Nishino, H.; Tsuda, H.; Okuyama, T. Isoliquiritigenin, a flavonoid from licorice, reduces prostaglandin E2 and nitric oxide, causes apoptosis, and suppresses aberrant crypt foci development. *Cancer Sci.* **2004**, *95*, 448–453. [CrossRef] [PubMed]
237. Antunes-Ricardo, M.; Guardado-Félix, D.; Rocha-Pizaña, M.; Garza-Martínez, J.; Acevedo-Pacheco, L.; Gutiérrez-Uribe, J.; Villela-Castrejón, J.; López-Pacheco, F.; Serna-Saldívar, S. Opuntia ficus-indica Extract and Isorhamnetin-3-O-Glucosyl-Rhamnoside Diminish Tumor Growth of Colon Cancer Cells Xenografted in Immune-Suppressed Mice through the Activation of Apoptosis Intrinsic Pathway. *Plant Foods Hum. Nutr.* **2021**, *76*, 434–441. [CrossRef]
238. Saud, S.M.; Young, M.R.; Jones-Hall, Y.L.; Ileva, L.; Evbuomwan, M.O.; Wise, J.; Colburn, N.H.; Kim, Y.S.; Bobe, G. Chemopreventive Activity of Plant Flavonoid Isorhamnetin in Colorectal Cancer Is Mediated by Oncogenic Src and β-CateninIsorhamnetin-Induced CSK Inhibits Colorectal Cancer. *Cancer Res.* **2013**, *73*, 5473–5484. [CrossRef]
239. Nirmala, P.; Ramanathan, M. Effect of kaempferol on lipid peroxidation and antioxidant status in 1, 2-dimethyl hydrazine induced colorectal carcinoma in rats. *Eur. J. Pharmacol.* **2011**, *654*, 75–79. [CrossRef]
240. Hassan, E.S.; Hassanein, N.M.; Ahmed, H.M.S. Probing the chemoprevention potential of the antidepressant fluoxetine combined with epigallocatechin gallate or kaempferol in rats with induced early stage colon carcinogenesis. *J. Pharmacol. Sci.* **2021**, *145*, 29–41. [CrossRef]

241. Hassanein, N.M.; Hassan, E.S.; Hegab, A.M.; Elahl, H.M.S. Chemopreventive effect of sulindac in combination with epigallocatechin gallate or kaempferol against 1, 2-dimethyl hydrazine-induced preneoplastic lesions in rats: A comparative study. *J. Biochem. Mol. Toxicol.* **2018**, *32*, e22198. [CrossRef]
242. Osman, N.H.; Said, U.Z.; El-Waseef, A.M.; Ahmed, E.S. Luteolin supplementation adjacent to aspirin treatment reduced dimethylhydrazine-induced experimental colon carcinogenesis in rats. *Tumor Biol.* **2015**, *36*, 1179–1190. [CrossRef]
243. Pandurangan, A.K.; Kumar, S.A.S.; Dharmalingam, P.; Ganapasam, S. Luteolin, a bioflavonoid inhibits azoxymethane-induced colon carcinogenesis: Involvement of iNOS and COX-2. *Pharmacogn. Mag.* **2014**, *10*, S306. [PubMed]
244. Pandurangan, A.K.; Ananda Sadagopan, S.K.; Dharmalingam, P.; Ganapasam, S. Luteolin, a bioflavonoid inhibits Azoxymethane-induced colorectal cancer through activation of Nrf2 signaling. *Toxicol. Mech. Methods* **2014**, *24*, 13–20. [CrossRef] [PubMed]
245. Kim, H.Y.; Jung, S.K.; Byun, S.; Son, J.E.; Oh, M.H.; Lee, J.; Kang, M.J.; Heo, Y.S.; Lee, K.W.; Lee, H.J. Raf and PI3K are the molecular targets for the anti-metastatic effect of Luteolin. *Phytother. Res.* **2013**, *27*, 1481–1488. [CrossRef] [PubMed]
246. Pandurangan, A.; Dharmalingam, P.; Sadagopan, S.; Ganapasam, S. Luteolin inhibits matrix metalloproteinase 9 and 2 in azoxymethane-induced colon carcinogenesis. *Hum. Exp. Toxicol.* **2014**, *33*, 1176–1185. [CrossRef]
247. Yao, Y.; Rao, C.; Zheng, G.; Wang, S. Luteolin suppresses colorectal cancer cell metastasis via regulation of the miR-384/pleiotrophin axis. *Oncol. Rep.* **2019**, *42*, 131–141. [CrossRef]
248. Xiao, B.; Qin, Y.; Ying, C.; Ma, B.; Wang, B.; Long, F.; Wang, R.; Fang, L.; Wang, Y. Combination of oncolytic adenovirus and luteolin exerts synergistic antitumor effects in colorectal cancer cells and a mouse model. *Mol. Med. Rep.* **2017**, *16*, 9375–9382. [CrossRef] [PubMed]
249. Gao, Z.; Jiang, J.; Hou, L.; Ji, F. Lysionotin Induces Ferroptosis to Suppress Development of Colorectal Cancer via Promoting Nrf2 Degradation. *Oxidative Med. Cell. Longev.* **2022**, *2022*, 1366957. [CrossRef]
250. Yu, H.; Yin, S.; Zhou, S.; Shao, Y.; Sun, J.; Pang, X.; Han, L.; Zhang, Y.; Gao, X.; Jin, C. Magnolin promotes autophagy and cell cycle arrest via blocking LIF/Stat3/Mcl-1 axis in human colorectal cancers. *Cell Death Dis.* **2018**, *9*, 702. [CrossRef]
251. Chen, R.; Zhang, L. Morin inhibits colorectal tumor growth through inhibition of NF-κB signaling pathway. *Immunopharmacol. Immunotoxicol.* **2019**, *41*, 622–629. [CrossRef]
252. Sharma, S.H.; Thulasingam, S.; Chellappan, D.R.; Chinnaswamy, P.; Nagarajan, S. Morin and Esculetin supplementation modulates c-myc induced energy metabolism and attenuates neoplastic changes in rats challenged with the procarcinogen 1, 2-dimethylhydrazine. *Eur. J. Pharmacol.* **2017**, *796*, 20–31. [CrossRef]
253. Lori, G.; Paoli, P.; Femia, A.P.; Pranzini, E.; Caselli, A.; Tortora, K.; Romagnoli, A.; Raugei, G.; Caderni, G. Morin-dependent inhibition of low molecular weight protein tyrosine phosphatase (LMW-PTP) restores sensitivity to apoptosis during colon carcinogenesis: Studies in vitro and in vivo, in an Apc-driven model of colon cancer. *Mol. Carcinog.* **2019**, *58*, 686–698. [CrossRef] [PubMed]
254. Vennila, S.; Nalini, N. Modifying effects of morin on the development of aberrant crypt foci and bacterial enzymes in experimental colon cancer. *Food Chem. Toxicol.* **2009**, *47*, 309–315.
255. Sharma, S.H.; Kumar, J.S.; Chellappan, D.R.; Nagarajan, S. Molecular chemoprevention by morin–A plant flavonoid that targets nuclear factor kappa B in experimental colon cancer. *Biomed. Pharmacother.* **2018**, *100*, 367–373. [CrossRef]
256. Sreedharan, V.; Venkatachalam, K.K.; Namasivayam, N. Effect of morin on tissue lipid peroxidation and antioxidant status in 1, 2-dimethylhydrazine induced experimental colon carcinogenesis. *Investig. New Drugs* **2009**, *27*, 21–30. [CrossRef] [PubMed]
257. Nirmala, P.; Ramanathan, M. Effect of myricetin on 1, 2 dimethylhydrazine induced rat colon carcinogenesis. *J. Exp. Ther. Oncol.* **2011**, *9*, 101–108.
258. Li, Y.; Cui, S.-X.; Sun, S.-Y.; Shi, W.-N.; Song, Z.-Y.; Wang, S.-Q.; Yu, X.-F.; Gao, Z.-H.; Qu, X.-J. Chemoprevention of intestinal tumorigenesis by the natural dietary flavonoid myricetin in APCMin/+ mice. *Oncotarget* **2016**, *7*, 60446. [CrossRef]
259. Zhang, M.-J.; Su, H.; Yan, J.-Y.; Li, N.; Song, Z.-Y.; Wang, H.-J.; Huo, L.-G.; Wang, F.; Ji, W.-S.; Qu, X.-J. Chemopreventive effect of Myricetin, a natural occurring compound, on colonic chronic inflammation and inflammation-driven tumorigenesis in mice. *Biomed. Pharmacother.* **2018**, *97*, 1131–1137. [CrossRef]
260. Wang, F.; Song, Z.-Y.; Qu, X.-J.; Li, F.; Zhang, L.; Li, W.-B.; Cui, S.-X. M10, a novel derivative of Myricetin, prevents ulcerative colitis and colorectal tumor through attenuating robust endoplasmic reticulum stress. *Carcinogenesis* **2018**, *39*, 889–899. [CrossRef]
261. Leonardi, T.; Vanamala, J.; Taddeo, S.S.; Davidson, L.A.; Murphy, M.E.; Patil, B.S.; Wang, N.; Carroll, R.J.; Chapkin, R.S.; Lupton, J.R. Apigenin and naringenin suppress colon carcinogenesis through the aberrant crypt stage in azoxymethane-treated rats. *Exp. Biol. Med.* **2010**, *235*, 710–717. [CrossRef]
262. Dou, W.; Zhang, J.; Sun, A.; Zhang, E.; Ding, L.; Mukherjee, S.; Wei, X.; Chou, G.; Wang, Z.-T.; Mani, S. Protective effect of naringenin against experimental colitis via suppression of Toll-like receptor 4/NF-κB signalling. *Br. J. Nutr.* **2013**, *110*, 599–608. [CrossRef]
263. Li, H.; Zhu, F.; Chen, H.; Cheng, K.W.; Zykova, T.; Oi, N.; Lubet, R.A.; Bode, A.M.; Wang, M.; Dong, Z. 6-C-(E-phenylethenyl)-Naringenin Suppresses Colorectal Cancer Growth by Inhibiting Cyclooxygenase-16CEPN Suppresses Colon Cancer by Inhibiting COX-1. *Cancer Res.* **2014**, *74*, 243–252. [CrossRef]
264. Sequetto, P.L.; Oliveira, T.T.; Maldonado, I.R.; Augusto, L.E.F.; Mello, V.J.; Pizziolo, V.R.; Almeida, M.R.; Silva, M.E.; Novaes, R.D. Naringin accelerates the regression of pre-neoplastic lesions and the colorectal structural reorganization in a murine model of chemical carcinogenesis. *Food Chem. Toxicol.* **2014**, *64*, 200–209. [CrossRef]

265. Zhang, Y.-S.; Wang, F.; Cui, S.-X.; Qu, X.-J. Natural dietary compound naringin prevents azoxymethane/dextran sodium sulfate-induced chronic colorectal inflammation and carcinogenesis in mice. *Cancer Biol. Ther.* **2018**, *19*, 735–744. [CrossRef] [PubMed]
266. Vanamala, J.; Leonardi, T.; Patil, B.S.; Taddeo, S.S.; Murphy, M.E.; Pike, L.M.; Chapkin, R.S.; Lupton, J.R.; Turner, N.D. Suppression of colon carcinogenesis by bioactive compounds in grapefruit. *Carcinogenesis* **2006**, *27*, 1257–1265. [CrossRef] [PubMed]
267. Miyamoto, S.; Yasui, Y.; Tanaka, T.; Ohigashi, H.; Murakami, A. Suppressive effects of nobiletin on hyperleptinemia and colitis-related colon carcinogenesis in male ICR mice. *Carcinogenesis* **2008**, *29*, 1057–1063. [CrossRef] [PubMed]
268. Thangaraj, K.; Vaiyapuri, M. Orientin, a C-glycosyl dietary flavone, suppresses colonic cell proliferation and mitigates NF-κB mediated inflammatory response in 1, 2-dimethylhydrazine induced colorectal carcinogenesis. *Biomed. Pharmacother.* **2017**, *96*, 1253–1266. [CrossRef]
269. Thangaraj, K.; Natesan, K.; Palani, M.; Vaiyapuri, M. Orientin, a flavanoid, mitigates 1, 2 dimethylhydrazine-induced colorectal lesions in Wistar rats fed a high-fat diet. *Toxicol. Rep.* **2018**, *5*, 977–987. [CrossRef]
270. Yang, X.; Zhang, F.; Wang, Y.; Cai, M.; Wang, Q.; Guo, Q.; Li, Z.; Hu, R. Oroxylin A inhibits colitis-associated carcinogenesis through modulating the IL-6/STAT3 signaling pathway. *Inflamm. Bowel Dis.* **2013**, *19*, 1990–2000. [CrossRef]
271. Ni, T.; He, Z.; Dai, Y.; Yao, J.; Guo, Q.; Wei, L. Oroxylin A suppresses the development and growth of colorectal cancer through reprogram of HIF1α-modulated fatty acid metabolism. *Cell Death Dis.* **2017**, *8*, e2865. [CrossRef]
272. Gan, C.; Li, Y.; Yu, Y.; Yu, X.; Liu, H.; Zhang, Q.; Yin, W.; Yu, L.; Ye, T. Natural product pectolinarigenin exhibits potent anti-metastatic activity in colorectal carcinoma cells in vitro and in vivo. *Bioorganic Med. Chem.* **2019**, *27*, 115089. [CrossRef]
273. Lim, S.; Xu, J.; Kim, J.; Chen, T.Y.; Su, X.; Standard, J.; Carey, E.; Griffin, J.; Herndon, B.; Katz, B. Role of anthocyanin-enriched purple-fleshed sweet potato p40 in colorectal cancer prevention. *Mol. Nutr. Food Res.* **2013**, *57*, 1908–1917. [CrossRef] [PubMed]
274. Han, L.; Yan, Y.; Fan, M.; Gao, S.; Zhang, L.; Xiong, X.; Li, R.; Xiao, X.; Wang, X.; Ni, L. Pt3R5G inhibits colon cancer cell proliferation through inducing ferroptosis by down-regulating SLC7A11. *Life Sci.* **2022**, *306*, 120859. [CrossRef]
275. Lin, S.-T.; Tu, S.-H.; Yang, P.-S.; Hsu, S.-P.; Lee, W.-H.; Ho, C.-T.; Wu, C.-H.; Lai, Y.-H.; Chen, M.-Y.; Chen, L.-C. Apple polyphenol phloretin inhibits colorectal cancer cell growth via inhibition of the type 2 glucose transporter and activation of p53-mediated signaling. *J. Agric. Food Chem.* **2016**, *64*, 6826–6837. [CrossRef]
276. Hao, X.; Xiao, H.; Ju, J.; Lee, M.-J.; Lambert, J.D.; Yang, C.S. Green tea polyphenols inhibit colorectal tumorigenesis in azoxymethane-treated F344 rats. *Nutr. Cancer* **2017**, *69*, 623–631. [CrossRef] [PubMed]
277. Gossé, F.; Guyot, S.; Roussi, S.; Lobstein, A.; Fischer, B.; Seiler, N.; Raul, F. Chemopreventive properties of apple procyanidins on human colon cancer-derived metastatic SW620 cells and in a rat model of colon carcinogenesis. *Carcinogenesis* **2005**, *26*, 1291–1295. [CrossRef] [PubMed]
278. Zhu, X.; Tian, X.; Yang, M.; Yu, Y.; Zhou, Y.; Gao, Y.; Zhang, L.; Li, Z.; Xiao, Y.; Moses, R.E. Procyanidin B2 promotes intestinal injury repair and attenuates colitis-associated tumorigenesis via suppression of oxidative stress in mice. *Antioxid. Redox Signal.* **2021**, *35*, 75–92. [CrossRef]
279. Tutino, V.; De Nunzio, V.; Tafaro, A.; Bianco, G.; Gigante, I.; Scavo, M.P.; D'ALESSANDRO, R.; Refolo, M.G.; Messa, C.; Caruso, M.G. Cannabinoid receptor-1 up-regulation in azoxymethane (AOM)-treated mice after dietary treatment with quercetin. *Anticancer Res.* **2018**, *38*, 4485–4491. [CrossRef]
280. Lin, C.; Yu, Y.; Zhao, H.-g.; Yang, A.; Yan, H.; Cui, Y. Combination of quercetin with radiotherapy enhances tumor radiosensitivity in vitro and in vivo. *Radiother. Oncol.* **2012**, *104*, 395–400. [CrossRef]
281. Warren, C.A.; Paulhill, K.J.; Davidson, L.A.; Lupton, J.R.; Taddeo, S.S.; Hong, M.Y.; Carroll, R.J.; Chapkin, R.S.; Turner, N.D. Quercetin may suppress rat aberrant crypt foci formation by suppressing inflammatory mediators that influence proliferation and apoptosis. *J. Nutr.* **2009**, *139*, 101–105. [CrossRef]
282. Lin, R.; Piao, M.; Song, Y.; Liu, C. Quercetin suppresses AOM/DSS-induced colon carcinogenesis through its anti-inflammation effects in mice. *J. Immunol. Res.* **2020**, *2020*, 9242601. [CrossRef]
283. Kee, J.-Y.; Han, Y.-H.; Kim, D.-S.; Mun, J.-G.; Park, J.; Jeong, M.-Y.; Um, J.-Y.; Hong, S.-H. Inhibitory effect of quercetin on colorectal lung metastasis through inducing apoptosis, and suppression of metastatic ability. *Phytomedicine* **2016**, *23*, 1680–1690. [CrossRef] [PubMed]
284. Li, Y.; Wang, Z.; Jin, J.; Zhu, S.-X.; He, G.-Q.; Li, S.-H.; Wang, J.; Cai, Y. Quercetin pretreatment enhances the radiosensitivity of colon cancer cells by targeting Notch-1 pathway. *Biochem. Biophys. Res. Commun.* **2020**, *523*, 947–953. [CrossRef]
285. Alonso-Castro, A.J.; Domínguez, F.; García-Carrancá, A. Rutin exerts antitumor effects on nude mice bearing SW480 tumor. *Arch. Med. Res.* **2013**, *44*, 346–351. [CrossRef] [PubMed]
286. Zeng, S.; Chen, L.; Sun, Q.; Zhao, H.; Yang, H.; Ren, S.; Liu, M.; Meng, X.; Xu, H. Scutellarin ameliorates colitis-associated colorectal cancer by suppressing Wnt/β-catenin signaling cascade. *Eur. J. Pharmacol.* **2021**, *906*, 174253. [CrossRef]
287. Xiong, L.-L.; Du, R.-L.; Xue, L.-L.; Jiang, Y.; Huang, J.; Chen, L.; Liu, J.; Wang, T.-H. Anti-colorectal cancer effects of scutellarin revealed by genomic and proteomic analysis. *Chin. Med.* **2020**, *15*, 1–5. [CrossRef] [PubMed]
288. Zeng, S.; Tan, L.; Sun, Q.; Chen, L.; Zhao, H.; Liu, M.; Yang, H.; Ren, S.; Ming, T.; Tang, S. Suppression of colitis-associated colorectal cancer by scutellarin through inhibiting Hedgehog signaling pathway activity. *Phytomedicine* **2022**, *98*, 153972. [CrossRef]
289. Yang, S.-H.; Lin, J.-K.; Huang, C.-J.; Chen, W.-S.; Li, S.-Y.; Chiu, J.-H. Silibinin inhibits angiogenesis via Flt-1, but not KDR, receptor up-regulation1. *J. Surg. Res.* **2005**, *128*, 140–146. [CrossRef]

290. Kauntz, H.; Bousserouel, S.; Gosse, F.; Marescaux, J.; Raul, F. Silibinin, a natural flavonoid, modulates the early expression of chemoprevention biomarkers in a preclinical model of colon carcinogenesis. *Int. J. Oncol.* **2012**, *41*, 849–854. [CrossRef]
291. Bao, H.; Zheng, N.; Li, Z.; Zhi, Y. Synergistic effect of tangeretin and atorvastatin for colon cancer combination therapy: Targeted delivery of these dual drugs using RGD Peptide decorated nanocarriers. *Drug Des. Dev. Ther.* **2020**, *14*, 3057. [CrossRef]
292. Razak, S.; Afsar, T.; Ullah, A.; Almajwal, A.; Alkholief, M.; Alshamsan, A.; Jahan, S. Taxifolin, a natural flavonoid interacts with cell cycle regulators causes cell cycle arrest and causes tumor regression by activating Wnt/β-catenin signaling pathway. *BMC Cancer* **2018**, *18*, 1–18. [CrossRef]
293. Yue, G.G.-L.; Gao, S.; Lee, J.K.-M.; Chan, Y.-Y.; Wong, E.C.-W.; Zheng, T.; Li, X.-X.; Shaw, P.-C.; Simmonds, M.S.; Lau, C.B.-S. A natural flavone tricin from grains can alleviate tumor growth and lung metastasis in colorectal tumor mice. *Molecules* **2020**, *25*, 3730. [CrossRef]
294. Oyama, T.; Yasui, Y.; Sugie, S.; Koketsu, M.; Watanabe, K.; Tanaka, T. Dietary tricin suppresses inflammation-related colon carcinogenesis in male Crj: CD-1 mice. *Cancer Prev. Res.* **2009**, *2*, 1031–1038. [CrossRef]
295. Vinothkumar, R.; Kumar, R.V.; Sudha, M.; Viswanathan, P.; Balasubramanian, T.; Nalini, N. Modulatory effect of troxerutin on biotransforming enzymes and preneoplasic lesions induced by 1, 2-dimethylhydrazine in rat colon carcinogenesis. *Exp. Mol. Pathol.* **2014**, *96*, 15–26. [CrossRef]
296. Bhardwaj, M.; Paul, S.; Jakhar, R.; Khan, I.; Kang, J.I.; Kim, H.M.; Yun, J.W.; Lee, S.-J.; Cho, H.J.; Lee, H.G. Vitexin confers HSF-1 mediated autophagic cell death by activating JNK and ApoL1 in colorectal carcinoma cells. *Oncotarget* **2017**, *8*, 112426. [CrossRef]
297. Bhardwaj, M.; Cho, H.J.; Paul, S.; Jakhar, R.; Khan, I.; Lee, S.-J.; Kim, B.-Y.; Krishnan, M.; Khaket, T.P.; Lee, H.G. Vitexin induces apoptosis by suppressing autophagy in multi-drug resistant colorectal cancer cells. *Oncotarget* **2018**, *9*, 3278. [CrossRef]
298. Yao, J.; Zhao, L.; Zhao, Q.; Zhao, Y.; Sun, Y.; Zhang, Y.; Miao, H.; You, Q.; Hu, R.; Guo, Q. NF-κB and Nrf2 signaling pathways contribute to wogonin-mediated inhibition of inflammation-associated colorectal carcinogenesis. *Cell Death Dis.* **2014**, *5*, e1283. [CrossRef]
299. Feng, Q.; Wang, H.; Pang, J.; Ji, L.; Han, J.; Wang, Y.; Qi, X.; Liu, Z.; Lu, L. Prevention of wogonin on colorectal cancer tumorigenesis by regulating p53 nuclear translocation. *Front. Pharmacol.* **2018**, *9*, 1356. [CrossRef]
300. You, W.; Di, A.; Zhang, L.; Zhao, G. Effects of wogonin on the growth and metastasis of colon cancer through the Hippo signaling pathway. *Bioengineered* **2022**, *13*, 2586–2597. [CrossRef]
301. Liu, H.; Zhang, L.; Li, G.; Gao, Z. Xanthohumol protects against Azoxymethane-induced colorectal cancer in Sprague-Dawley rats. *Environ. Toxicol.* **2020**, *35*, 136–144. [CrossRef]
302. Murillo, G.; Hirschelman, W.H.; Ito, A.; Moriarty, R.M.; Kinghorn, A.D.; Pezzuto, J.M.; Mehta, R.G. Zapotin, a phytochemical present in a Mexican fruit, prevents colon carcinogenesis. *Nutr. Cancer* **2007**, *57*, 28–37. [CrossRef]
303. Kang, N.J.; Lee, K.W.; Kim, B.H.; Bode, A.M.; Lee, H.-J.; Heo, Y.-S.; Boardman, L.; Limburg, P.; Lee, H.J.; Dong, Z. Coffee phenolic phytochemicals suppress colon cancer metastasis by targeting MEK and TOPK. *Carcinogenesis* **2011**, *32*, 921–928. [CrossRef]
304. Park, S.-R.; Kim, S.-R.; Hong, I.-S.; Lee, H.-Y. A novel therapeutic approach for colorectal cancer stem cells: Blocking the PI3K/Akt signaling axis with caffeic acid. *Front. Cell Dev. Biol.* **2020**, *8*, 585987. [CrossRef]
305. Chiang, E.-P.I.; Tsai, S.-Y.; Kuo, Y.-H.; Pai, M.-H.; Chiu, H.-L.; Rodriguez, R.L.; Tang, F.-Y. Caffeic acid derivatives inhibit the growth of colon cancer: Involvement of the PI3-K/Akt and AMPK signaling pathways. *PLoS ONE* **2014**, *9*, e99631. [CrossRef]
306. Tang, H.; Yao, X.; Yao, C.; Zhao, X.; Zuo, H.; Li, Z. Anti-colon cancer effect of caffeic acid p-nitro-phenethyl ester in vitro and in vivo and detection of its metabolites. *Sci. Rep.* **2017**, *7*, 1–11. [CrossRef]
307. Chen, C.; Kuo, Y.-H.; Lin, C.-C.; Chao, C.-Y.; Pai, M.-H.; Chiang, E.-P.I.; Tang, F.-Y. Decyl caffeic acid inhibits the proliferation of colorectal cancer cells in an autophagy-dependent manner in vitro and in vivo. *PLoS ONE* **2020**, *15*, e0232832. [CrossRef]
308. Tanaka, T.; Nishikawa, A.; Shima, H.; Sugie, S.; Shinoda, T.; Yoshimi, N.; Iwata, H.; Mori, H. Inhibitory effects of chlorogenic acid, reserpine, polyprenoic acid (E-5166), or coffee on hepatocarcinogenesis in rats and hamsters. *Basic Life Sci.* **1990**, *52*, 429–440.
309. Morishita, Y.; Yoshimi, N.; Kawabata, K.; Matsunaga, K.; Sugie, S.; Tanaka, T.; Mori, H. Regressive effects of various chemopreventive agents on azoxymethane-induced aberrant crypt foci in the rat colon. *Jpn. J. Cancer Res.* **1997**, *88*, 815–820. [CrossRef]
310. Rao, C.V.; Tokumo, K.; Rigotty, J.; Zang, E.; Kelloff, G.; Reddy, B.S. Chemoprevention of colon carcinogenesis by dietary administration of piroxicam, α-difluoromethylornithine, 16α-fluoro-5-androsten-17-one, and ellagic acid individually and in combination. *Cancer Res.* **1991**, *51*, 4528–4534.
311. Umesalma, S.; Sudhandiran, G. Chemomodulation of the antioxidative enzymes and peroxidative damage in the colon of 1, 2-dimethyl hydrazine-induced rats by ellagicacid. *Phytother. Res.* **2010**, *24*, S114–S119. [CrossRef]
312. Umesalma, S.; Sudhandiran, G. Differential inhibitory effects of the polyphenol ellagic acid on inflammatory mediators NF-κB, iNOS, COX-2, TNF-α, and IL-6 in 1, 2-dimethylhydrazine-induced rat colon carcinogenesis. *Basic Clin. Pharmacol. Toxicol.* **2010**, *107*, 650–655. [CrossRef]
313. Umesalma, S.; Sudhandiran, G. Ellagic acid prevents rat colon carcinogenesis induced by 1, 2 dimethyl hydrazine through inhibition of AKT-phosphoinositide-3 kinase pathway. *Eur. J. Pharmacol.* **2011**, *660*, 249–258. [CrossRef]
314. Kumar, K.N.; Raja, S.B.; Vidhya, N.; Devaraj, S.N. Ellagic acid modulates antioxidant status, ornithine decarboxylase expression, and aberrant crypt foci progression in 1, 2-dimethylhydrazine-instigated colon preneoplastic lesions in rats. *J. Agric. Food Chem.* **2012**, *60*, 3665–3672. [CrossRef]
315. Goyal, Y.; Koul, A.; Ranawat, P. Ellagic acid modulates cisplatin toxicity in DMH induced colorectal cancer: Studies on membrane alterations. *Biochem. Biophys. Rep.* **2022**, *31*, 101319. [CrossRef]

316. Kawabata, K.; Yamamoto, T.; Hara, A.; Shimizu, M.; Yamada, Y.; Matsunaga, K.; Tanaka, T.; Mori, H. Modifying effects of ferulic acid on azoxymethane-induced colon carcinogenesis in F344 rats. *Cancer Lett.* **2000**, *157*, 15–21. [CrossRef]
317. Han, B.S.; Park, C.B.; Takasuka, N.; Naito, A.; Sekine, K.; Nomura, E.; Taniguchi, H.; Tsuno, T.; Tsuda, H. A Ferulic Acid Derivative, Ethyl 3-(4′-Geranyloxy-3-methoxyphenyl)-2-propenoate, as a New Candidate Chemopreventive Agent for Colon Carcinogenesis in the Rat. *Jpn. J. Cancer Res.* **2001**, *92*, 404–409. [CrossRef]
318. Giftson, J.S.; Jayanthi, S.; Nalini, N. Chemopreventive efficacy of gallic acid, an antioxidant and anticarcinogenic polyphenol, against 1, 2-dimethyl hydrazine induced rat colon carcinogenesis. *Investig. New Drugs* **2010**, *28*, 251–259. [CrossRef]
319. Sanchez-Martin, V.; Plaza-Calonge, M.d.C.; Soriano-Lerma, A.; Ortiz-Gonzalez, M.; Linde-Rodriguez, A.; Perez-Carrasco, V.; Ramirez-Macias, I.; Cuadros, M.; Gutierrez-Fernandez, J.; Murciano-Calles, J. Gallic Acid: A Natural Phenolic Compound Exerting Antitumoral Activities in Colorectal Cancer via Interaction with G-Quadruplexes. *Cancers* **2022**, *14*, 2648. [CrossRef]
320. Jeong, J.H.; Kim, E.Y.; Choi, H.J.; Chung, T.W.; Kim, K.J.; Kim, S.Y.; Ha, K.T. Gallic acid inhibits STAT3 phosphorylation and alleviates DDS-induced colitis via regulating cytokine production. *J. Physiol. Pathol. Korean Med.* **2016**, *30*, 338–346. [CrossRef]
321. Lin, X.; Wang, G.; Liu, P.; Han, L.; Wang, T.; Chen, K.; Gao, Y. Gallic acid suppresses colon cancer proliferation by inhibiting SRC and EGFR phosphorylation. *Exp. Ther. Med.* **2021**, *21*, 1–11. [CrossRef]
322. Hong, Z.; Tang, P.; Liu, B.; Ran, C.; Yuan, C.; Zhang, Y.; Lu, Y.; Duan, X.; Yang, Y.; Wu, H. Ferroptosis-related genes for overall survival prediction in patients with colorectal cancer can be inhibited by gallic acid. *Int. J. Biol. Sci.* **2021**, *17*, 942. [CrossRef]
323. Senapathy, J.G.; Jayanthi, S.; Viswanathan, P.; Umadevi, P.; Nalini, N. Effect of gallic acid on xenobiotic metabolizing enzymes in 1, 2-dimethyl hydrazine induced colon carcinogenesis in Wistar rats–a chemopreventive approach. *Food Chem. Toxicol.* **2011**, *49*, 887–892. [CrossRef] [PubMed]
324. Zhou, L.-A.; Liu, T.-B.; Lü, H.-N. Geraniin inhibits proliferation and induces apoptosis through inhibition of phosphatidylinositol 3-kinase/Akt pathway in human colorectal cancer in vitro and in vivo. *Anti-Cancer Drugs* **2020**, *31*, 575–582. [CrossRef] [PubMed]
325. Sharma, S.H.; Chellappan, D.R.; Chinnaswamy, P.; Nagarajan, S. Protective effect of p-coumaric acid against 1, 2 dimethylhydrazine induced colonic preneoplastic lesions in experimental rats. *Biomed. Pharmacother.* **2017**, *94*, 577–588. [CrossRef] [PubMed]
326. Fang, W.; Zhu, S.; Niu, Z.; Yin, Y. The protective effect of syringic acid on dextran sulfate sodium-induced experimental colitis in BALB/c mice. *Drug Dev. Res.* **2019**, *80*, 731–740. [CrossRef]
327. Mihanfar, A.; Darband, S.G.; Sadighparvar, S.; Kaviani, M.; Mirza-Aghazadeh-Attari, M.; Yousefi, B.; Majidinia, M. In vitro and in vivo anticancer effects of syringic acid on colorectal cancer: Possible mechanistic view. *Chem.-Biol. Interact.* **2021**, *337*, 109337. [CrossRef]
328. Han, Y.-H.; Kee, J.-Y.; Kim, D.-S.; Mun, J.-g.; Jeong, M.-Y.; Park, S.-H.; Choi, B.-M.; Park, S.-J.; Kim, H.-J.; Um, J.-Y. Arctigenin inhibits lung metastasis of colorectal cancer by regulating cell viability and metastatic phenotypes. *Molecules* **2016**, *21*, 1135. [CrossRef]
329. Kang, K.; Oh, S.H.; Yun, J.H.; Jho, E.H.; Kang, J.-H.; Batsuren, D.; Tunsag, J.; Park, K.H.; Kim, M.; Nho, C.W. A novel topoisomerase inhibitor, daurinol, suppresses growth of HCT116 cells with low hematological toxicity compared to etoposide. *Neoplasia* **2011**, *13*, 1043–1057. [CrossRef]
330. Li, C.; Zhang, K.; Pan, G.; Ji, H.; Li, C.; Wang, X.; Hu, X.; Liu, R.; Deng, L.; Wang, Y. Dehydrodiisoeugenol inhibits colorectal cancer growth by endoplasmic reticulum stress-induced autophagic pathways. *J. Exp. Clin. Cancer Res.* **2021**, *40*, 1–15. [CrossRef]
331. Kee, J.-Y.; Han, Y.-H.; Mun, J.-G.; Park, S.-H.; Jeon, H.D.; Hong, S.-H. Gomisin a suppresses colorectal lung metastasis by inducing AMPK/P38-mediated apoptosis and decreasing metastatic abilities of colorectal cancer cells. *Front. Pharmacol.* **2018**, *9*, 986. [CrossRef]
332. Li, Q.; Ma, Y.; Liu, X.L.; Mu, L.; He, B.C.; Wu, K.; Sun, W.J. Anti-proliferative effect of honokiol on SW620 cells through upregulating BMP7 expression via the TGF-β1/p53 signaling pathway. *Oncol. Rep.* **2020**, *44*, 2093–2107. [CrossRef]
333. Won, S.J.; Yen, C.H.; Liu, H.S.; Wu, S.Y.; Lan, S.H.; Jiang-Shieh, Y.F.; Lin, C.N.; Su, C.L. Justicidin A-induced autophagy flux enhances apoptosis of human colorectal cancer cells via class III PI3K and Atg5 pathway. *J. Cell. Physiol.* **2015**, *230*, 930–946. [CrossRef] [PubMed]
334. Su, C.-M.; Weng, Y.-S.; Kuan, L.-Y.; Chen, J.-H.; Hsu, F.-T. Suppression of PKCδ/NF-κB Signaling and Apoptosis Induction through Extrinsic/Intrinsic Pathways Are Associated with Magnolol-Inhibited Tumor Progression in Colorectal Cancer In Vitro and In Vivo. *Int. J. Mol. Sci.* **2020**, *21*, 3527. [CrossRef] [PubMed]
335. Kang, Y.-J.; Park, H.J.; Chung, H.-J.; Min, H.-Y.; Park, E.J.; Lee, M.A.; Shin, Y.; Lee, S.K. Wnt/β-catenin signaling mediates the antitumor activity of magnolol in colorectal cancer cells. *Mol. Pharmacol.* **2012**, *82*, 168–177. [CrossRef]
336. Pu, Z.; Zhang, W.; Wang, M.; Xu, M.; Xie, H.; Zhao, J. Schisandrin B Attenuates colitis-associated colorectal cancer through SIRT1 linked SMURF2 signaling. *Am. J. Chin. Med.* **2021**, *49*, 1773–1789. [CrossRef] [PubMed]
337. Chen, T.; Wang, Z.; Zhong, J.; Zhang, L.; Zhang, H.; Zhang, D.; Xu, X.; Zhong, X.; Wang, J.; Li, H. Secoisolariciresinol diglucoside induces pyroptosis by activating caspase-1 to cleave GSDMD in colorectal cancer cells. *Drug Dev. Res.* **2022**, *83*, 1152–1166. [CrossRef]
338. Wang, Z.; Chen, T.; Yang, C.; Bao, T.; Yang, X.; He, F.; Zhang, Y.; Zhu, L.; Chen, H.; Rong, S. Secoisolariciresinol diglucoside suppresses Dextran sulfate sodium salt-induced colitis through inhibiting NLRP1 inflammasome. *Int. Immunopharmacol.* **2020**, *78*, 105931. [CrossRef]

339. Ohira, H.; Oikawa, D.; Kurokawa, Y.; Aoki, Y.; Omura, A.; Kiyomoto, K.; Nakagawa, W.; Mamoto, R.; Fujioka, Y.; Nakayama, T. Suppression of colonic oxidative stress caused by chronic ethanol administration and attenuation of ethanol-induced colitis and gut leakiness by oral administration of sesaminol in mice. *Food Funct.* **2022**, *13*, 9285–9298. [CrossRef]
340. Shin, M.-K.; Jeon, Y.-D.; Hong, S.-H.; Kang, S.-H.; Kee, J.-Y.; Jin, J.-S. In vivo and In vitro effects of Tracheloside on colorectal cancer cell proliferation and metastasis. *Antioxidants* **2021**, *10*, 513. [CrossRef] [PubMed]
341. Chen, J.; Zhong, J.; Liu, Y.; Huang, Y.; Luo, F.; Zhou, Y.; Pan, X.; Cao, S.; Zhang, L.; Zhang, Y. Purified vitexin compound 1, a new neolignan isolated compound, promotes PUMA-dependent apoptosis in colorectal cancer. *Cancer Med.* **2018**, *7*, 6158–6169. [CrossRef]
342. Kimura, Y. Long-term oral administration of piceatannol (3, 5, 3′, 4′-tetrahydroxystilbene) attenuates colon tumor growth induced by azoxymethane plus dextran sulfate sodium in C57BL/6J mice. *Nutr. Cancer* **2022**, *74*, 2184–2195. [CrossRef]
343. Jin, Y.; Zhan, X.; Zhang, B.; Chen, Y.; Liu, C.; Yu, L. Polydatin exerts an antitumor effect through regulating the miR-382/PD-L1 axis in colorectal cancer. *Cancer Biother. Radiopharm.* **2020**, *35*, 83–91. [CrossRef] [PubMed]
344. Chiou, Y.-S.; Tsai, M.-L.; Wang, Y.-J.; Cheng, A.-C.; Lai, W.-M.; Badmaev, V.; Ho, C.-T.; Pan, M.-H. Pterostilbene inhibits colorectal aberrant crypt foci (ACF) and colon carcinogenesis via suppression of multiple signal transduction pathways in azoxymethane-treated mice. *J. Agric. Food Chem.* **2010**, *58*, 8833–8841. [CrossRef]
345. Paul, S.; DeCastro, A.J.; Lee, H.J.; Smolarek, A.K.; So, J.Y.; Simi, B.; Wang, C.X.; Zhou, R.; Rimando, A.M.; Suh, N. Dietary intake of pterostilbene, a constituent of blueberries, inhibits the β-catenin/p65 downstream signaling pathway and colon carcinogenesis in rats. *Carcinogenesis* **2010**, *31*, 1272–1278. [CrossRef] [PubMed]
346. Chiou, Y.-S.; Tsai, M.-L.; Nagabhushanam, K.; Wang, Y.-J.; Wu, C.-H.; Ho, C.-T.; Pan, M.-H. Pterostilbene is more potent than resveratrol in preventing azoxymethane (AOM)-induced colon tumorigenesis via activation of the NF-E2-related factor 2 (Nrf2)-mediated antioxidant signaling pathway. *J. Agric. Food Chem.* **2011**, *59*, 2725–2733. [CrossRef] [PubMed]
347. Zhang, Y.; Li, Y.; Sun, C.; Chen, X.; Han, L.; Wang, T.; Liu, J.; Chen, X.; Zhao, D. Effect of pterostilbene, a natural derivative of resveratrol, in the treatment of colorectal cancer through Top1/Tdp1-mediated DNA repair pathway. *Cancers* **2021**, *13*, 4002. [CrossRef]
348. Suh, N.; Paul, S.; Hao, X.; Simi, B.; Xiao, H.; Rimando, A.M.; Reddy, B.S. Pterostilbene, an active constituent of blueberries, suppresses aberrant crypt foci formation in the azoxymethane-induced colon carcinogenesis model in rats. *Clin. Cancer Res.* **2007**, *13*, 350–355. [CrossRef]
349. Ji, Q.; Liu, X.; Han, Z.; Zhou, L.; Sui, H.; Yan, L.; Jiang, H.; Ren, J.; Cai, J.; Li, Q. Resveratrol suppresses epithelial-to-mesenchymal transition in colorectal cancer through TGF-β1/Smads signaling pathway mediated Snail/E-cadherin expression. *BMC Cancer* **2015**, *15*, 1–12. [CrossRef]
350. Saud, S.M.; Li, W.; Morris, N.L.; Matter, M.S.; Colburn, N.H.; Kim, Y.S.; Young, M.R. Resveratrol prevents tumorigenesis in mouse model of Kras activated sporadic colorectal cancer by suppressing oncogenic Kras expression. *Carcinogenesis* **2014**, *35*, 2778–2786. [CrossRef]
351. Alfaras, I.; Juan, M.E.; Planas, J.M. trans-Resveratrol reduces precancerous colonic lesions in dimethylhydrazine-treated rats. *J. Agric. Food Chem.* **2010**, *58*, 8104–8110. [CrossRef]
352. Majumdar, A.P.; Banerjee, S.; Nautiyal, J.; Patel, B.B.; Patel, V.; Du, J.; Yu, Y.; Elliott, A.A.; Levi, E.; Sarkar, F.H. Curcumin synergizes with resveratrol to inhibit colon cancer. *Nutr. Cancer* **2009**, *61*, 544–553. [CrossRef]
353. Sudha, T.; El-Far, A.H.; Mousa, D.S.; Mousa, S.A. Resveratrol and its nanoformulation attenuate growth and the angiogenesis of xenograft and orthotopic colon cancer models. *Molecules* **2020**, *25*, 1412. [CrossRef] [PubMed]
354. Hu, W.-H.; Chan, G.K.-L.; Duan, R.; Wang, H.-Y.; Kong, X.-P.; Dong, T.T.-X.; Tsim, K.W.-K. Synergy of ginkgetin and resveratrol in suppressing VEGF-induced angiogenesis: A therapy in treating colorectal cancer. *Cancers* **2019**, *11*, 1828. [CrossRef] [PubMed]
355. Sepporta, M.V.; Fuccelli, R.; Rosignoli, P.; Ricci, G.; Servili, M.; Fabiani, R. Oleuropein prevents Azoxymethane-induced Colon crypt dysplasia and leukocytes DNA damage in a/J mice. *J. Med. Food* **2016**, *19*, 983–989. [CrossRef] [PubMed]
356. Zeng, Q.; Che, Y.; Zhang, Y.; Chen, M.; Guo, Q.; Zhang, W. Thymol Isolated from Thymus vulgaris L. inhibits colorectal cancer cell growth and metastasis by suppressing the Wnt/β-catenin pathway. *Drug Des. Dev. Ther.* **2020**, *14*, 2535. [CrossRef] [PubMed]
357. Zhou, L.; Feng, Y.; Jin, Y.; Liu, X.; Sui, H.; Chai, N.; Chen, X.; Liu, N.; Ji, Q.; Wang, Y. Verbascoside promotes apoptosis by regulating HIPK2–p53 signaling in human colorectal cancer. *BMC Cancer* **2014**, *14*, 1–11. [CrossRef] [PubMed]
358. Singh, S.; Meena, A.; Luqman, S. Baicalin mediated regulation of key signaling pathways in cancer. *Pharmacol. Res.* **2021**, *164*, 105387. [CrossRef]
359. Patel, V.B.; Misra, S.; Patel, B.B.; Majumdar, A.P. Colorectal cancer: Chemopreventive role of curcumin and resveratrol. *Nutr. Cancer* **2010**, *62*, 958–967. [CrossRef]
360. Prasad, S.; Aggarwal, B.B. Turmeric, the golden spice. In *Herbal Medicine: Biomolecular and Clinical Aspects*, 2nd ed.; CRC Press/Taylor & Francis: Boca Raton, FL, USA, 2011; pp. 263–288.
361. Wang, Y.; Bu, C.; Wu, K.; Wang, R.; Wang, J. Curcumin protects the pancreas from acute pancreatitis via the mitogen-activated protein kinase signaling pathway. *Mol. Med. Rep.* **2019**, *20*, 3027–3034. [CrossRef]
362. Mishra, S.; Palanivelu, K. Thread Rating. *Ann. Indian Acad. Neurol.* **2008**, *11*, 13–19. [CrossRef]
363. Zorena, K.; Jachimowicz-Duda, O.; Ślęzak, D.; Robakowska, M.; Mrugacz, M. Adipokines and obesity. Potential link to metabolic disorders and chronic complications. *Int. J. Mol. Sci.* **2020**, *21*, 3570. [CrossRef]

364. Achari, A.E.; Jain, S.K. Adiponectin, a therapeutic target for obesity, diabetes, and endothelial dysfunction. *Int. J. Mol. Sci.* **2017**, *18*, 1321. [CrossRef] [PubMed]
365. Weidinger, C.; Ziegler, J.F.; Letizia, M.; Schmidt, F.; Siegmund, B. Adipokines and their role in intestinal inflammation. *Front. Immunol.* **2018**, *9*, 1974. [CrossRef] [PubMed]
366. Kelesidis, T.; Kelesidis, I.; Chou, S.; Mantzoros, C.S. Narrative review: The role of leptin in human physiology: Emerging clinical applications. *Ann. Intern. Med.* **2010**, *152*, 93–100. [CrossRef] [PubMed]
367. Iikuni, N.; Kwan Lam, Q.L.; Lu, L.; Matarese, G.; Cava, A.L. Leptin and inflammation. *Curr. Immunol. Rev.* **2008**, *4*, 70–79. [CrossRef] [PubMed]
368. Aggarwal, V.; Tuli, H.S.; Tania, M.; Srivastava, S.; Ritzer, E.E.; Pandey, A.; Aggarwal, D.; Barwal, T.S.; Jain, A.; Kaur, G. Molecular mechanisms of action of epigallocatechin gallate in cancer: Recent trends and advancement. *Semin. Cancer Biol.* **2022**, *80*, 256–275. [CrossRef]
369. Musial, C.; Kuban-Jankowska, A.; Gorska-Ponikowska, M. Beneficial properties of green tea catechins. *Int. J. Mol. Sci.* **2020**, *21*, 1744. [CrossRef]
370. Kim, J.S.; Kim, J.-M.; Jeong-Ja, O.; Jeon, B.S. Inhibition of inducible nitric oxide synthase expression and cell death by (−)-epigallocatechin-3-gallate, a green tea catechin, in the 1-methyl-4-phenyl-1, 2, 3, 6-tetrahydropyridine mouse model of Parkinson's disease. *J. Clin. Neurosci.* **2010**, *17*, 1165–1168. [CrossRef]
371. Kim, M.; Murakami, A.; Miyamoto, S.; Tanaka, T.; Ohigashi, H. The modifying effects of green tea polyphenols on acute colitis and inflammation-associated colon carcinogenesis in male ICR mice. *Biofactors* **2010**, *36*, 43–51. [CrossRef]
372. De Oliveira, G.A.; Cheng, R.Y.; Ridnour, L.A.; Basudhar, D.; Somasundaram, V.; McVicar, D.W.; Monteiro, H.P.; Wink, D.A. Inducible nitric oxide synthase in the carcinogenesis of gastrointestinal cancers. *Antioxid. Redox Signal.* **2017**, *26*, 1059–1077. [CrossRef]
373. Cianchi, F.; Cortesini, C.; Fantappiè, O.; Messerini, L.; Schiavone, N.; Vannacci, A.; Nistri, S.; Sardi, I.; Baroni, G.; Marzocca, C. Inducible nitric oxide synthase expression in human colorectal cancer: Correlation with tumor angiogenesis. *Am. J. Pathol.* **2003**, *162*, 793–801. [CrossRef]
374. Mandal, P. Molecular signature of nitric oxide on major cancer hallmarks of colorectal carcinoma. *Inflammopharmacology* **2018**, *26*, 331–336. [CrossRef] [PubMed]
375. Sheng, J.; Sun, H.; Yu, F.-B.; Li, B.; Zhang, Y.; Zhu, Y.-T. The role of cyclooxygenase-2 in colorectal cancer. *Int. J. Med. Sci.* **2020**, *17*, 1095. [CrossRef] [PubMed]
376. Greenhough, A.; Smartt, H.J.; Moore, A.E.; Roberts, H.R.; Williams, A.C.; Paraskeva, C.; Kaidi, A. The COX-2/PGE 2 pathway: Key roles in the hallmarks of cancer and adaptation to the tumour microenvironment. *Carcinogenesis* **2009**, *30*, 377–386. [CrossRef]
377. Tuli, H.S.; Tuorkey, M.J.; Thakral, F.; Sak, K.; Kumar, M.; Sharma, A.K.; Sharma, U.; Jain, A.; Aggarwal, V.; Bishayee, A. Molecular mechanisms of action of genistein in cancer: Recent advances. *Front. Pharmacol.* **2019**, *10*, 1336. [CrossRef] [PubMed]
378. Chen, X.; Gu, J.; Wu, Y.; Liang, P.; Shen, M.; Xi, J.; Qin, J. Clinical characteristics of colorectal cancer patients and anti-neoplasm activity of genistein. *Biomed. Pharmacother.* **2020**, *124*, 109835. [CrossRef]
379. Pintova, S.; Dharmupari, S.; Moshier, E.; Zubizarreta, N.; Ang, C.; Holcombe, R.F. Genistein combined with FOLFOX or FOLFOX–Bevacizumab for the treatment of metastatic colorectal cancer: Phase I/II pilot study. *Cancer Chemother. Pharmacol.* **2019**, *84*, 591–598. [CrossRef] [PubMed]
380. Felice, M.R.; Maugeri, A.; De Sarro, G.; Navarra, M.; Barreca, D. Molecular Pathways Involved in the Anti-Cancer Activity of Flavonols: A Focus on Myricetin and Kaempferol. *Int. J. Mol. Sci.* **2022**, *23*, 4411. [CrossRef]
381. Lin, Y.; Shi, R.; Wang, X.; Shen, H.-M. Luteolin, a flavonoid with potential for cancer prevention and therapy. *Curr. Cancer Drug Targets* **2008**, *8*, 634–646. [CrossRef]
382. Ganai, S.A.; Sheikh, F.A.; Baba, Z.A.; Mir, M.A.; Mantoo, M.A.; Yatoo, M.A. Anticancer activity of the plant flavonoid luteolin against preclinical models of various cancers and insights on different signalling mechanisms modulated. *Phytother. Res.* **2021**, *35*, 3509–3532. [CrossRef]
383. Xiao, Y.; Yang, H.; Lu, J.; Li, D.; Xu, C.; Risch, H.A. Serum gamma-glutamyltransferase and the overall survival of metastatic pancreatic cancer. *BMC Cancer* **2019**, *19*, 1–7. [CrossRef]
384. Ribatti, D.; Crivellato, E. Mast cells, angiogenesis, and tumour growth. *Biochim. Biophys. Acta BBA Mol. Basis Dis.* **2012**, *1822*, 2–8. [CrossRef] [PubMed]
385. Wang, Y.-X.; Chen, Y.-R.; Liu, S.-S.; Ye, Y.-P.; Jiao, H.-L.; Wang, S.-Y.; Xiao, Z.-Y.; Wei, W.-T.; Qiu, J.-F.; Liang, L. MiR-384 inhibits human colorectal cancer metastasis by targeting KRAS and CDC42. *Oncotarget* **2016**, *7*, 84826. [CrossRef] [PubMed]
386. Kong, Y.; Bai, P.-S.; Nan, K.-J.; Sun, H.; Chen, N.-Z.; Qi, X.-G. Pleiotrophin is a potential colorectal cancer prognostic factor that promotes VEGF expression and induces angiogenesis in colorectal cancer. *Int. J. Color. Dis.* **2012**, *27*, 287–298. [CrossRef]
387. Zhu, M.-L.; Zhang, P.-M.; Jiang, M.; Yu, S.-W.; Wang, L. Myricetin induces apoptosis and autophagy by inhibiting PI3K/Akt/mTOR signalling in human colon cancer cells. *BMC Complement. Med. Ther.* **2020**, *20*, 1–9. [CrossRef]
388. Rauf, A.; Shariati, M.A.; Imran, M.; Bashir, K.; Khan, S.A.; Mitra, S.; Emran, T.B.; Badalova, K.; Uddin, M.; Mubarak, M.S. Comprehensive review on naringenin and naringin polyphenols as a potent anticancer agent. *Environ. Sci. Pollut. Res.* **2022**, *29*, 31025–31041. [CrossRef] [PubMed]
389. Ghanbari-Movahed, M.; Jackson, G.; Farzaei, M.H.; Bishayee, A. A Systematic Review of the Preventive and Therapeutic Effects of Naringin against Human Malignancies. *Front. Pharmacol.* **2021**, *12*, 250. [CrossRef] [PubMed]

390. Gao, R.; Wang, L.; Yang, Y.; Ni, J.; Zhao, L.; Dong, S.; Guo, M. Simultaneous determination of oleanolic acid, ursolic acid, quercetin and apigenin in Swertia mussotii Franch by capillary zone electrophoresis with running buffer modifier. *Biomed. Chromatogr.* **2015**, *29*, 402–409. [CrossRef] [PubMed]
391. Khan, F.; Niaz, K.; Maqbool, F.; Ismail Hassan, F.; Abdollahi, M.; Nagulapalli Venkata, K.C.; Nabavi, S.M.; Bishayee, A. Molecular targets underlying the anticancer effects of quercetin: An update. *Nutrients* **2016**, *8*, 529. [CrossRef]
392. Terzić, J.; Grivennikov, S.; Karin, E.; Karin, M. Inflammation and colon cancer. *Gastroenterology* **2010**, *138*, 2101–2114.e2105. [CrossRef]
393. Long, A.G.; Lundsmith, E.T.; Hamilton, K.E. Inflammation and colorectal cancer. *Curr. Color. Cancer Rep.* **2017**, *13*, 341–351. [CrossRef]
394. Nouri, Z.; Fakhri, S.; Nouri, K.; Wallace, C.E.; Farzaei, M.H.; Bishayee, A. Targeting multiple signaling pathways in cancer: The rutin therapeutic approach. *Cancers* **2020**, *12*, 2276. [CrossRef] [PubMed]
395. Chua, L.S. A review on plant-based rutin extraction methods and its pharmacological activities. *J. Ethnopharmacol.* **2013**, *150*, 805–817. [CrossRef] [PubMed]
396. Negahdari, R.; Bohlouli, S.; Sharifi, S.; Maleki Dizaj, S.; Rahbar Saadat, Y.; Khezri, K.; Jafari, S.; Ahmadian, E.; Gorbani Jahandizi, N.; Raeesi, S. Therapeutic benefits of rutin and its nanoformulations. *Phytother. Res.* **2021**, *35*, 1719–1738. [CrossRef]
397. Pan, M.-H.; Chen, W.-J.; Lin-Shiau, S.-Y.; Ho, C.-T.; Lin, J.-K. Tangeretin induces cell-cycle G1 arrest through inhibiting cyclin-dependent kinases 2 and 4 activities as well as elevating Cdk inhibitors p21 and p27 in human colorectal carcinoma cells. *Carcinogenesis* **2002**, *23*, 1677–1684. [CrossRef]
398. He, L.; Lu, N.; Dai, Q.; Zhao, Y.; Zhao, L.; Wang, H.; Li, Z.; You, Q.; Guo, Q. Wogonin induced G1 cell cycle arrest by regulating Wnt/β-catenin signaling pathway and inactivating CDK8 in human colorectal cancer carcinoma cells. *Toxicology* **2013**, *312*, 36–47. [CrossRef]
399. Tan, H.; Li, X.; Yang, W.-H.; Kang, Y. A flavone, Wogonin from Scutellaria baicalensis inhibits the proliferation of human colorectal cancer cells by inducing of autophagy, apoptosis and G2/M cell cycle arrest via modulating the PI3K/AKT and STAT3 signalling pathways. *J. BUON* **2019**, *24*, 1143–1149. [PubMed]
400. Alam, M.; Ahmed, S.; Elasbali, A.M.; Adnan, M.; Alam, S.; Hassan, M.I.; Pasupuleti, V.R. Therapeutic implications of caffeic acid in cancer and neurological diseases. *Front. Oncol.* **2022**, *12*, 860508. [CrossRef]
401. Banerjee, N.; Kim, H.; Krenek, K.; Talcott, S.T.; Mertens-Talcott, S.U. Mango polyphenolics suppressed tumor growth in breast cancer xenografts in mice: Role of the PI3K/AKT pathway and associated microRNAs. *Nutr. Res.* **2015**, *35*, 744–751. [CrossRef]
402. Boghossian, S.; Hawash, A. Chemoprevention in colorectal cancer-where we stand and what we have learned from twenty year's experience. *Surgeon* **2012**, *10*, 43–52. [CrossRef]
403. Ko, J.-H.; Sethi, G.; Um, J.-Y.; Shanmugam, M.K.; Arfuso, F.; Kumar, A.P.; Bishayee, A.; Ahn, K.S. The role of resveratrol in cancer therapy. *Int. J. Mol. Sci.* **2017**, *18*, 2589. [CrossRef]
404. Bishayee, A. Cancer Prevention and Treatment with Resveratrol: From Rodent Studies to Clinical TrialsResveratrol and Cancer: In vivo and Clinical Studies. *Cancer Prev. Res.* **2009**, *2*, 409–418. [CrossRef] [PubMed]
405. Arslan, A.K.K.; Uzunhisarcıklı, E.; Yerer, M.B.; Bishayee, A. The golden spice curcumin in cancer: A perspective on finalized clinical trials during the last 10 years. *J. Cancer Res. Ther.* **2022**, *18*, 19–26.
406. Singh, A.P.; Singh, R.; Verma, S.S.; Rai, V.; Kaschula, C.H.; Maiti, P.; Gupta, S.C. Health benefits of resveratrol: Evidence from clinical studies. *Med. Res. Rev.* **2019**, *39*, 1851–1891. [CrossRef] [PubMed]
407. Wu, X.-Y.; Zhai, J.; Huan, X.-K.; Xu, W.-W.; Tian, J.; Farhood, B. A Systematic Review of the Therapeutic Potential of Resveratrol During Colorectal Cancer Chemotherapy. *Mini Rev. Med. Chem.* **2022**. [CrossRef]
408. Ma, Z.; Wang, N.; He, H.; Tang, X. Pharmaceutical strategies of improving oral systemic bioavailability of curcumin for clinical application. *J. Control. Release* **2019**, *316*, 359–380. [CrossRef]
409. Seufferlein, T.; Ettrich, T.J.; Menzler, S.; Messmann, H.; Kleber, G.; Zipprich, A.; Frank-Gleich, S.; Algül, H.; Metter, K.; Odemar, F. Green tea extract to prevent colorectal adenomas, results of a randomized, placebo-controlled clinical trial. *Off. J. Am. Coll. Gastroenterol. ACG* **2022**, *117*, 884–894. [CrossRef]
410. Farsad-Naeimi, A.; Alizadeh, M.; Esfahani, A.; Aminabad, E.D. Effect of fisetin supplementation on inflammatory factors and matrix metalloproteinase enzymes in colorectal cancer patients. *Food Funct.* **2018**, *9*, 2025–2031. [CrossRef]
411. Ganesan, K.; Jayachandran, M.; Xu, B. Diet-derived phytochemicals targeting colon cancer stem cells and microbiota in colorectal cancer. *Int. J. Mol. Sci.* **2020**, *21*, 3976. [CrossRef]
412. Greiner, A.K.; Papineni, R.V.; Umar, S. Chemoprevention in gastrointestinal physiology and disease. Natural products and microbiome. *Am. J. Physiol.-Gastrointest. Liver Physiol.* **2014**, *307*, G1–G15. [CrossRef]
413. Dacrema, M.; Ali, A.; Ullah, H.; Khan, A.; Di Minno, A.; Xiao, J.; Martins, A.M.C.; Daglia, M. Spice-Derived Bioactive Compounds Confer Colorectal Cancer Prevention via Modulation of Gut Microbiota. *Cancers* **2022**, *14*, 5682. [CrossRef]
414. O'keefe, S.J. Diet, microorganisms and their metabolites, and colon cancer. *Nat. Rev. Gastroenterol. Hepatol.* **2016**, *13*, 691–706. [CrossRef] [PubMed]

cancers

MDPI

Article

Gnetin C Intercepts MTA1-Associated Neoplastic Progression in Prostate Cancer

Prashanth Parupathi [1,†], Gisella Campanelli [1,†], Rabab Al Deabel [2,‡], Anand Puaar [1], Lakshmi Sirisha Devarakonda [1], Avinash Kumar [1] and Anait S. Levenson [3,*]

1 Division of Pharmaceutical Sciences, Arnold & Marie Schwartz College of Pharmacy and Health Sciences, Long Island University, Brooklyn, NY 11201, USA
2 Department of Biomedical Sciences, School of Health Professions and Nursing, Long Island University, Brookville, NY 11548, USA
3 Department of Biomedical Sciences, College of Veterinary Medicine, Long Island University, Brookville, NY 11548, USA
* Correspondence: anait.levenson@liu.edu
† These authors contributed equally to this work and are joint first authors.
‡ Current address: Department of Immunology, Regional Laboratory & Blood Bank, Ministry of Health, Dammam 34223, Saudi Arabia.

Simple Summary: The incidence of prostate cancer is increasing because of the aging population. Evidence suggests that diets rich in bioactive polyphenols can reduce the incidence of prostate cancer. The aim of this work was to investigate the potential of gnetin C, a compound found in the melinjo plant and commonly used in Indonesian foods, to block prostate cancer progression. To this end, we evaluated the anticancer efficacy of gnetin C-supplemented diets in a unique and adequate high-risk premalignant prostate cancer transgenic mouse model. Our results indicate that a gnetin C-supplemented diet reduces the progression of prostate cancer by reducing the proliferation of cells, inflammation, and the formation of blood vessels. The finding that a gnetin C-supplemented diet effectively blocks tumor progression in a preclinical mouse model may be exploited to initiate chemoprevention trials for novel nutritional interception for untreated patients under active surveillance.

Abstract: Nutritional chemoprevention is particularly suitable for prostate cancer. Gnetin C, a resveratrol dimer found abundantly in the melinjo plant (*Gnetum gnemon*), may possess more potent biological properties compared to other stilbenes. We examined the effects of gnetin C in a high-risk premalignant transgenic mouse model overexpressing tumor-promoting metastasis-associated protein 1 (MTA1) on the background of *Pten* heterozygosity ($R26^{MTA1}$; $Pten^{+/f}$; $Pb\text{-}Cre^{+}$). Mice were fed diets supplemented with the following compounds: pterostilbene (70 mg/kg diet); gnetin C, high dose (70 mg/kg diet); and gnetin C, low dose (35 mg/kg diet). Prostate tissues were isolated after 17 weeks and examined for histopathology and molecular markers. Serum was analyzed for cytokine expression. Gnetin C-supplemented diets substantially delayed the progression of preneoplastic lesions compared to other groups. Prostate tissues from gnetin C-fed mice showed favorable histopathology, with decreased severity and number of prostatic intraepithelial neoplasia (PIN) foci, reduced proliferation, and angiogenesis. A decreased level of MTA1, concurrent with the trend of increasing phosphatase and tensin homolog expression and reduced interleukin 2 (IL-2) levels in sera, were also detected in gnetin C-fed mice. Importantly, gnetin C did not exert any visible toxicity in mice. Our findings demonstrate that a gnetin C-supplemented diet effectively blocks MTA1-promoted tumor progression activity in high-risk premalignant prostate cancer, which indicates its potential as a novel form of nutritional interception for prostate cancer chemoprevention.

Keywords: gnetin C; diet supplementation; transgenic mice; targeted interception; MTA1; prostate cancer

Citation: Parupathi, P.; Campanelli, G.; Deabel, R.A.; Puaar, A.; Devarakonda, L.S.; Kumar, A.; Levenson, A.S. Gnetin C Intercepts MTA1-Associated Neoplastic Progression in Prostate Cancer. *Cancers* **2022**, *14*, 6038. https://doi.org/10.3390/cancers14246038

Academic Editor: Anupam Bishayee

Received: 13 October 2022
Accepted: 3 December 2022
Published: 8 December 2022

1. Introduction

Prostate cancer remains the second highest type of cancer-related mortality in men [1]. According to the American Cancer Society, prostate cancer accounts for about 14% of newly diagnosed cancers, and about 5.7% of all cancer deaths in the United States. Although prostate cancer incidence remained stable over the past few years, there was an annual 4–6% increase in advanced prostate cancer, which accounted for the rise in cases of metastatic disease [2]. Recent updates from the National Comprehensive Cancer Network guidelines for prostate cancer highlight a new risk categorization system for patients with prostate cancer, which demands different approaches for the management of the disease [3]. For the three categories defined as "very low", "low", and "intermediate" risk groups, there is no treatment strategy in current practice to prevent prostate cancer progression. It has been accepted that diverse clinical lesions in these groups are represented by "large gland" morphology, including high-grade prostatic intraepithelial neoplasia (PIN) and PIN-like carcinoma, which are main precursors to invasive carcinoma [4]. We believe that nutritional interception may represent the most adequate intervention to protect not only the general population, but also the moderate- or high-risk subpopulation of patients under active surveillance.

Epidemiological studies have continually supported the argument that naturally occurring dietary polyphenols with anti-inflammatory, antioxidant, and anticancer properties may be considered for prostate cancer chemoprevention [5–8]. It is well-established that natural polyphenols of different classes have pleiotropic effects through various signaling pathways, including epigenetic mechanisms, in inhibiting the progression of prostate cancer [9–11]. Specifically, the potential application of stilbene polyphenols acting through multiple mechanisms in prostate cancer chemoprevention and treatment was demonstrated and summarized by several groups [12–17].

It is imperative to establish a relevant and adequate preclinical model system that represents heterogeneous lesions observed in the clinic, in which to determine the efficacy of natural compounds [18]. In our previous studies, we have shown that stilbenes, such as resveratrol and pterostilbene, can act through metastasis-associated protein 1 (MTA1)-mediated mechanisms to prevent the progression of premalignant prostate cancer to adenocarcinoma [19–27]. MTA1 is a chromatin modifier and transcriptional regulator, and plays a cancer-promoting role in all stages of prostate cancer [19,27–29]. Aberrant alterations in the molecular levels of MTA1 trigger several downstream targets with significant roles in inflammation, cell survival, and invasion, ultimately causing metastasis [22,26,30,31]. Among the downstream pathways affected by the changes in MTA1 levels is the phosphatase and tensin homolog/v-akt murine thymoma viral oncogene (protein kinase B) (PTEN/Akt) pathway, the deregulation of which plays an essential role in prostate cancer [22,32,33]. We have previously shown an inverse association of MTA1 with PTEN, and a direct correlation of MTA1 with p-Akt [22,34]. In fact, we have demonstrated that MTA1 inhibition by resveratrol and pterostilbene promotes the acetylation and activity of PTEN, which in turn inhibits the activity of Akt [22,34]. Given that MTA1 can be targeted by stilbene polyphenols, these compounds are of great interest. We have recently reported that a pterostilbene-supplemented diet exerted beneficial effects by diminishing inflammatory pathways and accelerated PIN progression in $R26^{MTA1}$; $Pten^{+/f}$ mice [27]. Since we have also previously demonstrated the more potent MTA1-targeted inhibitory activity of gnetin C, a dimer resveratrol (Figure 1A), compared to resveratrol and pterostilbene, both in vitro and in prostate cancer xenografts [31,35], we sought to determine the efficacy of gnetin C in an adequate preclinical model of prostate cancer.

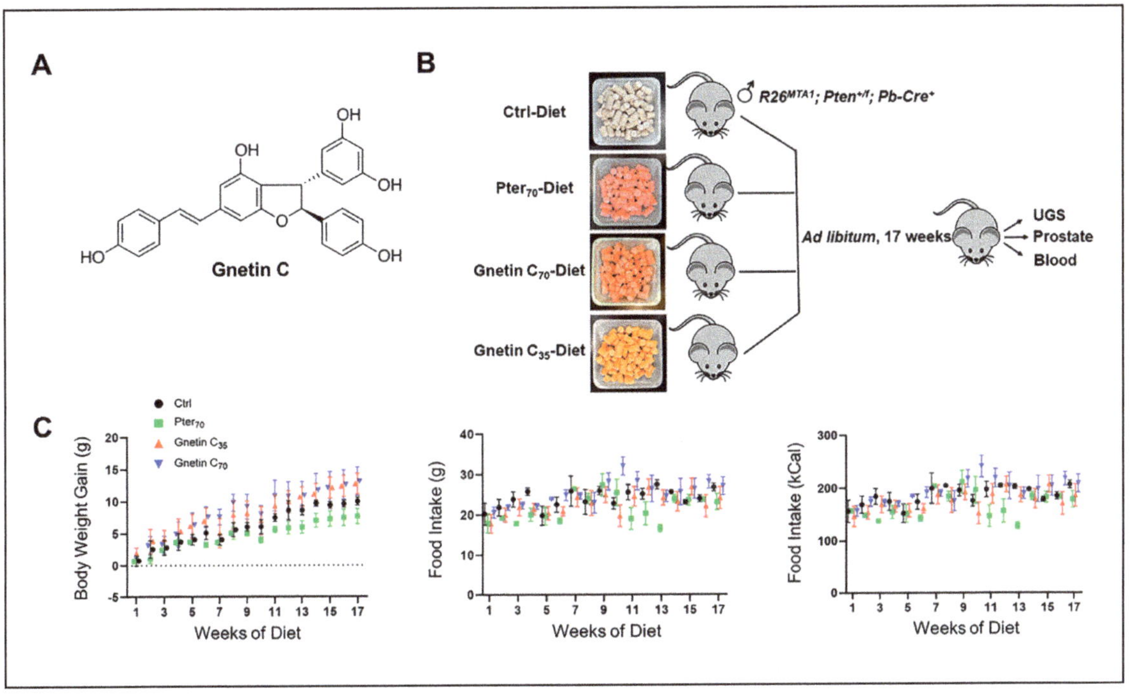

Figure 1. (**A**) Chemical structure of gnetin C, a resveratrol dimer, isolated from melinjo plant (*Gnetum gnemon*). (**B**) Schema showing the experimental design used for prostate cancer chemoprevention by diet supplementation in a precancerous *R26^{MTA1}*; *Pten$^{+/f}$*; *Cre^{+}* murine model. In total, 24 mice were fed with the control diet or diets supplemented with Pter$_{70}$ (70 mg/kg diet), Gnetin C$_{70}$ (70 mg/kg diet), or Gnetin C$_{35}$ (35 mg/kg diet). At sacrifice, urogenital system and prostate tissues were isolated for histological and molecular analysis. Blood was also collected. (**C**) Effects of different diets on average body weight gain and food intake in mice. Values are mean ± SD, *n* = 6 per group.

We hypothesized that gnetin C may possess more potent biological effects compared to pterostilbene in a transgenic model of prostate cancer. Therefore, the current study was undertaken to examine the promising MTA1/PTEN/Akt-mediated chemopreventive and interceptive properties of gnetin C, a dimeric stilbenoid, using a clinically relevant model of murine prostate cancer representing high-risk premalignant neoplasia.

2. Results

2.1. Effects of Gnetin C-Supplemented Diet on Prostate Cancer Progression

For the current study we accumulated twenty-four *R26^{MTA1}*; *Pten$^{+/f}$* mice and randomized them into four groups (*n* = 6 per group) on the respective diets ad libitum for 17 weeks (Figure 1B), after which prostate tissues and blood samples were collected for analysis. Diet supplementation with either pterostilbene or gnetin C did not have any significant effect on either the body weight gain or food intake in these mice (Figure 1C). The effect of such treatment on the gross anatomy of the urogenital system (UGS) over this period is shown in Figure 2A, *upper panel*. Gnetin C-supplemented diets decreased the appearance of the prostate compared to the pterostilbene diet (Pter$_{70}$-Diet)- and control diet (Ctrl-Diet)-fed mice. Consistent with our previous study [27], *R26^{MTA1}*; *Pten$^{+/f}$* mice in all the groups developed high-grade PIN characterized by disorganized glandular structures with pseudostratified epithelium and hyperproliferation, but with an intact basal layer of smooth muscle actin (SMA)-positive cells (Figure 2A). However, there were significant differences in pathological features, and some morphological differences, among the groups. As shown in Figure 2A, presenting hematoxylin and eosin (H&E) images, mice fed diets supplemented with compounds demonstrated favorable histopathology, with restored normal ductal structures and fewer glands involved in PIN compared to mice on the Ctrl-Diet (Figure 2B, *top*). Moreover, mice on the gnetin C high-concentration diet (Gnetin C_{70}-Diet) exhibited a significantly reduced number of glands involved in PIN compared to the $Pter_{70}$-Diet, suggesting a more potent efficacy of gnetin C in restoring the histopathology of the prostate when used at the same concentration in the diet. The gnetin C low-concentration diet (Gnetin C_{35}-Diet) worked at the same level as the $Pter_{70}$-Diet, demonstrating, once more, the greater biological potency of gnetin C compared to pterostilbene. The changes in histopathology were accompanied by a corresponding reduction in proliferation and angiogenesis in treatment groups. Analysis of prostate tissues for the cellular protein marker of proliferation (Ki67) and cluster of differentiation (CD31) markers revealed a significant reduction in corresponding positively stained cells in all treatment groups compared to control mice (Figure 2A, *lower panels*). Importantly, once again, the differences between reduced proliferation and angiogenesis in mice of the Gnetin C_{70}-Diet and $Pter_{70}$-Diet groups were statistically significant (Figure 2B, *lower panels*). Notably, gnetin C at half concentration (Gnetin C_{35}-Diet) showed either the same or more potency compared to $Pter_{70}$-Diet, indicating that gnetin C is more efficacious than pterostilbene. However, there were no significant differences in the anticancer histopathological activities between the lower and higher concentrations of gnetin C diets. Taken together, our data indicate a more potent anticancer activity of gnetin C compared to pterostilbene when provided as dietary supplementation in mice with premalignant neoplasia.

2.2. *Gnetin C Effectively Inhibits the MTA1-Associated PTEN/Akt Axis in a Transgenic Mouse Model of Early-Stage Prostate Cancer*

Our earlier studies using gnetin C in prostate cancer cell lines and xenografts had shown potent inhibition of the MTA1 and MTA1-associated downstream signaling targets, including proto-oncogene 2 (ETS2), Cyclin D1, and Notch 2 [31,35]. To further strengthen our previous in vivo findings on the effects of stilbenes on the MTA1/PTEN/p-Akt axis [22,34], we evaluated the expression of MTA1 and PTEN/pAkt in prostate tissues from $R26^{MTA1}$; $Pten^{+/f}$ mice fed gnetin C diets. We found that MTA1 protein levels were significantly reduced in prostate tissues by diets supplemented with both pterostilbene and gnetin C (Figure 3A *top*, B). Specifically, both pterostilbene and gnetin C diets inhibited MTA1 expression in prostate tissues compared to control prostates with high significance ($p < 0.0001$) (Figure 3B). Moreover, despite the heterogeneity of MTA1-stained tissues in the $Pter_{70}$-Diet group, the differences between $Pter_{70}$-Diet and Gnetin C_{70}-Diet groups were statistically significant. Furthermore, cytoplasmic PTEN and p-Akt staining of tissues showed a concomitant PTEN increase and p-Akt reduction in mice fed with supplemented diets compared to mice fed the control diet. Subtle differences in PTEN and p-Akt levels between the treatment groups are also evident in selected immunochemistry (IHC) images (Figure 3A, *middle and bottom panels*).

Next, we evaluated the response to treatments by measuring levels of MTA1, PTEN, and p-Akt/Akt in prostate tissue lysates. The expression MTA1 protein levels in prostate tissues from mice fed diets supplemented with stilbenes was significantly reduced compared to control mice (Figure 4A,B). We were also able to detect differences among treatment groups, indicating the trend towards gnetin C's greater potency. In contrast to the inhibitory effects on MTA1, diets supplemented with pterostilbene and gnetin C restored PTEN levels in prostate tissues (Figure 4A,B). In general, prostate tissues from mice in the same treatment group demonstrated an expected trend compared to control mice, however, with noticeable heterogeneity, particularly with respect to p-Akt/Akt in mice in the $Gnetin_{35}$-Diet group (Figure 4A, *right*) (Supplementary Figure S1). At the messenger RNA (mRNA) level, MTA1 and PTEN were respectively inhibited and upregulated by stilbene-supplemented diets compared to control mice (Figure 4C). The differences among treatments groups were not significant.

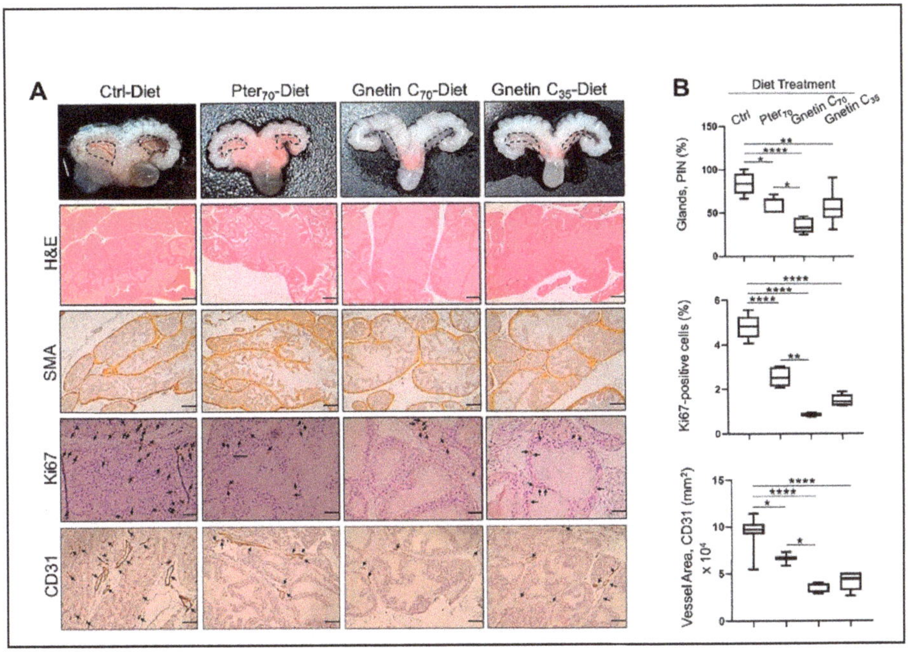

Figure 2. (**A**) *Top*, Representative images of UGS of mice from different groups: The anterior prostates (marked) in mice fed regular diet were larger compared to the treatment groups, but there were no differences in size between treatment groups. Representative images of H&E (scale bar, 100 µm), SMA (scale bar, 50 µm), and Ki67- and CD31-stained sections (scale bar, 20 µm) of the prostate tissues from mice in different groups. (**B**) *Top*, Quantitation of prostate glands involved in PIN formation: The glands were quantified in five randomly selected areas per sample (n = 3 per group), and the average count is expressed as a percent. *Middle*, Quantitative analysis of Ki67 immunostaining, expressed as a percent, showing the drastic effect of gnetin C supplementation on cell proliferation. *Bottom*, Quantitative analysis of CD31 immunostaining, expressed as area, showing the strong effect of gnetin C supplementation on angiogenesis. Values are mean ± SEM analyzed from five separate areas per sample. * $p < 0.05$; ** $p < 0.01$; **** $p < 0.0001$ (one-way ANOVA).

We have chosen the human prostate cancer cell line 22Rv1 that expresses wild-type PTEN for our in vitro experiments. Treatment of these cells for 24 h with the same equipotent concentrations resulted in a statistically significant reduction in MTA1 by gnetin C ($p < 0.05$) and an insignificant increase in PTEN by both compounds compared to control untreated cells, revealing, once again, the more potent activity of gnetin C compared to pterostilbene (Figure 5A,B). Inhibition of p-Akt/Akt under the treatments followed the same trend as MTA1.

Collectively, these data demonstrate a more potent MTA1/PTEN/Akt response to gnetin C than to pterostilbene treatment, both in a murine prostate model of early-stage prostate cancer and in a prostate cancer cell line. This emphasizes that MTA1-targeted interception by diet supplemented with gnetin C may have greater potential benefits compared to pterostilbene supplementation, which we have recently reported for prostate cancer chemoprevention [27].

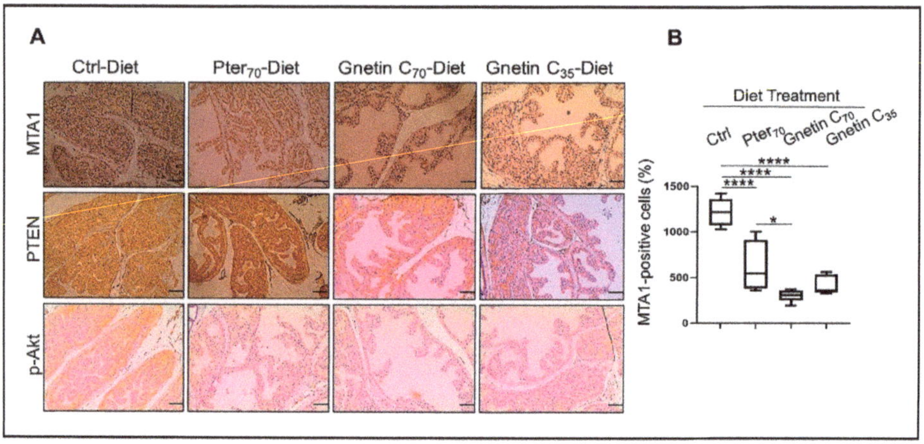

Figure 3. (**A**) Representative images of MTA1 (*top*), PTEN (*middle*), and p-Akt (*bottom*)-stained sections of the prostate tissues from mice in different groups ($n = 3$ per group). Images are 20× (scale bar, 50 μm). (**B**) Quantitative analysis of MTA1 immunostaining. Values are mean ± SEM of cells counted in five separate areas per sample, and the average count is expressed as a percent. * $p < 0.05$; **** $p < 0.0001$ (one-way ANOVA).

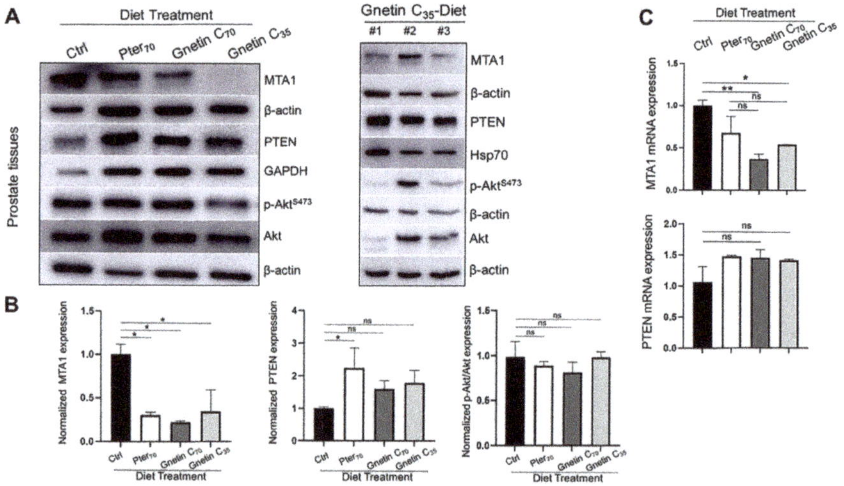

Figure 4. (**A**) Representative immunoblot images of MTA1, PTEN, and p-Akt/Akt levels in the prostate tissues from mice in different treatment groups ($n = 3$ per group). β-actin, GAPDH, or Hsp70 were used as loading controls (*left*). Immunoblot images of MTA1, PTEN, and pAkt/Akt levels in tissues from three mice (#1–3) of the Gnetin C_{35}-Diet group (*right*). (**B**) Quantitation of the relative expression of these markers in prostate tissues from mice in different treatment groups (*left*). Values are mean ± SEM of data from three or more independent experiments. * $p < 0.05$; ** $p < 0.01$; (one-way ANOVA). (**C**) Quantitation of relative MTA1 and PTEN mRNA levels in prostate tissues from mice in different treatment groups. β-actin amplification was used as a normalization control. Changes in mRNA expression were calculated by the $2^{-\Delta\Delta Ct}$ method. Values are mean ± SEM of data from three independent experiments. * $p < 0.05$; ** $p < 0.01$; (one-way ANOVA). ns, not significant.

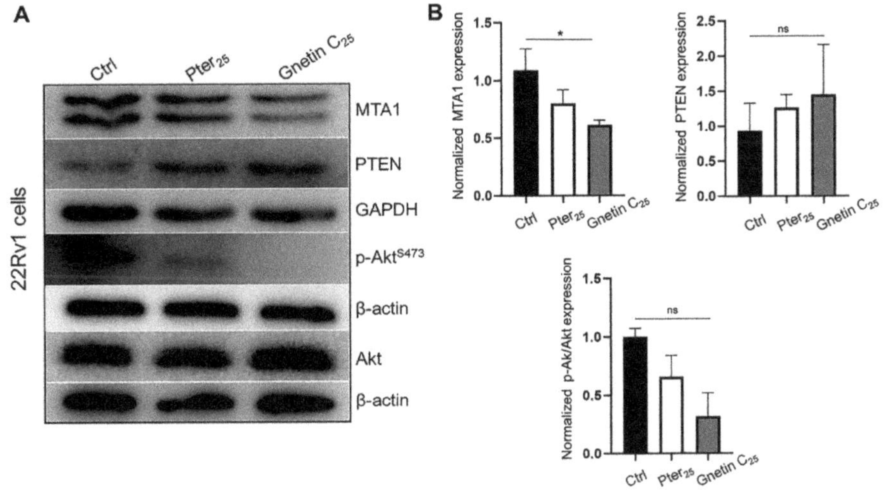

Figure 5. (**A**) Representative immunoblot images of MTA1, PTEN, and p-Akt/Akt levels in 22Rv1 prostate cancer cells treated with pterostilbene and gnetin C at 25 μM concentration. β-actin was used as a loading control. (**B**) Quantitation of the relative expression of these markers in prostate cancer cells. Values are mean ± SEM of data from three independent experiments. * $p < 0.05$; (one-way ANOVA). ns, not significant.

2.3. *Effects of Gnetin C-Supplemented Diet on Pro-Inflammatory Interleukin 2 (IL-2) and Interleukin 6 (IL-6) Cytokine Levels in Murine Serum*

To evaluate the systemic efficacy of gnetin C dietary intervention, we determined pro-inflammatory IL-2 and IL-6 levels in mouse sera by enzyme-linked immunosorbent assay (ELISA). Our results show significantly reduced levels of circulating IL-2 in sera of mice fed supplemented diets compared to control mice (68.34% reduction for Gnetin C_{70}-Diet and 93.86% reduction for Gnetin C_{35}-Diet) (Figure 6A). Interestingly, gnetin C supplementation at the lower 35 mg/kg diet concentration secured a greater attenuation of IL-2 levels compared to both $Pter_{70}$ and Gnetin C_{70} diets. Moreover, the Gnetin C_{35} diet also inhibited IL-6 levels, while Gnetin C_{70}-Diet mice showed a paradoxical increase in the levels of pro-inflammatory IL-6 (Supplementary Figure S2). In agreement with our previous data, which revealed that high-concentration pterostilbene supplementation (100 mg/kg diet) reduced serum IL-6 significantly ($p < 0.01$) [27], we now observe a downregulation of IL-6 in mice treated with $Pter_{70}$-Diet, albeit without significance. Nevertheless, these data suggest that systemic inflammation was decreased in mice fed the low-concentration gnetin C-supplemented diet (Gnetin C_{35}-Diet), which should ensure the beneficial anti-inflammatory effects of gnetin C, and validate the utilization of sera as a liquid biopsy strategy for the evaluation of gnetin C responsive, prognostic, and predictive noninvasive biomarkers.

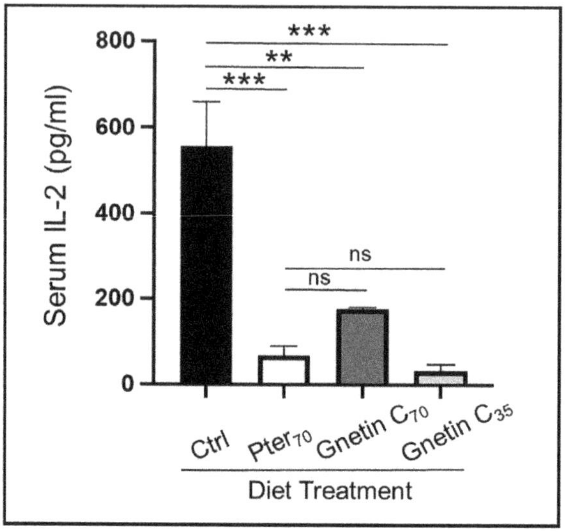

Figure 6. Effects of diets supplemented with gnetin C on circulating IL-2 cytokine levels **measured by ELISA in murine sera** (n = 3–4 per group) Data represent the mean ± SEM of three independent experiments performed in duplicate. ** $p < 0.01$; *** $p < 0.001$; (one-way ANOVA). ns, not significant.

3. Discussion

Naturally occurring resveratrol oligomers, including gnetin C, have been proposed as potential cancer chemopreventive compounds [36]. Antitumor activities of gnetin C, a resveratrol dimer, have been reported in acute myeloid leukemia [37], colon cancer [17], and neuroblastoma [38]. Accumulated data indicate that gnetin C exhibits potent antitumor activity in prostate cancer. Using a panel of human prostate cancer cell lines (PC3, LNCaP, and DU145) and mouse prostate cancer cells derived from the adenocarcinoma of PTEN null mice (PTEN-CaP8), Narayanan et al. [17] first reported the significant proliferation inhibitory effects of gnetin C in cancer cells without affecting normal prostate epithelial RWPE-1 cells. Moreover, gnetin C was significantly more potent in inhibiting cell proliferation and apoptosis in prostate cancer cells compared to resveratrol [17]. Our own published in vitro studies with DU145 and PC3M cells showed more potent inhibition of cell proliferation with lower IC_{50} values for gnetin C compared to pterostilbene and resveratrol [35]. In fact, we have repeatedly shown gnetin C-concentration-dependent cell survival inhibition in a panel of prostate cancer cells (Supplemental Figure S3). Moreover, we have demonstrated that gnetin C was more potent in causing apoptosis and inhibiting metastatic potential of prostate cancer cells than resveratrol and pterostilbene [35]. In addition, we also demonstrated that gnetin C is a lead compound among stilbenes for effectively blocking tumor progression in immunodeficient mice implanted with PC3M [35]. Importantly, in a recent paper using genetically modified DU145 and PC3M prostate cancer cells, gnetin C was shown to have more potent MTA1-mediated cytotoxicity, apoptosis, inhibition of clonogenic cell survival, and motility compared to resveratrol and pterostilbene [31]. To evaluate gnetin C's clinical potential, in the current study, we assessed the efficacy of gnetin C-supplemented diets as MTA1-targeted interception using a unique transgenic mouse model ($R26^{MTA1}$; $Pten^{+/f}$; $Pb\text{-}Cre^{+}$) representing high-risk early-stage prostate cancer.

The clinical significance of MTA1 in prostate cancer progression and metastasis has been reported [28–30,39]. We have also demonstrated that MTA1 is a molecular target for stilbene polyphenols, such as resveratrol, pterostilbene, and gnetin C, in prostate cancer, in vitro and in vivo [22,24–26,34,35,40,41]. Our group has tested the MTA1-targeted chemopreventive and therapeutic potential of stilbenes and grape extracts in murine prostate cancer models [22,24,27,42]. Particularly, our recent report showed that a pterostilbene-supplemented diet fed to mice with early-stage prostate cancer can block the progression of prostate cancer through the inhibition of MTA1-mediated signaling [27]. Since gnetin C showed improved pharmacokinetic parameters in mouse and human studies compared to both resveratrol and pterostilbene [35,43–46], we sought to compare, for the first time, the MTA1-targeted inhibitory efficacy of gnetin C and pterostilbene supplemented diets in a transgenic mouse model of early-stage prostate cancer.

For this study, we fed prostate-specific *R26*^{MTA1}; *Pten*$^{+/f}$ mice reference diets (Ctrl-Diet and Pter-Diet) along with gnetin C-supplemented diets, and asked two major questions: (1) whether gnetin C at the same diet concentration has a more potent MTA1-mediated effect than pterostilbene; and (2) whether gnetin C at half diet concentration has beneficial efficacy in this model.

While both pterostilbene- and gnetin C-supplemented diets showed expected beneficial effects compared to Ctrl-Diet, the differences between Pter-Diet and Gnetin C-Diet (s) were considerable: mice treated with Gnetin C-Diet(s) exhibited favorable histopathology compared to mice fed Pter-Diet. Immunohistochemical results showed a statistically significant decrease in epithelial cancer cell proliferation and angiogenesis in mice fed Gnetin C-Diet(s) compared to the Pter-Diet. Furthermore, gnetin C at both concentrations had potent anticancer activity through targeting MTA1, and this effect was statistically significant compared to the $Pter_{70}$-Diet group. In addition, consistent with apparent trends in inhibiting MTA1 expression after gnetin C treatment, levels of PTEN were increased and p-Akt were decreased in Gnetin C-Diet groups. Further analysis of prostate tissues and prostate cancer cell lines confirmed the potent MTA1 inhibitory potential of gnetin C compared to pterostilbene. The more potent biological effects of gnetin C could be explained by its improved pharmacokinetics [44].

It has been reported that stilbenoids can regulate cytokine expression in different cellular systems [47–49]. With regards to cytokine-mediated anti-inflammatory effects in cancer, resveratrol was found to inhibit metastasis and angiogenesis by reducing inflammatory cytokines, such as tumor necrosis factor α (TNFα), IL-6, and interleukin 1 beta (IL-1β), in vitro and in vivo in oral cancer [50], and decreasing levels of the pro-inflammatory cytokines in rat colon carcinogenesis [51]. In prostate cancer, we have shown the inhibitory effects of orally administered resveratrol, trimethoxy-resveratrol, and piceatannol on circulating IL-6 levels in LNCaP xenografts [41]. In addition, the inhibitory effects of dietary pterostilbene on IL-6 levels were also detected in sera from *R26*^{MTA1}; *Pten*$^{+/f}$ transgenic mice [27]. The inhibitory effects of grape extract diet supplementation and pterostilbene treatment on the levels of pro-inflammatory and pro-angiogenic IL-1β were also reported in prostate-specific *Pten*-deficient mouse models [26,42].

Here, murine serum was used to evaluate the systemic cytokine-mediated immune response to the gnetin C-supplemented diets. Our results show that, consistent with our previous observations [27], pterostilbene reduced the levels of IL-6 compared to the control. However, interesting results were obtained with gnetin C: low diet concentration of gnetin C (35 mg/kg diet) significantly suppressed levels of pro-inflammatory IL-2, and to a lesser extent, levels of IL-6. Curiously, the effectiveness of high-concentration gnetin C (70 mg/kg diet) was profoundly diminished for both cytokines, even resulting in a rather opposite effect by drastically increasing levels of IL-6. Our unexpected results on the systemic anti-inflammatory effects of gnetin C are consistent with some reports that natural products or individual polyphenols at lower doses exert more potent anti-inflammatory/anticancer effects than at higher doses in vivo [17,52–54]. Relevant to our study, a low dose of melinjo seed extract (MSE) that contains gnetin C had more profound effects on tumor growth and angiogenesis in mice with colon tumors than it did at double the dose [17]. Further studies are needed to clarify the dose-and-effect relationship of natural polyphenols as anticancer and anti-inflammatory agents.

Melinjo fruit is consumed as a food in Southeast Asia as well as being traditional medicine [55]. Importantly, nontoxic effects of MSE and gnetin C in nonmalignant cells in culture [17,36,37,56] and in vivo toxicity studies in mice [17] and rats [57] has been demonstrated. Crucially, MSE and gnetin C appear to be safe in humans, as it has been demonstrated in clinical trials [44,45,58,59].

Based on an average food consumption of 4g diet per day for each mouse (Figure 1C, middle panel), doses in the current study were 0.28 mg per day for the Gnetin C_{70} diet and $Pter_{70}$ diet, and was 0.14 mg per day for the Gnetin C_{35} diet. There are no other in vivo studies with these compounds in transgenic mouse models, except our own studies [22,26,27]. The dose that we used in our study is in line with the safe doses used in human studies.

In summary, to the best of our knowledge, the current study is the first to demonstrate the in vivo anticancer activity of gnetin C-supplemented diets in a clinically relevant transgenic mouse model of prostate cancer. Due to the known safety of gnetin C, and its improved bioavailability compared to pterostilbene and resveratrol, lower doses of gnetin C may become one of the most promising targeted strategies for prostate cancer interception. Our study also suggests that the evaluation of pro-inflammatory cytokines in the blood may provide noninvasive prognostic and predictive biomarkers. The curious mixture of gnetin C's ability to inhibit cancer cell proliferation and simultaneously have a complex immunomodulatory response at high concentrations needs further investigation.

4. Materials and Methods

4.1. Animals

We have previously generated prostate-specific MTA1-overexpressing mice ($R26^{MTA1}$; $Pb\text{-}Cre^{+}$) [27]. The generation of prostate-specific MTA1 overexpression on the background of *Pten* heterozygous mice was achieved by breeding our MTA1 transgenic mice ($R26^{MTA1}$) with a C57BL/6J female mouse homozygous for the "floxed" *Pten* allele, which was purchased from Jackson Laboratories (Bar Harbor, ME, USA). Transgenic $R26^{MTA1}$; $Pten^{+/f}$; $Pb\text{-}Cre^{+}$ male mice (hereafter $R26^{MTA1}$; $Pten^{+/f}$) for this study were confirmed by PCR-based tail genomic DNA genotyping using primers, as previously described [27]. The animals were housed in cages with corn cob bedding in a temperature-controlled room with a 12 h light–dark cycle. Mice had free access to drinking water and designated irradiated AIN-76A diets (Envigo Teklad, Boyertown, PA, USA). All animal protocols were approved in advance by the Institutional Animal Care and Use Committee (IACUC) at Long Island University in accordance with the NIH Guidelines for the Care and Use of Laboratory Animals. Mice were monitored daily for their general health and signs of toxicity.

4.2. Diets and Study Design

Gnetin C was a generous gift from Hosoda SHC Co., Ltd. (Fukui, Japan). The purity of gnetin C and pterostilbene (Pter) (Sigma Aldrich, St. Louis, MO, USA) was determined to be $\geq$99%. Gnetin C and Pter powders were shipped to Envigo Teklad Diets (Boyertown, PA, USA) for the formulation of three different supplemented diets on the basis of an AIN-76A control diet (Ctrl-Diet). Based on our previous experience with a Pter diet at a concentration of 100 mg/kg diet [27], we formulated the following diets with gnetin C and pterostilbene, as a reference diet: gnetin C, high concentration, 70 mg/kg diet (Gnetin C_{70}-Diet); gnetin C, low concentration, 35 mg/kg diet (Gnetin C_{35}-Diet); and pterostilbene at 70 mg/kg diet ($Pter_{70}$-Diet). For our calculations, we used the following formula: DD = (SD $\times$ BW)/FI (Research Diets Inc., New Brunswick, NJ, USA), where DD is diet dose (mg compound/kg Diet); SD is single dose (mg compound/kg bw/day); BW is body weight (g bw/animal), and FI is daily food intake (g Diet/day). For prospective clinical relevance of the doses used in this study, we determined equivalent doses for humans using the following human equivalent dose (HED) formula: HED (mg/kg) = Animal dose (mg/kg) $\times$ km ratio, where the Km ratio for mice is 0.081 [60]. Considering that the average human male BW is 70 kg, the doses used in this study for mice approximately translate into 53.2 mg/day (Gnetin C_{70}-Diet), 26.6 mg/day (Gnetin C_{35}-Diet), and 53.2 mg/day ($Pter_{70}$-Diet) in humans. All these doses are well tolerated and safe in humans, as shown in respective clinical trials [45,58,59,61]. The diets were stored at 4 °C and protected from light.

Fresh diets were weighed each week and added to cages. The nutritional composition of diets was published previously [27].

Treatment groups: Twenty-four 3-week-old $R26^{MTA1}$; $Pten^{+/f}$ mice were randomized into four major groups, $n = 6$ per group: Ctrl-Diet; $Pter_{70}$-Diet; Gnetin C_{70}-Diet; and Gnetin C_{35}-Diet. All mice were fed ad libitum. The animals were weighed weekly and monitored regularly for their food intake and general health. After 17 weeks on their respective diet, mice were euthanized by CO_2 inhalation and cervical dislocation. Due to small proportions of mouse prostate, animals from the same treatment group were used for different purposes. From six mice in each treatment group, we used three mice for the UGS (seminal vesicle, prostate, and the urinary bladder) isolation to be processed for histology and IHC. The remaining three mice were used for the isolation of prostate tissues for molecular analysis (protein and RNA isolation). Prostate tissues were dissected, snap frozen, and kept at −80 °C until use for further molecular analyses. Blood was collected by cardiac puncture upon sacrifice at week 17; serum samples were prepared and stored at −80 °C.

4.3. Histopathology and Immunohistochemistry

Urogenital system tissues were fixed in 10% neutral-buffered formalin, processed, and embedded in paraffin, cut into 4 μm sections, and mounted onto slides (Reveal Biosciences, San Diego, CA, USA). H&E-stained sections were assessed for mouse PIN and/or adenocarcinoma. Slides were subjected to IHC analysis as described previously [22,27], using antibodies from Abcam (Boston, MA, USA) for Ki67 (1:50) and SMA (1:700), and from Cell Signaling Technology (Beverly, MA, USA) for CD31 (1:500), MTA1 (1:50), PTEN (1:150), and $pAkt^{Ser473}$ (1:50). Images were taken using an EVOS XL Core microscope (Thermo Fisher Scientific, Somerset, NJ, USA). Ki67, MTA1, and CD31 positively stained cells were quantified in five randomly selected areas using Image J software.

4.4. Tissue Processing and Western Blot Analysis

Frozen prostate tissues were homogenized in RIPA buffer (Thermo Fisher Scientific, Somerset, NJ, USA), and Western blots were performed as described previously [22,26,27,42]. Briefly, samples were separated using 10–15% polyacrylamide gels, and transferred onto polyvinylidene difluoride membranes. Membranes were blocked with 5% milk/TBS/0.1% Tween, and then probed with primary antibodies for MTA1 (1:2500); PTEN (1:1000); and Akt and $p\text{-}Akt^{S473}$ (1:1000) from Cell Signaling Technology (Beverly, MA, USA). B-actin (1:5000), Hsp70 (1:1000), and GAPDH (1:1000) were purchased from Santa Cruz Biotechnology (Dallas, TX, USA), and were used as loading controls. Signals were detected using enhanced chemiluminescence (Thermo Fisher Scientific, Somerset, NJ, USA). Band intensity was measured using Image J.

4.5. Tissue Processing and Real-Time RT-PCR

Total RNA was isolated from prostate tissues that were stored in RNAlater (Thermo Fisher Scientific, Somerset, NJ, USA) immediately after tissue extraction using an miRNeasy mini kit (Qiagen, Germantown, MD, USA) as recently described [27]. The quality of RNA was evaluated on a NanoDrop spectrophotometer (Shimadzu Scientific Instruments, Kyoto, Japan). Quantitative RT-PCR was performed on a Lightcycler 480 II Real-Time PCR instrument (Roche Diagnostics, Indianapolis, IN, USA) using murine primers specific for MTA1 (forward: 5′-AGC TAC GAG CAG CAC AAC GGG GT-3′; reverse: 5′-CAC GCT TGG TTT CCG AGG AT-3′) and PTEN (forward: 5′-GAT TAC AGA CCC GTG GCA CT-3′; reverse: 5′-GGG TCC TGA ATT GGA AT-3′. β-actin was used for normalization (forward: 5′-CGT GGG CCG CCC TAG GCA CCA-3′; reverse: 5′-TTG GCT TAG GGT TCA GGG GGG-3′) (Integrated DNA Technologies, Coralville, IA, USA). Fold changes in mRNA expression were estimated by the $2^{-\Delta\Delta Ct}$ method.

4.6. ELISA

Serum IL-2 levels were analyzed using commercially available mouse IL-2 and IL-6 ELISA kits (Abcam, Boston, MA, USA) as per the manufacturer's instructions. Samples (50 μL) or standards were added to the pre-coated 96-well strip microplates covered with an anti-tag antibody, followed by the antibody mix, and incubated for 1 h at room temperature. After washing, 3, 3′,5,5′-tetramethylbenzidine substrate was added for 10 min at room temperature, followed by the stop solution, to each well. The reaction was read at 450 nm using a Tecan Sunrise Absorbance microplate reader (Tecan, Mannedorf, Switzerland). Using the standard titration curve, a concentration of IL-2 and IL-6 in serum was calculated based on their absorbance.

4.7. Cell Culture, Reagents, and Treatment

Prostate cancer 22Rv1 cells (ATCC, Manassas, VA, USA) were grown and maintained in RPMI-1640 media containing 10% FBS, as described previously [27,62]. Cells were validated for mycoplasma-free condition using the Universal Mycoplasma Detection Kit (ATCC, Manassas, VA, USA). Gnetin C was a generous gift from Hosoda SHC Co., Ltd. (Fukui, Japan). Pterostilbene was purchased from Sigma-Aldrich (St. Louis, MO, USA). Compounds were dissolved in pure dimethyl sulfoxide (DMSO, 0.1% final concentration) and stored in the dark at −20 °C until use. At approximately 60% confluency, cells were treated with pterostilbene and gnetin C at the same concentration of 25 μM for 24 h, after which, protein lysates were isolated for Western blot analysis, as described above. The dilutions for antibodies used in cell lines were the same as those used for tissues.

4.8. Statistical Analysis

The data from each group of mice were summarized as the mean ± SD/SEM. The statistical significance of differences between groups was determined by a one-way ANOVA (Prism v9, GraphPad Software, San Diego, CA, USA). A p-value of ≤ 0.05 was considered statistically significant.

5. Conclusions

In conclusion, our results established the MTA1/PTEN/p-Akt axis as a suitable target for gnetin C interception in early-stage prostate cancer in mice. The clinical usage of gnetin C may be a valuable tool for the management of prostate cancer progression in selected patients under active surveillance. We intend to use synthetic chemistry to produce gnetin C analogs with higher potency that can be used as pharmaceuticals. The development of natural and synthetic MTA1 inhibitors with improved pharmacokinetic profiles will secure the utilization of these new and targeted drugs not only for interception during early-stage prostate cancer, but also in the treatment of more advanced stages and metastatic disease.

Supplementary Materials: The following supporting information can be downloaded at: https://www.mdpi.com/article/10.3390/cancers14246038/s1, Figure S1: Screening of prostate tissues for molecular markers from mice fed different diets; Figure S2: Effects of diets supplemented with Gnetin C on the levels of circulating inflammatory IL-6 cytokine detected in murine serum by ELISA; Figure S3: Gnetin C inhibits proliferation of prostate cancer cells in a dose-dependent manner.

Author Contributions: Conceptualization, A.S.L.; methodology, A.K. and A.S.L.; formal analysis, P.P., G.C., A.K. and A.S.L.; investigation, P.P., G.C., R.A.D., A.P. and L.S.D.; resources. A.S.L. and A.K.; writing-original draft preparation, A.S.L.; writing—review and editing, G.C., A.K. and A.S.L.; visualization, P.P., G.C. and L.S.D.; supervision, A.K. and A.S.L.; funding acquisition, A.S.L. All authors have read and agreed to the published version of the manuscript.

Funding: This research and the APC was funded by the National Cancer Institute of the National Institutes of Health Grant Number R15CA216070.

Institutional Review Board Statement: The animal study protocol was approved by the Institutional Animal Care and Use Committee of the LONG ISLAND UNIVERSITY BROOKLYN (ID # 2022-011, 10 March 2022).

Informed Consent Statement: Not applicable.

Data Availability Statement: Not applicable.

Acknowledgments: The study was partly supported by the National Cancer Institute of the National Institutes of Health under Award Number R15CA216070 to A.S. Levenson. The content is solely the responsibility of the author and does not necessarily represent the official views of the National Institutes of Health. The authors are grateful to Dicky Gunawan, Hosoda SHC Co., Ltd., Fukui, Japan for providing Gnetin C for this study and to Noah Waxner, College of Veterinary Medicine, LIU, NY for his contribution to this study.

Conflicts of Interest: The authors declare no conflict of interest.

Abbreviations

Akt	v-Akt murine thymoma viral oncogene (protein kinase B)
ANOVA	Analysis of variance
AR	Androgen receptor
CD31	Cluster of differentiation 31
DMSO	Dimethyl sulfoxide
DNA	Deoxyribonucleic acid
DU145	Human prostate cancer cell line
Ctrl-Diet	Control Diet
ELISA	Enzyme-linked immunosorbent Assay
ETS2	ETS proto-oncogene 2, transcription factor
GAPDH	Glyceraldehyde 3-phosphate dehydrogenase
+/f	*Pten* gene flanked by two loxP sites in one allele
Gnetin C_{70}-Diet	Gnetin C high dose diet (70 mg/kg)
Gnetin C_{35}-Diet	Gnetin C low dose diet (35 mg/kg)
H&E	Hematoxylin and eosin
Hsp70	Heat shock protein 70
IACUC	Institutional Animal Care and Use Committee
IHC	Immunohistochemistry
IL-1β	Interleukin 1 beta
IL-2	Interleukin 2
IL-6	Interleukin 6
kCal	Kilocalorie
Ki67	Cellular protein marker of proliferation
LIU	Long Island University
LNCaP	Human prostate cancer cell line
MSE	Melinjo seed extract
mRNA	Messenger RNA
MTA1	Metastasis-associated protein 1
Notch2	Transmembrane protein
NS	Nonsignificant
NuRD	Nucleosome remodeling and deacetylase complex
p-Akt	Phosphorylated Akt
p-Akt^{S473}	Phosphorylation of serine 473 in C-terminus of Akt
Pb-Cre^{+}	Probasin promoter directing expression of epithelial Cre recombinase
PC3	Human prostate cancer cell line
PC3M	Human prostate cancer cell line
PCR	Polymerase chain reaction
PIN	Prostate intraepithelial neoplasia
PTEN	Phosphatase and tensin homolog
$Pten^{+/f}$	*Pten* heterozygous mice
Pter	Pterostilbene
$Pter_{70}$-Diet	Pterostilbene 70 mg/kg diet
PVDF	Polyvinylidene fluoride
qRT-PCR	Quantitative reverse transcriptase polymerase chain reaction
RNA	Ribonucleic acid

RPMI-1640	Roswell Park Memorial Institute 1640 cell culture media
RWPE-1	Immortalized human prostatic epithelial cell line
22Rv1	Human prostate cancer cell line
R26	Rosa26 loci in the mouse genome
SD	Standard deviation
SEM	Standard error of mean
SMA	Smooth muscle actin
TNFα	Tumor necrosis factor alpha
UGS	Urogenital system

References

1. Rawla, P. Epidemiology of Prostate Cancer. *World J. Oncol.* **2019**, *10*, 63–89. [CrossRef]
2. Siegel, R.L.; Miller, K.D.; Fuchs, H.E.; Jemal, A. Cancer statistics, 2022. *CA Cancer J. Clin.* **2022**, *72*, 7–33. [CrossRef]
3. Mohler, J.L.; Kantoff, P.W.; Armstrong, A.J.; Bahnson, R.R.; Cohen, M.; D'Amico, A.V.; Eastham, J.A.; Enke, C.A.; Farrington, T.A.; Higano, C.S.; et al. Prostate cancer, version 2.2014. *J. Natl. Compr. Cancer Netw.* **2014**, *12*, 686–718. [CrossRef] [PubMed]
4. Zhou, M. High-grade prostatic intraepithelial neoplasia, PIN-like carcinoma, ductal carcinoma, and intraductal carcinoma of the prostate. *Mod. Pathol.* **2018**, *31*, S71–S79. [CrossRef] [PubMed]
5. Fontana, F.; Raimondi, M.; Marzagalli, M.; Di Domizio, A.; Limonta, P. Natural Compounds in Prostate Cancer Prevention and Treatment: Mechanisms of Action and Molecular Targets. *Cells* **2020**, *9*, 460–491. [CrossRef] [PubMed]
6. Mokbel, K.; Wazir, U.; Mokbel, K. Chemoprevention of Prostate Cancer by Natural Agents: Evidence from Molecular and Epidemiological Studies. *Anticancer Res.* **2019**, *39*, 5231–5259. [CrossRef]
7. Pejcic, T.; Tosti, T.; Dzamic, Z.; Gasic, U.; Vuksanovic, A.; Dolicanin, Z.; Tesic, Z. The Polyphenols as Potential Agents in Prevention and Therapy of Prostate Diseases. *Molecules* **2019**, *24*, 3982. [CrossRef]
8. Schoonen, W.M.; Salinas, C.A.; Kiemeney, L.A.; Stanford, J.L. Alcohol consumption and risk of prostate cancer in middle-aged men. *Int. J. Cancer* **2005**, *113*, 133–140. [CrossRef]
9. Oczkowski, M.; Dziendzikowska, K.; Pasternak-Winiarska, A.; Wlodarek, D.; Gromadzka-Ostrowska, J. Dietary Factors and Prostate Cancer Development, Progression, and Reduction. *Nutrients* **2021**, *13*, 496. [CrossRef]
10. Izzo, S.; Naponelli, V.; Bettuzzi, S. Flavonoids as Epigenetic Modulators for Prostate Cancer Prevention. *Nutrients* **2020**, *12*, 1010. [CrossRef]
11. Kumar, A.; Butt, N.A.; Levenson, A.S. Natural epigenetic-modifying molecules in medical therapy. In *Medical Epigenetics;* Tollefsbol, T., Ed.; Elsevier: Oxford, UK, 2006; pp. 747–798.
12. Jayasooriya, R.G.; Lee, Y.G.; Kang, C.H.; Lee, K.T.; Choi, Y.H.; Park, S.Y.; Hwang, J.K.; Kim, G.Y. Piceatannol inhibits MMP-9-dependent invasion of tumor necrosis factor-alpha-stimulated DU145 cells by suppressing the Akt-mediated nuclear factor-kappaB pathway. *Oncol. Lett.* **2013**, *5*, 341–347. [CrossRef] [PubMed]
13. Chakraborty, S.; Kumar, A.; Butt, N.A.; Zhang, L.; Williams, R.; Rimando, A.M.; Biswas, P.K.; Levenson, A.S. Molecular insight into the differential anti-androgenic activity of resveratrol and its natural analogs: In silico approach to understand biological actions. *Mol. Biosyst.* **2016**, *12*, 1702–1709. [CrossRef] [PubMed]
14. Benitez, D.A.; Pozo-Guisado, E.; Alvarez-Barrientos, A.; Fernandez-Salguero, P.M.; Castellon, E.A. Mechanisms involved in resveratrol-induced apoptosis and cell cycle arrest in prostate cancer-derived cell lines. *J. Androl.* **2007**, *28*, 282–293. [CrossRef] [PubMed]
15. Zaffaroni, N.; Beretta, G.L. Resveratrol and Prostate Cancer: The Power of Phytochemicals. *Curr. Med. Chem.* **2021**, *28*, 4845–4862. [CrossRef]
16. Levenson, A.S.; Kumar, A. Pterostilbene as a potent chemopreventive agent in cancer. In *Natural Products for Chemoprevention: Single Compounds and Combinations*; Pezzuto, J.M., Vang, O., Eds.; Springer Nature: Cham, Switzerland, 2020; pp. 49–108.
17. Narayanan, N.K.; Kunimasa, K.; Yamori, Y.; Mori, M.; Mori, H.; Nakamura, K.; Miller, G.; Manne, U.; Tiwari, A.K.; Narayanan, B. Antitumor activity of melinjo (*Gnetum gnemon* L.) seed extract in human and murine tumor models in vitro and in a colon-26 tumor-bearing mouse model in vivo. *Cancer Med.* **2015**, *4*, 1767–1780. [CrossRef]
18. Lamb, D.J.; Zhang, L. Challenges in prostate cancer research: Animal models for nutritional studies of chemoprevention and disease progression. *J. Nutr.* **2005**, *135*, 3009S–3015S. [CrossRef]
19. Levenson, A.S.; Kumar, A.; Zhang, X. MTA family of proteins in prostate cancer: Biology, significance, and therapeutic opportunities. *Cancer Metastasis Rev.* **2014**, *33*, 929–942. [CrossRef]
20. Levenson, A.S. Metastasis-associated protein 1-mediated antitumor and anticancer activity of dietary stilbenes for prostate cancer chemoprevention and therapy. *Semin. Cancer Biol.* **2020**, *80*, 107–117. [CrossRef]
21. Dhar, S.; Kumar, A.; Rimando, A.M.; Zhang, X.; Levenson, A.S. Resveratrol and pterostilbene epigenetically restore PTEN expression by targeting oncomiRs of the miR-17 family in prostate cancer. *Oncotarget* **2015**, *6*, 27214–27226. [CrossRef]
22. Dhar, S.; Kumar, A.; Zhang, L.; Rimando, A.M.; Lage, J.M.; Lewin, J.R.; Atfi, A.; Zhang, X.; Levenson, A.S. Dietary pterostilbene is a novel MTA1-targeted chemopreventive and therapeutic agent in prostate cancer. *Oncotarget* **2016**, *7*, 18469–18484. [CrossRef]
23. Kumar, A.; Dhar, S.; Rimando, A.M.; Lage, J.M.; Lewin, J.R.; Zhang, X.; Levenson, A.S. Epigenetic potential of resveratrol and analogs in preclinical models of prostate cancer. *Ann. N. Y. Acad. Sci.* **2015**, *1348*, 1–9. [CrossRef] [PubMed]

24. Li, K.; Dias, S.J.; Rimando, A.M.; Dhar, S.; Mizuno, C.S.; Penman, A.D.; Lewin, J.R.; Levenson, A.S. Pterostilbene acts through metastasis-associated protein 1 to inhibit tumor growth, progression and metastasis in prostate cancer. *PLoS ONE* **2013**, *8*, e57542. [CrossRef] [PubMed]
25. Kai, L.; Samuel, S.K.; Levenson, A.S. Resveratrol enhances p53 acetylation and apoptosis in prostate cancer by inhibiting MTA1/NuRD complex. *Int. J. Cancer* **2010**, *126*, 1538–1548. [CrossRef]
26. Butt, N.A.; Kumar, A.; Dhar, S.; Rimando, A.M.; Akhtar, I.; Hancock, J.C.; Lage, J.M.; Pound, C.R.; Lewin, J.R.; Gomez, C.R.; et al. Targeting MTA1/HIF-1alpha signaling by pterostilbene in combination with histone deacetylase inhibitor attenuates prostate cancer progression. *Cancer Med.* **2017**, *6*, 2673–2685. [CrossRef]
27. Hemani, R.; Patel, I.; Inamdar, N.; Campanelli, G.; Donovan, V.; Kumar, A.; Levenson, A.S. Dietary Pterostilbene for MTA1-Targeted Interception in High-Risk Premalignant Prostate Cancer. *Cancer Prev. Res.* **2022**, *15*, 87–100. [CrossRef]
28. Dias, S.J.; Zhou, X.; Ivanovic, M.; Gailey, M.P.; Dhar, S.; Zhang, L.; He, Z.; Penman, A.D.; Vijayakumar, S.; Levenson, A.S. Nuclear MTA1 overexpression is associated with aggressive prostate cancer, recurrence and metastasis in African Americans. *Sci. Rep.* **2013**, *3*, 2331–2341. [CrossRef] [PubMed]
29. Hofer, M.D.; Kuefer, R.; Varambally, S.; Li, H.; Ma, J.; Shapiro, G.I.; Gschwend, J.E.; Hautmann, R.E.; Sanda, M.G.; Giehl, K.; et al. The role of metastasis-associated protein 1 in prostate cancer progression. *Cancer Res.* **2004**, *64*, 825–829. [CrossRef]
30. Kumar, A.; Dhar, S.; Campanelli, G.; Butt, N.A.; Schallheim, J.M.; Gomez, C.R.; Levenson, A.S. MTA1 drives malignant progression and bone metastasis in prostate cancer. *Mol. Oncol.* **2018**, *12*, 1596–1607. [CrossRef]
31. Kumar, A.; Dholakia, K.; Sikorska, G.; Martinez, L.A.; Levenson, A.S. MTA1-Dependent Anticancer Activity of Gnetin C in Prostate Cancer. *Nutrients* **2019**, *11*, 2096. [CrossRef]
32. Morgan, T.M.; Koreckij, T.D.; Corey, E. Targeted therapy for advanced prostate cancer: Inhibition of the PI3K/Akt/mTOR pathway. *Curr. Cancer Drug. Targets* **2009**, *9*, 237–249. [CrossRef]
33. Chang, L.; Graham, P.H.; Ni, J.; Hao, J.; Bucci, J.; Cozzi, P.J.; Li, Y. Targeting PI3K/Akt/mTOR signaling pathway in the treatment of prostate cancer radioresistance. *Crit. Rev. Oncol. Hematol.* **2015**, *96*, 507–517. [CrossRef] [PubMed]
34. Dhar, S.; Kumar, A.; Li, K.; Tzivion, G.; Levenson, A.S. Resveratrol regulates PTEN/Akt pathway through inhibition of MTA1/HDAC unit of the NuRD complex in prostate cancer. *Biochim. Biophys. Acta* **2015**, *1853*, 265–275. [CrossRef] [PubMed]
35. Gadkari, K.; Kolhatkar, U.; Hemani, R.; Campanelli, G.; Cai, Q.; Kumar, A.; Levenson, A.S. Therapeutic Potential of Gnetin C in Prostate Cancer: A Pre-Clinical Study. *Nutrients* **2020**, *12*, 3631–3642. [CrossRef] [PubMed]
36. Espinoza, J.L.; Inaoka, P.T. Gnetin-C and other resveratrol oligomers with cancer chemopreventive potential. *Ann. New York Acad. Sci.* **2017**, *1403*, 5–14. [CrossRef]
37. Espinoza, J.L.; Elbadry, M.I.; Taniwaki, M.; Harada, K.; Trung, L.Q.; Nakagawa, N.; Takami, A.; Ishiyama, K.; Yamauchi, T.; Takenaka, K.; et al. The simultaneous inhibition of the mTOR and MAPK pathways with Gnetin-C induces apoptosis in acute myeloid leukemia. *Cancer Lett.* **2017**, *400*, 127–136. [CrossRef]
38. Seino, S.; Kimoto, T.; Yoshida, H.; Tanji, K.; Matsumiya, T.; Hayakari, R.; Seya, K.; Kawaguchi, S.; Tsuruga, K.; Tanaka, H.; et al. Gnetin C, a resveratrol dimer, reduces amyloid-beta 1–42 (Abeta42) production and ameliorates Abeta42-lowered cell viability in cultured SH-SY5Y human neuroblastoma cells. *Biomed. Res.* **2018**, *39*, 105–115. [CrossRef]
39. Kai, L.; Wang, J.; Ivanovic, M.; Chung, Y.T.; Laskin, W.B.; Schulze-Hoepfner, F.; Mirochnik, Y.; Satcher, R.L., Jr.; Levenson, A.S. Targeting prostate cancer angiogenesis through metastasis-associated protein 1 (MTA1). *Prostate* **2011**, *71*, 268–280. [CrossRef]
40. Dhar, S.; Kumar, A.; Gomez, C.R.; Akhtar, I.; Hancock, J.C.; Lage, J.M.; Pound, C.R.; Levenson, A.S. MTA1-activated Epi-microRNA-22 regulates E-cadherin and prostate cancer invasiveness. *FEBS Lett.* **2017**, *591*, 924–933. [CrossRef]
41. Dias, S.J.; Li, K.; Rimando, A.M.; Dhar, S.; Mizuno, C.S.; Penman, A.D.; Levenson, A.S. Trimethoxy-resveratrol and piceatannol administered orally suppress and inhibit tumor formation and growth in prostate cancer xenografts. *Prostate* **2013**, *73*, 1135–1146. [CrossRef]
42. Joshi, T.; Patel, I.; Kumar, A.; Donovan, V.; Levenson, A.S. Grape Powder Supplementation Attenuates Prostate Neoplasia Associated with Pten Haploinsufficiency in Mice Fed High-Fat Diet. *Mol. Nutr. Food Res.* **2020**, *64*, e2000326. [CrossRef]
43. Kapetanovic, I.M.; Muzzio, M.; Huang, Z.; Thompson, T.N.; McCormick, D.L. Pharmacokinetics, oral bioavailability, and metabolic profile of resveratrol and its dimethylether analog, pterostilbene, in rats. *Cancer Chemother. Pharmacol.* **2011**, *68*, 593–601. [CrossRef] [PubMed]
44. Tani, H.; Hikami, S.; Iizuna, S.; Yoshimatsu, M.; Asama, T.; Ota, H.; Kimura, Y.; Tatefuji, T.; Hashimoto, K.; Higaki, K. Pharmacokinetics and safety of resveratrol derivatives in humans after oral administration of melinjo (*Gnetum gnemon* L.) seed extract powder. *J. Agric. Food Chem.* **2014**, *62*, 1999–2007. [CrossRef] [PubMed]
45. Nakagami, Y.; Suzuki, S.; Espinoza, J.L.; Vu Quang, L.; Enomoto, M.; Takasugi, S.; Nakamura, A.; Nakayama, T.; Tani, H.; Hanamura, I.; et al. Immunomodulatory and Metabolic Changes after Gnetin-C Supplementation in Humans. *Nutrients* **2019**, *11*, 1403. [CrossRef] [PubMed]
46. Ota, H.; Akishita, M.; Tani, H.; Tatefuji, T.; Ogawa, S.; Iijima, K.; Eto, M.; Shirasawa, T.; Ouchi, Y. trans-Resveratrol in Gnetum gnemon protects against oxidative-stress-induced endothelial senescence. *J. Nat. Prod.* **2013**, *76*, 1242–1247. [CrossRef]
47. Kato, H.; Samizo, M.; Kawabata, R.; Takano, F.; Ohta, T. Stilbenoids from the melinjo (*Gnetum gnemon* L.) fruit modulate cytokine production in murine Peyer's patch cells ex vivo. *Planta Med.* **2011**, *77*, 1027–1034. [CrossRef] [PubMed]
48. Lee, J.; Jung, E.; Lim, J.; Lee, J.; Hur, S.; Kim, S.S.; Lim, S.; Hyun, C.G.; Kim, Y.S.; Park, D. Involvement of nuclear factor-kappaB in the inhibition of pro-inflammatory mediators by pinosylvin. *Planta Med.* **2006**, *72*, 801–806. [CrossRef]

49. Clarke, J.O.; Mullin, G.E. A review of complementary and alternative approaches to immunomodulation. *Nutr. Clin. Pract.* **2008**, *23*, 49–62. [CrossRef] [PubMed]
50. Pradhan, R.; Chatterjee, S.; Hembram, K.C.; Sethy, C.; Mandal, M.; Kundu, C.N. Nano formulated Resveratrol inhibits metastasis and angiogenesis by reducing inflammatory cytokines in oral cancer cells by targeting tumor associated macrophages. *J. Nutr. Biochem.* **2021**, *92*, 108624. [CrossRef]
51. Vo, N.T.; Madlener, S.; Bago-Horvath, Z.; Herbacek, I.; Stark, N.; Gridling, M.; Probst, P.; Giessrigl, B.; Bauer, S.; Vonach, C.; et al. Pro- and anticarcinogenic mechanisms of piceatannol are activated dose dependently in MCF-7 breast cancer cells. *Carcinogenesis* **2010**, *31*, 2074–2081. [CrossRef]
52. Kresty, L.A.; Morse, M.A.; Morgan, C.; Carlton, P.S.; Lu, J.; Gupta, A.; Blackwood, M.; Stoner, G.D. Chemoprevention of esophageal tumorigenesis by dietary administration of lyophilized black raspberries. *Cancer Res.* **2001**, *61*, 6112–6119.
53. Narisawa, T.; Fukaura, Y.; Hasebe, M.; Nomura, S.; Oshima, S.; Inakuma, T. Prevention of N-methylnitrosourea-induced colon carcinogenesis in rats by oxygenated carotenoid capsanthin and capsanthin-rich paprika juice. *Proc. Soc. Exp. Biol. Med.* **2000**, *224*, 116–122. [CrossRef]
54. Bouayed, J.; Bohn, T. Exogenous antioxidants–Double-edged swords in cellular redox state: Health beneficial effects at physiologic doses versus deleterious effects at high doses. *Oxid. Med. Cell Longev.* **2010**, *3*, 228–237. [CrossRef] [PubMed]
55. Kato, E.; Tokunaga, Y.; Sakan, F. Stilbenoids isolated from the seeds of Melinjo (*Gnetum gnemon* L.) and their biological activity. *J. Agric. Food Chem.* **2009**, *57*, 2544–2549. [CrossRef] [PubMed]
56. Kunimasa, K.; Ohta, T.; Tani, H.; Kato, E.; Eguchi, R.; Kaji, K.; Ikeda, K.; Mori, H.; Mori, M.; Tatefuji, T.; et al. Resveratrol derivative-rich melinjo (*Gnetum gnemon* L.) seed extract suppresses multiple angiogenesis-related endothelial cell functions and tumor angiogenesis. *Mol. Nutr. Food Res.* **2011**, *55*, 1730–1734. [CrossRef] [PubMed]
57. Tatefuji, T.; Yanagihara, M.; Fukushima, S.; Hashimoto, K. Safety assessment of melinjo (*Gnetum gnemon* L.) seed extract: Acute and subchronic toxicity studies. *Food Chem. Toxicol.* **2014**, *67*, 230–235. [CrossRef]
58. Konno, H.; Kanai, Y.; Katagiri, M.; Watanabe, T.; Mori, A.; Ikuta, T.; Tani, H.; Fukushima, S.; Tatefuji, T.; Shirasawa, T. Melinjo (*Gnetum gnemon* L.) Seed Extract Decreases Serum Uric Acid Levels in Nonobese Japanese Males: A Randomized Controlled Study. *Evid. Based. Complement. Alternat. Med.* **2013**, *2013*, 589169. [CrossRef]
59. Espinoza, J.L.; An, D.T.; Trung, L.Q.; Yamada, K.; Nakao, S.; Takami, A. Stilbene derivatives from melinjo extract have antioxidant and immune modulatory effects in healthy individuals. *Integr. Mol. Med.* **2015**, *2*, 405–413.
60. Nair, A.B.; Jacob, S. A simple practice guide for dose conversion between animals and human. *J. Basic Clin. Pharm.* **2016**, *7*, 27–31. [CrossRef]
61. Riche, D.M.; McEwen, C.L.; Riche, K.D.; Sherman, J.J.; Wofford, M.R.; Deschamp, D.; Griswold, M. Analysis of safety from a human clinical trial with pterostilbene. *J. Toxicol.* **2013**, *2013*, 463595. [CrossRef]
62. Kumar, A.; Lin, S.-Y.; Dhar, S.; Rimando, A.M.; Levenson, A.S. Stilbenes inhibit androgen receptor expression in 22Rv1 castrate-resistant prostate cancer cells. *J. Med. Act. Plants* **2014**, *3*, 1–8.

cancers

MDPI

Review

Spice-Derived Bioactive Compounds Confer Colorectal Cancer Prevention via Modulation of Gut Microbiota

Marco Dacrema [1,†], Arif Ali [2,†], Hammad Ullah [1], Ayesha Khan [3], Alessandro Di Minno [1,4], Jianbo Xiao [5,6], Alice Maria Costa Martins [7] and Maria Daglia [1,6,*]

1 Department of Pharmacy, University of Napoli Federico II, Via D. Montesano 49, 80131 Naples, Italy
2 Postgraduate Program in Pharmacology, Federal University of Ceará, Fortaleza 60430372, Brazil
3 Department of Medicine, Combined Military Hospital Nowshera, Nowshera 24110, Pakistan
4 CEINGE-Biotecnologie Avanzate, Via Gaetano Salvatore 486, 80145 Naples, Italy
5 Department of Analytical and Food Chemistry, Faculty of Sciences, Universidade de Vigo, 32004 Ourense, Spain
6 International Research Center for Food Nutrition and Safety, Jiangsu University, Zhenjiang 212013, China
7 Department of Clinical and Toxicological Analysis, Federal University of Ceará, Fortaleza 60430372, Brazil
* Correspondence: maria.daglia@unina.it
† These authors contributed equally to this work.

Simple Summary: Colorectal cancer (CRC) is a highly prevalent form of cancer, and represents a serious, global, health threat. Available therapeutic approaches have failed to provide control over the increasing prevalence and incidence of CRC. In this context, CRC prevention may provide a fruitful strategy. Edible plants have the potential to alter numerous molecular pathways, which may fight against the pathogenesis of CRC, and the gut microbiota could represent this link between dietary factors and CRC incidence. Spices and their active principles are reported to alter the balance of gut microbial species by increasing eubiotic and decreasing dysbiotic strains. The present study is designed to highlight the cancer prevention potential of spices while focusing mainly on gut microbial modulation. Although several spices and their active components have shown CRC-preventing properties via gut microbial modulation, the literature is still very limited, and expanding the literature going forward is essential before any conclusion can be drawn.

Abstract: Colorectal cancer (CRC) is the second most frequent cause of cancer-related mortality among all types of malignancies. Sedentary lifestyles, obesity, smoking, red and processed meat, low-fiber diets, inflammatory bowel disease, and gut dysbiosis are the most important risk factors associated with CRC pathogenesis. Alterations in gut microbiota are positively correlated with colorectal carcinogenesis, as these can dysregulate the immune response, alter the gut's metabolic profile, modify the molecular processes in colonocytes, and initiate mutagenesis. Changes in the daily diet, and the addition of plant-based nutraceuticals, have the ability to modulate the composition and functionality of the gut microbiota, maintaining gut homeostasis and regulating host immune and inflammatory responses. Spices are one of the fundamental components of the human diet that are used for their bioactive properties (i.e., antimicrobial, antioxidant, and anti-inflammatory effects) and these exert beneficial effects on health, improving digestion and showing anti-inflammatory, immunomodulatory, and glucose- and cholesterol-lowering activities, as well as possessing properties that affect cognition and mood. The anti-inflammatory and immunomodulatory properties of spices could be useful in the prevention of various types of cancers that affect the digestive system. This review is designed to summarize the reciprocal interactions between dietary spices and the gut microbiota, and highlight the impact of dietary spices and their bioactive compounds on colorectal carcinogenesis by targeting the gut microbiota.

Keywords: dietary spices; gut microbiota; colorectal cancer; prevention

Citation: Dacrema, M.; Ali, A.; Ullah, H.; Khan, A.; Di Minno, A.; Xiao, J.; Martins, A.M.C.; Daglia, M. Spice-Derived Bioactive Compounds Confer Colorectal Cancer Prevention via Modulation of Gut Microbiota. *Cancers* **2022**, *14*, 5682. https://doi.org/10.3390/cancers14225682

Academic Editor: Anupam Bishayee

Received: 27 July 2022
Accepted: 17 November 2022
Published: 19 November 2022

1. Introduction

Colorectal cancer (CRC) is the most prevalent form of carcinoma, and represents a leading component of the global health burden. Advancements in treatment methods, colonoscopy, and avoidance of risk factors, such as smoking and red meat consumption, have contributed to a decline in CRC cases over the last three decades in the United States [1,2]. However, similar declines have only been observed in developed countries [3]. Despite innovative strategies of treatment and diagnosis, CRC remains the third most common cancer and the second leading cause of mortality across the globe. In the year 2018 alone, 1.8 million new CRC cases were recorded including 881,000 deaths [4]. CRC cases may rise to 2.5 million by the year 2035 [3]. The modifiable risk factors for CRC include obesity [5], cigarette smoking [6], heavy alcohol use [7], poor diet [8], and a sedentary lifestyle [9]. The genetic contribution towards CRC is in the range of 12–35% as demonstrated in twin and family studies [10,11]. While 60–65% of cases arise sporadically without any family history of CRC [12]. This sizeable sporadic contribution to the instigation of CRC shows the significance of environmental factors, which play a large role in causing CRC [13]. Among environmental factors, infectious agents are responsible for 15 percent of all cancers [14]. Colorectal carcinogenesis is a process involving years of development, possibly taking decades. In such scenarios, early life risk factors and lifestyle modification are pertinent contributors [15]. The current rise of CRC in the young adult population in the US is alarming [2], and this supports the concept that early life risk factors provide a major impact on CRC carcinogenesis [16].

The human microflora counts around thirty trillion bacteria without considering fungi and viruses. The microbiota is not only altered by the environment but also by the relationship between the host and the symbiotic organisms [17]. The total number of microbial cells is 10 times greater than that of human somatic cells [18–22] and these include over 1000 different species of bacteria populating our gut. Most of these belong to the *Firmicutes* and *Bacteroides* phyla and are linked to the protection of the host, as they can produce metabolites and bioproducts promoting a protective effect against different pathologies. The dietary compounds and vitamins produced by these bacteria are considered protective elements against the infiltration of gut pathogens and the development of pathologies [23–25]. The impairment of the microbiota could lead to dysbiosis, and several studies sustain this link between tumorigenesis and microbiome diversity, thanks to the combination of next-generation sequencing and computational analysis [26–31]. A well-regulated microbiome is essential for maintaining the homeostasis of the metabolism and immune response, in fact, several clinical studies underline how the immunotherapeutic response could be influenced by the gut microbiome, suggesting that treatments could be enhanced or depressed according to the gut microbiota status [31–34].

Another important role of the microbiome is the recognition of the conserved regions of Gram-negative pathogenic bacteria after the production of immunoglobin G antibodies [35,36]. However, the composition and the alteration of the microbiota are also related to different host life stages and diets [37–41]. It is calculated that 20% of all cancers are related to dysbiosis, and with this perspective, probiotics could be used as therapeutic agents to re-establish the normal microbial environment, enhancing the immune response to counteract tumor growth. Literature data have shown that gut microbiota may provide the missing link between dietary factors and CRC incidence [42]. Some dietary components, such as saturated fats, processed carbohydrates, red meat, and ultra-processed food can affect the gut microbiota and lead to inflammation [43], and inflammation is a known factor for 20–30% of CRC cases and is acknowledged as the principal driver of tumorigenesis [44–46].

While chemotherapy and radiotherapy are the key approaches employed for the treatment of patients with cancer, both are associated with serious adverse events that may outweigh their therapeutic benefits in certain cases. Drug resistance is another concern that is very common for anticancer therapies and may result in failure of the treatment [47]. Nature has provided a range of preventive and therapeutic agents with the potential to fight against the most devastating chronic disorders including cancer [48,49]. Edible plants containing phytochemicals are known to alter numerous molecular pathways that may impact anticancer effects (i.e., oxidative stress, inflammatory cascade, apoptosis, epigenetic regulation, p53 signaling pathway, nuclear factor kappa-light-chain-enhancer of activated B cells (NF-kB) pathway, mitogen-activated protein kinases (MAPKs), proteasome pathway, insulin-like growth factor-I mediated signal transduction pathway, matrix metalloproteinases (MMPs), vascular endothelial growth factor, Hippo signaling pathway, phosphoinositide 3-kinase–protein kinase B–mammalian target of a rapamycin signaling pathway (PI3K/Akt/mTOR), cyclooxygenase-2, and the Janus kinase–signal transducer and activator of transcription signaling pathway) [50–57].

Some spices such as turmeric, black cumin, ginger, ginseng, garlic, saffron, and black pepper, are potential sources of cancer prevention owing to their natural bioactive compounds (curcumin, thymoquinone, piperine, and capsaicin) [58–60]. About 80% of the world population is currently relying on phytomedicine for their primary healthcare [61], in fact, these natural products are commonly considered a safer alternative for patients, if compared to systematic chemotherapeutic drugs although their scientific validity and efficacy are currently under analysis [62,63]. These spices and herbs have been used for thousands of years in small amounts thanks to their beneficial effects. In particular, curcuma, ginger, garlic, clove, chili pepper, saffron, and flaxseed seem to inhibit CRC growth thanks to their chemotherapeutic roles [58,64–66]. CRC development is sustained by cancer stem cells (CSC), which are self-renewal and pluripotent stem cells able to promote carcinogenesis and the formation of heterogeneous tumors [67]. Increasing evidence sustains the link between microbiota alterations and mature tumor formation. In particular, their metabolome [68] can promote pro or anti-carcinogenic actions. The preservation of the CSC is essential and mediated by several phytochemicals such as curcumin, quercetin, lycopene, cinnamic acid, resveratrol, sibilin, and epigallocatechin-3-gallate [EGCG] [69]. The main pathways involved in the regulation of the CSC phenotype are Hedgehog, Notch, and Wnt/β-catenin [70], which are modulated thanks to the colonic microbiota transformation of phytochemicals. At the same time, these substances can modify the microbiota population. Thus, the diet can change the colonic bacteria and vice versa in a triangular rapport where is involved CRC formation.

The previous similar reviews [71,72] focused their attention on the molecular basis of CRC linking the antioxidant/anti-inflammatory activities of these spices or other diet-derived phytochemicals and CRC pathogenesis. In some cases, recent articles also considered the relationship between the dietary compounds and the gut microbiota-derived metabolites without considering that these two aspects are essential for CRC prevention. In fact, year after year, it is clear how new discoveries on CRC lead to the hypothesis that the anti-inflammatory and antioxidant activities of herbs and spices, normally consumed in the diet, are not the only mechanism of action that intervenes in CRC prevention. The role of microbiota, in fact, seems to be crucial in the modulation of the microbiome and control of the CSC population. The aim of this review is to focus on spice-derived bioactive compounds influencing gut microbiota strains, with special reference to CRC prevention.

2. Gut Dysbiosis and Carcinogenesis

The maintenance of healthy gut microbiota during an individual's lifespan, and any potential loss of diversity, is strictly connected with their diet. The progression of a disease could also involve the long-term depletion of specific groups of bacteria, which could be induced by lifestyle changes and other societal factors [37,38]. Healthy conditions are completely different from those of patients affected by dysbiosis. In the first case, the immune system can easily recognize pathogenic microbes, promoting their consequent elimination [73], most gut bacteria are non-pathogenic, and they offer an important defense role in inhibiting colonization by pathogens. The immune cells (i.e., dendritic cells, macrophages, and phagocytes) are involved in the gut microbiome and are essential for the recognition of pathogenic bacteria [74]. Healthy individuals could suffer either mild or severe issues if bacteria translocate across the epithelial mucosa. Kupffer cells may be involved, after the production of endotoxins and viable or dead bacteria. However, in the case of dysbiosis, the commensal bacteria may also spread into extra-intestinal sites and tissues. Obviously, this event can promote septic shocks, sepsis, organ failure, and death [75] over short-term periods. The dysregulation of the microbiota is associated with various pathologies, and this could be also induced using antibiotics which are known to reduce microbiotal diversity. The state of the art sustains that diabetes types 1 and 2, obesity, arthritis, Crohn's disease, arthritis, and celiac disease are linked with the deregulation of the microbiotal metabolism and inflammation, which promotes the incidence of these pathologies [75–80].

Obviously, the microbiota is strongly involved in the absorption and metabolization of nutrients, thanks to the expression of a great number of genes, which are not expressed in our own organism. The impairment and the downregulation of these processes can promote inflammation, which may also lead to cancer in the longer-term [81,82]. The increased incidence and prevalence of cancer over recent decades are mainly due to a higher exposure to cancer-causing molecules, but also to high-fat diets, which promote dysbiosis and the inflammation process [78]. The microbial alteration could be one of the main factors, which contribute to carcinogenesis [83], in fact, different studies have supported the importance of the relationship between carcinogenesis and lifestyle. The inflammation process remains a driving force in the progression of cancer, promoting its development through the production of inflammatory cytokines [84], with microbial dysbiosis leading to increased concentrations of interleukin (IL)-1, 6, 10, and tumor necrosis factor alpha (TNF-α). The production of IL-10 is essential for the body's elimination of cancer, in fact it is considered the most effective anti-inflammatory cytokine involved in tumorigenesis [85–87]. Wnt signaling is involved with NF-kB and MAPKs, which together can lead to an increase in oxidative stress and inhibition of apoptosis [88,89]. Animal and human studies have shown that bacteria such as *Fusobacteria, Alistipes, Porphyromonadaceae, Coriobacteridae, Staphylococcaceae, Akkermansia* species and *Methanobacteriales* are predominantly increased in CRC, while *Lactobacillus, Bifidobacterium, Faecalibacterium species, Treponema, Roseburia,* and *Ruminococcus* are known to reduce [90].

The production of toxins can also influence the tumorigenesis process, with *Helicobacter pylori, Escherichia coli,* and *Shigella flexneri,* for example, inducing double-strand DNA cuts causing apoptosis or alteration of the cell cycle [91]. Starting from *E. coli*, colibactin and cytolethal distengin toxins induce genomic instability, promoting breaks in the host's DNA and tumorigenesis [89]. *S. Flexneri* instead produces cysteine proteases, such as virulence gene A and the inisitol phosphate phosphatase D, with the final response, in this case, being necrosis, with the development of cancer and cell death due to the degradation of the *p53* gene and host damage [92]. *Fusobacterium nucleatum* disrupts the junction of β-catenin through the effector adhesin A (FadA); moreover, it is responsible for the production of virulence factor (Fap2) but in this case, it is through the mediation of blocks of natural killer cells (NK cells) through the binding of the NK inhibitory receptor [92–94]. *Bacteroides fragilis* produces a toxin responsible for DNA damage after the production of reactive oxygen species and hydrogen peroxide [95], the same is the case for *Enterococcus fecalis*, which is responsible for the production of extracellular superoxide, able to trigger mutations in host DNA [55]. Finally, *Lactobacillus casei* is responsible for the production of the ferrichrome siderophore, which activates c-Jun N-terminal kinase (JNK) signaling and consequent apoptosis [96].

3. Gut Microbial Alteration, Chemotherapy, and Cancer Prevention

Our gut contains trillions of microorganisms interacting with the host, and it is important to underline their essential role in bodily function. Digestion, secretion of metabolites, and the intervention of the immune system as cited above, are strictly related to the microbiota. Bacteria-free mouse models underline how dysbiosis is related to immunoglobulin A, lymphadenitis, and the absence of mucus [97,98]. Cancers very often become resistant to the drugs most used for their treatment [99,100], and unfortunately in 90% of cases, this phenomenon is responsible for the patient's death [101–103]. Obviously, this problem requires attention and time to promote the development of new treatments, and the gut microbiota in particular may also influence the efficacy of antitumor therapies [104].

The negative impact of the absence of a microbiota is becoming clearer year after year, with different studies on mice treated with antibiotics underlining the efficacy of chemotherapy and immunotherapy [105]. Moreover, it is possible that the efficacy of chemotherapy treatments may be heightened under normal conditions, promoting the destruction of cancer through the intervention of T-lymphocytes and myeloid cells. The antibiotic treatments applied in certain mice studies [106] can impair the presence of bacteria and the production of cytokines, however further clinical studies are required to confirm these preliminary findings. The combination of metabolomics and metagenomics underlines the importance of the gut-brain axis [107], which regulates the composition of the gut flora through the production of neuro-hormones and hormones. The case of cyclophosphamide is particularly interesting, a chemotherapeutic drug able to promote the T-cell immune response in the presence of commensal microbiota, which translocates from the spleen to the lymph nodes promoting their anticancer effect [94,108]. It appears that *Bifidobacterium* can enhance dendritic cells, promoting the activation of T CD8-positive cells and enhancing the efficiency of anti-programmed death ligand (PDL-1) therapy [109]. The five-year survival rate was found to have increased by 80% for 1000 sarcoma patients treated with killed microorganism activate (*Serratia* and *Streptococcus*) [110]. The T lymphocytes associated with antigen 4 (CTLA-4) seem to have anticancer effects, promoting the production of CTLA-4 inhibitors. In the absence of CTLA-4, germ-free mice registered a positive response against cancer following an exposure to *Bacteroides* [111] underlying the anticancer effects of these molecules.

Only a few studies to date appear to sustain the relationship between cancer prevention and the microbiota. The production of short-chain fatty acids (SCFAs) by microbiota (i.e., *Propionibacteria* such as *P. freudenreichii*) [112–114] has an anti-cancer effect [115], inhibiting the deacetylases of cancer cells. Indeed, a lower concentration of butyrate is registered in cancer patients. The production of SCFAs stimulates the production of IL-18, promoting the healing process in mucosal tissues [116]. Probiotic administration also exhibits interesting effects, as it seems to trigger the immune response with an antitumor effect. Gram-negative bacteria activate TLR4 and T-cells, with *Salmonella enterica,* for example, appearing to be very effective against cervical cancer [117]. Finally, *L. casei* stimulates apoptosis in cancer cells thanks to ferricrome production, through the activation of the JNK signaling pathway [89].

4. Spice-Derived Phytochemicals and CRC Prevention by Modulating Gut Bacteria for In Vivo Studies

Predominantly used as flavoring, coloring, and aromatic agents in beverages and foods, spices are gaining attention for their potential health benefits. The nutritional, antioxidant, anti-inflammatory, antimicrobial, and other medicinal uses of spices have paramount importance [118]. Numerous health benefits of these food adjuncts have been recognized by pioneering experimental studies involving both in vitro and in vivo studies over the past few decades, including their antioxidant and anti-inflammatory potential, digestive stimulant effects, hypolipidemic actions, anti-lithogenic properties, antidiabetic influence, antimutagenic, and anticarcinogenic potentials [119]. Studies have shown that spices and their bioactive compounds may inhibit or even activate pathways related to cell division, proliferation, and detoxification, in addition to immunomodulatory and anti-inflammatory effects [120]. The chemopreventive properties of spice-derived phytochemicals are mainly attributed to the regulation of B-cell leukemia/lymphoma 2 protein, K-ras, MMP pathways, apoptotic pathway, and caspase activation [71]. Considering the scope of the current review, a link between gut microbial modulation by spices and the prevention of CRC pathogenesis has been comprehensively discussed in the sections below. Table 1 summarizes these studies, highlighting the effects of spice-derived phytochemicals on gut microbiota and their ultimate effect on intestinal health. Figures 1 and 2 illustrate the modulation of gut microbes with spices as part of CRC prevention.

Table 1. Summary of anti-colon cancer effects of spice phytocompounds/phytocomplex by modulation of gut microbiota in in vivo studies.

Spice-Derived Compounds	In vivo Study Model	Dose	Treatment Duration	Effect on Gut Microbiota	Comments	References
Curcumin	Mice/Human	100 mg/kg	15 days	↑*Lactobacilli* and *Bifidobacterium*; ↓*Enterococci*, *Enterobacteria*, *Prevotellaceae*, and *Coriobacterales*	May produce immune modulation and anti-tumor effects in the colon	[121]
Curcumin	Mice	NA (meta-analysis)	NA	↑*Bacteroides*, *Rikenellaceae*, *Alistipes*, and *Bacteroidaceae*; ↓*Prevotella* and *Prevotellaceae*	*Prevotella* has been observed as higher in patients with CRC	[122]
Curcumin	Pilot study	1000 mg of curcumin + 1.25 mg black pepper	8 weeks	↓*Ruminococus* and *Blautia*; ↑*Clostridium* and *Enterobacter*	*Ruminococus* species have been observed as higher in patients with CRC	[123]
Curcumin nanoparticles	Mice	0.2 *w*/*w*	7 days	↑number of butyrate-producing bacteria and feal butyrate levels; ↓NF-kB activation in colonic epithelial cells	Increased SCFA production may reduce inflammatory processes and intestinal mucosa and promote antitumor effects	[124]
Curcumin	Mice	8 mg/kg/day–162 mg/kg/day	20 days	↓*Coriobacterales*; ↑*Lactobacillales*	Decreased oxidative and inflammatory stresses, and hyper-immune activation	[125]
Curcumin	Mice	20 mg/kg, 100 mg/kg, and 200 mg/kg	10 days	↓*Enterobacteria* and *Enterococci*; ↑*Lactobacilli* and *Bifidobacteria*	Suppressed pro-inflammatory processes and promoted anti-inflammatory effects	[126]
Ginger	Mice	500 mg/kg daily	7 days	↓*Lactobacillus murinus*, *Lachnospiraceae bacterium*, and *Ruminiclostridium* specie KB18	Reduced the expression of mRNA of IL-6 and iNOS	[127]

Table 1. *Cont.*

Spice-Derived Compounds	In vivo Study Model	Dose	Treatment Duration	Effect on Gut Microbiota	Comments	References
Ginger	Mice	50 mg/kg	4 weeks	Altered the abundance of *Helicobacter* and *Peptococcaceae* species	Ameliorated weight loss, colon shortening, inflammatory processes, intestinal barrier dysfunction, and gut dysbiosis	[128]
Daikenchuto, Japanese traditional herbal medicine (processed ginger, ginseng, and Chinese or Japanese pepper)	Human colonic microbiota	0.5% wt	48 h	↑*Bifidobacterium adolescentis*	Bifidogenic effects may have beneficial effects on colon	[129]
Ginger polysaccharides	Mice	200 mg/Kg	1,3,5,7 and 9-day dose	Balancing *Firmicutes/Bacteroidetes* ratio; ↑*Lactobacillus* and *Verrucomicrobiota;* ↓*Proteobacteria* and *Bacteroides*	Reduced the level of colonic pro-inflammatory mediators (TNF-α, IL-6, IL-1β, IL-17A, and IFN-γ), restored gut barrier function, and restrained apoptosis	[130]
Ginger juice	Healthy volunteers	500 mg/Kg/day	7 days	↓*Ruminococcus_1* and *Ruminococcus_2* and *Prevotella/Bacteroides* ratio; ↑*Proteobacteria, Faecalibacterium*, and *Firmicutes/Bacteroidetes* ratio	Promoted anti-inflammatory effects in intestinal mucosa	[131]
Garlic polysaccharides	Mice	NA (systematic review)	NA	↑*Bacteroidetes* and *Actinobacteria;* ↓*Firmicutes/Bacteroidetes* ratio	Inhibited the expression of inflammatory mediators (TNF-α, IL-1β, and IL-6); Increased colon length and decrease in the disease activity and histological score of colitis	[132]

Table 1. *Cont.*

Spice-Derived Compounds	In vivo Study Model	Dose	Treatment Duration	Effect on Gut Microbiota	Comments	References
Propyl-propane thiosulfonate	Mice	0.01, 0.05, 0.1, 0.5, 1, and 10 mg/kg day	5 days	↑*Firmicutes/Bacteroidetes* ratio; ↓*Actinobacteria*	Improved intestinal epithelial barrier integrity and reduced the expression of pro-inflammatory mediators (TNF-α, IL-1β, IL-8, IL-17, and iNOS)	[133]
Clove oil	Quails	0.75 and 1.5 mL/Kg	42 days	↓*Eescherechia coli*, and *Salmonella* species	Improved body weight, activities of antioxidant enzymes, lipid profile, and intestinal bacterial diversity	[134]
Capsaicin	Healthy adults	10 mg/day	6 weeks	↑*Firmicutes/Bacteriodes* ratio and *Faecalibacterium* abundance	Decreased inflammatory processes and risk factors for CRC	[135]
Crocin-I	Mice	20 mg/kg and 40 mg/kg	3 weeks	↓*Firmicutes*; ↑*Bacteroidetes*	Increased α-diversity of microbes in the cecal contents	[136]
Crocetin	Mice	10 mg/kg	1 week	↑*Mediterraneibacter* and *Akkermansia*; ↓*Dubosiella*, *Muribaculaceae*, *Paramuribaculum*, *Allobaculum*, *Parasutterella*, *Duncaniella*, *Stoquefichus*, *Coriobacteriaceae* UCG-002, and *Candidatus*.	Promoted inflammation with disturbed intestinal homeostasis	[137]
Saffron	Amnion of the *Gallus gallus* eggs	1% CFWE, 2% CFWE, 5% CFWE, 10% CFWE.	Incubation until 21 days	↓*Lactobacillus* and *Clostridium*	Disrupted cecal microbiome and brush border membrane functionality	[138]
Flaxseed	Mice	10% FS diet	1 week	↓*Akkermansia muciniphila*; ↑*Prevotella* species	Decreased susceptibility to gut-associated diseases including inflammatory pathologies and cancer	[139]

Table 1. *Cont.*

Spice-Derived Compounds	In vivo Study Model	Dose	Treatment Duration	Effect on Gut Microbiota	Comments	References
Flaxseed oligosaccharides	Mice	50 mg/kg day, 100 mg/kg day, and 200 mg/kg day	14 days	↓*Clostridiales*	Increased colon length, improved colonic histology, decreased oxidative stress markers (malondialdehyde and myeloperoxidase), suppressed pro-inflammatory cytokines (TNF-α, IL-1β, and IL-6), and increased anti-inflammatory cytokine (IL-10); Increased propionic and butyric acids	[140]
Flaxseed oil	Pigs	Flaxseed oil (FO, purity ≥ 98%)	3 weeks	↓*Spirochaetes*; ↑*Actinobacteria*, *Bifidobacterium* and *Blautia*	Decreased intestinal expression of MyD88, NF-κB, TNF-α, and IL-10 genes	[141]
Flaxseed	Mice		12 weeks	↑*Prevotella*, *Ruminococcus*, *Clostridiales*, and *Paraprevotella*	Increased butyrate concentration; Ameliorated the adherent-invasive *E. coli* induced intestinal inflammation	[142]

Colorectal cancer, CRC; short chain fatty acids, SCFAs; nuclear factor kappa-light-chain-enhancer of activated B cells, NF-kB; tumor necrosis factor alpha, TNF-α; interleukin-6, IL-6; interleukin-1β, IL-1β; interleukin-17A, IL-17A; interferon-γ, IFN-γ; inducible nitric oxide synthase, iNOS.

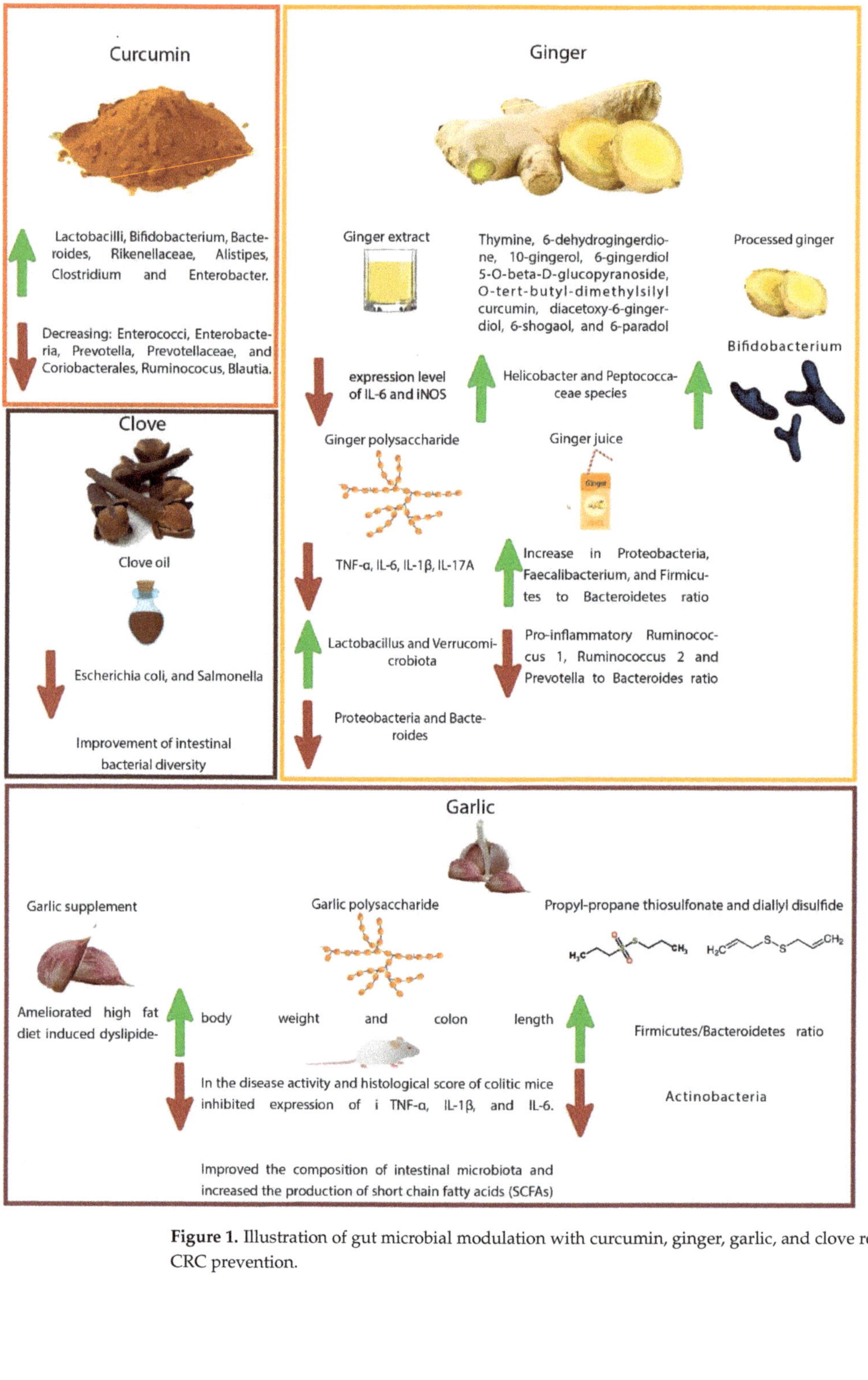

Figure 1. Illustration of gut microbial modulation with curcumin, ginger, garlic, and clove regards to CRC prevention.

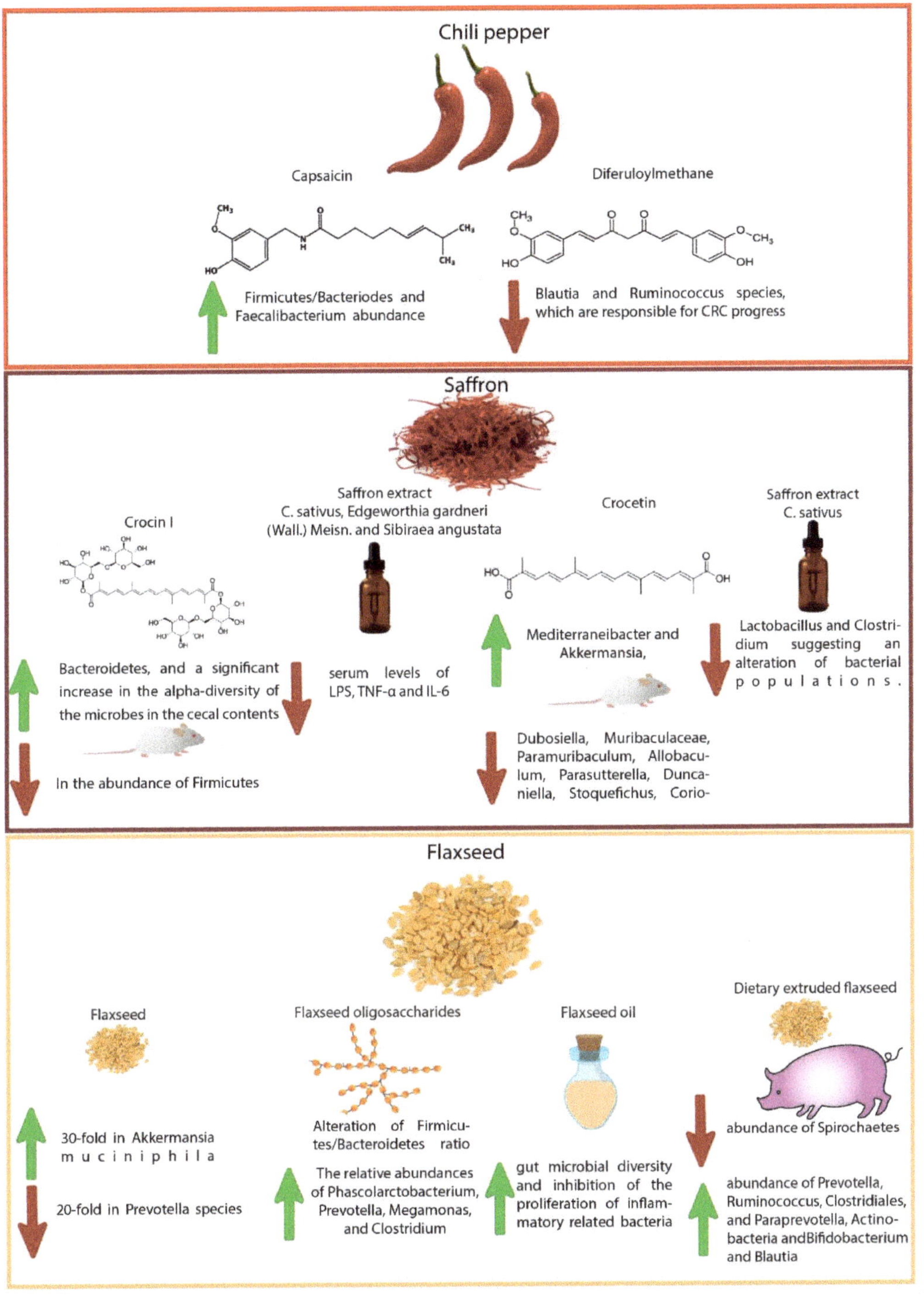

Figure 2. Illustration of gut microbial modulation with chili pepper, saffron, and flaxseed regards to CRC prevention.

4.1. Turmeric-Derived Compounds

Curcumin, derived from the roots of the plant known as *Curcuma longa* L., is a natural product that has been extensively studied for the prevention and treatment of cancer [143,144]. Curcumin exerts its anticancer action via various mechanisms, e.g., by inducing apoptosis, thereby inhibiting cell proliferation of cancerous cells, activating caspase, and inducing the expression of anti-oncogenes such as *p53* [145,146]. Interruptions in mucosal barrier function play a significant role in CRC. The persistent inflammation of, and oxidative stress within, intestinal epithelial cells are the most evident causes of colorectal carcinogenesis. Dysfunctions in the mucosal barrier further synergize with this vicious progression of carcinogenesis [147]. The circulating lipopolysaccharide (LPS), due to dysfunction in the gut microbiota, may be a possible cause for the development of chronic inflammatory disorders. The translocation of LPS into systemic circulation occurs due to a dysfunction in the intestinal barrier [148]. The western style diet has been reported to increase intestinal permeability and may be responsible for intestinal barrier dysfunction [149]. Many studies have demonstrated that pretreatment with curcumin attenuates LPS-induced inflammatory cytokines by modulating the p38 MAPK pathway. Curcumin exerts this action most likely on intestinal epithelial cells, thereby reducing intestinal barrier dysfunction [150,151].

The higher concentration of curcumin in the gastrointestinal tract after oral administration suggests that it may regulate the gut microbiota, resulting in various pharmacological actions despite its low systemic bioavailability [121,152]. The present data suggest that curcumin is metabolized by the gut microbiota into different metabolites through diverse pathways, including demethoxylation, hydroxylation, and demethylation. Moreover, these metabolites have been found to be more active compared to the parent molecule curcumin. The higher concentration of curcumin in the gastrointestinal tract after oral administration shows its preferential impact on gut microbiota composition. On the other hand, the processing of the parent molecule transforms it into its bioactive metabolites, resulting in its various therapeutic and pharmacological actions [153].

As evidenced in many studies, curcumin shows a direct influence on gut microbiota by increasing the ratio of beneficial bacteria compared to pathological ones [154–156]. An in vivo study has shown a significant effect of curcumin on numerous bacterial families in the gut including *Prevotellaceae*, *Rikenellaceae*, and *Bacteroidaceae* [155]. Curcumin administration considerably alters the ratios of beneficial and pathogenic intestinal microflora by enhancing the number and diversity of *Lactobacilli* and *Bifidobacterium*, and decreasing the bacterial load of *Enterococci*, *Enterobacteria*, *Prevotellaceae*, and *Coriobacterales*, thus explaining its immune modulation and anti-tumor effects in the colon [121]. Curcumin administration to mice significantly increased the number of *Bacteroides*, *Rikenellaceae*, *Alistipes*, and *Bacteroidaceae* while decreasing the number of *Prevotella* and *Prevotellaceae* [122]. The number of *Prevotella* has been observed to be higher in patients with CRC, compared to cancer-free patients [157].

In patients with CRC, increased levels of *Ruminococus* species of bacteria have been noticed in the gut microbiota [158,159]. Interestingly, a pilot study elucidated that curcumin, when used as a dietary supplement, reduced *Ruminococus* and *Blautia* bacterial species, and increased the population of *Clostridium* and *Enterobacter* in gut microbiota [123]. The suppressive activity of curcumin on gut microbiotal species shows its anticancer potential in preventing CRC. Through modulating gut microbiota, the administration of nanoparticles of curcumin in mice has demonstrated increased numbers of butyrate-producing bacteria, increased fecal butyrate levels, and suppressed NF-kB activation, in colonic epithelial cells. Moreover, it also downregulated the expression of mucosal mRNA in inflammatory mediators [124].

Supplementation of rats with curcumin showed improvements in fecal microbes (reduced *Coriobacterales* and increased *Lactobacillales*), resulting in the regulation of the host immune system, which in turn lowered oxidative and inflammatory stresses, and hyper-immune activation, which may lower the incidence of inflammatory gastrointestinal disorders such as inflammatory bowel disease (IBD) [125]. Literature also reported the eradication of *H. pylori* production with curcumin treatment and its attachment to the human gastric adenocarcinoma cell lines die to its anti-adhesion properties [160–162]. Treatment of animals (infected with *Toxoplasma gondii*) with curcumin not only reduced the number of pro-inflammatory *Enterobacteria* and *Enterococci*, but also increased the abundance of anti-inflammatory *Lactobacilli* and *Bifidobacteria* [126]. Oral supplementation of curcumin alleviated acute inflammation of the small intestine by downregulating the Th1-type immune response and preventing bacterial translocation by maintaining the intestinal-barrier function [149]. It inhibited mRNA expression on the mucosa on inflammatory mediators and activated NF-kB in colon epithelial cells accompanied by enhanced butyrate-producing bacteria and fecal butyrate levels.

4.2. Ginger-Derived Compounds

Ginger rhizome (*Zingiber officinale* Roscoe) belonging to the plant family *Zingiberaceae*, is extensively used as a hot dietary spice in foods and drinks because of its distinctive flavor [163]. Ginger rhizome has a rich chemistry, containing phenolic compounds, terpenes, polysaccharides, organic acids, and raw fibers [164]. The volatile oil components of ginger include sesquiterpenes, zingerberene, curcumene, farnesene, and 40 different monoterpenoid hydrocarbons [165] while the main non-volatile active compounds of ginger include geingerols, shogoals, paradols and zingerone [166,167]. The active constituents [6]-shogaol and [6]-gingerol have shown anti-proliferative activity against various forms of gastrointestinal cancer [167].

As evidenced by numerous studies, ginger extract has a protective activity against ulcerative colitis, a chronic IBD of unknown pathology [168–170]. Recently Guo et al. [127] identified the mechanism by which ginger ameliorates dextran sulfate sodium (DSS) induced ulcerative colitis. They found that oral administration of ginger extract modulates the gut microbiota, where it reduces the population of pathogenic bacteria such as *Lactobacillus murinus*, *Lachnospiraceae bacterium 615*, and *Ruminiclostridium_sp. KB18*. Moreover, the ginger extract also reduces the expression level of mRNA of inflammatory cytokines, such as IL-6 and inducible nitric oxide synthase. These studies show that ginger most likely modulates the gut microbiota to reduce inflammation, consequently preventing CRC.

An in vivo study demonstrated a decrease in susceptibility to DSS-induced colitis in mice with ginger extract (containing 16-compounds including thymine, 6-dehydrogingerdione, 10-gingerol, 6-gingerdiol 5-O-β-D-glucopyranoside, O-tert-butyl-dimethylsilyl curcumin, diacetoxy-6-gingerdiol, 6-shogaol, and 6-paradol) following antibiotic exposure in early life [128]. Supplementation to mice with ginger extract for 4-weeks ameliorated weight loss, colon shortening, inflammatory cascade, intestinal barrier dysfunction, and gut dysbiosis. It increased the bacterial diversity and altered the abundance of *Helicobacter* and *Peptococcaceae* species, modulating gut microbial structure and composition adversely affected by antibiotic exposure. A Japanese traditional herbal medicine (Daikenchuto), containing processed ginger, ginseng, and Chinese or Japanese pepper, significantly promoted the growth of *Bifidobacterium adolescentis*, but not that of *E. coli* and *Fusobacterium nucleatum*, in human fecal samples, suggesting an in vitro bifidogenic effect that may contribute to the beneficial effects on colon [129]. Ginger polysaccharides relieved DSS-induced ulcerative colitis in mice via gut microbial modulation, maintaining intestinal barrier integrity [130]. Ginger polysaccharides reduced the level of colonic pro-inflammatory mediators such as TNF-α, IL-6, IL-1β, IL-17A, and interferon (IFN)-γ. In addition, ginger polysaccharides restored gut barrier function, restrained apoptosis, and modulated gut microbiota (by balancing *Firmicutes/Bacteroidetes* ratio, increasing *Lactobacillus* and *Verrucomicrobiota*, and decreasing *Proteobacteria* and *Bacteroides*). An intervention with ginger juice in healthy adults decreased the relative abundance of pro-inflammatory *Ruminococcus_1* and *Ruminococcus_2* and *Prevotella* to *Bacteroides* ratio, with an increase in *Proteobacteria*, *Faecalibacterium*, and *Firmicutes* to *Bacteroidetes* ratio [131].

4.3. Garlic-Derived Compounds

Garlic (*Allium sativum* L.), belonging to the plant family *Liliaceae*, is a widespread dietary spice consumed around the globe [171,172]. Garlic consists of various bioactive compounds such as saponins, phenolic compounds, organosulfur compounds, and polysaccharides [173]. The presence of bioactive organosulfur compounds in garlic raises the possibility of anticancer activity [174–177]. Garlic has a paradoxical effect on the gut microbiota, however, whole garlic supplementation has revealed that it increases the α-diversity of the gut microbiota and as a result ameliorated high-fat diet-induced dyslipidemia [178]. Similarly, the GarGIC Trial results showed that the administration of Kyolic aged garlic extract lowered blood pressure in hypertensive patients by reducing arterial stiffness, inflammation and improving the gut microbiotal profile [179]. The anticancer action of garlic has been explored by its interaction with multiple pathways in carcinogenesis. More experimental and clinical trials are necessary to identify the role of garlic in cancer and particularly in CRC via gut microbiota modulation.

A. sativum polysaccharides (200 or 400 mg/kg/day) demonstrated anti-inflammatory activities via modulation of gut microbiota in an experimental model of DSS-induced colitis [132]. Garlic polysaccharides increased body weight and colon length with a decrease in disease activity and histological scores of colitic mice as well as inhibiting the expression of inflammatory mediators i.e., TNF-α, IL-1β, and IL-6. Moreover, they improved the composition of intestinal microbiota and increased the production of SCFAs. The key intestinal microbial strains associated with the inflammatory intestinal conditions identified were *Muribaculaceae*, *Lachnospiraceae* NK4A136 group, *Lachnospiraceae*, *Helicobacter*, *Mucispirillum*, *Ruminococcus 1*, and *Ruminiclostridium 5*. Propyl-propane thiosulfonate (one of the biologically active compounds present in *A. sativum*) modulated immune responses, contributing to anti-inflammatory effects in experimental colitis [133]. The immunomodulatory effects of propyl-propane thiosulfonate were supported by reducing the in vitro production of pro-inflammatory cytokines (TNF-α, IL-1β, and IL-6) and downstream regulation of MAPK-signaling pathways (p44/42 ERK and p38), and in vivo by improving the intestinal epithelial barrier integrity, reducing the expression of pro-inflammatory mediators (TNF-α, IL-1β, IL-8, IL-17, and iNOS), and restoration of gut microbial alteration induced by DSS exposure (increased *Firmicutes/Bacteroidetes* ratio and decreased *Actinobacteria*). On the contrary, another study showed alteration of gut microbiota with diallyl disulfide and induction of fatty liver in the same fashion as caused by a high-fat diet [180].

4.4. Clove-Derived Compounds

Clove (*Syzygium aromaticum* (L.) Merr. and L.M.Perry) belongs to the *Myrtaceae* plant family, and is one of the oldest and most valuable dietary spices [181]. The major bioactive constituents of clove oil are eugenol (70–90%) eugenyl acetate, β-caryophyllene, and various sesquiterpenes [182]. Other phytochemicals from clove include bicornin, eugenitin, myricetin, gallic acid, methyl salicylate, methyl amayl ketone, vanillin, ellagic acid, kaempferol, stigmasterol, oleanolic acid, β-caryophyllene and crategolic acid [183]. Considering the broad phytochemistry and biological activities of clove, it has the therapeutic potential to prevent various types of cancers and other diseases [184].

Regarding the effect of clove against CRC, an active fraction of clove extract has demonstrated an anti-proliferative effect against CRC (HCT-116) cells. The active fraction of clove extract induced apoptosis in HCT-116 cell lines, autophagy and inhibited the phosphorylation of the PI3K/Akt/mTOR signaling pathway [185]. In another study, ethyl acetate extract of cloves demonstrated antitumor activity both in in vivo and in vitro models. The clove extract shows dose-dependent induction of apoptosis and has downregulated cell cycle proteins. The authors suggested that clove extract has the potential to be used as a therapeutic herb for treating CRC [186]. Similarly, eugenol has anti-inflammatory effects as observed in mice with DSS-induced colitis, where eugenol treatment has ameliorated the colonic inflammation and oxidative stress in the DSS group [187].

An intake of *S. aromaticum* oil 1.5 mL/kg in the diet administered to quails led to an improvement in body weight, activities of antioxidant enzymes, lipid profile, and intestinal bacterial diversity [134]. The coliforms, *E. coli*, and *Salmonella* species were found to be lowered in the ileal contents of quails supplemented with *S. aromaticum* oil, suggesting a reduction in intestinal pathogens, aiming to promote a healthy intestinal status.

4.5. Chili Pepper-Derived Compounds

Chili pepper belongs to the *Capsicum* genus, a member of the family Solanaceae. The use of chilies as complementary and alternative medicine in developing countries is rapidly increasing. Alkaloids are the most active compounds present in *Capsicum*, known as capsaicinoids, such as capsaicin, dihydrocapsaicin, nordihydrocapsaicin, norcapsaicin, nornordihydrocapsaicin, homocapsaicin and homodihydrocapsaicin [188]. To date, no clinical investigation has confirmed the effects of capsaicin in human colon cancer, and few studies are focused on the relationship between capsaicin consumption and microbiota alterations [189].

A recent study on 512,000 adults revealed that consumption of spices is associated with a lower risk of GI cancer after 5 years of consumption, however, capsaicin also seems to have a negative effect on human health, even if most studies underline that only high doses seem to be harmful. An inverse association was found between spicy food consumption and CRC risk for those who never/rarely consumed and consumed monthly, 1–2 days/week, 3–5 days/week, and 6–7 days/week [190]. This could be related to an increase in butyrogenic bacteria and a decrease in LPS-producing bacteria. Another study found that consumption of 5 mg/d or 10 mg/day capsaicin on a regular basis increased *Firmicutes/Bacteriodes* and *Faecalibacterium* abundance. This event leads to an increase in glucagon-like peptide 1 and gastric inhibitory polypeptide with a decrease in ghrelin [135]. Diferuloylmethane is another interesting compound, which can influence the progress of CRC by changing the gut microbiome. Different studies registered lower intestinal inflammation through a reduction in NF-kB in colonic epithelial cells. Another positive effect is the growth of T cells in CD4+ Foxp3+ DSS colitis models and the reduction of *Blautia* and *Ruminococcus* species, which are responsible for CRC progress [191].

4.6. Saffron-Derived Compounds

Saffron (*Crocus sativus*, L) belongs to the plant family *Iridaceae*, and has been used as a food additive for centuries [192,193]. The phytochemistry of saffron reveals more than 150 compounds, principally comprising flavonoids, apocarotenoids (picrocrocin, crocin, and crocetin), safranal, terpenes, aromatic hydrocarbons, alkaloids, and amino acids [194]. Saffron and its bioactive constituents have the potential to prevent and treat various types of cancer, as evidenced by multiple studies [195]. Crocin significantly prevented DSS and azoxymethane-induced colitis by reducing the level of mRNA expression, inflammatory cytokines, and NF-κB, in colorectal mucosa [196]. Similarly, in another in vivo study, crocin synergized the anti-proliferative action of 5-flurouracil via Wnt/PI3K pathway in CRC mice, associated with colitis [197].

In a recent study, saffron extract was administered to CRC cells for anti-proliferation and anti-motility progression by targeting MET transcriptional regulator (MACC1) expression [198]. This accumulating evidence shows the therapeutic potential of saffron in the prevention of CRC via gut microbiota modulation. Crocin-I ameliorated the disruption of gut dysbiosis in mice induced by chronic corticosterone administration. High-throughput sequencing of 16s rRNA demonstrated that crocin-I could mitigate gut dysbiosis through significant decreases in the abundance of *Firmicutes* and an increase of *Bacteroidetes*, and a significant increase in the α-diversity of the microbes in the cecal contents [136]. An herbal formula containing *C. sativus*, *Edgeworthia gardneri* (Wall.) Meisn., and *Sibiraea angustata* modulated gut microbiota with the regulation of gut-liver axis in Zucker diabetic fatty rats [199]. The formula modulated the dysbiosis of gut microbiota and maintained intestinal epithelial homeostasis, resulting in the reduction of serum levels of LPS, TNF-α, and IL-6.

Some pieces of recently published literature have also reported the negative effects of saffron and crocetin on gastrointestinal diseases such as colitis. While investigating the effects of crocetin on the regulation of intestinal barrier function and intestinal microbiota composition in mice, Feng et al. [137] observed prolonged recovery of colitis due to the promotion of inflammation with disturbed intestinal homeostasis under crocetin (10 mg/kg/day for 21-days) with an altered composition of gut microflora and its metabolic products compared to the DSS group. The 16s rDNA sequencing analysis of the feces samples showed a higher abundance of *Mediterraneibacter* and *Akkermansia*, and a lower abundance of *Dubosiella*, *Muribaculaceae*, *Paramuribaculum*, *Allobaculum*, *Parasutterella*, *Duncaniella*, *Stoquefichus*, *Coriobacteriaceae* UCG-002, and *Candidatus*. In addition, crocetin intake also reduced the levels of bile acids including 7-ketodeoxycholic acid, 12-ketodeoxycholic acid, 3-sulfodeoxycholic acid, chenodeoxycholate, 6-ethylchenodeoxycholic acid, glycochenodeoxycholate-7-sulfate, sulfolithocholic acid, and glycocholate in the colon. Another study showed disruption of the cecal microbiome and brush border membrane functionality with *C. sativus* flower water extract [138]. The *C. sativus* extract (1%, 2%, 5%, and 10%) was administered in the amnion of the *Gallus gallus* eggs and was allowed to be consumed by the developing embryo over the next few days. The hatchlings were euthanized, and blood, duodenum, and cecum were harvested for assessment, which showed a significant increase in Mucin 2 gene expression and Paneth cell number proportional to the increase in extract concentration, accompanied by a dose-dependent reduction of *Lactobacillus* and *Clostridium* suggesting an alteration of bacterial populations.

4.7. Flaxseed-Derived Compounds

Flaxseed (*Linum usitatissimum* L.) belonging to the Linaceae, is one of the richest dietary sources of omega-3 fatty acids. Other compounds identified in flaxseed include dietary fibers, lignans, and phenolics [200]. Flaxseed is already being extensively used in animal studies to treat cancers of different origins. Numerous studies have demonstrated the prevention of colon carcinogenesis in preclinical studies due to the consumption of flaxseed. Flaxseed possesses immunomodulatory effects, possibly due to prebiotic effects. It maintains the integrity of the intestinal epithelial barrier, inhibiting inflammatory responses and promoting the proliferation of beneficial phyla that may help in preventing CRC development and pathogenesis [201]. Dietary flaxseed supplementation in healthy C57Bl/6 male mice exhibited an alteration in fecal microbial community structure (i.e., a 30-fold decrease in *Akkermansia muciniphila* abundance and a 20-fold increase in *Prevotella* species) along with a significant increase in fecal branched-chain fatty acids, thus decreasing susceptibility to gut-associated diseases including inflammatory pathologies and cancer [139].

Flaxseed polysaccharides may reach the colon intact (without being degraded) where changes in carbohydrate contents, reducing sugars, and culture pH suggest that these polysaccharides may be broken down and used by gut microbiota. Zhou et al. [202] observed a modulation of the structure and composition of gut microbiota with flaxseed polysaccharides through the alteration of the *Firmicutes/Bacteroidetes* ratio, and enhanced relative abundances of *Phascolarctobacterium*, *Prevotella*, *Megamonas*, and *Clostridium*, which can degrade polysaccharides. Moreover, the fermentation of flaxseed polysaccharides increased the concentration of SCFAs, particularly propionate and butyrate. Flaxseed oligosaccharides alleviated DSS-induced colitis via the modulation of gut microbiota and repairing of the intestinal barrier in mice [140]. Flaxseed oligosaccharides (200 mg/kg/day) resulted in the improvement of colonic histology, downregulation of oxidative stress markers (malondialdehyde and myeloperoxidase), and suppressed pro-inflammatory cytokines (TNF-α, IL-1β, and IL-6) while increasing the levels of an anti-inflammatory cytokine (IL-10). The 16S rDNA gene high-throughput sequencing indicated an increase in gut microbial diversity and inhibition of the proliferation of inflammatory-related bacteria (*Clostridiales*). An increase in propionic and butyric acids was also observed in mice treated with flaxseed oligosaccharides.

Flaxseed oil supplementation in pigs with intrauterine growth retardation improved intestinal function and immunity (downregulated intestinal expression of MyD88, NF-κB, TNF-α, and IL-10 genes) associated with altered colonic microflora, by decreasing the abundance of *Spirochaetes* and increasing phylum *Actinobacteria*, and genera *Bifidobacterium* and *Blautia* [141]. Treatment of CEABAC10 transgenic mice (with Crohn's disease) with dietary extruded flaxseed for 12 weeks ameliorated the adherent-invasive *E. coli*-induced intestinal inflammation [142]. Analysis of mucosa-associated microbiota showed a higher abundance of *Prevotella*, *Ruminococcus*, *Clostridiales*, and *Paraprevotella*, in addition to higher butyrate concentration in mice treated with flaxseed. Conversely, ground flaxseeds (rich in omega-3 fatty acids, lignans, and fibers) exacerbated *Citrobacter rodentium*-induced colitis in C57BL/6 mice despite the higher levels of omega-3 fatty acids and cecal SCFAs [203].

5. Conclusions

The available literature data suggest that spices and their phytochemicals could be one of the dietary factors that may prevent the risk of CRC development by affecting tumor behavior and targeting numerous molecular mechanisms. Many processes (i.e., oxidative stress, inflammatory cascade, apoptosis, and proliferation) can be influenced by one or more spice-derived phytochemicals. Studies on gut microbial modulation by spice-derived phytochemicals in CRC are still very limited, as spice-derived phytochemicals have been studied in this regard. Thus, the exploration of other spice-derived phytochemicals is essential to provide further insights into the interesting relationship between spice-derived phytochemicals and gut microbiota in CRC. Certain spice-derived phytochemicals have been found to exacerbate gut dysbiosis and intestinal inflammation, such as diallyl disulfide, saffron, crocetin, and ground flaxseeds. So, further confirmation is required on whether this phenomenon will affect the CRC-preventing activity of other spices such as garlic and flaxseed. Additionally, the data reviewed from the literature has mainly been based on preclinical studies, thus robust clinical trials are needed to determine who will benefit from an adequate intake of spice-derived phytochemicals, and what interactions (both positive and negative) may exist among spices with other dietary components or medications (that an individual with CRC may regularly consume). Moreover, the testing of phytochemicals, both in cell cultures and animal studies, at much higher doses than would be regularly ingested, represents pharmacological therapeutic intervention rather than a dietary preventive approach, and thus spice-derived phytochemicals must be tested within the range of dietary doses to assess the actual potential of dietary spices to prevent CRC via gut microbial modulation.

Author Contributions: Conceptualization, M.D. (Maria Daglia) and H.U.; writing original draft, M.D. (Marco Dacrema), A.A., H.U. and A.K.; writing—review and editing, H.U., A.A., A.K., A.D.M., J.X. and A.M.C.M.; supervision, M.D. (Maria Daglia). All authors have read and agreed to the published version of the manuscript.

Funding: This research received no external funding.

Conflicts of Interest: The authors declare no conflict of interest.

Abbreviations

CRC	colorectal cancer
CSC	cancer stem cells
CTLA-4	T lymphocytes associated with antigen 4
DSS	dextran sulfate sodium
IBD	inflammatory bowel disease
IL-1	interleukin-1
JNK pathway	c-Jun N-terminal kinase pathway
LPS	Lipopolysaccharide
MAPKs	mitogen activated protein kinases

MMPs	matrix metalloproteinases
NF-kB	nuclear factor kappa-light-chain-enhancer of activated B cells
NK cells	natural killer cells
SCFAs	short chain fatty acids
TNF-α	tumor necrosis factor alpha

References

1. Vogelaar, I.; van Ballegooijen, M.; Schrag, D.; Boer, R.; Winawer, S.J.; Habbema, J.D.F.; Zauber, A.G. How Much Can Current Interventions Reduce Colorectal Cancer Mortality in the US? Mortality Projections for Scenarios of Risk-factor Modification, Screening, and Treatment. *Cancer* **2006**, *107*, 1624–1633. [CrossRef] [PubMed]
2. Siegel, R.L.; Miller, K.D.; Fedewa, S.A.; Ahnen, D.J.; Meester, R.G.; Barzi, A.; Jemal, A. Colorectal Cancer Statistics, 2017. *CA Cancer J. Clin.* **2017**, *67*, 177–193. [CrossRef] [PubMed]
3. Dekker, E.; Tanis, P.J.; Vleugels, J.L.; Kasi, P.M.; Wallace, M.B. Colorectal Cancer. *Lancet* **2019**, *10207*, 1467–1480. [CrossRef]
4. Bray, F.; Ferlay, J.; Soerjomataram, I.; Siegel, R.L.; Torre, L.A.; Jemal, A. Global Cancer Statistics 2018: GLOBOCAN Estimates of Incidence and Mortality Worldwide for 36 Cancers in 185 Countries. *CA Cancer J. Clin.* **2018**, *68*, 394–424. [CrossRef]
5. Dong, Y.; Zhou, J.; Zhu, Y.; Luo, L.; He, T.; Hu, H.; Liu, H.; Zhang, Y.; Luo, D.; Xu, S.; et al. Abdominal Obesity and Colorectal Cancer Risk: Systematic Review and Meta-Analysis of Prospective Studies. *Biosci. Rep.* **2017**, *37*, BSR20170945. [CrossRef]
6. Liang, P.S.; Chen, T.Y.; Giovannucci, E. Cigarette Smoking and Colorectal Cancer Incidence and Mortality: Systematic Review and Meta-analysis. *Int. J. Cancer* **2009**, *124*, 2406–2415. [CrossRef]
7. McNabb, S.; Harrison, T.A.; Albanes, D.; Berndt, S.I.; Brenner, H.; Caan, B.J.; Campbell, P.T.; Cao, Y.; Chang-Claude, J.; Chan, A.; et al. Meta-analysis of 16 Studies of the Association of Alcohol with Colorectal Cancer. *Int. J. Cancer* **2020**, *146*, 861–873. [CrossRef]
8. Zheng, X.; Hur, J.; Nguyen, L.H.; Liu, J.; Song, M.; Wu, K.; Smith-Warner, S.A.; Ogino, S.; Willett, W.C.; Chan, A.T.; et al. Comprehensive Assessment of Diet Quality and Risk of Precursors of Early-Onset Colorectal Cancer. *J. Natl. Cancer Inst.* **2021**, *113*, 543–552. [CrossRef]
9. de Rezende, L.F.M.; de Sá, T.H.; Markozannes, G.; Rey-López, J.P.; Lee, I.M.; Tsilidis, K.K.; Ioannidis, J.P.; Eluf-Neto, J. Physical Activity and Cancer: An Umbrella Review of the Literature Including 22 Major Anatomical Sites and 770,000 Cancer Cases. *Br. J. Sports Med.* **2018**, *52*, 826–833. [CrossRef]
10. Lichtenstein, P.; Holm, N.V.; Verkasalo, P.K.; Iliadou, A.; Kaprio, J.; Koskenvuo, M.; Pukkala, E.; Skytthe, A.; Hemminki, K. Environmental and Heritable Factors in the Causation of Cancer—Analyses of Cohorts of Twins from Sweden, Denmark, and Finland. *N. Engl. J. Med.* **2000**, *343*, 78–85. [CrossRef]
11. Graff, R.E.; Möller, S.; Passarelli, M.N.; Witte, J.S.; Skytthe, A.; Christensen, K.; Tan, Q.; Adami, H.O.; Czene, K.; Harris, J.R.; et al. Familial Risk and Heritability of Colorectal Cancer in the Nordic Twin Study of Cancer. *Clin. Gastroenterol. Hepatol.* **2017**, *15*, 1256–1264. [CrossRef] [PubMed]
12. Jasperson, K.W.; Tuohy, T.M.; Neklason, D.W.; Burt, R.W. Hereditary and Familial Colon Cancer. *Gastroenterology* **2010**, *138*, 2044–2058. [CrossRef] [PubMed]
13. Wong, S.H.; Yu, J. Gut Microbiota in Colorectal Cancer: Mechanisms of Action and Clinical Applications. *Nat. Rev. Gastroenterol. Hepatol.* **2019**, *16*, 690–704. [CrossRef] [PubMed]
14. Plummer, M.; de Martel, C.; Vignat, J.; Ferlay, J.; Bray, F.; Franceschi, S. Global Burden of Cancers Attributable to Infections in 2012: A Synthetic Analysis. *Lancet Glob. Health* **2016**, *4*, e609–e616. [CrossRef]
15. Hughes, L.A.; van den Brandt, P.A.; Goldbohm, R.A.; de Goeij, A.F.; de Bruïne, A.P.; van Engeland, M.; Weijenberg, M.P. Childhood and Adolescent Energy Restriction and Subsequent Colorectal Cancer Risk: Results from the Netherlands Cohort Study. *Int. J. Epidemiol.* **2010**, *39*, 1333–1344. [CrossRef]
16. Nimptsch, K.; Wu, K. Is Timing Important? The Role of Diet and Lifestyle during Early Life on Colorectal Neoplasia. *Curr. Colorectal Cancer Rep.* **2018**, *14*, 1–11. [CrossRef]
17. Ursell, L.K.; Metcalf, J.L.; Parfrey, L.W.; Knight, R. Defining the Human Microbiome. *Nutr. Rev.* **2012**, *70*, S38–S44. [CrossRef]
18. Bull, M.J.; Plummer, N.T. Part 1: The Human Gut Microbiome in Health and Disease. *Integr. Med.* **2014**, *13*, 17–22.
19. Sender, R.; Fuchs, S.; Milo, R. Revised Estimates for the Number of Human and Bacteria Cells in the Body. *PLoS Biol.* **2016**, *14*, e1002533. [CrossRef] [PubMed]
20. Gao, R.; Gao, Z.; Huang, L.; Qin, H. Gut Microbiota and Colorectal Cancer. *Eur. J. Clin. Microbiol. Infect. Dis.* **2017**, *36*, 757–769. [CrossRef] [PubMed]
21. Valdes, A.M.; Walter, J.; Segal, E.; Spector, T.D. Role of the Gut Microbiota in Nutrition and Health. *BMJ* **2018**, *361*, k2179. [CrossRef] [PubMed]
22. Leeming, E.R.; Louca, P.; Gibson, R.; Menni, C.; Spector, T.D.; le Roy, C.I. The Complexities of the Diet-Microbiome Relationship: Advances and Perspectives. *Genome Med.* **2021**, *13*, 10. [CrossRef] [PubMed]
23. Vaishnava, S.; Behrendt, C.L.; Ismail, A.S.; Eckmann, L.; Hooper, L.V. Paneth Cells Directly Sense Gut Commensals and Maintain Homeostasis at the Intestinal Host-Microbial Interface. *Proc. Natl. Acad. Sci. USA* **2008**, *105*, 20858–20863. [CrossRef] [PubMed]
24. Belkaid, Y.; Naik, S. Compartmentalized and Systemic Control of Tissue Immunity by Commensals. *Nat. Immunol.* **2013**, *14*, 646–653. [CrossRef] [PubMed]

25. Magnúsdóttir, S.; Ravcheev, D.; de Crécy-Lagard, V.; Thiele, I. Systematic Genome Assessment of B-Vitamin Biosynthesis Suggests Co-Operation among Gut Microbes. *Front. Genet.* **2015**, *6*, 148. [CrossRef]
26. Grice, E.A.; Segre, J.A. The Human Microbiome: Our Second Genome. *Annu. Rev. Genomics Hum. Genet.* **2012**, *13*, 151–170. [CrossRef] [PubMed]
27. Geva-Zatorsky, N.; Sefik, E.; Kua, L.; Pasman, L.; Tan, T.G.; Ortiz-Lopez, A.; Yanortsang, T.B.; Yang, L.; Jupp, R.; Mathis, D.; et al. Mining the Human Gut Microbiota for Immunomodulatory Organisms. *Cell* **2017**, *168*, 928–943. [CrossRef] [PubMed]
28. Haber, A.L.; Biton, M.; Rogel, N.; Herbst, R.H.; Shekhar, K.; Smillie, C.; Burgin, G.; Delorey, T.M.; Howitt, M.R.; Katz, Y.; et al. A Single-Cell Survey of the Small Intestinal Epithelium. *Nature* **2017**, *551*, 333–339. [CrossRef]
29. Rothschild, D.; Weissbrod, O.; Barkan, E.; Kurilshikov, A.; Korem, T.; Zeevi, D.; Costea, P.I.; Godneva, A.; Kalka, I.N.; Bar, N.; et al. Environment Dominates over Host Genetics in Shaping Human Gut Microbiota. *Nature* **2018**, *555*, 210–215. [CrossRef] [PubMed]
30. Korem, T.; Zeevi, D.; Suez, J.; Weinberger, A.; Avnit-Sagi, T.; Pompan-Lotan, M.; Matot, E.; Jona, G.; Harmelin, A.; Cohen, N.; et al. Growth Dynamics of Gut Microbiota in Health and Disease Inferred from Single Metagenomic Samples. *Science (1979)* **2015**, *349*, 1101–1106. [CrossRef] [PubMed]
31. Gopalakrishnan, V.; Helmink, B.A.; Spencer, C.N.; Reuben, A.; Wargo, J.A. The Influence of the Gut Microbiome on Cancer, Immunity, and Cancer Immunotherapy. *Cancer Cell* **2018**, *33*, 570–580. [CrossRef] [PubMed]
32. Shindo, Y.; Hazama, S. Novel Biomarkers for Personalized Cancer Immunotherapy. *Cancers* **2019**, *11*, 1223. [CrossRef] [PubMed]
33. Picardo, S.L.; Coburn, B.; Hansen, A.R. The Microbiome and Cancer for Clinicians. *Crit. Rev. Oncol. Hematol.* **2019**, *141*, 1–12. [CrossRef] [PubMed]
34. Wilson, I.D.; Nicholson, J.K. Gut Microbiome Interactions with Drug Metabolism, Efficacy, and Toxicity. *Transl. Res.* **2017**, *179*, 204–222. [CrossRef]
35. Brenchley, J.M.; Douek, D.C. Microbial Translocation across the GI Tract. *Annu. Rev. Immunol.* **2012**, *30*, 149. [CrossRef]
36. Zeng, M.Y.; Cisalpino, D.; Varadarajan, S.; Hellman, J.; Warren, H.S.; Cascalho, M.; Inohara, N.; Núñez, G. Gut Microbiota-Induced Immunoglobulin G Controls Systemic Infection by Symbiotic Bacteria and Pathogens. *Immunity* **2016**, *44*, 647–658. [CrossRef]
37. David, L.A.; Maurice, C.F.; Carmody, R.N.; Gootenberg, D.B.; Button, J.E.; Wolfe, B.E.; Ling, A.V.; Devlin, A.S.; Varma, Y.; Fischbach, M.A.; et al. Diet Rapidly and Reproducibly Alters the Human Gut Microbiome. *Nature* **2014**, *505*, 559–563. [CrossRef]
38. Xu, Z.; Knight, R. Dietary Effects on Human Gut Microbiome Diversity. *Br. J. Nutr.* **2015**, *113*, S1–S5. [CrossRef]
39. Sonnenburg, E.D.; Smits, S.A.; Tikhonov, M.; Higginbottom, S.K.; Wingreen, N.S.; Sonnenburg, J.L. Diet-Induced Extinctions in the Gut Microbiota Compound over Generations. *Nature* **2016**, *529*, 212–215. [CrossRef]
40. Bhatt, A.P.; Redinbo, M.R.; Bultman, S.J. The Role of the Microbiome in Cancer Development and Therapy. *CA Cancer J. Clin.* **2017**, *67*, 326–344. [CrossRef]
41. David, L.A.; Materna, A.C.; Friedman, J.; Campos-Baptista, M.I.; Blackburn, M.C.; Perrotta, A.; Erdman, S.E.; Alm, E.J. Host Lifestyle Affects Human Microbiota on Daily Timescales. *Genome Biol.* **2014**, *15*, R89. [CrossRef] [PubMed]
42. De Filippo, C.; Cavalieri, D.; di Paola, M.; Ramazzotti, M.; Poullet, J.B.; Massart, S.; Collini, S.; Pieraccini, G.; Lionetti, P. Impact of Diet in Shaping Gut Microbiota Revealed by a Comparative Study in Children from Europe and Rural Africa. *Proc. Natl. Acad. Sci. USA* **2010**, *107*, 14691–14696. [CrossRef] [PubMed]
43. Shi, Z. Gut Microbiota: An Important Link between Western Diet and Chronic Diseases. *Nutrients* **2019**, *11*, 2287. [CrossRef]
44. Brennan, C.A.; Garrett, W.S. Gut Microbiota, Inflammation, and Colorectal Cancer. *Annu. Rev. Microbiol.* **2016**, *70*, 395. [CrossRef] [PubMed]
45. Choi, C.H.R.; Bakir, I.A.; Hart, A.L.; Graham, T.A. Clonal Evolution of Colorectal Cancer in IBD. *Nat. Rev. Gastroenterol. Hepatol.* **2017**, *14*, 218–229. [CrossRef] [PubMed]
46. Lasry, A.; Zinger, A.; Ben-Neriah, Y. Inflammatory Networks Underlying Colorectal Cancer. *Nat. Immunol.* **2016**, *17*, 230–240. [CrossRef]
47. Alam, W.; Ullah, H.; Santarcangelo, C.; di Minno, A.; Khan, H.; Daglia, M.; Arciola, C.R. Micronutrient Food Supplements in Patients with Gastro-Intestinal and Hepatic Cancers. *Int. J. Mol. Sci.* **2021**, *22*, 8014. [CrossRef]
48. Kim, D.H.; Khan, H.; Ullah, H.; Hassan, S.T.S.; Šmejkal, K.; Efferth, T.; Mahomoodally, M.F.; Xu, S.; Habtemariam, S.; Filosa, R.; et al. MicroRNA Targeting by Quercetin in Cancer Treatment and Chemoprotection. *Pharmacol. Res.* **2019**, *147*, 104346. [CrossRef]
49. Shankar, E.; Kanwal, R.; Candamo, M.; Gupta, S. Dietary Phytochemicals as Epigenetic Modifiers in Cancer: Promise and Challenges. *Semin. Cancer Biol.* **2016**, *40*, 82–99. [CrossRef]
50. Khan, H.; Ullah, H.; Martorell, M.; Valdes, S.E.; Belwal, T.; Tejada, S.; Sureda, A.; Kamal, M.A. Flavonoids Nanoparticles in Cancer: Treatment, Prevention and Clinical Prospects. *Semin. Cancer Biol.* **2021**, *69*, 200–211. [CrossRef]
51. Khan, H.; Reale, M.; Ullah, H.; Sureda, A.; Tejada, S.; Wang, Y.; Zhang, Z.J.; Xiao, J. Anti-Cancer Effects of Polyphenols via Targeting P53 Signaling Pathway: Updates and Future Directions. *Biotechnol. Adv.* **2020**, *38*, 107385. [CrossRef] [PubMed]
52. Bose, S.; Banerjee, S.; Mondal, A.; Chakraborty, U.; Pumarol, J.; Croley, C.R.; Bishayee, A. Targeting the JAK/STAT Signaling Pathway Using Phytocompounds for Cancer Prevention and Therapy. *Cells* **2020**, *9*, 1451. [CrossRef] [PubMed]
53. Tewari, D.; Patni, P.; Bishayee, A.; Sah, A.N.; Bishayee, A. Natural Products Targeting the PI3K-Akt-MTOR Signaling Pathway in Cancer: A Novel Therapeutic Strategy. *Semin. Cancer Biol.* **2019**, *80*, 1–17. [CrossRef] [PubMed]
54. Moloudizargari, M.; Asghari, M.H.; Nabavi, S.F.; Gulei, D.; Berindan-Neagoe, I.; Bishayee, A.; Nabavi, S.M. Targeting Hippo Signaling Pathway by Phytochemicals in Cancer Therapy. *Semin. Cancer Biol.* **2020**, *80*, 183–194. [CrossRef]

55. Tewari, D.; Priya, A.; Bishayee, A.; Bishayee, A. Targeting Transforming Growth Factor-β Signalling for Cancer Prevention and Intervention: Recent Advances in Developing Small Molecules of Natural Origin. *Clin. Transl. Med.* **2022**, *12*, e795. [CrossRef] [PubMed]
56. Patra, S.; Mishra, S.R.; Behera, B.P.; Mahapatra, K.K.; Panigrahi, D.P.; Bhol, C.S.; Praharaj, P.P.; Sethi, G.; Patra, S.K.; Bhutia, S.K. Autophagy-Modulating Phytochemicals in Cancer Therapeutics: Current Evidences and Future Perspectives. *Semin. Cancer Biol.* **2020**, *80*, 205–217. [CrossRef] [PubMed]
57. Khan, H.; Ullah, H.; Castilho, P.C.M.F.; Gomila, A.S.; D'Onofrio, G.; Filosa, R.; Wang, F.; Nabavi, S.M.; Daglia, M.; Silva, A.S.; et al. Targeting NF-KB Signaling Pathway in Cancer by Dietary Polyphenols. *Crit. Rev. Food Sci. Nutr.* **2019**, *60*, 2790–2800. [CrossRef] [PubMed]
58. Zheng, J.; Zhou, Y.; Li, Y.; Xu, D.P.; Li, S.; Li, H.B. Spices for Prevention and Treatment of Cancers. *Nutrients* **2016**, *8*, 495. [CrossRef] [PubMed]
59. Chen, H.; Yang, H.; Fan, D.; Deng, J. The Anticancer Activity and Mechanisms of Ginsenosides: An Updated Review. *eFood* **2020**, *1*, 226–241. [CrossRef]
60. Jing, H. Black Garlic: Processing, Composition Change, and Bioactivity. *eFood* **2020**, *1*, 242–246. [CrossRef]
61. Ekor, M. The Growing Use of Herbal Medicines: Issues Relating to Adverse Reactions and Challenges in Monitoring Safety. *Front. Pharmacol.* **2014**, *4*, 177. [CrossRef] [PubMed]
62. Hossain, M.; Urbi, Z. Effect of Naphthalene Acetic Acid on the Adventitious Rooting in Shoot Cuttings of Andrographis paniculata (Burm. f.) Wall. Ex Nees: An Important Therapeutical Herb. *Int. J. Agron.* **2016**, *2016*, 1–6. [CrossRef]
63. Hossain, M.S.; Sharfaraz, A.; Dutta, A.; Ahsan, A.; Masud, M.A.; Ahmed, I.A.; Goh, B.H.; Urbi, Z.; Sarker, M.M.R.; Ming, L.C. A Review of Ethnobotany, Phytochemistry, Antimicrobial Pharmacology and Toxicology of *Nigella sativa* L. *Biomed. Pharmacother.* **2021**, *143*, 112182. [CrossRef]
64. DeLuca, J.A.; Garcia-Villatoro, E.L.; Allred, C.D. Flaxseed Bioactive Compounds and Colorectal Cancer Prevention. *Curr. Oncol. Rep.* **2018**, *20*, 59. [CrossRef]
65. Jaksevicius, A.; Carew, M.; Mistry, C.; Modjtahedi, H.; Opara, E.I. Inhibitory Effects of Culinary Herbs and Spices on the Growth of HCA-7 Colorectal Cancer Cells and Their COX-2 Expression. *Nutrients* **2017**, *9*, 1051. [CrossRef] [PubMed]
66. Narayanankutty, A. PI3K/Akt/MTOR Pathway as a Therapeutic Target for Colorectal Cancer: A Review of Preclinical and Clinical Evidence. *Curr. Drug Targets* **2019**, *20*, 1217–1226. [CrossRef] [PubMed]
67. Zheng, S.; Xin, L.; Liang, A.; Fu, Y. Cancer Stem Cell Hypothesis: A Brief Summary and Two Proposals. *Cytotechnology* **2013**, *65*, 505–512. [CrossRef] [PubMed]
68. Alexander, J.L.; Scott, A.J.; Pouncey, A.L.; Marchesi, J.; Kinross, J.; Teare, J. Colorectal Carcinogenesis: An Archetype of Gut Microbiota–Host Interaction. *Ecancermedicalscience* **2018**, *12*, 865. [CrossRef] [PubMed]
69. Scarpa, E.S.; Ninfali, P. Phytochemicals as Innovative Therapeutic Tools against Cancer Stem Cells. *Int. J. Mol. Sci.* **2015**, *16*, 15727–15742. [CrossRef] [PubMed]
70. Koury, J.; Zhong, L.; Hao, J. Targeting Signaling Pathways in Cancer Stem Cells for Cancer Treatment. *Stem Cells Int.* **2017**, *2017*, 1–10. [CrossRef] [PubMed]
71. Hossain, M.S.; Kader, M.A.; Goh, K.W.; Islam, M.; Khan, M.S.; Harun-Ar, M.R.; Ooi, J.; Melo, H.C.; Al-Worafi, Y.M.; Moshawih, S.; et al. Herb and Spices in Colorectal Cancer Prevention and Treatment: A Narrative Review. *Front. Pharmacol.* **2022**, *13*, 865801. [CrossRef] [PubMed]
72. Ganesan, K.; Jayachandran, M.; Xu, B. Diet-Derived Phytochemicals Targeting Colon Cancer Stem Cells and Microbiota in Colorectal Cancer. *Int. J. Mol. Sci.* **2020**, *21*, 3976. [CrossRef] [PubMed]
73. Jandhyala, S.M.; Talukdar, R.; Subramanyam, C.; Vuyyuru, H.; Sasikala, M.; Reddy, D.N. Role of the Normal Gut Microbiota. *World J. Gastroenterol.* **2015**, *21*, 8787–8803. [CrossRef] [PubMed]
74. Jiao, Y.; Wu, L.; Huntington, N.D.; Zhang, X. Crosstalk between Gut Microbiota and Innate Immunity and Its Implication in Autoimmune Diseases. *Front. Immunol.* **2020**, *11*, 282. [CrossRef] [PubMed]
75. Guarner, F.; Malagelada, J.R. Gut Flora in Health and Disease. *Lancet* **2003**, *361*, 512–519. [CrossRef]
76. Jeyamogan, S.; Khan, N.A.; Anwar, A.; Shah, M.R.; Siddiqui, R. Cytotoxic Effects of Benzodioxane, Naphthalene Diimide, Porphyrin and Acetamol Derivatives on HeLa Cells. *SAGE Open Med.* **2018**, *6*. [CrossRef]
77. Jeyamogan, S.; Khan, N.A.; Siddiqui, R. Application and Importance of Theranostics in the Diagnosis and Treatment of Cancer. *Arch. Med. Res.* **2021**, *52*, 131–142. [CrossRef] [PubMed]
78. Bultman, S.J. Emerging Roles of the Microbiome in Cancer. *Carcinogenesis* **2014**, *35*, 249–255. [CrossRef] [PubMed]
79. Siegel, R.L.; Miller, K.D.; Jemal, A. Cancer Statistics, 2015. *CA Cancer J. Clin.* **2015**, *65*, 5–29. [CrossRef] [PubMed]
80. Agrawal, B. New Therapeutic Targets for Cancer: The Interplay between Immune and Metabolic Checkpoints and Gut Microbiota. *Clin. Transl. Med.* **2019**, *8*, 23. [CrossRef] [PubMed]
81. Chen, W.; Liu, F.; Ling, Z.; Tong, X.; Xiang, C. Human Intestinal Lumen and Mucosa-Associated Microbiota in Patients with Colorectal Cancer. *PLoS One* **2012**, *7*, e39743. [CrossRef]
82. Wu, N.; Yang, X.; Zhang, R.; Li, J.; Xiao, X.; Hu, Y.; Chen, Y.; Yang, F.; Lu, N.; Wang, Z.; et al. Dysbiosis Signature of Fecal Microbiota in Colorectal Cancer Patients. *Microb. Ecol.* **2013**, *66*, 462–470. [CrossRef] [PubMed]
83. Khatoon, J.; Rai, R.P.; Prasad, K.N. Role of Helicobacter pylori in Gastric Cancer: Updates. *World J. Gastroenterol.* **2016**, *8*, 147. [CrossRef] [PubMed]

84. Hattori, N.; Ushijima, T. Epigenetic Impact of Infection on Carcinogenesis: Mechanisms and Applications. *Genome Med.* **2016**, *8*, 1–13. [CrossRef]
85. Arthur, J.C.; Perez-Chanona, E.; Mühlbauer, M.; Tomkovich, S.; Uronis, J.M.; Fan, T.J.; Campbell, B.J.; Abujamel, T.; Dogan, B.; Rogers, A.B.; et al. Intestinal Inflammation Targets Cancer-Inducing Activity of the Microbiota. *Science (1979)* **2012**, *338*, 120–123. [CrossRef]
86. Nougayrède, J.P.; Homburg, S.; Taieb, F.; Boury, M.; Brzuszkiewicz, E.; Gottschalk, G.; Buchrieser, C.; Hacker, J.; Dobrindt, U.; Oswald, E. Escherichia coli Induces DNA Double-Strand Breaks in Eukaryotic Cells. *Science (1979)* **2006**, *313*, 848–851. [CrossRef]
87. Dennis, K.L.; Blatner, N.R.; Gounari, F.; Gounari, F. Current Status of Interleukin-10 and Regulatory T-Cells in Cancer. *Curr. Opin. Oncol.* **2013**, *25*, 637–645. [CrossRef]
88. Al-Hebshi, N.N.; Borgnakke, W.S.; Johnson, N.W. The Microbiome of Oral Squamous Cell Carcinomas: A Functional Perspective. *Curr. Oral Health Rep.* **2019**, *6*, 145–160. [CrossRef]
89. Vivarelli, S.; Salemi, R.; Candido, S.; Falzone, L.; Santagati, M.; Stefani, S.; Torino, F.; Banna, G.L.; Tonini, G.; Libra, M. Gut Microbiota and Cancer: From Pathogenesis to Therapy. *Cancers (Basel)* **2019**, *11*, 38. [CrossRef]
90. Borges-Canha, M.; Portela-Cidade, J.P.; Dinis-Ribeiro, M.; Leite-Moreira, A.F.; Pimentel-Nunes, P. Role of Colonic Microbiota in Colorectal Carcinogenesis: A Systematic Review. *Rev. Esp. Enferm. Dig.* **2015**, *107*, 659–671. [CrossRef] [PubMed]
91. Klampfer, L. Cytokines, Inflammation and Colon Cancer. *Curr. Cancer Drug Targets* **2011**, *11*, 451–464. [CrossRef] [PubMed]
92. Bergounioux, J.; Elisee, R.; Prunier, A.L.; Donnadieu, F.; Sperandio, B.; Sansonetti, P.; Arbibe, L. Calpain Activation by the Shigella flexneri Effector VirA Regulates Key Steps in the Formation and Life of the Bacterium's Epithelial Niche. *Cell Host Microbe* **2012**, *11*, 240–252. [CrossRef] [PubMed]
93. Rubinstein, M.R.; Wang, X.; Liu, W.; Hao, Y.; Cai, G.; Han, Y.W. Fusobacterium nucleatum Promotes Colorectal Carcinogenesis by Modulating E-Cadherin/β-Catenin Signaling via Its FadA Adhesin. *Cell Host Microbe* **2013**, *14*, 195–206. [CrossRef]
94. Cheng, W.Y.; Wu, C.Y.; Yu, J. The Role of Gut Microbiota in Cancer Treatment: Friend or Foe? *Gut* **2013**, *69*, 1867–1876. [CrossRef]
95. Goodwin, A.C.; Shields, C.E.D.; Wu, S.; Huso, D.L.; Wu, X.; Murray-Stewart, T.R.; Hacker-Prietz, A.; Rabizadeh, S.; Woster, P.M.; Sears, C.L.; et al. Polyamine Catabolism Contributes to Enterotoxigenic Bacteroides fragilis-Induced Colon Tumorigenesis. *Proc. Natl. Acad. Sci. USA* **2011**, *108*, 15354–15359. [CrossRef] [PubMed]
96. Konishi, H.; Fujiya, M.; Tanaka, H.; Ueno, N.; Moriichi, K.; Sasajima, J.; Ikuta, K.; Akutsu, H.; Tanabe, H.; Kohgo, Y. Probiotic-Derived Ferrichrome Inhibits Colon Cancer Progression via JNK-Mediated Apoptosis. *Nat. Commun.* **2016**, *7*, 12365. [CrossRef] [PubMed]
97. Johansson, M.E.; Jakobsson, H.E.; Holmén-Larsson, J.; Schütte, A.; Ermund, A.; Rodríguez-Piñeiro, A.M.; Arike, L.; Wising, C.; Svensson, F.; Bäckhed, F.; et al. Normalization of Host Intestinal Mucus Layers Requires Long-Term Microbial Colonization. *Cell Host Microbe* **2015**, *18*, 582–592. [CrossRef]
98. Spiljar, M.; Merkler, D.; Trajkovski, M. The Immune System Bridges the Gut Microbiota with Systemic Energy Homeostasis: Focus on TLRs, Mucosal Barrier, and SCFAs. *Front. Immunol.* **2017**, *8*, 1353. [CrossRef] [PubMed]
99. Wang, Q.; Rao, Y.; Guo, X.; Liu, N.; Liu, S.; Wen, P.; Li, S.; Li, Y. Oral Microbiome in Patients with Oesophageal Squamous Cell Carcinoma. *Sci. Rep.* **2019**, *9*, 19055. [CrossRef]
100. Nair, M.; Sandhu, S.S.; Sharma, A.K. Cancer Molecular Markers: A Guide to Cancer Detection and Management. *Semin. Cancer Biol.* **2018**, *52*, 39–55. [CrossRef]
101. Housman, G.; Byler, S.; Heerboth, S.; Lapinska, K.; Longacre, M.; Snyder, N.; Sarkar, S. Drug Resistance in Cancer: An Overview. *Cancers (Basel)* **2014**, *6*, 1769–1792. [CrossRef]
102. Rueff, J.; Rodrigues, A.S. Cancer Drug Resistance: A Brief Overview from a Genetic Viewpoint. *Methods Mol. Biol.* **2016**, *1395*, 1–18. [PubMed]
103. Alfarouk, K.O.; Stock, C.-M.; Taylor, S.; Walsh, M.; Muddathir, A.K.; Verduzco, D.; Bashir, A.H.H.; Mohammed, O.Y.; Elhassan, G.O.; Harguindey, S.; et al. Resistance to Cancer Chemotherapy: Failure in Drug Response from ADME to P-Gp. *Cancer Cell Int.* **2015**, *15*, 71. [CrossRef] [PubMed]
104. Schwabe, R.F.; Jobin, C. The Microbiome and Cancer. *Nat. Rev. Cancer* **2013**, *13*, 800–812. [CrossRef] [PubMed]
105. Zitvogel, L.; Daillère, R.; Roberti, M.P.; Routy, B.; Kroemer, G. Anticancer Effects of the Microbiome and Its Products. *Nat. Rev. Microbiol.* **2017**, *15*, 465–478. [CrossRef] [PubMed]
106. Iida, N.; Dzutsev, A.; Stewart, C.; Smith, L.; Bouladoux, N.; Weingarten, R.; Molina, D.; Salcedo, R.; Back, T.; Cramer, S.; et al. Commensal Bacteria Control Cancer Response to Therapy by Modulating the Tumor Microenvironment. *Science (1979)* **2013**, *342*, 967–970. [CrossRef]
107. Kuwahara, A.; Matsuda, K.; Kuwahara, Y.; Asano, S.; Inui, T.; Marunaka, Y. Microbiota-Gut-Brain Axis: Enteroendocrine Cells and the Enteric Nervous System Form an Interface between the Microbiota and the Central Nervous System. *Biomed. Res.* **2020**, *41*, 199–216. [CrossRef]
108. Viaud, S.; Saccheri, F.; Mignot, G.; Yamazaki, T.; Daillère, R.; Hannani, D.; Enot, D.; Pfirschke, C.; Engblom, C.; Pittet, M.; et al. The Intestinal Microbiota Modulates the Anticancer Immune Effects of Cyclophosphamide. *Science (1979)* **2013**, *342*, 971–976. [CrossRef]
109. Sivan, A.; Corrales, L.; Hubert, N.; Williams, J.B.; Aquino-Michaels, K.; Earley, Z.M.; Benyamin, F.W.; Man Lei, Y.; Jabri, B.; Alegre, M.L.; et al. Commensal Bifidobacterium Promotes Antitumor Immunity and Facilitates Anti–PD-L1 Efficacy. *Science (1979)* **2015**, *350*, 1084–1089. [CrossRef]

110. Lin, C.; Cai, X.; Zhang, J.; Wang, W.; Sheng, Q.; Hua, H.; Zhou, X. Role of Gut Microbiota in the Development and Treatment of Colorectal Cancer. *Digestion* **2019**, *100*, 72–78. [CrossRef]
111. Vétizou, M.; Pitt, J.; Daillère, R.; Lepage, P.; Waldschmitt, N.; Flament, C.; Rusakiewicz, S.; Routy, B.; Roberti, M.; Duong, C.; et al. Anticancer Immunotherapy by CTLA-4 Blockade Relies on the Gut Microbiota. *Science (1979)* **2015**, *350*, 1079–1084. [CrossRef] [PubMed]
112. Jan, G.B.A.S.; Belzacq, A.S.; Haouzi, D.; Rouault, A.; Metivier, D.; Kroemer, G.; Brenner, C. Propionibacteria Induce Apoptosis of Colorectal Carcinoma Cells via Short-Chain Fatty Acids Acting on Mitochondria. *Cell Death Differ.* **2002**, *9*, 179–188. [CrossRef] [PubMed]
113. Wei, W.; Sun, W.; Yu, S.; Yang, Y.; Ai, L. Butyrate Production from High-Fiber Diet Protects against Lymphoma Tumor. *Leuk. Lymphoma* **2016**, *57*, 2401–2408. [CrossRef] [PubMed]
114. Zhang, J.; Xia, Y.; Sun, J. Breast and Gut Microbiome in Health and Cancer. *Genes Dis.* **2021**, *8*, 581–589. [CrossRef] [PubMed]
115. Sánchez-Alcoholado, L.; Ramos-Molina, B.; Otero, A.; Laborda-Illanes, A.; Ordóñez, R.; Medina, J.A.; Gómez-Millán, J.; Queipo-Ortuño, M.I. The Role of the Gut Microbiome in Colorectal Cancer Development and Therapy Response. *Cancers (Basel)* **2020**, *12*, 1406. [CrossRef]
116. Salcedo, R.; Worschech, A.; Cardone, M.; Jones, Y.; Gyulai, Z.; Dai, R.M.; Wang, E.; Ma, W.; Haines, D.; O'hUigin, C.; et al. MyD88-Mediated Signaling Prevents Development of Adenocarcinomas of the Colon: Role of Interleukin 18. *J. Exp. Med.* **2010**, *207*, 1625–1636. [CrossRef]
117. Paavonen, J.; Naud, P.; Salmerón, J.; Wheeler, C.; Chow, S.; Apter, D.; Kitchener, H.; Castellsague, X.; Teixeira, J.; Skinner, S.; et al. Efficacy of Human Papillomavirus (HPV)-16/18 AS04-Adjuvanted Vaccine against Cervical Infection and Precancer Caused by Oncogenic HPV Types (PATRICIA): Final Analysis of a Double-Blind, Randomised Study in Young Women. *Lancet* **2009**, *374*, 301–314. [CrossRef]
118. Shylaja, M.R.; Peter, K.V. Spices in the Nutraceutical and Health Food Industry. In *International Symposium on Medicinal and Nutraceutical Plants*; International Society for Horticultural Science: Macon, GA, USA, 2007; pp. 369–378.
119. Srinivasan, K. Role of Spices beyond Food Flavoring: Nutraceuticals with Multiple Health Effects. *Food Rev. Int.* **2005**, *21*, 167–188. [CrossRef]
120. Kaefer, C.M.; Milner, J.A. The Role of Herbs and Spices in Cancer Prevention. *J. Nutr. Biochem.* **2008**, *19*, 347–361. [CrossRef]
121. Shen, L.; Ji, H.F. Intestinal Microbiota and Metabolic Diseases: Pharmacological Implications. *Trends Pharmacol. Sci.* **2016**, *37*, 169–171. [CrossRef]
122. Shen, L.; Liu, L.; Ji, H.F. Alzheimer's Disease Histological and Behavioral Manifestations in Transgenic Mice Correlate with Specific Gut Microbiome State. *J. Alzheimer's Dis.* **2017**, *56*, 385–390. [CrossRef] [PubMed]
123. Peterson, C.T.; Vaughn, A.R.; Sharma, V.; Chopra, D.; Mills, P.J.; Peterson, S.N.; Sivamani, R.K. Effects of Turmeric and Curcumin Dietary Supplementation on Human Gut Microbiota: A Double-Blind, Randomized, Placebo-Controlled Pilot Study. *J. Evid. Based Integr. Med.* **2018**, *23*. [CrossRef] [PubMed]
124. Ohno, M.; Nishida, A.; Sugitani, Y.; Nishino, K.; Inatomi, O.; Sugimoto, M.; Kawahara, M.; Andoh, A. Nanoparticle Curcumin Ameliorates Experimental Colitis via Modulation of Gut Microbiota and Induction of Regulatory T Cells. *PLoS One* **2017**, *12*, e0185999. [CrossRef] [PubMed]
125. McFadden, R.M.T.; Larmonier, C.B.; Shehab, K.W.; Midura-Kiela, M.; Ramalingam, R.; Harrison, C.A.; Besselsen, D.G.; Chase, J.H.; Caporaso, J.G.; Jobin, C.; et al. The Role of Curcumin in Modulating Colonic Microbiota during Colitis and Colon Cancer Prevention. *Inflamm. Bowel Dis.* **2015**, *21*, 2483–2494. [CrossRef] [PubMed]
126. Bereswill, S.; Muñoz, M.; Fischer, A.; Plickert, R.; Haag, L.M.; Otto, B.; Kühl, A.A.; Loddenkemper, C.; Göbel, U.B.; Heimesaat, M.M. Anti-Inflammatory Effects of Resveratrol, Curcumin and Simvastatin in Acute Small Intestinal Inflammation. *PLoS One* **2010**, *5*, e15099. [CrossRef]
127. Guo, S.; Geng, W.; Chen, S.; Wang, L.; Rong, X.; Wang, S.; Wang, T.; Xiong, L.; Huang, J.; Pang, X.; et al. Ginger Alleviates DSS-Induced Ulcerative Colitis Severity by Improving the Diversity and Function of Gut Microbiota. *Front. Pharmacol.* **2021**, *12*, 632569. [CrossRef] [PubMed]
128. Zhou, X.; Liu, X.; He, Q.; Wang, M.; Lu, H.; You, Y.; Chen, L.; Cheng, J.; Li, F.; Fu, X.; et al. Ginger Extract Decreases Susceptibility to Dextran Sulfate Sodium-Induced Colitis in Mice Following Early Antibiotic Exposure. *Front. Med.* **2022**, *8*.
129. Sasaki, K.; Sasaki, D.; Sasaki, K.; Nishidono, Y.; Yamamori, A.; Tanaka, K.; Kondo, A. Growth Stimulation of Bifidobacterium from Human Colon Using Daikenchuto in an In Vitro Model of Human Intestinal Microbiota. *Sci. Rep.* **2021**, *22*, 4580. [CrossRef] [PubMed]
130. Hao, W.; Chen, Z.; Yuan, Q.; Ma, M.; Gao, C.; Zhou, Y.; Zhou, H.; Wu, X.; Wu, D.; Farag, M.A.; et al. Ginger Polysaccharides Relieve Ulcerative Colitis via Maintaining Intestinal Barrier Integrity and Gut Microbiota Modulation. *Int. J. Biol. Macromol.* **2022**, *219*, 730–739. [CrossRef]
131. Wang, X.; Zhang, D.; Jiang, H.; Zhang, S.; Pang, X.; Gao, S.; Zhang, H.; Zhang, S.; Xiao, Q.; Chen, L.; et al. Gut Microbiota Variation with Short-Term Intake of Ginger Juice on Human Health. *Front. Microbiol.* **2021**, *11*, 576061. [CrossRef]
132. Shao, X.; Sun, C.; Tang, X.; Zhang, X.; Han, D.; Liang, S.; Qu, R.; Hui, X.; Shan, Y.; Hu, L.; et al. Anti-Inflammatory and Intestinal Microbiota Modulation Properties of Jinxiang Garlic (*Allium sativum* L.) Polysaccharides toward Dextran Sodium Sulfate-Induced Colitis. *J. Agric. Food Chem.* **2020**, *68*, 12295–12309. [CrossRef] [PubMed]

133. Vezza, T.; Algieri, F.; Garrido-Mesa, J.; Utrilla, M.P.; Rodríguez-Cabezas, M.E.; Banos, A.; Guillamón, E.; García, F.; Rodríguez-Nogales, A.; Gálvez, J. The Immunomodulatory Properties of Propyl-propane Thiosulfonate Contribute to Its Intestinal Anti-inflammatory Effect in Experimental Colitis. *Mol. Nutr. Food Res.* **2019**, *63*, 1800653. [CrossRef]
134. Hussein, M.M.; Abd El-Hack, M.E.; Mahgoub, S.A.; Saadeldin, I.M.; Swelum, A.A. Effects of Clove (Syzygium aromaticum) Oil on Quail Growth, Carcass Traits, Blood Components, Meat Quality, and Intestinal Microbiota. *Poult. Sci.* **2019**, *98*, 319–329. [CrossRef] [PubMed]
135. Kang, C.; Zhang, Y.; Zhu, X.; Liu, K.; Wang, X.; Chen, M.; Wang, J.; Chen, H.; Hui, S.; Huang, L.; et al. Healthy Subjects Differentially Respond to Dietary Capsaicin Correlating with Specific Gut Enterotypes. *J. Clin. Endocrinol. Metab.* **2016**, *101*, 4681–4689. [CrossRef] [PubMed]
136. Xie, X.; Xiao, Q.; Xiong, Z.; Yu, C.; Zhou, J.; Fu, Z. Crocin-I Ameliorates the Disruption of Lipid Metabolism and Dysbiosis of the Gut Microbiota Induced by Chronic Corticosterone in Mice. *Food Funct.* **2019**, *10*, 6779–6791. [CrossRef]
137. Feng, P.; Li, Q.; Liu, L.; Wang, S.; Wu, Z.; Tao, Y.; Huang, P.; Wang, P. Crocetin Prolongs Recovery Period of DSS-Induced Colitis via Altering Intestinal Microbiome and Increasing Intestinal Permeability. *Int. J. Mol. Sci.* **2022**, *23*, 3832. [CrossRef]
138. Agarwal, N.; Kolba, N.; Jung, Y.; Cheng, J.; Tako, E. Saffron (*Crocus sativus* L.) Flower Water Extract Disrupts the Cecal Microbiome, Brush Border Membrane Functionality, and Morphology in Vivo (Gallus gallus). *Nutrients* **2022**, *14*, 220. [CrossRef]
139. Power, K.A.; Lepp, D.; Zarepoor, L.; Monk, J.M.; Wu, W.; Tsao, R.; Liu, R. Dietary Flaxseed Modulates the Colonic Microenvironment in Healthy C57Bl/6 Male Mice Which May Alter Susceptibility to Gut-Associated Diseases. *J. Nutr. Biochem.* **2016**, *28*, 61–69. [CrossRef]
140. Xu, Z.; Chen, W.; Deng, Q.; Huang, Q.; Wang, X.; Yang, C.; Huang, F. Flaxseed Oligosaccharides Alleviate DSS-Induced Colitis through Modulation of Gut Microbiota and Repair of the Intestinal Barrier in Mice. *Food Funct.* **2020**, *11*, 8077–8088. [CrossRef]
141. Che, L.; Zhou, Q.; Liu, Y.; Hu, L.; Peng, X.; Wu, C.; Zhang, R.; Tang, J.; Wu, F.; Fang, Z.; et al. Flaxseed Oil Supplementation Improves Intestinal Function and Immunity, Associated with Altered Intestinal Microbiome and Fatty Acid Profile in Pigs with Intrauterine Growth Retardation. *Food Funct.* **2019**, *10*, 8149–8160. [CrossRef]
142. Plissonneau, C.; Sivignon, A.; Chassaing, B.; Capel, F.; Martin, V.; Etienne, M.; Wawrzyniak, I.; Chausse, P.; Dutheil, F.; Mairesse, G.; et al. Beneficial Effects of Linseed Supplementation on Gut Mucosa-Associated Microbiota in a Physically Active Mouse Model of Crohn's Disease. *Int. J. Mol. Sci.* **2022**, *23*, 5891. [CrossRef]
143. Bachmeier, B.E.; Killian, P.H.; Melchart, D. The Role of Curcumin in Prevention and Management of Metastatic Disease. *Int. J. Mol. Sci.* **2018**, *19*, 1716. [CrossRef]
144. Mirzaei, H.; Bagheri, H.; Ghasemi, F.; Khoi, J.M.; Pourhanifeh, M.H.; Heyden, Y.V.; Mortezapour, E.; Nikdasti, A.; Jeandet, P.; Khan, H.; et al. Anti-Cancer Activity of Curcumin on Multiple Myeloma. *Anticancer Agents Med. Chem.* **2021**, *21*, 575–586. [CrossRef] [PubMed]
145. Duvoix, A.; Blasius, R.; Delhalle, S.; Schnekenburger, M.; Morceau, F.; Henry, E.; Dicato, M.; Diederich, M. Chemopreventive and Therapeutic Effects of Curcumin. *Cancer Lett.* **2005**, *223*, 181–190. [CrossRef] [PubMed]
146. Wong, S.C.; Kamarudin, M.N.A.; Naidu, R. Anticancer Mechanism of Curcumin on Human Glioblastoma. *Nutrients* **2021**, *13*, 950. [CrossRef] [PubMed]
147. Genua, F.; Raghunathan, V.; Jenab, M.; Gallagher, W.M.; Hughes, D.J. The Role of Gut Barrier Dysfunction and Microbiome Dysbiosis in Colorectal Cancer Development. *Front. Oncol.* **2021**, *11*, 6349. [CrossRef] [PubMed]
148. Wang, J.; Ghosh, S.S.; Ghosh, S. Curcumin Improves Intestinal Barrier Function: Modulation of Intracellular Signaling, and Organization of Tight Junctions. *Am. J. Physiol. Cell Physiol.* **2017**, *312*, C438–C445. [CrossRef]
149. Ghosh, S.S.; Bie, J.; Wang, J.; Ghosh, S. Oral Supplementation with Non-Absorbable Antibiotics or Curcumin Attenuates Western Diet-Induced Atherosclerosis and Glucose Intolerance in LDLR−/− Mice–Role of Intestinal Permeability and Macrophage Activation. *PLoS One* **2014**, *9*, e108577. [CrossRef]
150. Ghosh, S.S.; He, H.; Wang, J.; Gehr, T.W.; Ghosh, S. Curcumin-Mediated Regulation of Intestinal Barrier Function: The Mechanism Underlying Its Beneficial Effects. *Tissue Barriers* **2018**, *6*, e1425085. [CrossRef]
151. Wang, P.; Su, C.; Feng, H.; Chen, X.; Dong, Y.; Rao, Y.; Ren, Y.; Yang, J.; Shi, J.; Tian, J.; et al. Curcumin Regulates Insulin Pathways and Glucose Metabolism in the Brains of APPswe/PS1dE9 Mice. *Int. J. Immunopathol. Pharmacol.* **2017**, *30*, 25–43. [CrossRef]
152. Scazzocchio, B.; Minghetti, L.; D'Archivio, M. Interaction between Gut Microbiota and Curcumin: A New Key of Understanding for the Health Effects of Curcumin. *Nutrients* **2020**, *12*, 2499. [CrossRef]
153. Shen, L.; Ji, H.F. Bidirectional Interactions between Dietary Curcumin and Gut Microbiota. *Crit. Rev. Food Sci. Nutr.* **2019**, *59*, 2896–2902. [CrossRef]
154. Zhai, S.S.; Ruan, D.; Zhu, Y.W.; Li, M.C.; Ye, H.; Wang, W.C.; Yang, L. Protective Effect of Curcumin on Ochratoxin A–Induced Liver Oxidative Injury in Duck Is Mediated by Modulating Lipid Metabolism and the Intestinal Microbiota. *Poult. Sci.* **2020**, *99*, 1124–1134. [CrossRef] [PubMed]
155. Shen, L.; Liu, L.; Ji, H.F. Regulative Effects of Curcumin Spice Administration on Gut Microbiota and Its Pharmacological Implications. *Food Nutr. Res.* **2017**, *61*, 1361780. [CrossRef] [PubMed]
156. Feng, W.; Wang, H.; Zhang, P.; Gao, C.; Tao, J.; Ge, Z.; Zhu, D.; Bi, Y. Modulation of Gut Microbiota Contributes to Curcumin-Mediated Attenuation of Hepatic Steatosis in Rats. *Biochim. Biophys. Acta Gen. Subj.* **2017**, *1861*, 1801–1812. [CrossRef] [PubMed]

157. Greiner, A.K.; Papineni, R.V.; Umar, S. Chemoprevention in Gastrointestinal Physiology and Disease. Natural Products and Microbiome. *Am. J. Physiol. Gastrointest. Liver Physiol.* **2014**, *307*, G1–G15. [CrossRef] [PubMed]
158. Youssef, O.; Lahti, L.; Kokkola, A.; Karla, T.; Tikkanen, M.; Ehsan, H.; Carpelan-Holmström, M.; Koskensalo, S.; Böhling, T.; Rautelin, H.; et al. Stool Microbiota Composition Differs in Patients with Stomach, Colon, and Rectal Neoplasms. *Dig. Dis. Sci.* **2018**, *63*, 2950–2958. [CrossRef]
159. Mori, G.; Orena, B.S.; Cultrera, I.; Barbieri, G.; Albertini, A.M.; Ranzani, G.N.; Carnevali, I.; Tibiletti, M.G.; Pasca, M.R. Gut Microbiota Analysis in Postoperative Lynch Syndrome Patients. *Front. Microbiol.* **2019**, *10*, 1746. [CrossRef] [PubMed]
160. Kundu, P.; De, R.; Pal, I.; Mukhopadhyay, A.K.; Saha, D.R.; Swarnakar, S. Curcumin Alleviates Matrix Metalloproteinase-3 and-9 Activities during Eradication of Helicobacter pylori Infection in Cultured Cells and Mice. *PLoS One* **2011**, *6*, e16306. [CrossRef]
161. Haghi, A.; Azimi, H.; Rahimi, R. A Comprehensive Review on Pharmacotherapeutics of Three Phytochemicals, Curcumin, Quercetin, and Allicin, in the Treatment of Gastric Cancer. *J. Gastrointest. Cancer* **2017**, *48*, 314–320. [CrossRef] [PubMed]
162. Ullah, H.; di Minno, A.; Santarcangelo, C.; Khan, H.; Xiao, J.; Arciola, C.R.; Daglia, M. Vegetable Extracts and Nutrients Useful in the Recovery from Helicobacter pylori Infection: A Systematic Review on Clinical Trials. *Molecules* **2021**, *26*, 2272. [CrossRef] [PubMed]
163. Srinivasan, K. Ginger Rhizomes (Zingiber officinale): A Spice with Multiple Health Beneficial Potentials. *PharmaNutrition* **2017**, *5*, 18–28. [CrossRef]
164. Mao, Q.Q.; Xu, X.Y.; Cao, S.Y.; Gan, R.Y.; Corke, H.; Beta, T.; Li, H.B. Bioactive Compounds and Bioactivities of Ginger (Zingiber officinale Roscoe). *Foods* **2019**, *8*, 185. [CrossRef] [PubMed]
165. Govindarajan, V.S.; Connell, D.W. Ginger—Chemistry, Technology, and Quality Evaluation: Part 1. *Crit. Rev. Food Sci. Nutr.* **1983**, *17*, 1–96. [CrossRef] [PubMed]
166. Baliga, M.S.; Haniadka, R.; Pereira, M.M.; D'Souza, J.J.; Pallaty, P.L.; Bhat, H.P.; Popuri, S. Update on the Chemopreventive Effects of Ginger and Its Phytochemicals. *Crit. Rev. Food Sci. Nutr.* **2011**, *51*, 499–523. [CrossRef] [PubMed]
167. Prasad, S.; Tyagi, A.K. Ginger and Its Constituents: Role in Prevention and Treatment of Gastrointestinal Cancer. *Gastroenterol. Res. Pract.* **2015**, *2015*, 142979. [CrossRef] [PubMed]
168. El-Abhar, H.S.; Hammad, L.N.; Gawad, H.S.A. Modulating Effect of Ginger Extract on Rats with Ulcerative Colitis. *J. Ethnopharmacol.* **2008**, *118*, 367–372. [CrossRef] [PubMed]
169. Zhang, M.; Xu, C.; Liu, D.; Han, M.K.; Wang, L.; Merlin, D. Oral Delivery of Nanoparticles Loaded with Ginger Active Compound, 6-Shogaol, Attenuates Ulcerative Colitis and Promotes Wound Healing in a Murine Model of Ulcerative Colitis. *J. Crohns Colitis* **2018**, *12*, 217–229. [CrossRef]
170. Zhang, M.; Viennois, E.; Prasad, M.; Zhang, Y.; Wang, L.; Zhang, Z.; Han, M.K.; Xiao, B.; Xu, C.; Srinivasan, S.; et al. Edible Ginger-Derived Nanoparticles: A Novel Therapeutic Approach for the Prevention and Treatment of Inflammatory Bowel Disease and Colitis-Associated Cancer. *Biomaterials* **2016**, *101*, 321–340. [CrossRef] [PubMed]
171. Shang, A.; Cao, S.Y.; Xu, X.Y.; Gan, R.Y.; Tang, G.Y.; Corke, H.; Mavumengwana, V.; Li, H.B. Bioactive Compounds and Biological Functions of Garlic (*Allium sativum* L.). *Foods* **2019**, *8*, 246. [CrossRef]
172. Petropoulos, S.A.; di Gioia, F.; Polyzos, N.; Tzortzakis, N. Natural Antioxidants, Health Effects and Bioactive Properties of Wild Allium Species. *Curr. Pharm. Des.* **2020**, *26*, 1816–1837. [CrossRef]
173. Martins, N.; Petropoulos, S.; Ferreira, I.C. Chemical Composition and Bioactive Compounds of Garlic (*Allium sativum* L.) as Affected by Pre-and Post-Harvest Conditions: A Review. *Food Chem.* **2016**, *211*, 41–50. [CrossRef] [PubMed]
174. Miroddi, M.; Calapai, F.; Calapai, G. Potential Beneficial Effects of Garlic in Oncohematology. *Mini Rev. Med. Chem.* **2011**, *11*, 461–472. [CrossRef] [PubMed]
175. Zhang, Y.; Liu, X.; Ruan, J.; Zhuang, X.; Zhang, X.; Li, Z. Phytochemicals of Garlic: Promising Candidates for Cancer Therapy. *Biomed. Pharmacother.* **2020**, *123*, 109730. [CrossRef] [PubMed]
176. Mondal, A.; Banerjee, S.; Bose, S.; Mazumder, S.; Haber, R.A.; Farzaei, M.H.; Bishayee, A. Garlic Constituents for Cancer Prevention and Therapy: From Phytochemistry to Novel Formulations. *Pharmacol. Res.* **2022**, *175*, 105837. [CrossRef] [PubMed]
177. de Greef, D.; Barton, E.M.; Sandberg, E.N.; Croley, C.R.; Pumarol, J.; Wong, T.L.; Das, N.; Bishayee, A. Anticancer Potential of Garlic and Its Bioactive Constituents: A Systematic and Comprehensive Review. *Semin. Cancer Biol.* **2021**, *73*, 219–264. [CrossRef] [PubMed]
178. Chen, K.; Xie, K.; Liu, Z.; Nakasone, Y.; Sakao, K.; Hossain, M.A.; Hou, D.X. Preventive Effects and Mechanisms of Garlic on Dyslipidemia and Gut Microbiome Dysbiosis. *Nutrients* **2019**, *11*, 1225. [CrossRef]
179. Ried, K.; Travica, N.; Sali, A. The Effect of Kyolic Aged Garlic Extract on Gut Microbiota, Inflammation, and Cardiovascular Markers in Hypertensives: The GarGIC Trial. *Front. Nutr.* **2018**, *5*, 122. [CrossRef]
180. Yang, Y.; Yang, F.; Huang, M.; Wu, H.; Yang, C.; Zhang, X.; Yang, L.; Chen, G.; Li, S.; Wang, Q.; et al. Fatty Liver and Alteration of the Gut Microbiome Induced by Diallyl Disulfide. *Int. J. Mol. Med.* **2019**, *44*, 1908–1920. [CrossRef] [PubMed]
181. Kamatou, G.P.; Vermaak, I.; Viljoen, A.M. Eugenol—from the Remote Maluku Islands to the International Market Place: A Review of a Remarkable and Versatile Molecule. *Molecules* **2012**, *17*, 6953–6981. [CrossRef]
182. Chaieb, K.; Hajlaoui, H.; Zmantar, T.; Kahla-Nakbi, A.B.; Rouabhia, M.; Mahdouani, K.; Bakhrouf, A. The Chemical Composition and Biological Activity of Clove Essential Oil, Eugenia Caryophyllata (*Syzigium aromaticum* L. Myrtaceae): A Short Review. *Phytother. Res.* **2007**, *21*, 501–506. [CrossRef]

183. Pérez-Jiménez, J.; Neveu, V.; Vos, F.; Scalbert, A. Identification of the 100 Richest Dietary Sources of Polyphenols: An Application of the Phenol-Explorer Database. *Eur. J. Clin. Nutr.* **2010**, *64*, S112–S120. [CrossRef]
184. Gülçin, İ.; Elmastaş, M.; Aboul-Enein, H.Y. Antioxidant Activity of Clove Oil–A Powerful Antioxidant Source. *Arab. J. Chem.* **2012**, *5*, 489–499. [CrossRef]
185. Liu, M.; Zhao, G.; Zhang, D.; An, W.; Lai, H.; Li, X.; Cao, S.; Lin, X. Active Fraction of Clove Induces Apoptosis via PI3K/Akt/MTOR-Mediated Autophagy in Human Colorectal Cancer HCT-116 Cells. *Int. J. Oncol.* **2018**, *53*, 1363–1373. [CrossRef] [PubMed]
186. Liu, H.; Schmitz, J.C.; Wei, J.; Cao, S.; Beumer, J.H.; Strychor, S.; Cheng, L.; Liu, M.; Wang, C.; Wu, N.; et al. Clove Extract Inhibits Tumor Growth and Promotes Cell Cycle Arrest and Apoptosis. *Oncol. Res.* **2014**, *21*, 247–259. [CrossRef] [PubMed]
187. Chen, S.; Wu, X.; Tang, S.; Yin, J.; Song, Z.; He, X.; Yin, Y. Eugenol Alleviates Dextran Sulfate Sodium-Induced Colitis Independent of Intestinal Microbiota in Mice. *J. Agric. Food Chem.* **2021**, *69*, 10506–10514. [CrossRef] [PubMed]
188. Saleh, B.K.; Omer, A.; Teweldemedhin, B. Medicinal Uses and Health Benefits of Chili Pepper (Capsicum Spp.): A Review. *MOJ Food Process. Technol.* **2018**, *6*, 325–328. [CrossRef]
189. de Jong, P.R.; Takahashi, N.; Harris, A.R.; Lee, J.; Bertin, S.; Jeffries, J.; Jung, M.; Duong, J.; Triano, A.I.; Lee, J.; et al. Ion Channel TRPV1-Dependent Activation of PTP1B Suppresses EGFR-Associated Intestinal Tumorigenesis. *J. Clin. Invest.* **2014**, *124*, 3793–3806. [CrossRef]
190. Chan, W.C.; Millwood, I.Y.; Kartsonaki, C.; Du, H.; Guo, Y.; Chen, Y.; Bian, Z.; Walters, R.G.; Lv, J.; He, P.; et al. Spicy Food Consumption and Risk of Gastrointestinal-Tract Cancers: Findings from the China Kadoorie Biobank. *Int. J. Epidemiol.* **2021**, *50*, 199–211. [CrossRef]
191. Hayashi, K.; Shibata, C.; Nagao, M.; Sato, M.; Kakyo, M.; Kinouchi, M.; Saijo, F.; Miura, K.; Ogawa, H.; Sasaki, I. Intracolonic Capsaicin Stimulates Colonic Motility and Defecation in Conscious Dogs. *Surgery* **2010**, *147*, 789–797. [CrossRef]
192. Ashktorab, H.; Soleimani, A.; Singh, G.; Amin, A.; Tabtabaei, S.; Latella, G.; Stein, U.; Akhondzadeh, S.; Solanki, N.; Gondré-Lewis, M.C.; et al. Saffron: The Golden Spice with Therapeutic Properties on Digestive Diseases. *Nutrients* **2019**, *11*, 943. [CrossRef]
193. Melnyk, J.P.; Wang, S.; Marcone, M.F. Chemical and Biological Properties of the World's Most Expensive Spice: Saffron. *Food Res. Int.* **2010**, *43*, 1981–1989. [CrossRef]
194. Xing, B.; Li, S.; Yang, J.; Lin, D.; Feng, Y.; Lu, J.; Shao, Q. Phytochemistry, Pharmacology, and Potential Clinical Applications of Saffron: A Review. *J. Ethnopharmacol.* **2021**, *281*, 114555. [CrossRef] [PubMed]
195. Gezici, S. Comparative Anticancer Activity Analysis of Saffron Extracts and a Principle Component, Crocetin for Prevention and Treatment of Human Malignancies. *J. Food Sci. Technol.* **2019**, *56*, 5435–5443. [CrossRef] [PubMed]
196. Kawabata, K.; Tung, N.H.; Shoyama, Y.; Sugie, S.; Mori, T.; Tanaka, T. Dietary Crocin Inhibits Colitis and Colitis-Associated Colorectal Carcinogenesis in Male ICR Mice. *Evid. base Compl. Alternative Med.* **2012**, *2012*, 820415. [CrossRef] [PubMed]
197. Amerizadeh, F.; Rezaei, N.; Rahmani, F.; Hassanian, S.M.; Moradi-Marjaneh, R.; Fiuji, H.; Boroumand, N.; Nosrati-Tirkani, A.; Ghayour-Mobarhan, M.; Ferns, G.A.; et al. Crocin Synergistically Enhances the Antiproliferative Activity of 5-flurouracil through Wnt/PI3K Pathway in a Mouse Model of Colitis-associated Colorectal Cancer. *J. Cell. Biochem.* **2018**, *119*, 10250–10261. [CrossRef] [PubMed]
198. Güllü, N.; Kobelt, D.; Brim, H.; Rahman, S.; Timm, L.; Smith, J.; Soleimani, A.; di Marco, S.; Bisti, S.; Ashktorab, H.; et al. Saffron Crudes and Compounds Restrict MACC1-Dependent Cell Proliferation and Migration of Colorectal Cancer Cells. *Cells* **2020**, *9*, 1829. [CrossRef]
199. Li, M.; Ding, L.; Hu, Y.L.; Qin, L.L.; Wu, Y.; Liu, W.; Wu, L.L.; Liu, T.H. Herbal Formula LLKL Ameliorates Hyperglycaemia, Modulates the Gut Microbiota and Regulates the Gut-liver Axis in Zucker Diabetic Fatty Rats. *J. Cell. Mol. Med.* **2021**, *25*, 367–382. [CrossRef] [PubMed]
200. Shim, Y.Y.; Gui, B.; Arnison, P.G.; Wang, Y.; Reaney, M.J. Flaxseed (*Linum usitatissimum* L.) Bioactive Compounds and Peptide Nomenclature: A Review. *Trends Food Sci. Technol.* **2014**, *38*, 5–20. [CrossRef]
201. Mendonça, L.A.; dos Santos Ferreira, R.; de Cássia Avellaneda Guimarães, R.; de Castro, A.P.; Franco, O.L.; Matias, R.; Carvalho, C.M. The Complex Puzzle of Interactions among Functional Food, Gut Microbiota, and Colorectal Cancer. *Front. Oncol.* **2018**, *8*, 325. [CrossRef] [PubMed]
202. Zhou, X.; Zhang, Z.; Huang, F.; Yang, C.; Huang, Q. In Vitro Digestion and Fermentation by Human Fecal Microbiota of Polysaccharides from Flaxseed. *Molecules* **2020**, *25*, 4354. [CrossRef] [PubMed]
203. Määttänen, P.; Lurz, E.; Botts, S.R.; Wu, R.Y.; Yeung, C.W.; Li, B.; Abiff, S.; Johnson-Henry, K.C.; Lepp, D.; Power, K.A.; et al. Ground Flaxseed Reverses Protection of a Reduced-Fat Diet against Citrobacter rodentium-Induced Colitis. *Am. J. Physiol. Gastrointest. Liver Physiol.* **2018**, *315*, G788–G798. [CrossRef] [PubMed]

cancers

Article

Polygodial, a Sesquiterpene Dialdehyde, Activates Apoptotic Signaling in Castration-Resistant Prostate Cancer Cell Lines by Inducing Oxidative Stress

Reshmii Venkatesan [1,†], Mohamed Ali Hussein [1,†], Leah Moses [1], Jennifer S. Liu [2], Salman R. Khetani [2], Alexander Kornienko [3] and Gnanasekar Munirathinam [1,*]

1 Department of Biomedical Sciences, College of Medicine, University of Illinois, 1601 Parkview Avenue, Rockford, IL 61107, USA
2 Department of Biomedical Engineering, University of Illinois at Chicago, Chicago, IL 60607, USA
3 Department of Chemistry and Biochemistry, Texas State University, San Marcos, TX 78666, USA
* Correspondence: mgnanas@uic.edu; Tel.: +1-(815)-395-5773
† These authors contributed equally to this work.

Simple Summary: Prostate cancer (PCa) is the second leading cause of cancer death in men in the United States. The emergence of resistance to androgen deprivation therapy results in castration-resistant prostate cancer (CRPC) development. Taxanes are diterpene compounds approved to treat hormonal-resistant PCa. CRPC patients treated with taxanes show poor outcomes. Polygodial (PG) is a natural sesquiterpene compound isolated from water pepper (*Persicaria hydropiper*), Dorrigo pepper (*Tasmannia stipitata*), and mountain pepper (*Tasmannia lanceolata*), which has shown to exhibit anticancer properties. PG robustly inhibits the viability, colony formation, and migration of taxane-resistant CRPC (PC3-TXR and DU145-TXR) cell lines. Additionally, our data show that PG promotes anoikis and induces cell cycle arrest at the G0 phase in PCa cells. Our results reveal that PG induces oxidative stress and activates apoptosis in drug-resistant CRPC cell lines. Altogether, our data suggest that the anticancer activity of PG is via the induction of apoptosis in CRPC cells.

Abstract: Prostate cancer (PCa) is the second leading cause of cancer death among men in the United States. Surgery, radiation therapy, chemotherapy, and androgen deprivation therapy are currently the standard treatment options for PCa. These have poor outcomes and result in the development of castration-resistant prostate cancer (CRPC), which is the foremost underlying cause of mortality associated with PCa. Taxanes, diterpene compounds approved to treat hormonal refractory PCa, show poor outcomes in CRPC. Polygodial (PG) is a natural sesquiterpene isolated from water pepper (*Persicaria hydropiper*), Dorrigo pepper (*Tasmannia stipitata*), and mountain pepper (*Tasmannia lanceolata*). Previous reports show that PG has an anticancer effect. Our results show that PG robustly inhibits the cell viability, colony formation, and migration of taxane-resistant CRPC cell lines and induces cell cycle arrest at the G0 phase. A toxicity investigation shows that PG is not toxic to primary human hepatocytes, 3T3-J2 fibroblast co-cultures, and non-cancerous BPH-1 cells, implicating that PG is innocuous to healthy cells. In addition, PG induces oxidative stress and activates apoptosis in drug-resistant PCa cell lines. Our mechanistic evaluation by a proteome profiler–human apoptotic array in PC3-TXR cells shows that PG induces upregulation of cytochrome c and caspase-3 and downregulation of antiapoptotic markers. Western blot analysis reveals that PG activates apoptotic and DNA damage markers in PCa cells. Our results suggest that PG exhibits its anticancer effect by promoting reactive oxygen species generation and induction of apoptosis in CRPC cells.

Keywords: prostate cancer; castration-resistant prostate cancer; polygodial; taxane-resistant CRPC; anoikis; natural products

Citation: Venkatesan, R.; Hussein, M.A.; Moses, L.; Liu, J.S.; Khetani, S.R.; Kornienko, A.; Munirathinam, G. Polygodial, a Sesquiterpene Dialdehyde, Activates Apoptotic Signaling in Castration-Resistant Prostate Cancer Cell Lines by Inducing Oxidative Stress. *Cancers* **2022**, *14*, 5260. https://doi.org/10.3390/cancers14215260

Academic Editors: Anupam Bishayee and Marcos Roberto de Oliveira

Received: 19 September 2022
Accepted: 17 October 2022
Published: 26 October 2022

1. Introduction

Prostate cancer (PCa) is the most common cancer among men in the United States of America (USA), with an estimated 268,490 new cases in 2022, and it occupies the second place in causes of high mortality among men in the USA, after lung cancer [1,2]. One in eight men will have PCa during their lifetime, and the five-year relative survival rate for PCa is 96.8% [2]. The global burden of PCa is vastly increased worldwide, with PCa ranked fourth among the top five most common cancers, with 7.3% of all new cancer cases being PCa [3]. The incidence of PCa increases in older men aged above 50 years, men of African descent, men with a family history of the disease, and men with genetic risk factors [4]. The early stages of PCa are indolent and mostly asymptomatic; by the time it becomes symptomatic, it is aggressive and metastasizes to other parts of the body [4]. The heterogeneity of PCa is due to the disease's multifaceted nature, which mainly originates from the spatial, morphological, genetic, and molecular differences of PCa. The genetic and molecular aspects particularly show discrepancies due to intra-patient, inter-patient, and intra-tumoral variations, rendering PCa a complex disease and making targeted genetic therapy impermissible [5,6].

The current armamentarium in treating PCa includes the usage of different strategies such as surgery (surgical castration), radiation therapy (external beam radiotherapy), androgen deprivation therapy (ADT) inducing castration using luteinizing hormone-releasing hormone agonist or antagonist (leuprorelin and goserelin), antiandrogen (abiraterone, enzalutamide, and bicalutamide) and nonsteroidal antiandrogen (such as apalutamide), chemotherapy including carboplatin, and taxanes (paclitaxel, docetaxel, and cabazitaxel), immunotherapy (sipuleucel-T and pembrolizumab), or a combination of these treatment options [7,8]. Surgery and radiation therapy are the most preferable options for localized PCa [9–11]. ADT is used as a primary systematic treatment for regional or advanced PCa, or as an adjuvant/neoadjuvant therapy in combination with radiotherapy in locally advanced PCa [8]. Taxanes, including paclitaxel, docetaxel, and cabazitaxel, approved to treat advanced and hormonal refractory PCa, show poor outcomes in CRPC [12,13]. Resistance to ADT results in the attainment of castration-resistant prostate cancer (CRPC), which is identified as progression of the disease with a concomitant upsurge in the serum levels of the prostate-specific antigen (PSA), despite using ADT therapy [14]. The CRPC spectrum ranges from a surge in the PSA serum level alone, to an increase in the PSA level and metastasis, giving rise to a more progressive form called metastatic CRPC [15]. Predominantly, resistance to ADT therapy emerges within two to three years of treatment [16]. The current options available for the treatment of metastatic CRPC are ADT in combination with luteinizing hormone-releasing hormone agonist-antagonist, along with taxanes [8]. However, taxanes show poor outcomes, resistance, and severe side effects [17,18]. Therefore, there is an urgent need for a better treatment approach for men with CRPC.

Over the years, natural products or their derivatives have shown chemopreventive and chemotherapeutic benefits [19–21]. The indefinite diversity of natural products renders diverse biological functions that may be advantageous over conventional chemotherapeutic agents [22–24]. Several natural products have been shown to regulate the oncogene and tumor suppressor genes in cancer [25], epigenetic mechanisms [26], and tumor microenvironment [27]. Polygodial (PG) is a sesquiterpene isolated from water pepper (*Persicaria hydropiper*), Dorrigo pepper (*Tasmannia stipitata*), and mountain pepper (*Tasmannia lanceolata*) [28,29]. PG exhibits antibacterial activity against Gram-negative bacteria, such as *Escherichia coli* and *Salmonella choleraesuis*, and Gram-positive bacteria, such as *Bacillus subtilis* and *Staphylococcus aureus* [29]. PG also exhibits antifungal, anti-inflammatory, and anticancer activity [29–31]. Several studies have reported that PG and its derivatives, including isopolygodial, 9-epipolygodial (DR-P27), 1-β-(p-coumaroyloxy)-polygodial, and 1-β-(*p*-methoxycinnamoyl)-polygodial, exhibit anticancer activity in different cancers [32–35]. Dasari et al. [30] reported that DR-P27 possesses superior antiproliferative efficacy compared to PG in drug resistant cancer cells. In contrast, De La Chapa et al. [32] showed that DR-P27 is equipotent to PG in oral squamous cell carcinoma (OSCC) [32]. Our previous study has demonstrated that the PG derivative DR-P27 exhibits anticancer activity against androgen-sensitive PCa by inducing apoptosis in vitro [28]. In this study, we have examined the anticancer efficacy and the underlying anticancer mechanism of PG against the taxane-resistant CRPC using an in vitro model. In addition, our study revealed for the first time that PG treatment induces anoikis in CRPC cell lines.

2. Materials and Methods

2.1. Cell Lines

PCa cell lines (PC3-TXR and DU145-TXR) were generously donated by Dr. Evan Keller (University of Michigan, Ann Arbor, Michigan, USA). These cells were established from PC3 and DU145 through exposure to paclitaxel at regular intervals, as described by Takeda et al. [36]. The BPH-1 cell line was obtained from Dr. Simon W. Hayward (University of Chicago, Northshore Research Institute, Pritzker School of Medicine, Chicago, USA). The BPH-1 cells were cultured in RPMI-1640 media (Gibco, Grand Island, NY, USA) supplemented with 10% (*v/v*) fetal bovine serum (FBS), 1% (*v/v*) antimycotic (Sigma Aldrich, St. Louis, MO, USA), and 0.6% (*v/v*) gentamycin (Fisher Scientific, Waltham, MA, USA) and grown at 37 °C with 5% CO_2. Micropatterned co-cultures (MPCCs) of primary human hepatocytes and 3T3-J2 murine embryonic fibroblasts were created as described previously [37]. The cells were seeded into the micropatterned plates in a serum-free culture medium, consisting of 1X Dulbecco's modified Eagle's medium (DMEM, Corning Life Sciences, Corning, NY, USA) supplemented with 15 mM HEPES [4-(2-hydroxyethyl)-1-piperazineethane-sulfonic acid] buffer (Corning Life Sciences, Corning, NY, USA), 1% penicillin/streptomycin, 1% ITS+ (insulin, transferrin, selenous acid, linoleic acid, bovine serum albumin; Corning Life Sciences, Corning, New York, NY, USA), 7 ng mL-1 glucagon (Sigma-Aldrich, St. Louis, MO, USA), and 0.1 μM dexamethasone (Sigma-Aldrich, St. Louis, MO, USA). The hepatocytes preferentially attached to the circular collagen domains, leaving approximately 5000 primary human hepatocytes per 96 well plates. The 3T3-J2 murine embryonic fibroblasts were generously donated by Dr. Howard Green [38]. The cells were cultured in DMEM containing 10% bovine calf serum and 1% penicillin/streptomycin.

2.2. Chemicals and Antibodies

PG with ≥97% purity was obtained from Sigma-Aldrich (Sigma-Aldrich, St. Louis, MO, USA). The molecular weight of PG is 234.33 g/mol. The main stock of 10 mM was prepared by dissolving the drug in 0.1% dimethyl sulfoxide (DMSO), purchased from Fisher Scientific (Waltham, MA, USA). Further, different concentrations were prepared from the main stock and added to complete RPMI for treating cells. Necrostatin-1 (NEC), 3–4,5-dimethylthiazol-2-yl,2,5-diphenyl tetrazolium bromide (MTT), N-acetyl cysteine (NAC), propidium Iodide (PI), and 3-methyladenine (3MA) was obtained from Sigma-Aldrich, St. Louis, MO, USA. The pan caspase inhibitor (CI) Z-VAD-FMK was procured from APExBIO (Houston, TX, USA). The antibodies used were against PARP, pH2AX, Bcl-2, caspase-3, cleaved caspase-3, pro-caspase-3, XIAP, cIAP-2, and β-actin. HRP-conjugated anti-rabbit and HRP-conjugated anti-mouse antibodies were obtained from Cell Signaling Technology (Danvers, MA, USA).

2.3. Cell Viability Assay

To examine the effect of PG on the cell viability of PCa cell lines (PC3-TXR and DU145-TXR), cells were treated with various concentrations of PG. Cell viability was measured using MTT dye to determine the colorimetric dye reduction, according to van Meerloo et al. [39]. The PCa cells were seeded in 96 well plates at a cell density of 3×10^3/well in 100 μL of complete RPMI (10% FBS, 1% antimycotic, and 0.6% antibiotic) and maintained at 37 °C with 5% CO_2 humidity. Various concentrations of PG (5, 10, 20, and 50 μM) were used to treat the cells. Following treatment, 100 μL of MTT reagent was added to each well after 24, 48, and 72 h of treatment and incubated for 3 h at 37 °C. After incubation, the insoluble formazan crystals were solubilized with a 90% isopropanol

(Fisher Scientific, Waltham, MA, USA) and 10% Triton-X (Sigma-Aldrich, St. Louis, MO, USA) solution. The plates were kept on the shaker for 15 min to solubilize all the crystals completely, and absorbance was measured at 590 nm using a Biotek plate reader. The cell viability percentages were calculated according to the formula given below,

$$\%\ Cell\ viabilty = \frac{Avg.\ OD\ of\ experimental\ cells}{Avg.\ OD\ of\ control\ cells} \times 100$$

Moreover, to determine the cell death mechanism, a cell viability assay was performed using a combination of varying concentrations of PG and different inhibitors such as NAC, 3MA, NEC, and CI to block the PG effect. In addition, to test cytotoxicity and hepatotoxicity of PG, well-established MPCCs of primary human hepatocytes and supportive 3T3-J2 murine embryonic fibroblasts, as well as 3T3-J2 fibroblast-only monocultures, were created as previously described [40]. All cultures were functionally stabilized for 7 days and then treated for 6 days with fresh PG added to a serum-free culture medium every 2 days. Cell viability was assessed 2 days after every PG treatment (i.e., day 9, 11, and 13 of culture) via the PrestoBlue™ cell viability assay (Invitrogen, Waltham, MA, USA).

2.4. Colony Formation Assay

To assess the anchorage-independent cell growth of PG on PCa cell lines, a colony formation assay was used, according to Samy et al. [41]. The colony formation assay investigates the different capacities of a single cell to form a colony in treated cells compared with the untreated control. PCa cells were seeded in a 6-well plate with complete RPMI media containing approximately 500 cells per well, and cells were allowed to grow at 37 °C with 5% CO_2. After 24 h, the cells were treated with different concentrations of PG (5, 10, 20, and 50 μM) and incubated for 1–3 weeks. The media was changed every 3 days during incubation. To observe colony formation, the media was removed, and the cells were fixed with acetic acid and methanol in a ratio of 1:7 and incubated at room temperature for 5 min. The fixative agent was removed, and the cells were stained with 1 mL of 0.5% (*v/v*) crystal violet (Fisher Scientific, Waltham, MA, USA) and incubated for 2 h at room temperature. Then, the plates were washed with running tap water twice and allowed to dry for 5 days.

2.5. Wound Healing Assay

Wound healing assay is an in vitro method to study the migration ability of metastatic cancer cells. The assay evaluates the inhibitory effect of PG on cell migration characteristics in a PCa model [42]. The PCa cells were cultured in a 24-well plate and incubated at 37 °C with 5% CO_2. After the cell reached 100% confluency, the old media was removed, and the cells were treated with mitomycin C at a concentration of 15μM for 1 h. After that, each well was washed with 1 mL of 1X PBS, then a scratch (wound) was made on the surface of each well using a 200 μL pipet tip, and the wells were washed with PBS. Complete RPMI media was added to each well and treated with different concentrations of PG (5, 10, 20, and 50 μM). The wound closing of PCa cell line image was taken using a microscope (Olympus IX73) at 0, 24, 48, and 72 h after treatment. The percentage of open area over treatment data was analyzed using T scratch image software.

2.6. Apoptosis Assay by Immunofluorescence Analysis

To examine whether PG induces apoptosis in PCa cell lines, an apoptosis assay was performed using annexin V FITC/PI staining as per the protocol of Gong et al. [43]. In an 8-well chamber, PCa cells were seeded at a density of 10,000 cells per well in 250 μL of complete RPMI media and allowed to grow at 37 °C with 5% CO_2 for 48 h. The spent media were replaced with fresh complete RPMI media, and the cells were treated with different concentrations of PG (5, 10, 20, and 50 μM). After 48 h of incubation, each well was washed with 250 μL of 1X PBS and stained with 2.5 μL annexin V FITC and PI using the BD Annexin V: FITC apoptosis detection kit-I (BD Bioscience, San Jose, CA, USA). The plate was incubated in the dark at room temperature for 15 min. Again, the cells were washed with 250 μL of 1X PBS. After removing the chamber, a drop of fluorogel was added to each well and covered with a coverslip. The slides were imaged under an Olympus FV10i confocal microscope.

2.7. Apoptosis Assay by Flow Cytometry

To dissect the mechanism by which PG induces apoptosis in PCa cell lines, we performed flow cytometry analysis using annexin V FITC / PI staining as per the protocol of Wlodkowic et al. [44]. PCa cells were seeded at a density of 50,000 cells per well in a 6-well plate and incubated at 37 °C with 5% CO_2 for 48 h. The cells were treated with various concentrations of PG (5, 10, 20, and 50 μM). After 48 h of treatment, both live and dead cells were collected and stained with 2.5 μL of annexin V FITC/ PI using the annexin V: FITC apoptosis detection kit I, followed by incubation in the dark for 15 min at room temperature. The treated and untreated cells were then analyzed via flow cytometry (FACS Calibur; Becton Dickinson, Mountain View, CA, USA).

2.8. Anchorage-Dependent Cell Death Assay

Anchorage-dependent cell death assay, also known as anoikis, is a type of apoptosis that is induced by a lack of appropriate cell-extracellular matrix (ECM) adhesion. Healthy cells undergo cell death in the absence of ECM adhesion, whereas cancer cells evade anoikis to metastasize to another organ [45]. To evaluate whether PG promotes anoikis, the assay was performed by calcein-AM and EthD-1 staining, and the MTT assay was performed as per Kummrow et al. [45], with modifications. The plates were coated with poly-HEMA to prevent the cells from adhering to the plate, and approximately 10,000 PCa cells were seeded in each well and incubated at 37 °C with 5% CO_2. After 24 h of incubation, the cells were treated with varying concentrations of PG (1, 5, 1, 2, and 50 μM). After 24 h of treatment time, the cells were stained with calcein-AM (stains live cells) and EthD-1 (stains dead cells), observed under the immunofluorescence microscope (Olympus IX73), and images were acquired. In addition, we assessed cell viability by adding 10% MTT to each well in a 24-well anchorage resistant plate and incubating overnight as per Chinnapaka et al. [46]. The media was removed, leaving behind the purple formazan crystals, which were solubilized with a solubilizing agent. The absorbance was measured at 590 nm using a Biotek plate reader.

2.9. Quantitative Expression of Anchorage-Dependent Cell Death Markers by Real Time-qPCR Analysis

To confirm that PG promotes anoikis, PCa cells were treated with different concentrations of PG (5,10, 25, and 50μM) for 48 hrs. The cells were harvested, and total RNA was extracted using the TRIzol reagent (Invitrogen, Waltham, MA, USA), as per Dasari et al. [20]. The complementary DNA (cDNA) was synthesized using a high-capacity cDNA reverse transcription kit (Fisher Scientific, Waltham, MA, USA). Real-time PCR was performed using the Maxima SYBR green qPCR master mix (Fisher Scientific, Waltham, MA, USA). The expression level of β-actin, VIM, CDH1, SNAI1, SNAI2, TWIST1, and ZO-1 mRNA was quantified by real-time PCR QuantStudio 3 (Applied Biosystems, Waltham, CA, USA). β-actin was used as an endogenous control. The relative gene expression was analyzed using the fold change ($2^{(-\Delta(\Delta Ct))}$) of treated samples.

2.10. Cell Cycle Analysis by Flow Cytometry

To investigate whether PG promotes cell death by inducing cell cycle arrest in the PCa cell line, flow cytometry analysis was performed. The DNA was quantitatively analyzed using the DNA binding dye PI, as per Pozarowski et al. [47]. PCa cell lines were cultured in a 6-well plate at a density of 50,000 cells per well with complete RPMI media and allowed to grow at 37 °C with 5% CO_2 for 48 h. After 48 h of treatment with varying concentrations of PG, the cells were collected and fixed with ice-cold 70% ethanol and incubated overnight at 4 °C. The cells were washed with 1X PBS, treated with 100 μg/mL RNAase, and incubated at

37 °C for 30 min. After washing with 1X PBS, the cells were stained with 50 μg/mL PI, and the samples were incubated at room temperature for 30 min. The cells were then analyzed using flow cytometry (FACS Calibur; Becton Dickinson, Mountain View, CA, USA).

2.11. Reactive Oxygen Species Assay

Cancer cells exhibit a basal level of reactive oxygen species (ROS), which is a highly reactive molecule that causes proteins, lipids, and nucleic acid damage in high concentrations. Intracellular antioxidants detoxify excess ROS. ROS levels are elevated when the balance between ROS and antioxidants is disrupted, leading to oxidative stress-mediated cell death [48]. An ROS assay was performed to examine whether PG promotes ROS generation, mediating cell death in taxane-resistant CRPC cell lines, as per Casaburi et al. [49]. Approximately 10,000 cells were seeded with complete RMPI media in an 8-well chamber and incubated at 37 °C with 5% CO_2 for 48 h. The cells were treated with different concentrations of PG. After 6 h, the cells were washed with 1X PBS and stained with 2.5 μL of the ROS fluorescent dye 2′,7′-Dichlorodihydrofluorescein diacetate (DCFH2-DA) and incubated at room temperature in the dark for 15 min. The chambers were removed from the slide, then a drop of fluorogel was added to each well and covered with a coverslip. The cells were observed under the immunofluorescent microscope, and images were acquired.

2.12. Reactive Oxygen Species Analysis by Flow Cytometry

To affirm our results from the previous experiment, ROS production was analyzed by flow cytometry using DCFH2-DA. Approximately 10,000 cells were seeded with complete RMPI media in a 6-well chamber and incubated at 37 °C with 5% CO_2 for 48 h. At 70–80% confluence, cells were treated with 20 μM DCFH2-DA and incubated for 45 min. After incubation, cells were treated with different concentrations of PG for 4 h. After incubation, cells were centrifuged at 1000 rpm for 7 min and washed with 1X PBS. Fluorescence was measured using flow cytometry (FACS Calibur; Becton Dickinson, Mountain View, CA, USA).

2.13. Proteome Profiler-Human Apoptosis Array

To determine the expression profile of various apoptotic markers and to understand the mechanism of PG, a proteome profiler was performed using a human apoptosis array kit (R&D Systems Inc., Minneapolis, MN, USA). The PC3-TXR cells were cultured in 2 T-25 flasks and grown for 48 h at 37 °C with 5% CO_2. One flask was treated with PG 20 μM, and the other flask remained untreated and was incubated for 12 h. Using a cell lysis buffer, cell lysates were collected from untreated and treated flasks. Capture and control antibodies were spotted on the array (nitrocellulose membrane) provided along with the kit. The collected lysates (untreated and PG 20 μM) were incubated overnight with a nitrocellulose membrane array. After incubation, the array was washed 3 times with 1X wash buffer to remove the unbound proteins, followed by 1 h incubation with a cocktail of biotinylated detection antibodies on a rocking platform. The array was washed 3 times with 1X wash buffer and incubated in streptavidin HRP on a rocking platform. Again, the array was washed thrice with 1X wash buffer, chemiluminescent reagents were added, and the signals obtained as spots were captured using X-ray films. The spot intensity was analyzed using a Dot-Blot Protein Array Analyzer macro for Image J software developed by Carpentier in 2008 [50]. The macro is accessible at (https://imagej.nih.gov/ij/macros/toolsets/Dot%20Blot%20Analyzer.txt) (accessed on 4 April 2022) [50].

2.14. Western Blotting

Western blot analysis was performed to determine the anticancer mechanisms of PG and to depict the underlying pathway that induces cell death [51,52]. PCa cell lines were seeded in T25 flasks and grown at 37 °C with 5% CO_2 for 48 h. The cells were treated with varying concentrations of PG and incubated for a treatment period of 48 h. Cell lysates, protein estimation, and gel loading were performed as per Chinnapaka et al. [53]. After loading, the gels were run at 140 volts for 70 min, then transferred to the nitrocellulose membrane using the semi-dry transfer (Bio-Rad Laboratories, Inc., California, USA) at 25 volts for 60 min. The membrane was incubated with 5% skimmed milk in TBS for 1 h. After blocking, the membrane was washed thrice with tris-buffered saline tween 20 (TBST) every 10 min. The membrane was probed with respective primary antibodies and incubated overnight at 4 °C. Similarly, the blots were washed 3 times with TBST and probed with the HRP conjugated secondary antibody for 1 h. The signals were detected using the SuperSignal™ West Pico PLUS Chemiluminescent Substrate (Thermo Scientific, Waltham, MA, USA) and developed using X-ray films. The band intensities were analyzed using ImageJ software. Original blots see Supplementary File S1.

2.15. Statistical Analysis

Quantitative data were analyzed using the One-way, and Two-way analysis of variance (ANOVA) test followed by Tukey's multiple comparison test to determine the treatment significance between the PG treated and the controls within each cell line. A p-value ≤ 0.05 is considered to be statistically significant. GraphPad Prism version 9 was used for the statistical analysis.

3. Results

3.1. PG Is Less Toxic in Hepatocytes and 3T3-J2 Fibroblasts and Inhibits the Cell Viability of Taxane-Resistant CRPC Cell Lines in a Concentration-Dependent Manner

The cell viability assay is used to investigate the cytotoxic effect of the drug in cell lines. It is based on determining the colorimetric change resulting from the enzymatic conversion of the water-soluble MTT dye to water-insoluble formazan crystals by mitochondrial dehydrogenases in the live cells [54]. Hepatocyte/3T3-J2 fibroblast MPCCs and 3T3-J2 fibroblast-only monocultures were treated with increasing concentrations of PG. Our results show no significant fold change difference in the treated cells compared to the DMSO control (Figure 1A,B). This insinuates that PG exhibits an innocuous effect on normal cells.

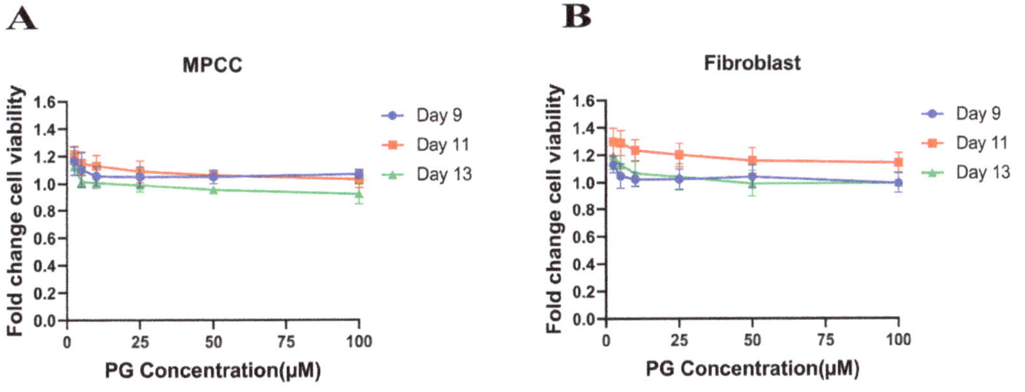

Figure 1. Polygodial (PG) treatments are not toxic to hepatocytes and fibroblasts. MPCCs and 3T3-J2 fibroblast-only monocultures were cultured for 7 days. Cells were treated with various concentrations of PG every other day for 6 days (i.e., three total treatments), and cell viability was measured on the 9th, 11th, and 13th day of culture. The results show that the cell viability of MPCC (**A**) and fibroblast (**B**) is not significantly affected by PG treatment.

Similarly, the PC3-TXR and DU145-TXR cell lines were treated with varying concentrations of PG. Our results reveal that PG significantly decreases cell viability with the increase in PG concentration, as shown in Figure 2A,B. In both the cell lines, the half maximal inhibitory concentration (IC50) is 20 μM, and the maximum inhibition of cell viability by PG is observed at 50 μM. Different time intervals (24, 48, and 72 h) show similar cell viability at higher PG concentrations. Furthermore, to study the potential mechanism of cell death caused by PG, cell viability–blocking experiments were performed. The assay was performed by several inhibitors, including 3MA, NEC, CI, and NAC. In PC3-TXR (Figure 2C), we find that NAC, CI, and 3MA significantly abrogate the cytotoxic effect of PG at a concentration of 10 µM. In addition, the cytotoxic effect of PG at a concentration of 20 µM is considerably inhibited by NAC, CI, 3MA, and NEC within 48 h of treatment.

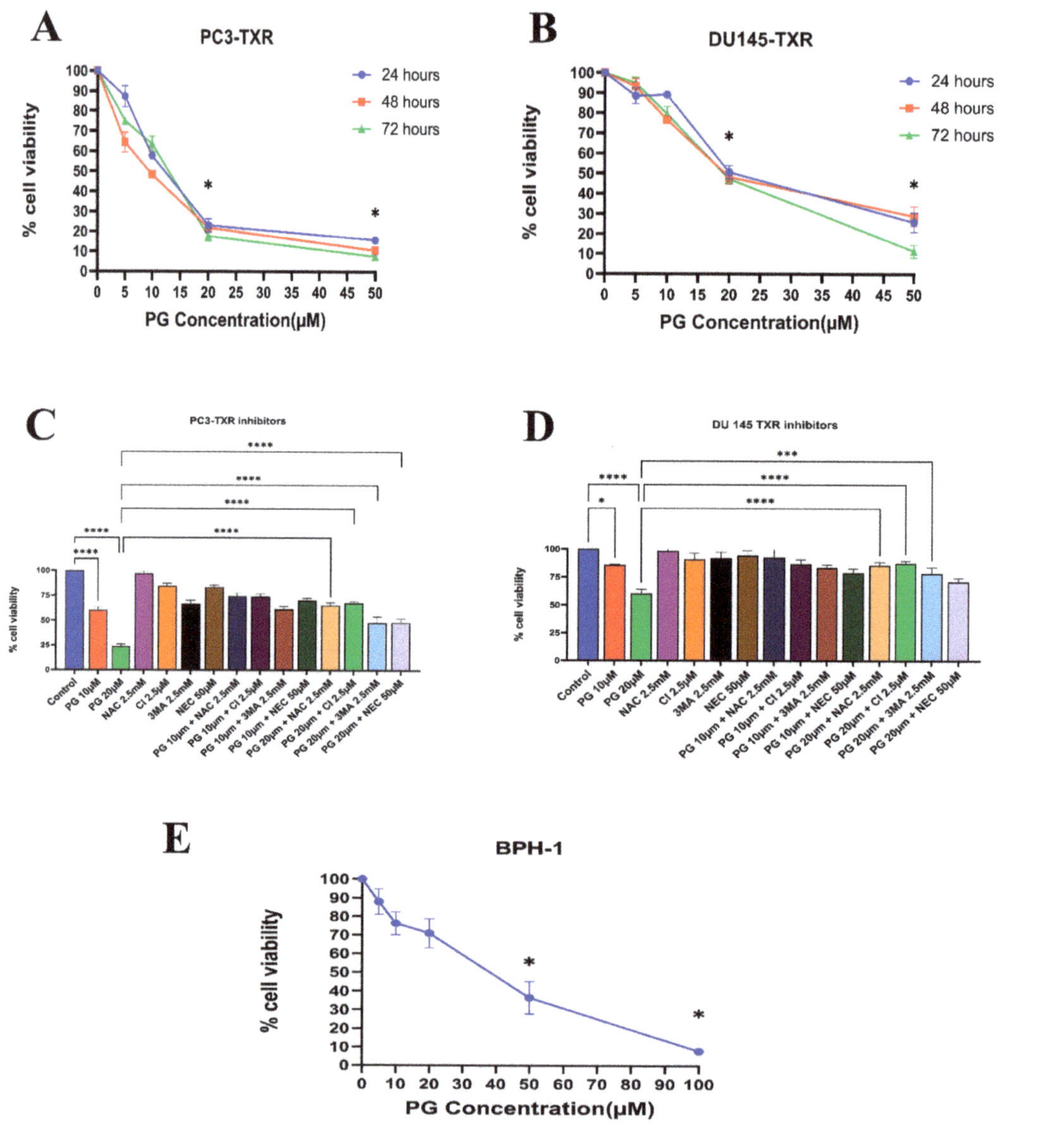

Figure 2. PG inhibits the cell viability of taxane-resistant PCa cell lines in a concentration-dependent manner. The taxane-resistant PCa cell lines (**A**) PC3-TXR and (**B**) DU145-TXR were treated with various concentrations of PG (treatment periods 24, 48, and 72 h). Viability was determined by MTT assay. (**C**) PC3-TXR and (**D**) DU145-TXR were treated with different inhibitors for 48 h. (**E**) depicts the effect of PG on the BPH-1 cell line. Data are represented as mean ± SD (n = 3) and describe three independent experiments performed in triplicate. * $p < 0.05$, *** $p < 0.01$, **** $p < 0.001$.

In contrast, in DU145-TXR (Figure 2D), we observed that NAC, CI, and 3MA significantly block the cytotoxic effect of PG at a concentration of 20 μM. Moreover, we examined the impact of PG on the non-malignant BPH-1 cell line compared to cancerous cell lines PC3-TXR and DU145-TXR. Our results show that PG has an innocuous effect on BPH-1 in low concentrations (Figure 2E). Overall, our data suggest that the taxane-resistant CRPC cell lines are sensitive to PG treatment, indicating that PG has a higher potential for targeting taxane-resistant CRPC. Moreover, the effect of PG was predominately blocked by the antioxidant NAC, implying that PG induces oxidative stress as a potential anticancer mechanism.

3.2. PG Inhibits Colony Formation in Taxane-Resistant CRPC Cell Lines

The clonogenic assay is used to evaluate the capability of a single cell to proliferate independently and form a colony. The assay was conducted to examine the effectiveness of the cytotoxic compounds in tumor-forming (colony formation), a characteristic of cancer in in vitro conditions [55]. We observed a substantial decrease in the number of colonies compared to those in the control in both PC3-TXR and DU145-TXR cells treated with PG (Figure 3A,B). In addition, we observed that NAC significantly abrogates the PG effect in both cell lines (Figure 3C,D). Collectively, our findings demonstrate that PG substantially decreases the number of colonies in taxane-resistant CRPC cell lines in a concentration-dependent manner.

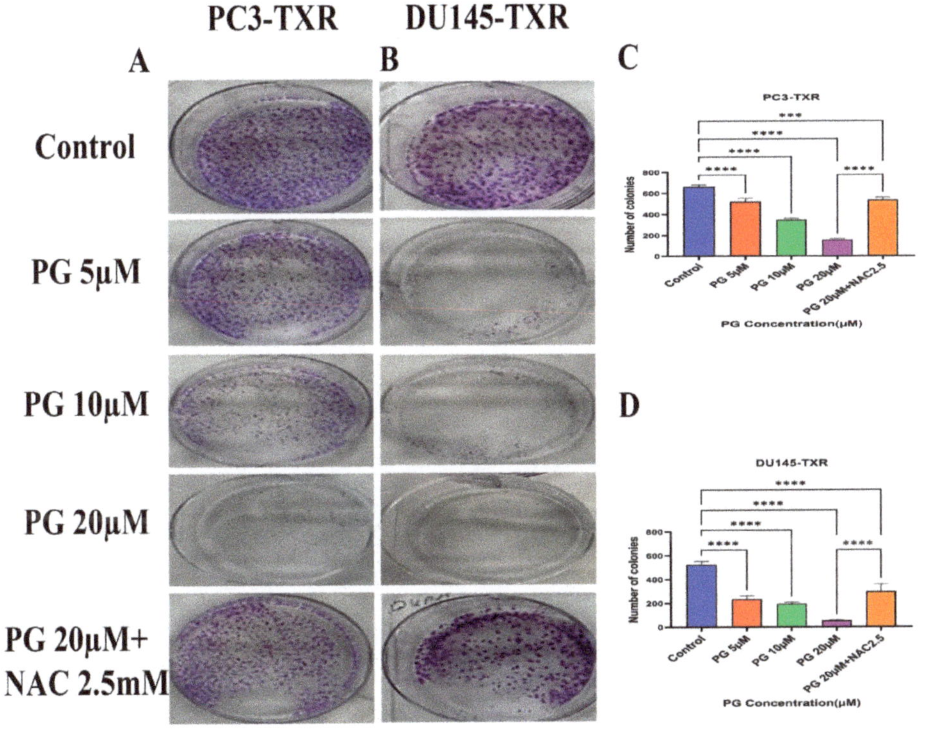

Figure 3. PG inhibits colony formation in taxane-resistant PCa cell lines. (**A**) PC3-TXR and (**B**) DU145-TXR represent images of colony formation after PG treatment. Compared to the control, a substantial decrease in the colonies' number is observed with PG treatment. (**C**) and (**D**) display the quantified results of the average number of colonies plotted against varying concentrations of PG. Data are represented as mean ± SD (n = 3) and represent three trials performed in triplicate independently. *** $p < 0.01$, and **** $p < 0.001$.

3.3. PG Inhibits In Vitro Migration Ability of Taxane-Resistant CRPC Cell Lines

The migration of cancer cells from the primary site to nearby tissues or distant organs is a hallmark of cancer [56]. For the cells to metastasize from one organ to another, the cells must dissociate from the primary site, enter circulatory and lymphatic systems, extravasate at distant capillaries, and invade other organs as a secondary tumor [57]. Wound healing is an inexpensive, robust, in vitro method that mimics the in vivo cell migration system. To investigate the effect of PG on migration, wound healing was performed. Our study demonstrates that taxane-resistant CRPC cell lines treated with varying concentrations of PG have a higher percentage of open wound area compared to the control when measured at different time intervals (0, 24, 48, and 72 h) (Figure 4). PC3-TXR cells treated with PG at 50 μM had 45.5% of the open area after 72 h, whereas in the control, the percentage was 0%. In the case of DU145-TXR, the percentage of the open area after 72 h was 34.7% in PG at 50 μM and 0% in the control (Figure 4D). Consistent with our results in the colony formation assay, our data also show that NAC blocks the effect of PG in both cell lines. Moreover, in both taxane-resistant CRPC cell lines, we observed that PG inhibits migration in a concentration-dependent manner. Hence, taxane-resistant CRPC cell lines are susceptible to the antimetastatic effect of PG.

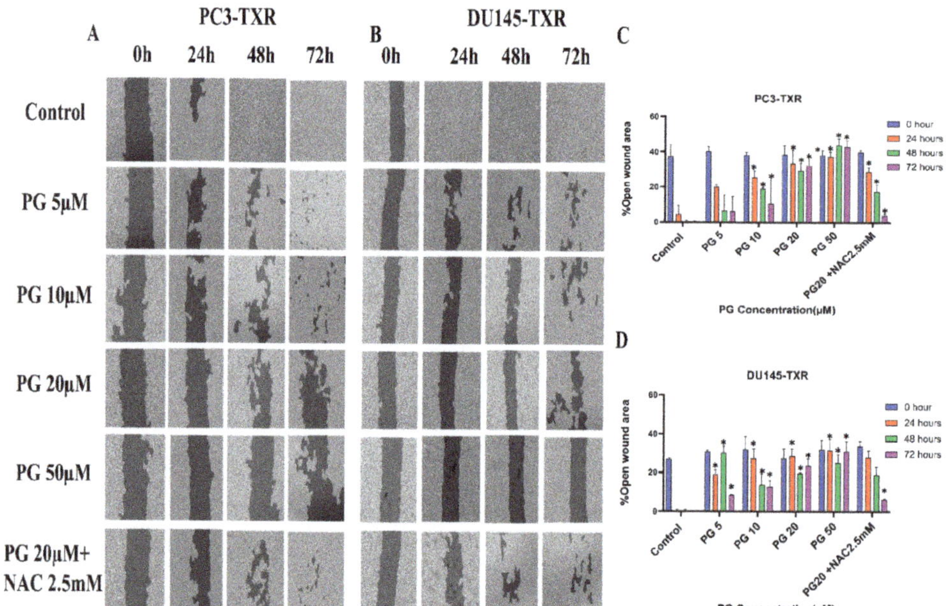

Figure 4. PG inhibits cell migration in taxane-resistant PCa cell lines. (**A**) PC3-TXR and (**B**) DU145-TXR cell line images were taken at 0, 24, 48, and 72 h and analyzed using T-scratch software. (**C**) and (**D**) represent the % open area plotted against varying concentrations of PG for PC3-TXR and DU145-TXR. Images were taken at 10× magnification. Data are represented as mean ± SD (n = 3), and three independent trials were conducted in triplicate. * $p < 0.05$.

3.4. PG Induces Programmed Cell Death in Taxane-Resistant CRPC Cell Lines

Programmed cell death, also well known as apoptosis, is a cellular process associated with maintaining the physiological balance between cell death and cell growth [58]. Cancer cells mostly evade apoptosis. The previous experiments reveal that PG inhibits cell viability, colony formation, and metastasis. We want to study whether PG induces apoptosis in taxane-resistant CRPC cell lines. Cells undergoing apoptosis evince a specific morphological change, such as loss of plasma membrane asymmetry, condensation of the nucleus and cytoplasm, and chromatin condensation. In early apoptosis, the membrane lipid molecule phosphatidylserine is flipped from the inner leaflet to the outer leaflet. To determine the apoptosis, we used annexin V conjugated to the green fluorescence dye FITC, which stains the cytoplasm, and propidium iodide (PI), which stains the DNA. Early apoptotic cells were stained with annexin V FITC (green fluorescence), whereas late apoptotic cells took both annexin V FITC (green fluorescence) and PI (red fluorescence) [44].

Figure 5A,B shows that PG induces apoptosis in PC3-TXR cells. At higher concentrations of PG (50 μM), we found a marked increase in the annexin V FITC green fluorescence, whereas, at lower concentrations of PG (5, 10, and 20 μM), we found weak, faint green fluorescence. Likewise, DU145-TXR cells treated with various concentrations of PG also showed apoptosis with a relative increase in FITC signal. PG concentrations of 20 and 50 μM showed a significant increase in green fluorescence, whereas PG 5 and 10 μM treatments displayed faint green fluorescence (Figure 5C,D). Together, these results indicate that PG induces apoptosis in taxane-resistant CRPC cell lines.

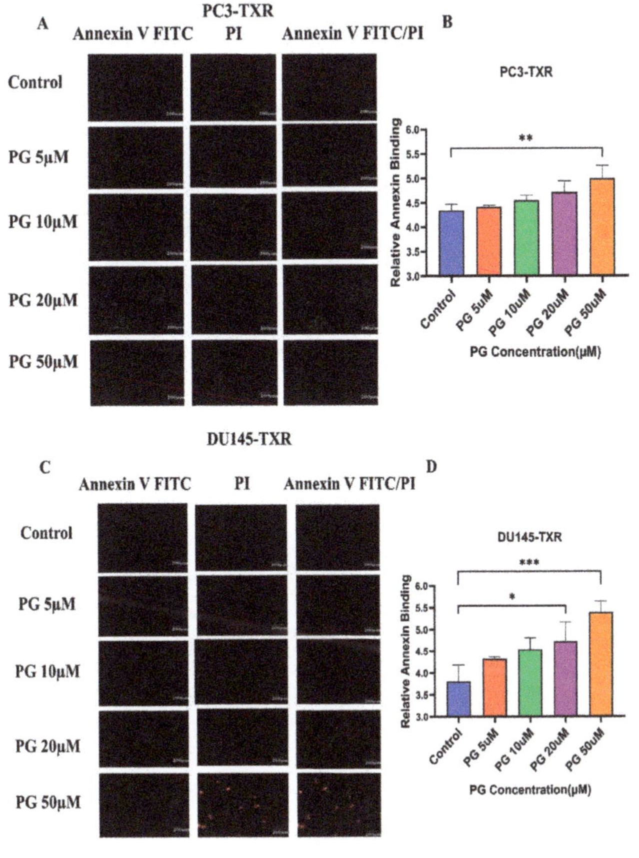

Figure 5. PG treatment elicits apoptosis in taxane-resistant PCa cell lines. (**A**) PC3-TXR and (**C**) DU145-TXR cell lines were treated with varying concentrations of PG for 48 h, and apoptosis was detected by annexin V FITC/PI staining. Images were taken via confocal microscopy and analyzed using ImageJ. In the taxane-resistant PCa cell lines, the relative annexin V FITC binding was higher in the treatment groups compared to that of controls. (**B**) and (**D**) show relative annexin V binding plotted against concentrations of PG for PC3-TXR and DU145-TXR, respectively. Images were taken at 60× magnification. Data are depicted as mean ± SD (n = 3) and represent three experiments performed in triplicate. * $p < 0.05$, ** $p < 0.01$, *** $p < 0.001$.

3.5. PG Promotes Apoptotic Cell Death in Taxane-Resistant CRPC Cell Lines

To further confirm the apoptotic-inducing potential and to quantitively examine whether PG initiates apoptosis in taxane-resistant CRPC cell lines, we assessed apoptosis using flow cytometry. The viable cells are negative for annexin V and PI stains, whereas early apoptotic cells are positive for annexin V only as plasma membrane integrity is not entirely lost; late apoptotic cells are positive for annexin V and PI. Figure 6 illustrates that taxane-resistant CRPC cell lines treated with varying concentrations of PG undergo apoptosis. PC3-TXR showed 42.32% of apoptosis (positive for annexin V and PI) at a concentration of 50 µM, whereas the control only showed 4.28% (Figure 6A,C). Likewise, in DU145-TXR, we found that the apoptosis percentage was 30.24% in treatment group and 4.59% in controls at a concentration of 50 µM (Figure 6B,D). Together, our results suggest that the percentage of apoptosis is significantly higher in treatment samples compared to that of controls, indicating that taxane-resistant CRPC cell lines are particularly susceptible to apoptosis induced by PG treatment.

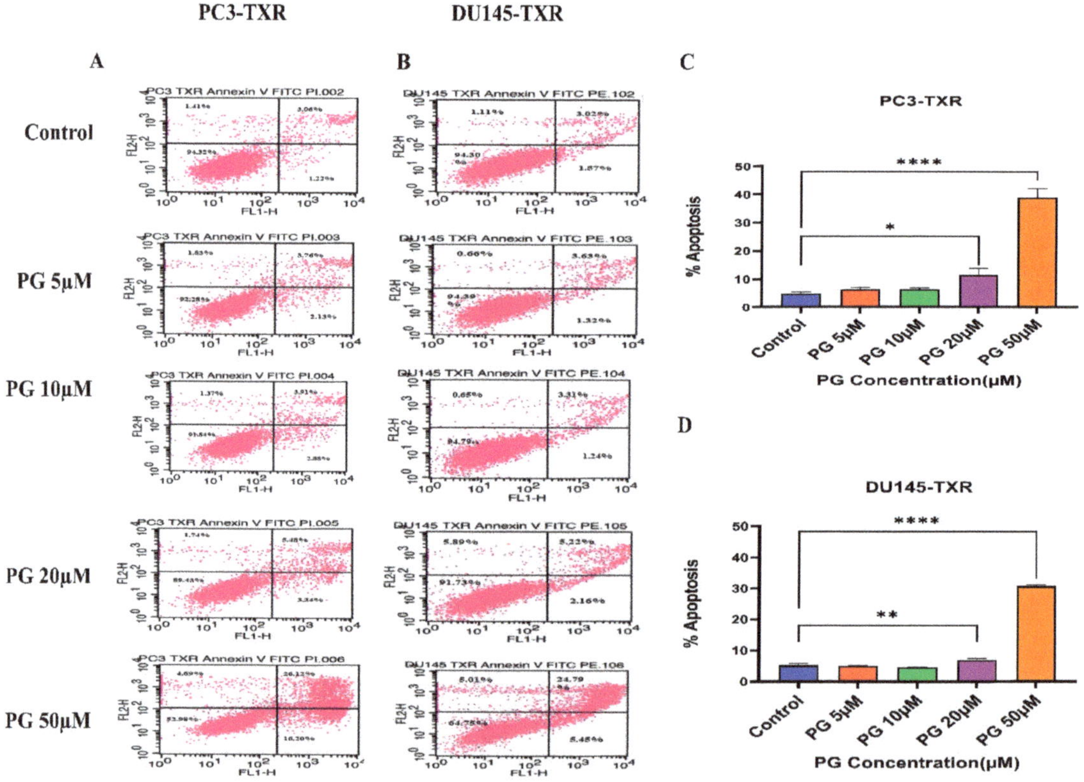

Figure 6. PG induces apoptosis in taxane-resistant PCa cell lines. (**A**) PC3-TXR and (**B**) DU145-TXR cell lines were treated with varying concentrations of PG, and apoptosis was detected by staining cells with annexin V FITC/PI followed by flow cytometry analysis. The results suggest that PG induces apoptosis in higher concentrations. (**C**) and (**D**) represent % apoptosis plotted against concentrations of PG for PC3-TXR and DU145-TXR. Data are shown as mean ± SD (n = 3) and denote three independent experiments in triplicate. * $p < 0.05$, ** $p < 0.01$, **** $p < 0.001$.

3.6. PG Promotes Anoikis in Taxane-Resistant CRPC Cell Lines

Anoikis is a self-defense mechanism that acts as a barrier to prevent metastasis. Healthy cells undergo death when they detach or lose contact with the ECM through an apoptotic process known as anoikis. Cancer cells have the ability to escape this mechanism. The cells can expand, invade, and disseminate throughout the body, causing metastasis. Anoikis has a vital role in modulating metastasis in cancer [58,59]. Therefore, we assessed the potential role of PG in promoting anoikis in taxane-resistant PCa cell lines. We treated taxane-resistant PCa cell lines with various concentrations of PG and stained the cells with calcein-AM and EthD-1. Calcein-AM, a green fluorescence dye, stains live cells, whereas EthD-1, a red fluorescence dye, stains cells undergoing anoikis. Using the immunofluorescence data of calcein-AM and EthD-1 of control and PG-treated cells, we observed that the number of dead cells stained with EthD-1 (red fluorescence) increased in association with the increase in PG concentration.

In contrast, the number of live cells stained with calcein-AM (green fluorescence) decreased, suggesting that PG promotes anoikis in taxane-resistant CRPC cell lines (Figure 7A,B). In the MTT assay, we observed that a higher concentration of PG (20 and 50μM) exhibited a robust reduction in the percentage of cell viability in PC3-TXR (Figure 7C), while PG exhibited a marked decrease in the percentage of cell viability at a concentration of 50 μM in DU145-TXR (Figure 7D). Altogether, our results reveal that PG treatment induces anoikis in taxane-resistant CRPC cell lines.

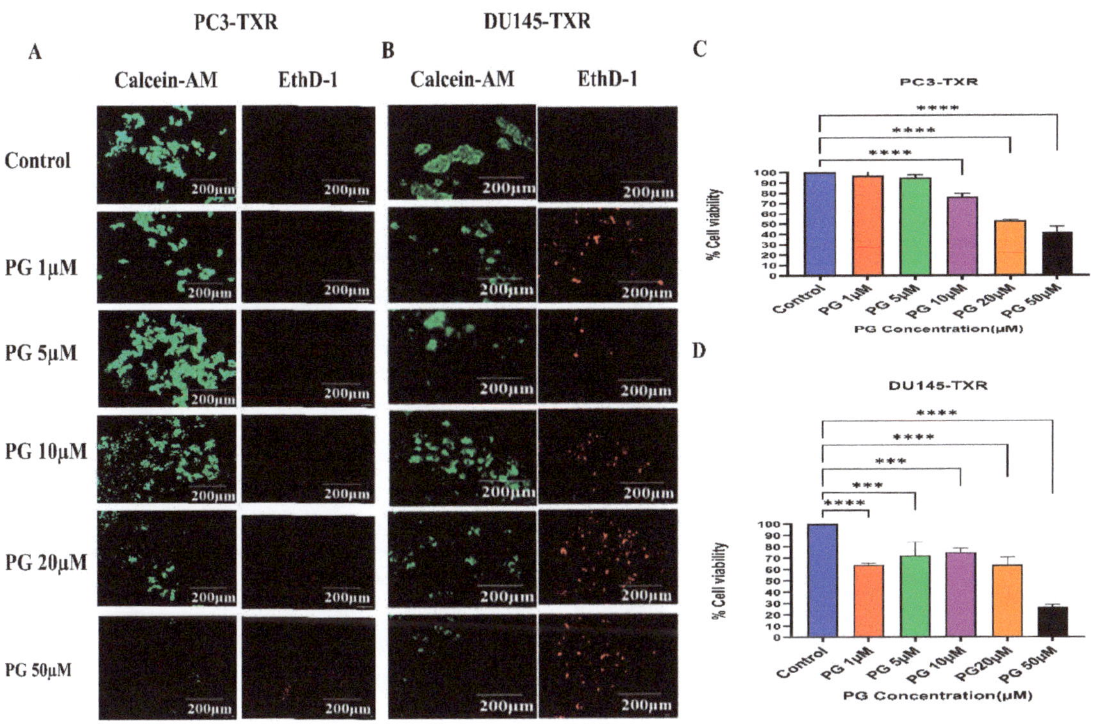

Figure 7. PG promotes anoikis in taxane-resistant PCa cell lines. (**A**) PC3-TXR and (**B**) DU145-TXR cell lines were treated with varying concentrations of PG for 48 h and stained with calcein AM and EthD-1 to detect anoikis. We observed that with the increase in the concentration of PG, the number of viable cells stained with calcein-AM (green fluorescence) decreased, and the number of dead cells stained with EthD-1 (red fluorescence) increased. (**C**) and (**D**) % cell viability plotted against various concentrations of PG for PC3-TXR and DU145-TXR, respectively. Images were taken at 10× magnification. Data are represented as mean ± SD (n = 3), and a total of three experiments were performed independently in triplicate. *** $p < 0.05$, **** $p < 0.01$.

3.7. PG Induces Anoikis in Taxane-Resistant CRPC Cell Lines via PTEN

Several studies have discussed the connection between PTEN and anoikis, showing that PTEN induces anoikis in several cancers [60–63]. Our previous results show that PG promotes anoikis in taxane-resistant PCa cell lines. Therefore, we examined the expression level of PTEN in taxane-resistant PCa cell lines PC3-TXR and DU145-TXR, respectively. Our data reveal that PG at a higher concentration of 20 μM significantly induces the expression of PTEN in both cell lines, indicating that PG induces anoikis in taxane-resistant CRPC cell lines (Figure 8A,B).

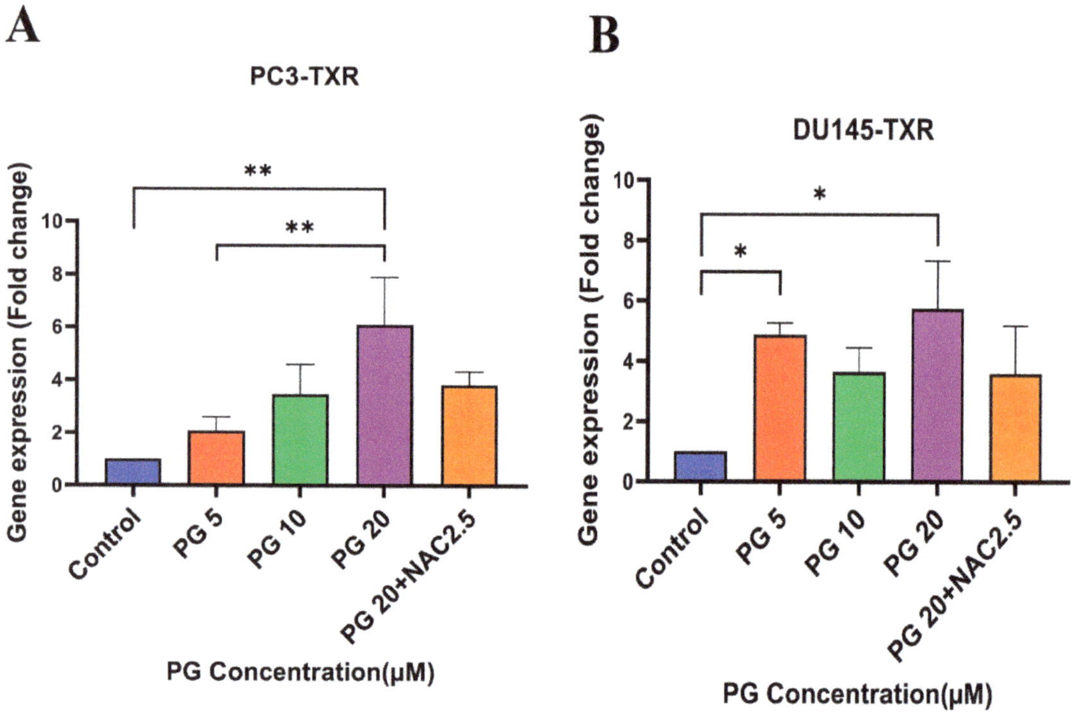

Figure 8. PG promotes anoikis in taxane-resistant PCa cell lines via the activation of PTEN. (**A**) PC3-TXR and (**B**) DU145-TXR cell lines. Our data illustrate that PG induces upregulation in the expression of *PTEN*. Data are represented as mean ± SD ($n = 3$), and a total of three experiments were performed independently in triplicate. * $p < 0.05$, ** $p < 0.01$.

3.8. PG Causes G0 Phase Cell Cycle Arrest in Taxane-Resistant CRPC Cell Lines

We investigated the effect of PG on the cell cycle of taxane-resistant CRPC cell lines using flow cytometry to examine whether PG treatment impacts cell cycle progression. In this technique, PI binds to the DNA, and the amount of DNA present correlates to the relative intensity of PI. In PC3-TXR, G0 phase cells in the control have 4.64% of total cells, whereas G0 phase cells in the treatment sample at a concentration of 50 μM have 67.08% of cells (Figure 9A,C). Similarly, in DU145-TXR, G0 phase cells in the control have 1.46% of cells. Interestingly, treatment with PG at a concentration of 50 μM significantly increases the proportion of G0 phase cells to 88.10% (Figure 9B,D). We did not detect significant differences with other concentrations (5, 10, and 20 μM). Overall, our results suggest that PG causes G0 phase cell cycle arrest in a concentration-dependent fashion.

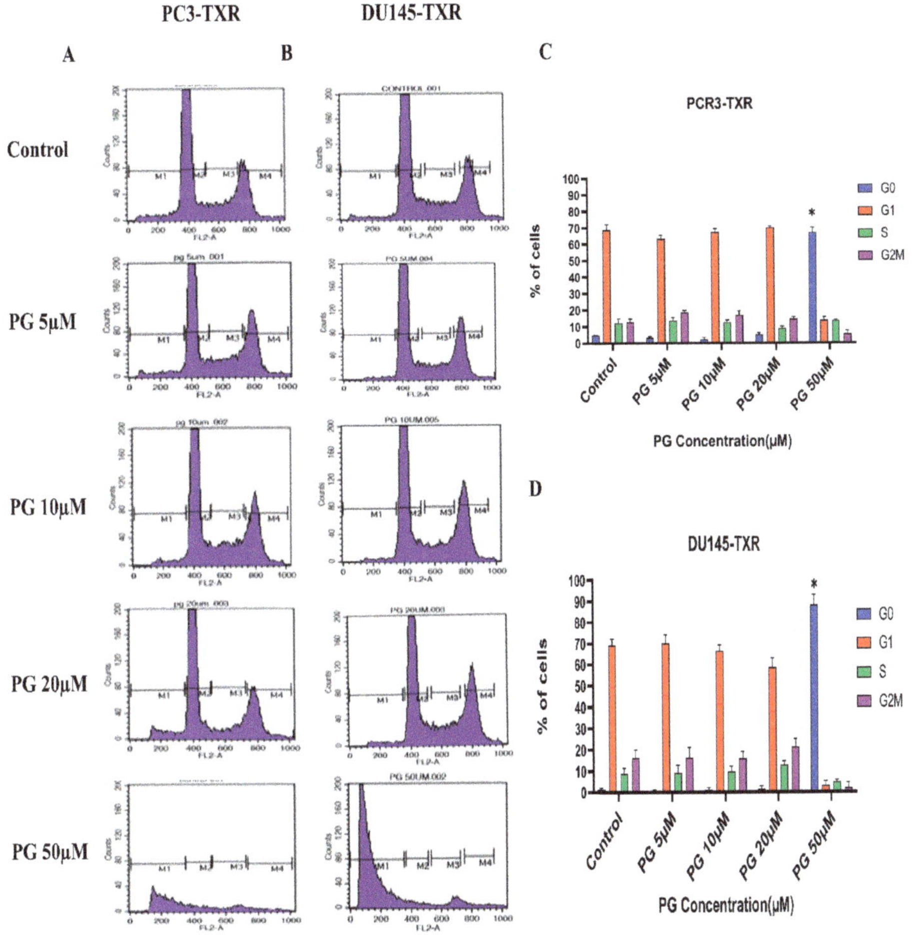

Figure 9. PG induces G0 phase cell cycle arrest in taxane-resistant PCa cell lines. (**A**) PC3-TXR and (**B**) DU145-TXR cell lines were treated with varying concentrations of PG for 48 h and stained with PI, and flow cytometry analysis was performed. We observed that PG 50 µM significantly blocks the cell cycle at the G0 phase in taxane-resistant PCa cell lines. (**C**) and (**D**) represent the quantified results of % of cells plotted against varying PG treatment of PC3-TXR and DU145-TXR. Data are represented as mean ± SD (n = 3), and three experiments were performed in triplicate. * $p < 0.05$.

3.9. PG Treatment Induces Oxidative Stress in Taxane-Resistant CRPC Cell Lines

Cancer cells exhibit elevated ROS levels; however, the cells produce high amounts of antioxidants to counteract the generated ROS and maintain intercellular balance to abrogate the high level of oxidative stress that drives the cell to commit apoptosis. Generally, a high percentage of chemotherapy drugs trigger cell death by promoting ROS generation, which results in elevated oxidative stress and cell death [64]. To investigate whether PG treatment could result in ROS generation and, subsequently, cell death, we performed a ROS assay. The relative ROS level was determined using ImageJ software, which correlates with the intensity of green fluorescence produced. As shown in Figure 10, our data illustrate an increase in green fluorescence upon using PG treatment at a concentration of PG 20 µM compared to the control. Nonetheless, PG at a concentration of 50 µM does not show a remarkable increase in green fluorescence compared to the control, possibly due to nonviable cells at higher concentrations. Our results suggest that PG induces ROS generation in taxane-resistant CRPC cell lines and subsequently promotes oxidative stress and cell death.

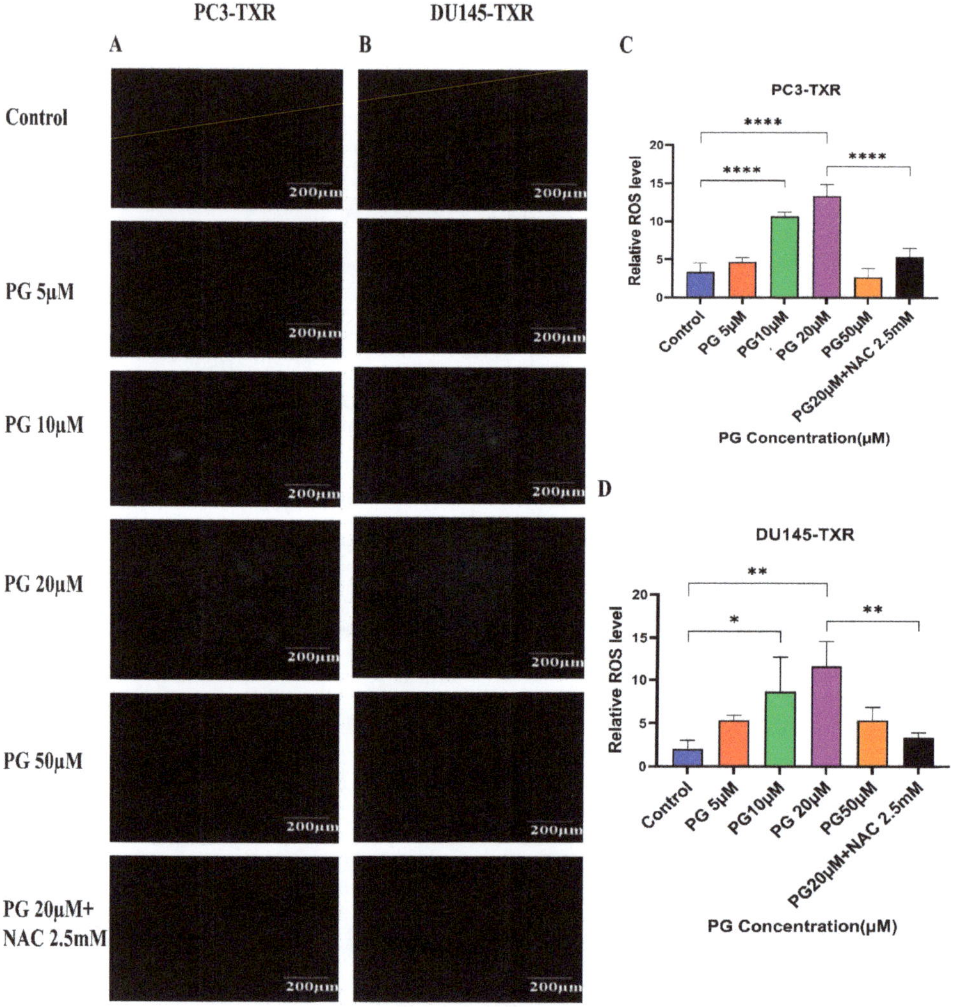

Figure 10. PG treatment induces ROS generation, leading to oxidative stress in taxane-resistant PCa cell lines. The taxane-resistant PCa cell lines were treated with varying concentrations of PG for 6 h and stained with DCFH2-DA. The images were taken and analyzed using ImageJ software. (**A**) PC3-TXR and (**B**) DU145-TXR show an increase in green fluorescence with an increase in PG treatment up to PG 20 μM compared to the control, but PG 50 μM shows slight green fluorescence. (**C**,**D**) represent the quantified results of relative ROS levels plotted against concentrations of PG of PC3-TXR and DU145-TXR. Images were taken at 40× magnification. Data are represented as mean ± SD ($n = 3$), and three experiments were carried out in triplicate. * $p < 0.05$, ** $p < 0.01$, **** $p < 0.001$.

Furthermore, to confirm our findings, we examined whether PG induces ROS production in taxane-resistant PCa cell lines by the means of flow cytometry. For this assay, we used the DCFH2-DA dye to detect ROS production. Our results demonstrate that in the PC3-TXR cell line (Figure 11A), PG significantly induces ROS production at a concentration of 20 μM. Similar results are also observed in DU145-TXR (Figure 11B). Moreover, our data show that NAC markedly blocks the effect of PG in both cell lines (Figure 11C,D). Collectively, our results indicate that PG promotes ROS production and consequently induces oxidative stress and cell death.

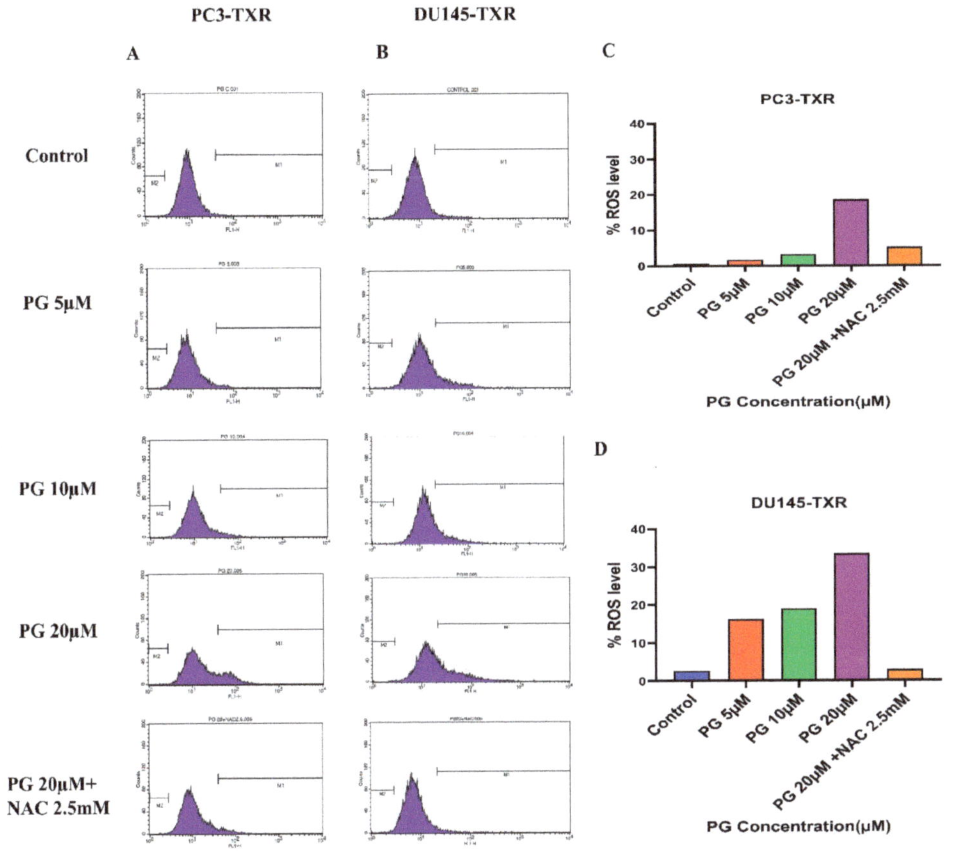

Figure 11. PG induces ROS production, resulting in oxidative stress in CRPC cells. PC3-TXR and DU145-TXR cells were stained with DCFH2-DA and then treated with different concentrations of PG for 4 h, followed by flow cytometry analysis. (**A**) PC3-TXR and (**B**) DU145-TXR show an increase in the amount of ROS generated with PG treatment compared to the control. (**C**) and (**D**) represent the quantified ROS levels' results plotted against PG concentrations of PC3-TXR and DU145-TXR compared to the untreated control.

3.10. PG Differentially Modulates the Expression of Various Apoptotic Markers in PC3-TXR

The previous experiments revealed that PG induces apoptosis in PC3-TXR cells. As a follow-up to previous investigations demonstrating PG apoptotic-inducing potential, we wanted to examine the specific expression of various apoptotic markers by an apoptosis profiler array, which is a rapid method to detect the expression of 35 apoptosis-related proteins in a single array (Figure 12). The principle behind this experiment remains the same as in a Western blot assay. For apoptosis marker profiling, we chose PC3-TXR cells as both PC3-TXR and DU145-TXR cell lines showed similar results in previous experiments. Proteome array results illustrated that PG modulates key apoptosis markers. Using PG at a concentration of 20 μM, our data show downregulation in the expression level of antiapoptotic proteins Bcl-2 and Bcl-xL. In addition, the expression level of the inhibitors of apoptosis (IAP) proteins cIAP-1, cIAP-2, survivin, and XIAP expressed downregulation as well. The IAP family endogenously inhibits apoptosis by binding to the caspases, abrogating programmed cell death, and enhancing tumor cell proliferation [65,66].

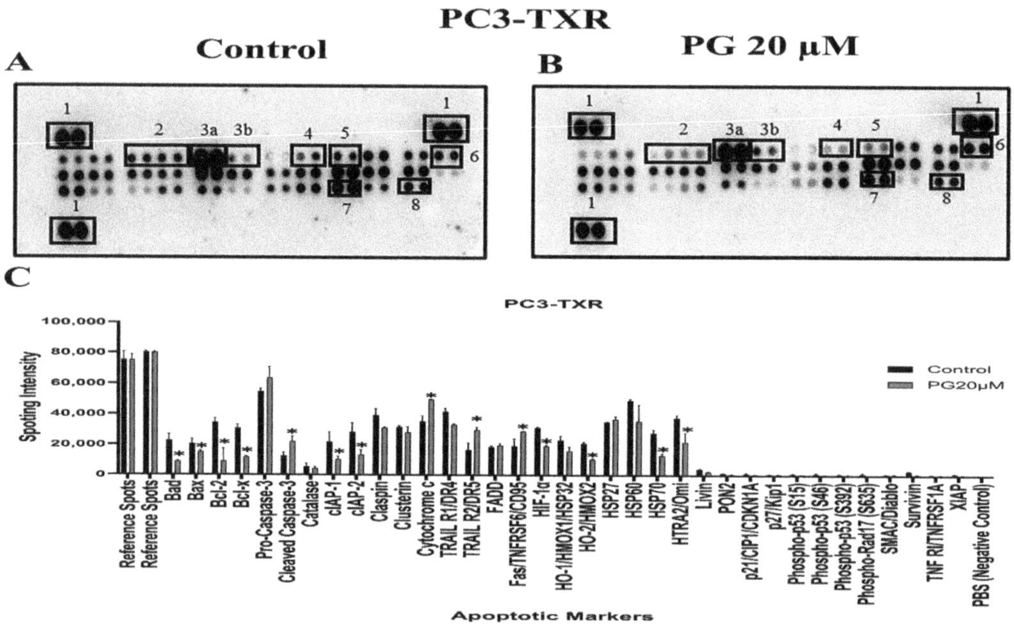

Figure 12. PG modulates the expression of various apoptotic markers in PC3-TXR. Figure (**A**) represents PC3-TXR control and (**B**) represents PC3-TXR treated with PG 20µM, in which the cells were seeded and treated with PG 20 µM for 48 h. Expression of the various apoptotic markers was found using a proteome profiler-human apoptosis array. PG promotes downregulation in the antiapoptotic markers Bcl-2, Bcl-xL, and IAP family, in addition to an upregulation in cytochrome c and cleaved-caspase-3. Numbers used to depict the expression of selected markers compared to reference spots: 1 = reference spot, 2 = Bcl family, 3a = pro-caspase 3, 3b = cleaved caspase 3, 4,5,8 = IAP family, 6 = cytochrome c, 7 = survivin. (**C**) represents the quantified results of the relative band intensities calculated using ImageJ, and relative expression levels were plotted against PG treatment. Data are represented as mean ± SD. * $p < 0.05$.

Furthermore, our results also show that the expression level of cytochrome c is elevated. In addition, pro-caspase-3 is downregulated, and cleaved caspase-3 is upregulated, indicating that PG induces cell death via the activation of the intrinsic apoptosis pathway. Cells undergo apoptosis via the intrinsic pathway characterized by the disruption of mitochondrial function, resulting in the release of cytochrome c and eventually caspase activation. Caspase-3 is an executioner among the caspases in programmed cell death [67]. In summary, our results suggest that PG treatment activates the intrinsic apoptosis pathway in CRPC cells.

PG Regulates the Expression of Key Apoptotic Markers and DNA Damage Markers in Taxane-Resistant CRPC Cell Lines

Based on the human apoptosis array results, it is evident that PG treatment modulates various apoptosis markers in PC3-TXR. To further study the mechanism of PG action, immunoblot analysis was conducted to substantiate the expression of apoptotic and DNA damage proteins. Immunoblot results (Figure 13) illustrate that PG treatment upregulates the expression of DNA damage response protein pH2AX in taxane-resistant CRPC cell lines. In addition, we also observed downregulation of PARP-1, pro-caspase-3, XIAP, and cIAP-2 in both cell lines, implicating apoptosis activation [68]. Moreover, to confirm that PG induces the cell to undergo apoptosis, we examined the expression of cleaved PARP-1 in both cell lines. Our data show that cleaved PARP-1 expression is upregulated while total PARP-1 is downregulated, indicating that cells commit apoptosis (Figure 13E,F). The expression of β-actin was observed to be homogeneous in treated as well as untreated samples. Taken together, our work shows that PG treatment causes apoptosis-mediated cell death.

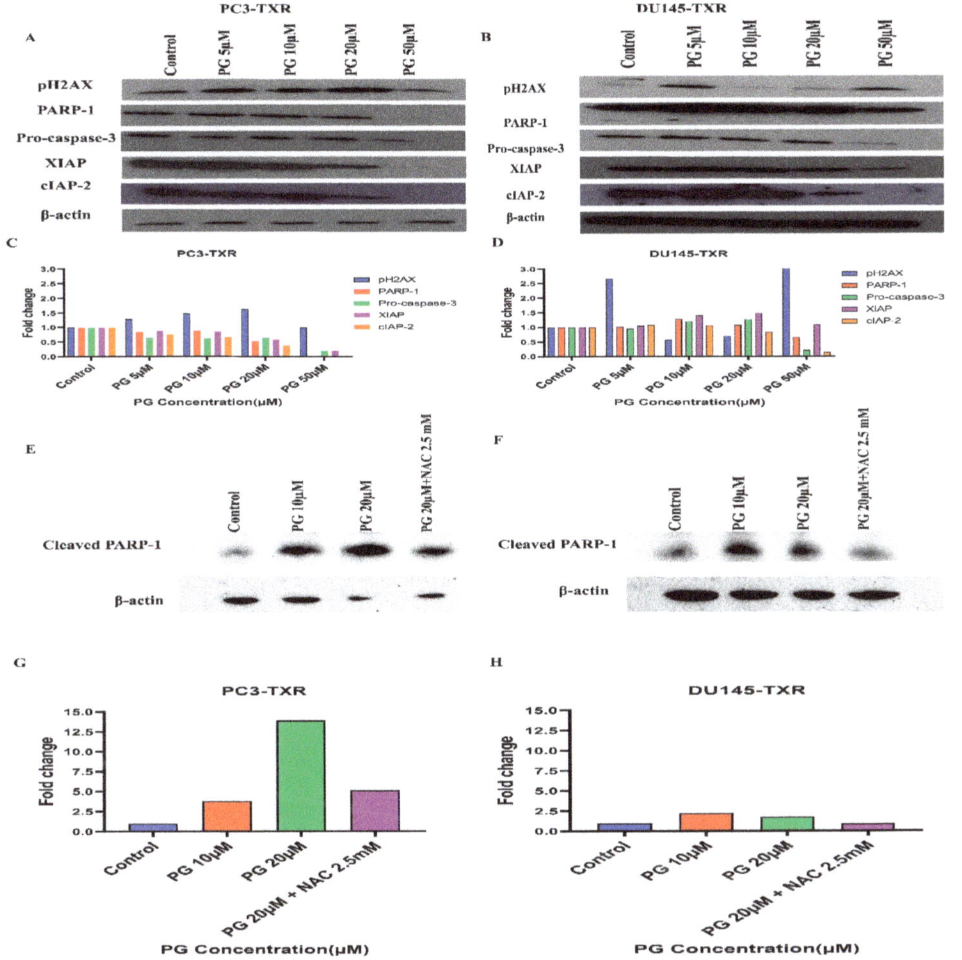

Figure 13. PG differentially modulates the expression of key apoptotic markers and DNA damage markers in taxane-resistant PCa cell lines. (**A**) PC3-TXR and (**B**) DU145-TXR cells were treated with varying concentrations of PG, and an immunoblot assay was performed. PG induces downregulation of various apoptotic markers, such as pro-caspase-3, XIAP, and cIAP-2. We also observed that the DNA damage marker pH2AX is upregulated, and PARP-1 is downregulated. (**C**) and (**D**) represent the quantified results of relative band intensities calculated using ImageJ, and relative expression levels were plotted against PG treatment. (**E**) and (**F**) depict the expression of cleaved PARP-1 in PC3-TXR and DU145-TXR, respectively, confirming that PG induces taxane-resistant PCa cell lines to commit apoptosis. (**G**) and (**H**) are graphical representations of the relative band intensities calculated using ImageJ, and fold change in expression levels were plotted against various PG treatments.

4. Discussion

PCa is the most frequent cancer among males in the United States. Surgery, chemotherapy, radiation therapy, and ADT are the currently available treatment options for PCa. Although there have been recent advancements in treatment strategies, challenges still obstruct the chances of curing PCa. One of these challenges is the development of resistance to ADT therapy and, consequently, the development of CRPC after 18–24 months [14,15]. In this study, we wanted to explore the potential of PG as an alternative and natural therapeutic anticancer agent against taxane-resistant CRPC. Our results show that PG is not toxic to primary human hepatocytes, 3T3-J2 fibroblast co-cultures, and non-cancerous BPH-1 cell lines, implicating that PG is innocuous to healthy cells. Importantly, PG significantly inhibits the cell viability of taxane-resistant CRPC cell lines in a concentration-dependent manner at 24 h and 48 h time intervals. Our previous work showed that DR-P27, a derivative of PG, had antiproliferative properties against several cancer types, including apoptosis-resistant human glioblastoma U373, human SKMEL-28 melanoma, apoptosis-sensitive human Hs683 anaplastic oligodendroglioma, human A549 non-small cell lung cancer, and human MCF-7 breast cancer [30]. Similarly, our current study affirms that PG inhibits the proliferation of taxane-resistant CRPC cell lines.

Colony formation and metastasis are essential properties for tumor survival and progression. A study on piperine, an alkaloid from black pepper, revealed that piperine inhibited colon cancer's colony formation ability in the HT-29 cell line and the growth of colon cancer spheroids [69]. Besides, Zhang et al. [70] substantiated that piperine attenuates cell migration of HOS and U2OS osteosarcoma cell lines. PG is a natural compound present in water pepper, Dorrigo pepper, and mountain pepper. Our study demonstrates high efficacy in reducing the colony size as well as the number of colonies proportionally to an increase in the concentration of PG in taxane-resistant CRPC cell lines. In addition, our wound healing data demonstrate a significant decrease in the gap closure percentage of taxane-resistant CRPC cell lines in a concentration-dependent manner, and at different time intervals compared to the control. Moreover, our data show that NAC abrogates the effect of PG, indicating that PG induces cell death by promoting oxidative stress and ROS generation. Our work suggests that PG has an antimetastatic potential impact against taxane-resistant CRPC cell lines.

Our previous work has indicated that a PG analog DR-P27 induces apoptosis in LNCaP PCa cells [28]. In this study, we examined the anticancer properties of PG by using various cellular assays. Our work demonstrates that PG induces apoptosis in taxane-resistant CRPC cell lines, and we found a significant increase in the apoptosis percentage upon using PG at a concentration of 50 μM. Moreover, anoikis is a known form of programmed cell death that ensues when a cell detaches from the ECM [58]. Cancerous cells are resistant to this mechanism, which helps in metastatic dissemination. Our data show that PG induces anoikis in taxane-resistant PCa cell lines (Figure 7).

Moreover, PTEN has been shown to induce anoikis in various cancers. To affirm our finding, we examined the gene expression of *PTEN*, and our results demonstrate that PG treatment expedites anoikis in taxane-resistant CRPC cell lines through PTEN activation (Figure 8). Similarly, another study showed that curcumin, a primary compound from the spice turmeric, promoted anoikis in non-small lung cancer [71], indicating that natural products could be a valuable strategy to vanquish the cancer resistance dilemma.

The cell cycle checkpoints do not allow cells with DNA damage to duplicate or divide; instead, the cells undergo apoptosis. However, mutated cells escape different checkpoints, resulting in uncontrolled cell growth and, subsequently, cancer development. Piperine has been shown to induce cell cycle arrest at the G0/G1 phase and apoptosis in melanoma cells [72]. Our results reveal that PG instigates G0 phase arrest at a concentration of 50 μM, indicating that PG exterminates taxane-resistant CRPC via apoptosis. In contrast, De La Chapa et al. [32] demonstrated that PG induces cell cycle arrest in the S phase in OSCC, indicating that PG might elicit different mechanisms according to the cancer type [32]. To further investigate the underlying mechanism of cell death, we have examined ROS production in taxane-resistant CRPC. Cancer cells express elevated levels of ROS; however, antioxidants present in the cancer cells detoxify ROS. This promotes cell growth progression and development. When the intercellular ROS and antioxidant balance is disrupted, the intracellular ROS threshold level increases, leading to oxidative stress–mediating apoptotic death. Our recent study has reported that DR-P27, a derivative of PG, induced ROS generation, leading to oxidative stress–mediated cell death of androgen-sensitive human PCa cells [28]. In this study, we found that PG gradually increased ROS generation from 5 to 20 μM.

Interestingly, a higher concentration of PG (50 μM) significantly increased cell death. However, we observed relatively low ROS generation. The lower levels of ROS detected at 50 μM PG treatment suggest the possibility of rapid ROS generation earlier than 6 h of treatment, resulting in ROS exhaustion. In addition, our results reveal that NAC blocks the effect of PG in both cell lines. Based on our data, we suggest that PG induces robust ROS generation, leading to oxidative stress in taxane-resistant CRPC cell lines. Previous studies have shown that the compound alantolactone, a plant-derived sesquiterpene lactone, activates apoptosis via ROS generation leading to the disruption of mitochondrial membrane potential, the release of apoptotic factor cytochrome c, the downregulation of antiapoptotic proteins, and the activation of apoptosis executioner caspase-3 in glioblastoma cells [73].

We wanted to confirm that PG induces apoptosis; therefore, we used a proteome profiler-human apoptosis array with several spotted apoptotic markers to ascertain the mechanism of action of PG in taxane-resistant CRPC. This study used only PC3-TXR cells as both the taxane-resistant CRPC cell lines exhibited indistinguishable potency with PG treatment. Apoptotic proteome array analysis revealed an increase in cytochrome c levels. Here, we postulate that PG treatment induces ROS generation leading to disruption of mitochondrial membrane potential and further activating cytochrome c release, subsequently activating different caspases.

Tumor cells depend on the Bcl-2 family of proteins to protect them from stress-induced apoptotic death. Bcl-2 and Bcl-xL are antiapoptotic proteins and essential regulators of apoptosis [65]. In our study, the proteome profiler-human apoptosis array also reveals the expression of Bcl-2 and Bcl-xL, along with the downregulated expression of the IAP group of antiapoptotic proteins such as XIAP, survivin, cIAP-1, and cIAP-2. These results substantiate that PG induces apoptosis. Since PG treatment stimulates cytochrome c upregulation, we believe this leads to cell death through the intrinsic apoptosis pathway via mitochondrial depolarization. We further investigated the expression of caspase-3 and found that pro-caspase-3 was downregulated in Western blot results, while cleaved caspase-3 was upregulated in proteome array results in PC3-TXR cells. Moreover, the expression levels of the antiapoptotic markers cIAP-2 and XIAP were also downregulated.

DR-P27 induced ROS generation and apoptosis along with the cleavage of PARP-1 and the activation of γH2AX, leading us to conclude that DR-P27 induces DNA damage response in androgen-sensitive human PCa cells [28]. Our study found that PG treatment downregulates PARP-1 expression implicating apoptosis activation. Further, in Western blot analysis, we observed an upregulation of pH2AX, another crucial DNA damage response marker associated with apoptosis or cell cycle arrest, suggesting that PG induces DNA damage response in taxane-resistant CRPC cell lines. Collectively, these results confirm our hypothesis that PG induces ROS generation leading to the disruption of the mitochondrial membrane and the upregulation of cytochrome c, followed by apoptosis/anoikis and the inhibition of various antiapoptotic factors. In addition, our data suggest that PG effectively targets taxane-resistant CRPC cell lines by activating apoptotic cell death and inhibiting antiapoptotic signaling, suggesting that PG endows similar efficacy to DR-P27 in drug resistant cancer in vitro models.

Moreover, PG also showed significant antiproliferative potency comparable to DR-P27 in Cal27-derived tumors in a xenograft model of athymic nude mice [32]. However, this is the only study that addresses PG antitumor efficacy using an in vivo model, and further investigations are warranted. Figure 14 highlights the proposed anticancer mechanism of PG against taxane-resistant CRPC cell lines.

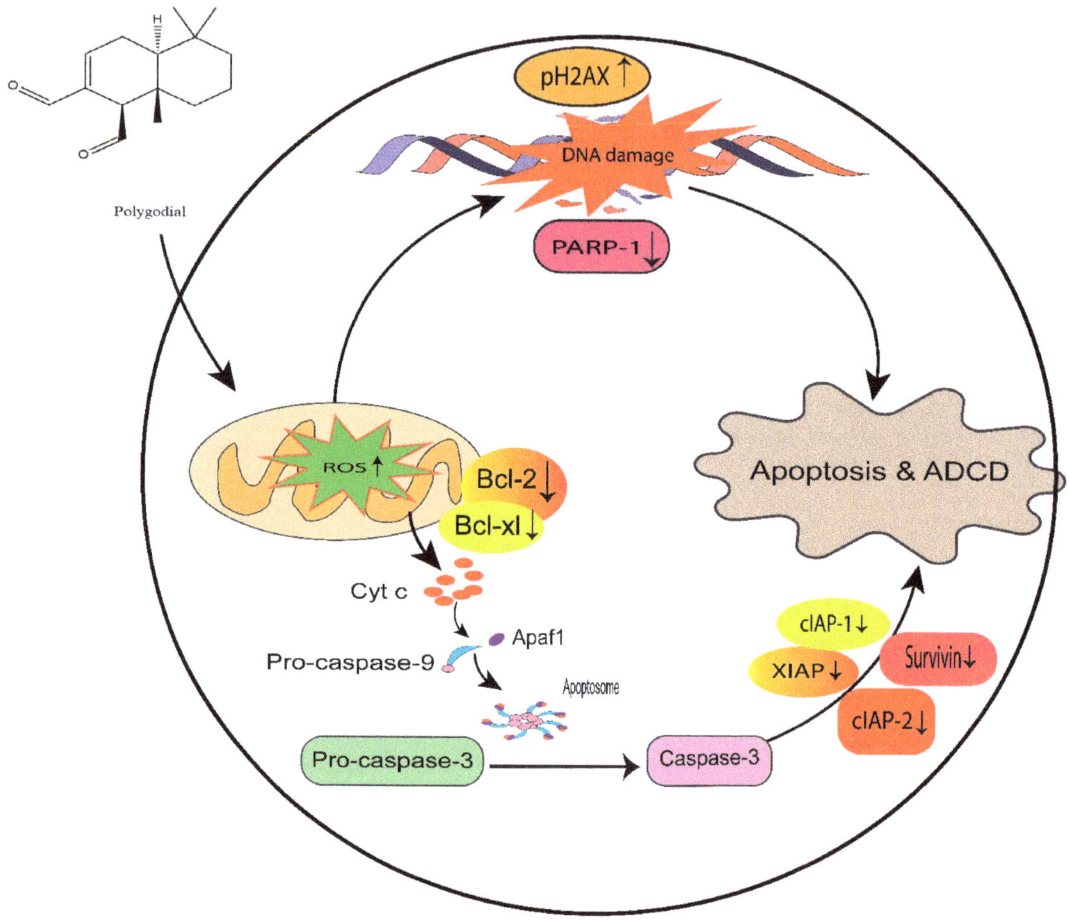

Figure 14. Proposed mechanism of PG action in taxane-resistant CRPC cell lines. We identified that ROS generation by PG induces DNA damage and apoptosis by the intrinsic signaling apoptosis pathway, indicating that PG has a potential therapeutic effect on taxane-resistant PCa.

5. Conclusions and Future Perspective

This study confirms that PG has promising therapeutic potential in taxane-resistant CRPC cell lines. PG effectively inhibits the cell viability, cell cycle progression, and migration properties of CRPC cells, suggesting that PG endows tumor growth suppression and metastasis inhibition potential. Furthermore, PG induces ROS generation, disrupting the mitochondrial membrane and upregulating cytochrome c, which activates the intrinsic death pathway and anoikis. The mechanistic study confirmed that PG induces DNA damage response and apoptosis in the taxane-resistant CRPC cell lines. However, additional work is needed to unveil the detailed anticancer mechanism of PG, and further in vivo studies are warranted to ascertain the therapeutic or chemopreventive usefulness of PG in managing CRPC.

Supplementary Materials: The following supporting information can be downloaded at: https://www.mdpi.com/article/10.3390/cancers14215260/s1, File S1: Original blots.

Author Contributions: Conceptualization, R.V., M.A.H., A.K. and G.M.; methodology, R.V., M.A.H., L.M., J.S.L., S.R.K. and G.M.; writing—Original draft preparation, R.V. and M.A.H., writing—Review and editing, R.V., M.A.H., L.M., J.S.L., S.R.K., A.K. and G.M.; supervision, G.M. All authors have read and agreed to the published version of the manuscript.

Funding: This research received no external funding.

Institutional Review Board Statement: Not applicable.

Informed Consent Statement: Not applicable.

Data Availability Statement: The data represented in this article are available on request from the corresponding author.

Conflicts of Interest: The authors declare no conflict of interest.

Abbreviations

3MA	3-methyladenine
ADT	androgen deprivation therapy
ANOVA	analysis of variance
CI	pan-caspase inhibitor
CRPC	castration-resistant prostate cancer
DCFH2-DA	2′,7′-Dichlorodihydrofluorescein diacetate
DMEM	Dulbecco's modified Eagle's medium
DMSO	dimethyl sulfoxide
DR-P27	9-epipolygodial
ECM	extracellular matrix
IAP	inhibitors of apoptosis
MPCCs	micropatterned co-cultures
MTT	3–4,5-dimethylthiazol-2-yl,2,5-diphenyl tetrazolium bromide
NAC	N-acetyl cysteine
NEC	necrostatin-1
OSCC	oral squamous cell carcinoma
PCa	prostate cancer
PG	polygodial
PI	propidium Iodide
PSA	prostate-specific antigen
ROS	reactive oxygen species
TBST	tris-buffered saline tween

References

1. Siegel, R.L.; Miller, K.D.; Fuchs, H.E.; Jemal, A. Cancer statistics, 2022. *CA Cancer J. Clin.* **2022**, *72*, 7–33. [CrossRef] [PubMed]
2. American Cancer Society. Key Statistics for Prostate Cancer | Prostate Cancer Facts. Available online: https://www.cancer.org/cancer/prostate-cancer/about/key-statistics.html (accessed on 30 April 2022).
3. Sung, H.; Ferlay, J.; Siegel, R.L.; Laversanne, M.; Soerjomataram, I.; Jemal, A.; Bray, F. Global Cancer Statistics 2020: GLOBOCAN Estimates of Incidence and Mortality Worldwide for 36 Cancers in 185 Countries. *CA Cancer J. Clin.* **2021**, *71*, 209–249. [CrossRef] [PubMed]
4. Pernar, C.H.; Ebot, E.M.; Wilson, K.M.; Mucci, L.A. The Epidemiology of Prostate Cancer. *Cold Spring Harb. Perspect. Med.* **2018**, *8*, a030361. [CrossRef] [PubMed]
5. Tolkach, Y.; Kristiansen, G. The Heterogeneity of Prostate Cancer: A Practical Approach. *Pathobiology* **2018**, *85*, 108–116. [CrossRef]
6. Wu, B.; Lu, X.; Shen, H.; Yuan, X.; Wang, X.; Yin, N.; Sun, L.; Shen, P.; Hu, C.; Jiang, H.; et al. Intratumoral heterogeneity and genetic characteristics of prostate cancer. *Int. J. Cancer* **2020**, *146*, 3369–3378. [CrossRef]
7. Teo, M.Y.; Rathkopf, D.E.; Kantoff, P. Treatment of Advanced Prostate Cancer. *Annu. Rev. Med.* **2019**, *70*, 479–499. [CrossRef]
8. Mohler, J.L.; Antonarakis, E.S.; Armstrong, A.J.; D'Amico, A.V.; Davis, B.J.; Dorff, T.; Eastham, J.A.; Enke, C.A.; Farrington, T.A.; Higano, C.S.; et al. Prostate Cancer, Version 2.2019, NCCN Clinical Practice Guidelines in Oncology. *J. Natl. Compr. Canc. Netw.* **2019**, *17*, 479–505. [CrossRef]

9. Keyes, M.; Crook, J.; Morton, G.; Vigneault, E.; Usmani, N.; Morris, W.J. Treatment options for localized prostate cancer. *Can. Fam. Phys.* **2013**, *59*, 1269–1274.
10. Naitoh, J.; Zeiner, R.L.; Dekernion, J.B. Diagnosis and treatment of prostate cancer. *Am. Fam. Phys.* **1998**, *57*, 1531–1539.
11. Dunn, M.W.; Kazer, M.W. Prostate cancer overview. *Semin. Oncol. Nurs.* **2011**, *27*, 241–250. [CrossRef]
12. Parker, C.; Castro, E.; Fizazi, K.; Heidenreich, A.; Ost, P.; Procopio, G.; Tombal, B.; Gillessen, S. Prostate cancer: ESMO Clinical Practice Guidelines for diagnosis, treatment and follow-up. *Ann. Oncol.* **2020**, *31*, 1119–1134. [CrossRef] [PubMed]
13. Cassinello, J.; Carballido Rodriguez, J.; Anton Aparicio, L. Role of taxanes in advanced prostate cancer. *Clin. Transl. Oncol.* **2016**, *18*, 972–980. [CrossRef] [PubMed]
14. Saad, F.; Hotte, S.J. Guidelines for the management of castrate-resistant prostate cancer. *Can. Urol. Assoc. J.* **2010**, *4*, 380–384. [CrossRef] [PubMed]
15. Hotte, S.J.; Saad, F. Current management of castrate-resistant prostate cancer. *Curr. Oncol.* **2010**, *17* (Suppl. 2), S72–S79. [CrossRef]
16. Wadosky, K.M.; Koochekpour, S. Molecular mechanisms underlying resistance to androgen deprivation therapy in prostate cancer. *Oncotarget* **2016**, *7*, 64447–64470. [CrossRef]
17. Nader, R.; El Amm, J.; Aragon-Ching, J.B. Role of chemotherapy in prostate cancer. *Asian J. Androl* **2018**, *20*, 221–229. [CrossRef]
18. Gjyrezi, A.; Xie, F.; Voznesensky, O.; Khanna, P.; Calagua, C.; Bai, Y.; Kung, J.; Wu, J.; Corey, E.; Montgomery, B.; et al. Taxane resistance in prostate cancer is mediated by decreased drug-target engagement. *J. Clin. Investig.* **2020**, *130*, 3287–3298. [CrossRef]
19. Newman, D.J.; Cragg, G.M. Natural Products as Sources of New Drugs from 1981 to 2014. *J. Nat. Prod.* **2016**, *79*, 629–661. [CrossRef]
20. Dasari, S.; Bakthavachalam, V.; Chinnapaka, S.; Venkatesan, R.; Samy, A.; Munirathinam, G. Neferine, an alkaloid from lotus seed embryo targets HeLa and SiHa cervical cancer cells via pro-oxidant anticancer mechanism. *Phytother. Res.* **2020**, *34*, 2366–2384. [CrossRef]
21. Huang, M.; Lu, J.J.; Ding, J. Natural Products in Cancer Therapy: Past, Present and Future. *Nat. Prod. Bioprospect.* **2021**, *11*, 5–13. [CrossRef]
22. Swetha, M.; Keerthana, C.K.; Rayginia, T.P.; Anto, R.J. Cancer Chemoprevention: A Strategic Approach Using Phytochemicals. *Front. Pharmacol.* **2021**, *12*, 809308. [CrossRef]
23. Haque, A.; Brazeau, D.; Amin, A.R. Perspectives on natural compounds in chemoprevention and treatment of cancer: An update with new promising compounds. *Eur. J. Cancer* **2021**, *149*, 165–183. [CrossRef] [PubMed]
24. Atanasov, A.G.; Zotchev, S.B.; Dirsch, V.M.; International Natural Product Sciences, T.; Supuran, C.T. Natural products in drug discovery: Advances and opportunities. *Nat. Rev. Drug Discov.* **2021**, *20*, 200–216. [CrossRef]
25. Zuckerman, V.; Wolyniec, K.; Sionov, R.V.; Haupt, S.; Haupt, Y. Tumour suppression by p53: The importance of apoptosis and cellular senescence. *J. Pathol.* **2009**, *219*, 3–15. [CrossRef] [PubMed]
26. Chen, L.; Li, Q.; Jiang, Z.; Li, C.; Hu, H.; Wang, T.; Gao, Y.; Wang, D. Chrysin Induced Cell Apoptosis Through H19/let-7a/COPB2 Axis in Gastric Cancer Cells and Inhibited Tumor Growth. *Front. Oncol.* **2021**, *11*, 651644. [CrossRef]
27. Dias, A.S.; Helguero, L.; Almeida, C.R.; Duarte, I.F. Natural Compounds as Metabolic Modulators of the Tumor Microenvironment. *Molecules* **2021**, *26*, 3494. [CrossRef]
28. Dasari, S.; Samy, A.; Narvekar, P.; Dontaraju, V.S.; Dasari, R.; Kornienko, A.; Munirathinam, G. Polygodial analog induces apoptosis in LNCaP prostate cancer cells. *Eur. J. Pharmacol.* **2018**, *828*, 154–162. [CrossRef]
29. Kubo, I.; Fujita, K.; Lee, S.H.; Ha, T.J. Antibacterial activity of polygodial. *Phytother. Res.* **2005**, *19*, 1013–1017. [CrossRef]
30. Dasari, R.; De Carvalho, A.; Medellin, D.C.; Middleton, K.N.; Hague, F.; Volmar, M.N.; Frolova, L.V.; Rossato, M.F.; De La Chapa, J.J.; Dybdal-Hargreaves, N.F.; et al. Synthetic and Biological Studies of Sesquiterpene Polygodial: Activity of 9-Epipolygodial against Drug-Resistant Cancer Cells. *ChemMedChem* **2015**, *10*, 2014–2026. [CrossRef]
31. Kubo, I.; Fujita, K.; Lee, S.H. Antifungal mechanism of polygodial. *J. Agric. Food Chem.* **2001**, *49*, 1607–1611. [CrossRef]
32. De La Chapa, J.; Singha, P.K.; Sallaway, M.; Self, K.; Nasreldin, R.; Dasari, R.; Hart, M.; Kornienko, A.; Just, J.; Smith, J.A.; et al. Novel polygodial analogs P3 and P27: Efficacious therapeutic agents disrupting mitochondrial function in oral squamous cell carcinoma. *Int. J. Oncol.* **2018**, *53*, 2627–2636. [CrossRef] [PubMed]
33. Russo, A.; Cardile, V.; Graziano, A.C.E.; Avola, R.; Montenegro, I.; Cuellar, M.; Villena, J.; Madrid, A. Antigrowth activity and induction of apoptosis in human melanoma cells by Drymis winteri forst extract and its active components. *Chem. Biol. Interact.* **2019**, *305*, 79–85. [CrossRef] [PubMed]
34. Fratoni, E.; de Athayde, A.E.; da Silva Machado, M.; Zermiani, T.; Venturi, I.; Correa Dos Santos, M.; Lobato, F.; Cechinel Filho, V.; Franchi, G.C., Jr.; Nowill, A.E.; et al. Antiproliferative and toxicological properties of drimanes obtained from Drimys brasiliensis stem barks. *Biomed. Pharmacother.* **2018**, *103*, 1498–1506. [CrossRef] [PubMed]
35. Maslivetc, V.; Laguera, B.; Chandra, S.; Dasari, R.; Olivier, W.J.; Smith, J.A.; Bissember, A.C.; Masi, M.; Evidente, A.; Mathieu, V.; et al. Polygodial and Ophiobolin A Analogues for Covalent Crosslinking of Anticancer Targets. *Int. J. Mol. Sci.* **2021**, *22*, 11256. [CrossRef]
36. Takeda, M.; Mizokami, A.; Mamiya, K.; Li, Y.Q.; Zhang, J.; Keller, E.T.; Namiki, M. The establishment of two paclitaxel-resistant prostate cancer cell lines and the mechanisms of paclitaxel resistance with two cell lines. *Prostate* **2007**, *67*, 955–967. [CrossRef]
37. Berger, D.R.; Ware, B.R.; Davidson, M.D.; Allsup, S.R.; Khetani, S.R. Enhancing the functional maturity of induced pluripotent stem cell-derived human hepatocytes by controlled presentation of cell-cell interactions in vitro. *Hepatology* **2015**, *61*, 1370–1381. [CrossRef]
38. Rheinwald, J.G.; Green, H. Serial cultivation of strains of human epidermal keratinocytes: The formation of keratinizing colonies from single cells. *Cell* **1975**, *6*, 331–343. [CrossRef]

39. van Meerloo, J.; Kaspers, G.J.; Cloos, J. Cell sensitivity assays: The MTT assay. *Methods Mol. Biol.* **2011**, *731*, 237–245. [CrossRef]
40. Khetani, S.R.; Bhatia, S.N. Microscale culture of human liver cells for drug development. *Nat. Biotechnol.* **2008**, *26*, 120–126. [CrossRef]
41. Samy, A.; Bakthavachalam, V.; Vudutha, M.; Vinjamuri, S.; Chinnapaka, S.; Munirathinam, G. Eprinomectin, a novel semi-synthetic macrocylic lactone is cytotoxic to PC3 metastatic prostate cancer cells via inducing apoptosis. *Toxicol. Appl. Pharmacol.* **2020**, *401*, 115071. [CrossRef]
42. Liang, C.C.; Park, A.Y.; Guan, J.L. In vitro scratch assay: A convenient and inexpensive method for analysis of cell migration in vitro. *Nat. Protoc.* **2007**, *2*, 329–333. [CrossRef] [PubMed]
43. Gong, J.; Zheng, Y.; Wang, Y.; Sheng, W.; Li, Y.; Liu, X.; Si, S.; Shao, R.; Zhen, Y. A new compound of thiophenylated pyridazinone IMB5043 showing potent antitumor efficacy through ATM-Chk2 pathway. *PLoS ONE* **2018**, *13*, e0191984. [CrossRef] [PubMed]
44. Wlodkowic, D.; Skommer, J.; Darzynkiewicz, Z. Flow cytometry-based apoptosis detection. *Methods Mol. Biol.* **2009**, *559*, 19–32. [CrossRef] [PubMed]
45. Kummrow, A.; Frankowski, M.; Bock, N.; Werner, C.; Dziekan, T.; Neukammer, J. Quantitative assessment of cell viability based on flow cytometry and microscopy. *Cytom. A* **2013**, *83*, 197–204. [CrossRef] [PubMed]
46. Chinnapaka, S.; Zheng, G.; Chen, A.; Munirathinam, G. Nitro aspirin (NCX4040) induces apoptosis in PC3 metastatic prostate cancer cells via hydrogen peroxide (H2O2)-mediated oxidative stress. *Free Radic. Biol. Med.* **2019**, *143*, 494–509. [CrossRef]
47. Pozarowski, P.; Darzynkiewicz, Z. Analysis of cell cycle by flow cytometry. *Methods Mol. Biol.* **2004**, *281*, 301–311. [CrossRef]
48. Nakamura, H.; Takada, K. Reactive oxygen species in cancer: Current findings and future directions. *Cancer Sci.* **2021**, *112*, 3945–3952. [CrossRef]
49. Casaburi, I.; Avena, P.; De Luca, A.; Sirianni, R.; Rago, V.; Chimento, A.; Trotta, F.; Campana, C.; Rainey, W.E.; Pezzi, V. GPER-independent inhibition of adrenocortical cancer growth by G-1 involves ROS/Egr-1/BAX pathway. *Oncotarget* **2017**, *8*, 115609–115619. [CrossRef]
50. Carpentier, G. Dot-Blot Protein Array Analyzer Macro for Image J Software. Available online: https://imagej.nih.gov/ij/macros/toolsets/Dot%20Blot%20Analyzer.txt (accessed on 4 April 2022).
51. Mahmood, T.; Yang, P.C. Western blot: Technique, theory, and trouble shooting. *N. Am. J. Med. Sci.* **2012**, *4*, 429–434. [CrossRef]
52. Kaur, J.; Bachhawat, A.K. A modified Western blot protocol for enhanced sensitivity in the detection of a membrane protein. *Anal. Biochem.* **2009**, *384*, 348–349. [CrossRef]
53. Chinnapaka, S.; Bakthavachalam, V.; Munirathinam, G. Repurposing antidepressant sertraline as a pharmacological drug to target prostate cancer stem cells: Dual activation of apoptosis and autophagy signaling by deregulating redox balance. *Am. J. Cancer Res.* **2020**, *10*, 2043–2065. [PubMed]
54. Kumar, P.; Nagarajan, A.; Uchil, P.D. Analysis of Cell Viability by the MTT Assay. *Cold Spring Harb. Protoc.* **2018**, *2018*. [CrossRef] [PubMed]
55. Rafehi, H.; Orlowski, C.; Georgiadis, G.T.; Ververis, K.; El-Osta, A.; Karagiannis, T.C. Clonogenic assay: Adherent cells. *J. Vis. Exp.* **2011**, e2573. [CrossRef]
56. Hanahan, D.; Weinberg, R.A. Hallmarks of cancer: The next generation. *Cell* **2011**, *144*, 646–674. [CrossRef] [PubMed]
57. Seyfried, T.N.; Huysentruyt, L.C. On the origin of cancer metastasis. *Crit. Rev. Oncog.* **2013**, *18*, 43–73. [CrossRef]
58. Kim, Y.N.; Koo, K.H.; Sung, J.Y.; Yun, U.J.; Kim, H. Anoikis resistance: An essential prerequisite for tumor metastasis. *Int. J. Cell Biol.* **2012**, *2012*, 306879. [CrossRef]
59. Guadamillas, M.C.; Cerezo, A.; Del Pozo, M.A. Overcoming anoikis–pathways to anchorage-independent growth in cancer. *J. Cell Sci.* **2011**, *124*, 3189–3197. [CrossRef]
60. Lei, Q.Y.; Wang, L.Y.; Dai, Z.Y.; Zha, X.L. The relationship between PTEN expression and anoikis in human lung carcinoma cell lines. *Sheng Wu Hua Xue Yu Sheng Wu Wu Li Xue Bao (Shanghai)* **2002**, *34*, 463–468. [PubMed]
61. Yang, Z.F.; Yi, J.L.; Li, X.R.; Xie, D.X.; Liao, X.F. PTEN induces anoikis through its phosphatase activity in hepatocellular carcinoma cells. *Zhonghua Zhong Liu Za Zhi* **2005**, *27*, 273–275.
62. Vitolo, M.I.; Weiss, M.B.; Szmacinski, M.; Tahir, K.; Waldman, T.; Park, B.H.; Martin, S.S.; Weber, D.J.; Bachman, K.E. Deletion of PTEN promotes tumorigenic signaling, resistance to anoikis, and altered response to chemotherapeutic agents in human mammary epithelial cells. *Cancer Res.* **2009**, *69*, 8275–8283. [CrossRef]
63. Lu, Y.; Lin, Y.Z.; LaPushin, R.; Cuevas, B.; Fang, X.; Yu, S.X.; Davies, M.A.; Khan, H.; Furui, T.; Mao, M.; et al. The PTEN/MMAC1/TEP tumor suppressor gene decreases cell growth and induces apoptosis and anoikis in breast cancer cells. *Oncogene* **1999**, *18*, 7034–7045. [CrossRef] [PubMed]
64. Kumari, S.; Badana, A.K.; Malla, R. Reactive Oxygen Species: A Key Constituent in Cancer Survival. *Biomark. Insights* **2018**, *13*, 1177271918755391. [CrossRef] [PubMed]
65. Silke, J.; Meier, P. Inhibitor of apoptosis (IAP) proteins-modulators of cell death and inflammation. *Cold Spring Harb. Perspect. Biol.* **2013**, *5*, a008730. [CrossRef]
66. Deveraux, Q.L.; Reed, J.C. IAP family proteins–suppressors of apoptosis. *Genes Dev.* **1999**, *13*, 239–252. [CrossRef] [PubMed]
67. Porter, A.G.; Janicke, R.U. Emerging roles of caspase-3 in apoptosis. *Cell Death Differ.* **1999**, *6*, 99–104. [CrossRef]
68. D'Amours, D.; Sallmann, F.R.; Dixit, V.M.; Poirier, G.G. Gain-of-function of poly(ADP-ribose) polymerase-1 upon cleavage by apoptotic proteases: Implications for apoptosis. *J. Cell Sci.* **2001**, *114*, 3771–3778. [CrossRef]

69. Yaffe, P.B.; Power Coombs, M.R.; Doucette, C.D.; Walsh, M.; Hoskin, D.W. Piperine, an alkaloid from black pepper, inhibits growth of human colon cancer cells via G1 arrest and apoptosis triggered by endoplasmic reticulum stress. *Mol. Carcinog.* **2015**, *54*, 1070–1085. [CrossRef]
70. Zhang, J.; Zhu, X.; Li, H.; Li, B.; Sun, L.; Xie, T.; Zhu, T.; Zhou, H.; Ye, Z. Piperine inhibits proliferation of human osteosarcoma cells via G2/M phase arrest and metastasis by suppressing MMP-2/-9 expression. *Int. Immunopharmacol.* **2015**, *24*, 50–58. [CrossRef]
71. Pongrakhananon, V.; Nimmannit, U.; Luanpitpong, S.; Rojanasakul, Y.; Chanvorachote, P. Curcumin sensitizes non-small cell lung cancer cell anoikis through reactive oxygen species-mediated Bcl-2 downregulation. *Apoptosis* **2010**, *15*, 574–585. [CrossRef]
72. Fofaria, N.M.; Kim, S.H.; Srivastava, S.K. Piperine causes G1 phase cell cycle arrest and apoptosis in melanoma cells through checkpoint kinase-1 activation. *PLoS ONE* **2014**, *9*, e94298. [CrossRef]
73. Khan, M.; Yi, F.; Rasul, A.; Li, T.; Wang, N.; Gao, H.; Gao, R.; Ma, T. Alantolactone induces apoptosis in glioblastoma cells via GSH depletion, ROS generation, and mitochondrial dysfunction. *IUBMB Life* **2012**, *64*, 783–794. [CrossRef] [PubMed]

cancers

Review

Advances in Dietary Phenolic Compounds to Improve Chemosensitivity of Anticancer Drugs

Abdelhakim Bouyahya [1,†], Nasreddine El Omari [2,†], Saad Bakrim [3], Naoufal El Hachlafi [4], Abdelaali Balahbib [5], Polrat Wilairatana [6,*] and Mohammad S. Mubarak [7,*]

1 Laboratory of Human Pathologies Biology, Department of Biology, Faculty of Sciences, Mohammed V University, Rabat 10106, Morocco
2 Laboratory of Histology, Embryology, and Cytogenetic, Faculty of Medicine and Pharmacy, Mohammed V University, Rabat 10100, Morocco
3 Geo-Bio-Environment Engineering and Innovation Laboratory, Molecular Engineering, Biotechnologies, and Innovation Team, Polydisciplinary Faculty of Taroudant, Ibn Zohr University, Agadir 80000, Morocco
4 Microbial Biotechnology and Bioactive Molecules Laboratory, Sciences and Technologies Faculty, Sidi Mohmed Ben Abdellah University, Fez 30050, Morocco
5 Laboratory of Biodiversity, Ecology, and Genome, Faculty of Sciences, Mohammed V University, Rabat 10056, Morocco
6 Department of Clinical Tropical Medicine, Faculty of Tropical Medicine, Mahidol University, Bangkok 10400, Thailand
7 Department of Chemistry, The University of Jordan, Amman 11942, Jordan
* Correspondence: polrat.wil@mahidol.ac.th (P.W.); mmubarak@ju.edu.jo (M.S.M.)
† These authors contributed equally to this work.

Simple Summary: Several dietary phenolic compounds isolated from medicinal plants exert significant anticancer effects via several mechanisms. They induce apoptosis, autophagy, telomerase inhibition, and angiogenesis. Certain dietary phenolic compounds increase the effectiveness of drugs used in conventional chemotherapy. Some clinical uses of dietary phenolic compounds for treating certain cancers have shown remarkable therapeutic results, suggesting effective incorporation in anticancer treatments in combination with traditional chemotherapeutic agents.

Abstract: Despite the significant advances and mechanistic understanding of tumor processes, therapeutic agents against different types of cancer still have a high rate of recurrence associated with the development of resistance by tumor cells. This chemoresistance involves several mechanisms, including the programming of glucose metabolism, mitochondrial damage, and lysosome dysfunction. However, combining several anticancer agents can decrease resistance and increase therapeutic efficacy. Furthermore, this treatment can improve the effectiveness of chemotherapy. This work focuses on the recent advances in using natural bioactive molecules derived from phenolic compounds isolated from medicinal plants to sensitize cancer cells towards chemotherapeutic agents and their application in combination with conventional anticancer drugs. Dietary phenolic compounds such as resveratrol, gallic acid, caffeic acid, rosmarinic acid, sinapic acid, and curcumin exhibit remarkable anticancer activities through sub-cellular, cellular, and molecular mechanisms. These compounds have recently revealed their capacity to increase the sensitivity of different human cancers to the used chemotherapeutic drugs. Moreover, they can increase the effectiveness and improve the therapeutic index of some used chemotherapeutic agents. The involved mechanisms are complex and stochastic, and involve different signaling pathways in cancer checkpoints, including reactive oxygen species signaling pathways in mitochondria, autophagy-related pathways, proteasome oncogene degradation, and epigenetic perturbations.

Keywords: cancer; chemotherapy; drugs resistance; dietary phenolic compounds; drugs sensibilization; combination treatment

Citation: Bouyahya, A.; Omari, N.E.; Bakrim, S.; Hachlafi, N.E.; Balahbib, A.; Wilairatana, P.; Mubarak, M.S. Advances in Dietary Phenolic Compounds to Improve Chemosensitivity of Anticancer Drugs. *Cancers* **2022**, *14*, 4573. https://doi.org/10.3390/cancers14194573

Academic Editor: Anupam Bishayee

Received: 4 July 2022
Accepted: 16 September 2022
Published: 21 September 2022

1. Introduction

Cancer is a significant issue for physicians in multidisciplinary health care facilities. It is a complex and multifactorial pathology in which normal cells develop mutations in their genetic structure, resulting in continued cell growth, colonization, and metastasis to other organs such as the liver, prostate, breast, lungs, brain, and colon. The transformation mechanisms range from genetic and hormonal disturbances to environmental inducers and metabolic deregulations. This divergence of risk factors gives rise to various forms of cancer and, sometimes, implies therapeutic specificity even for the same type of cancer [1–3]. In this regard, searching for anticancer treatments requires screening several chemical molecules with functional diversity. Among the candidate molecules studied are phenolic compounds. Chemically defined as having a phenolic structure, phenolic compounds are well recognized for their extensive pharmacological properties such as anti-inflammatory, antibiotic, antiseptic, antitumor, antiallergic, cardioprotective, etc. Phenolic compounds are derived from edible plants, particularly medicinal and aromatic plants, in many food products such as vegetables, cereals, legumes, fruits, nuts, and certain beverages. Indeed, this chemical family constitutes a group of substances frequently present in the metabolism of medicinal plants and contains several subclasses, such as acids, flavonoids, and tannins, which are the most abundant molecules [4–6]. Various investigations have focused on phenolic compounds as anticancer bioactive compounds. These groups of molecules exert anticancer properties by acting on the multiple checkpoints of cancerous cells and can induce apoptosis, autophagy, and cell cycle arrest with high specificity [7,8].

In addition, phenolic compounds exert other actions such as inhibiting telomeres, blocking their expression and inhibiting angiogenesis and metastases. On the other hand, phenolic compounds have recently been shown to act in combination with other bioactive compounds used in chemotherapy, sometimes with a potent synergistic mechanism. Recent investigations have also highlighted the sensitization action of cancer cells to chemotherapeutic treatments [9,10]. Indeed, dietary phenolic compounds can induce chemosensitivity of human cancers towards used drugs in chemotherapy via different molecular mechanisms, which include reducing the expression of a transcription factor regulating the expression of cytoprotective genes, the down-regulation of the phosphatidylinositol 3-kinase and Akt protein kinase B (PI3K/Ak) pathway, reducing p53 activation, enhancing the cytotoxicity of used drugs, decreasing Bcl-2 expression and mitochondrial membrane potential ($\Delta\Psi m$) while inhibiting tumor growth, enhancing the cytotoxicity of used drugs, reducing Bcl-2 expression and mitochondrial membrane potential ($\Delta\Psi m$) while inhibiting tumor growth, suppressing the expression of hypoxia-inducible factor (HIF-1α) and P-glycoprotein (P-gp) responsible for multidrug resistance, and increasing cellular apoptosis with down-regulation of p-Akt expression and up-regulation of phosphatase and tensin homolog (PTEN) expression [9,10]. Based on the previous discussion, this study aims to investigate and demonstrate the potential benefits of dietary sources, notably phenolic compounds, in managing and preventing cancer. Additionally, the current review aims to examine combining chemotherapeutic drugs with phenolic compounds and their sensitizing effects on cancer treatments to improve the effectiveness and diminish the harmful effects of anticancer bioactive compounds.

2. Dietary Phenolic Compounds Improving the Chemosensitivity of Anticancer Drugs

Recent research findings showed that cancer cells could develop resistance to used drugs in chemotherapy. This resistance is related to different molecular mechanisms which give cancer cells a selective advantage in resisting drugs administered during cancer chemotherapy (Figure 1).

2.1. *Flavonoids*

Resistance to various anti-cancer treatments, whether chemotherapy or radiotherapy, remains a significant obstacle in the management of cancer patients. Therefore, the use of chemo- and radio-sensitizers of plant origin has attracted the attention of scientists to replace synthetic drugs to improve tumor sensitivity. One example of these natural compounds is flavonoids. Food products containing high levels of flavonoids include blueberries and other berries, parsley, onions, bananas, green and black tea, citrus fruits, sea buckthorn, *Ginkgo biloba*, and dark chocolate.

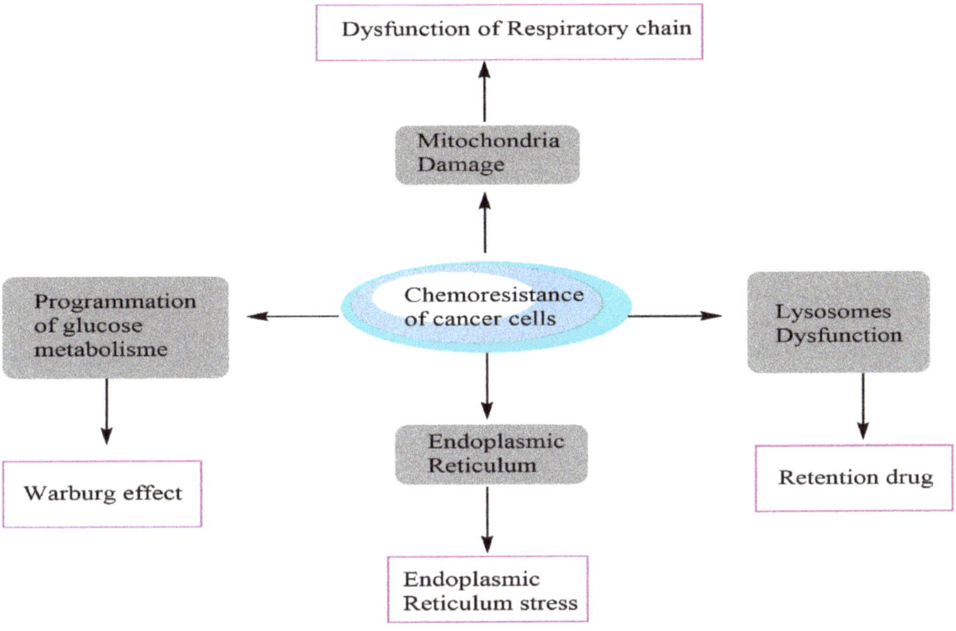

Figure 1. Mechanisms of chemoresistance of cancer cells against anticancer drugs.

Combinatorial treatment with flavonoids has been suggested in several studies as a potential therapeutic approach to avoid drug resistance and enhance their antitumor properties. Table 1 lists flavonoids (Figure 2) that improve the chemosensitivity of chemotherapeutic drugs in cancer.

Table 1. Flavonoids improve the chemosensitivity of chemotherapeutic drugs in cancer.

Molecules	Origins	Experimental Approaches	Key Results	References
Apigenin	Synthetized	MDA435/LCC6 and P388 cells Cell proliferation assay ATPase assay	Enhanced the cytotoxicity of paclitaxel (PTX), doxorubicin (Dox), daunomycin (DM), vincristine (VCR), and vinblastine, resulting in a reduction of IC_{50} by 5–50 times	[11]
	Purchased	Parental human HCC cells (BEL-7402) and BEL-7402/ADM cells MTT assay Cell cycle analysis Real-time quantitative PCR Western blot analysis In vivo xenograft studies	Sensitized Dox-resistant BEL-7402 (BEL- 7402/ADM) cells to Dox Increased intracellular concentration of Dox Reduced Nrf2 expression APG + Dox (in vivo) inhibited tumor growth, reduced cell proliferation, and induced apoptosis more substantially when compared with Dox treatment alone	[12]
	Purchased	Human pancreatic cancer cell line BxPC-3 Human pancreatic ductal epithelium (HPDE) cells Western blot analysis MTS cell proliferation assay	APG (13 μM) + gemcitabine (Gem) (13 μM) inhibited cell proliferation APG (11–19 μM) + Gem (10 μM) inhibited growth by 59–73% Enhanced the anti-proliferative activity of chemotherapeutic drugs	[13]

Table 1. *Cont.*

Molecules	Origins	Experimental Approaches	Key Results	References
	Purchased	Human pancreatic cancer cell lines AsPc-1, Panc-1, and MiaPaCa-2 MTT assay Cell apoptosis assay Western blot analysis In vitro IKK-β kinase activity assay Xenograft model	Reduced cell growth Induced cell apoptosis Down-regulated the TNF-α-induced NF-κB DNA binding activity Suppressed pancreatic cancer growth and IKK-β activation in nude mice xenograft	[14]
	Purchased	Laryngeal carcinoma Hep-2 cell line RT-PCR Cell counting Kit-8 (CCK-8) system Western blot analysis	Enhanced the cisplatin (CP)-induced suppression of Hep-2 cell growth in a concentration- and time-dependent manner Reduced the levels of GLUT-1 mRNA and GLUT-1 and p-Akt proteins in CP-treated Hep-2 cells in a concentration and time-dependent manner	[15]
	Purchased	Laryngeal hep-2 carcinoma cell line Nude mouse model of laryngeal carcinoma Western blot analysis	Improved xenograft radio-sensitivity Reduced the expression of PI3K mRNA, Akt, and GLUT-1 after X-ray radiation	[16]
	Purchased	Tumor xenografts in nude mice SK-Hep-1 and BEL-7402 cells MTT assay Annexin V/PI assay Western blotting analysis Cellular ROS detection	Enhanced the cytotoxicity of 5-FU in HCC cells APG + 5-fluorouracil (5-FU) (in vivo) inhibited HCC xenograft tumor growth APG + 5-FU increased the levels of reactive oxygen species (ROS) APG + 5-FU decreased the mitochondrial membrane potential (ΔΨm) APG + 5-FU decreased Bcl-2 expression	[17]
	Purchased	Human renal proximal tubular epithelial (HK-2) cells MTT assay Analysis of cell morphology and cell cycleCaspase-3 activity assay Western blot analysis ROS production assay	Inhibited the CP-induced apoptosis of HK-2 cells Induced cell cycle arrest Inhibited caspase-3 activity and PARP cleavage Reduced CP-induced phosphorylation and expression of p53 Promoted the CP-induced Akt phosphorylation	[18]
	Purchased	80 Swiss albino male mice ELISA Quantitative real-time RT-PCR Histopathological and immunohistochemical analysis	APG alone or combined with 5-FU Increased Beclin-1 levels, caspase-3 and -9, and JNK activities, decreased tumor volume, Mcl-1expression, and total antioxidant capacity, alleviated histopathological changes, and decreased Ki-67 proliferation index	[19]
	Not reported	BEL-7402 and BEL-7402/ADM cells TUNEL assay qRT-PCR Annexin V-FITC/PI apoptosis assay Western blot analysis	Reversed Dox sensitivity Induced the caspase-dependent apoptosis in BEL-7402/ADM cells Induced the miR-101 expression	[20]
	Not reported	Human hepatocellular carcinoma (HCC) and adjacent normal tissue specimens qRT-PCR MTT assay Western blot analysis In vivo xenograft studies	Enhanced Dox sensitivity Induced miR-520b expression Inhibited ATG7-dependent autophagy in BEL-7402/ADM cells Inhibited hepatocellular carcinoma xenograft growth	[21]
	Purchased	Ovarian cancer-sensitive cell line SKOV3 Ovarian cancer drug-resistant cell line SKOV3/DDP MTT assay PCR test Western blot test Apoptosis test	Enhanced the chemosensitivity of ovarian cancer-sensitive cells and drug-resistant cells Induced the apoptosis of ovarian cancer cells by down-regulating the Mcl-1 gene	[22]

Table 1. *Cont.*

Molecules	Origins	Experimental Approaches	Key Results	References
Quercetin	Purchased	DB-1 melanoma and SK Mel 28 cell lines Western blot analysis Annexin V-FITC staining RNA isolation and RT-PCR Immunocytochemistry siRNA transfection	Induced a redistribution of ΔNp73 in the cytoplasm and nucleus Que + temozolomide (TMZ) abolished drug insensitivity and caused a more than additive induction of apoptosis	[23]
	Not reported	Human esophageal cancer cells (EC9706 and Eca109) MTT assay Annexin V-FITC/propidium iodide (PI)-stained fluorescence-activated cell sorting (FACS) Western blot analysis	Que + 5-FU inhibited growth and stimulated apoptosis in EC9706 and Eca109 esophageal cancer cells compared to Que	[24]
	Purchased	MCF-7 and MCF-7/Dox cells MTT assay Flow cytometry Matrigel invasion assay Western blot analysis	Increased intracellular concentration of Dox Improved Dox cytotoxicity Que + Dox inhibited cell proliferation and invasion and suppressed HIF-1α and P-gp expression	[25]
	Not reported	Human ovarian cancer cell lines, SKOV-3, EFO27, OVCAR-3, and A2780P Evaluation of quercetin toxicity SRB staining	Inhibited proliferation and increased sensitivity of ovarian cancer cells to CP and PTX	[26]
	Purchased	U251 and U87 human glioblastoma cells MTT assay Flow cytometry Western blot analysis	Que (30 μmol/L) + TMZ (100 μmol/L) inhibited cell viability and enhanced TMZ inhibition Que did not affect the caspase-3 activity and cell apoptosis, whereas combined with TMZ, it increased the caspase-3 activity and induced cell apoptosis.	[27]
	Purchased	MCF-7 cells and MCF-7/Dox cells MTT assay Flow cytometry	Que + Dox inhibited cell proliferation and invasion Que + Dox increased cell apoptosis Que + Dox up-regulated PTEN expression Que + Dox down-regulated p-Akt expression	[28]
	Purchased	Lung cancer cells (A549 and H460 cells) Western blot analysis	Reduced cell viability Suppressed HSP70 expression Improved Gem-induced cell death linked to increased caspase-3 and caspase-9 activities Que + Gem down-regulated HSP70 expression more significantly than treatment with Que or Gem alone	[29]
	Not reported	BEL-7402 and multidrug-resistant cell line BEL/5-FU MTT assay Flow cytometry Real-time PCR Western blot analysis	Increased intracellular accumulation of Dox Increased sensitivity of BEL/5-FU cells to chemotherapeutic drugs Down-regulated the expressions of ABCB1, ABCC1, and ABCC2 Inhibited the functions and expressions of ABCB1, ABCC1, and ABCC2 efflux pump	[30]
	Purchased	Human prostate cancer cell line PC3 MTT assay Western blot analysis Flow cytometry	Inhibited c-met expression and the downstream PI3K/AKT pathway Que + Dox promoted the Dox-induced cell apoptosis through the mitochondrial/ROS pathway	[31]
	Purchased	Human pancreatic cancer cell lines Transfection of small interfering RNA MTT assay Western blot analysis Cell cycle measurement	Attenuated RAGE expression to facilitate cell cycle arrest, autophagy, apoptosis, and GEM chemosensitivity in MIA Paca-2 GEMR cells	[32]

Table 1. *Cont.*

Molecules	Origins	Experimental Approaches	Key Results	References
	Purchased	Human prostate cancer (PC-3) cell lines Nude male BALB/c mice MTT assay Intracellular ROS content assays RNA extraction and qRT-PCR Western blot analysis Immunohistochemistry	Que + PTX inhibited cell proliferation, increased apoptosis, arrested cell cycle at the G_2/M phase, inhibited cell migration, induced ER stress, and increased ROS generation Que + PTX exerted the most beneficial therapeutic effects (in vivo) Increased the cancer cell-killing effects of PTX (in vivo)	[33]
	Not reported	MCF 7 cells MTT assay Flow cytometry qRT-PCR ELISA	Quer + 5-FU improved apoptosis by increasing the gene expression of Bax and p53 and caspase-9 activity and decreasing Bcl2 gene expression Quer + 5-FU decreased colony formation	[34]
	Purchased	MDA-MB-231 human breast cancer cell line MTT assay Flow cytometry qRT-PCR Western blot analysis	Decreased cell viability Que (95 μM) + docetaxel (7 nM) up-regulated p53, increased BAX levels, and decreased levels of BCL2, pERK1/2, AKT, and STAT3 proteins	[35]
Kaempferol	Purchased	Human myelogenous leukemia K562 cells and the adriamycin-resistant variant K562/A cells MTT assay Annexin V/PI analysis PCR array	Kae + Que inhibited the growth of both cells Kae + Que increased the sensitivity of both cells Kae + Que induced apoptosis Kae + Que influenced the expression of drug transporter genes	[36]
	Purchased	LS174 colon cancer cells MTT assay Colony formation assay Spheroid generation Sensitization assay Measurement of ROS Western blot analysis qRT-PCR	Chemo-sensitized 5-FU-resistant LS174-R cells Blocked the production of ROS and modulated the expression of JAK/STAT3, MAPK, PI3K/AKT, and NF-κBKae + 5-FU exerted a synergistic inhibitory effect on cell viability Kae + 5-FU enhanced apoptosis and induced cell cycle arrest in chemo-resistant and sensitive cells	[37]
	Purchased	Human colorectal cancer cell line HCT8 5-FU-resistant cell line HCT8-R CCK-8 assay qPCR assay Western blot analysis Clonogenic assay	Reversed the drug resistance of HCT8-R cells to 5-FU Reduced glucose uptake and lactic acid production in drug-resistant colorectal cancer cells Promoted the expression of microRNA-326 in colon cancer cells Reversed the resistance of colorectal cancer cells to 5-FU	[38]
Myricetin	Purchased	Esophageal carcinoma EC9706 cells Colony formation assays Flow cytometry Western blot analysis Nude mouse tumor xenograft model	MYR + 5-FU suppressed cell survival fraction and proliferation, and increased cell apoptosis MYR + 5-FU decreased survivin, cyclin D, and Bcl-2, and increased the expression level of caspase-3 and p53 MYR + 5-FU reduced the growth rate of tumor xenografts in mice	[39]
	Purchased	A2780 and OVCAR3 ovarian cancer cells MTT assay Apoptosis assay Boyden chamber assay Western blot analysis	Induced cytotoxicity, with an IC_{50} value of 25 μM Induced cell apoptosis, accompanied by the modulation of certain pro- and anti-apoptotic markers Increased paclitaxel cytotoxicity	[40]
Rutin	Purchased	Human breast cancer MDA- MB-231 cellsCalcein acetoxymethyl accumulation assayRhodamine-123 uptake assay Annexin V and 7-aminoactinomycin D Propidium iodide staining	Increased the anticancer activity of both chemotherapeutic agents Decreased the activity of adenosine triphosphate binding cassette transporters RTN (20 μM) enhanced cytotoxicity related to cyclophosphamide and methotrexate RTN (20 and 50 μM) arrested the cell cycle at the G_2/M and G_0/G_1 phases, respectively, thus promoting cell apoptosis	[41]

Table 1. *Cont.*

Molecules	Origins	Experimental Approaches	Key Results	References
	Purchased	Human HCC cell lines qRT-PCR Luciferase reporter assay Cell viability assay Flow cytometry In vivo tumor xenograft	Attenuated autophagy and BANCR expression in SO-resistant cells Decreased the number of autophagosomes in HepG2/SO and HCCLM3/SO cells Enhanced the efficacy of SO in a xenograft model of HCC in nude mice	[42]
Hispidulin	Not reported	Human gallbladder carcinoma cell line GBC-SD MTT assay Western blot analysis Flow cytometry Caspase-3 activity assay qRT-PCR In vivo xenograft experiments	Inhibited the growth of GBC cells Promoted apoptosis in GBC cells Induced cell arrest at the G_0/G_1 phase Exerted antitumor effect mediated through HIF-1α inhibition Repressed the transactivation activity and expression of HIF-1α Suppressed the HIF-1α expression via AMPK signaling	[43]

2.1.1. Flavones

Apigenin is a natural product found in numerous fruits and vegetables, but it is particularly abundant in chamomile tea, parsley, celery, propolis, and garlic oil. It was among the most investigated flavonoids in this field. In 2006, Chan, et al. [11] synthesized a series of apigenin dimers that increased the chemo-sensitivity of leukemic and breast cells, known to be multidrug-resistant (MDR), to numerous anticancer drugs, such as vinblastine (VBL), vincristine (VCR), daunomycin (DM), doxorubicin (DOX), and paclitaxel (PTX) [11]. Seven years later, the chemo-sensitive mechanism by which apigenin acts on DOX has been investigated [12]. The mechanism involves reducing the expression of a transcription factor regulating the expression of cytoprotective genes, called Nrf2, at the levels of proteins and messenger RNA by down-regulating the PI3K/Akt pathway. Compared to DOX treatment alone, the combination treatment of apigenin with DOX showed anticancer effects by inducing apoptosis, reducing cell proliferation, and inhibiting tumor growth.

Johnson and Mejia [13] evaluated the interaction effect between this flavonoid and one of the known chemotherapeutic drugs, gemcitabine (GEM), on human pancreatic cancer cells. This interaction inhibited cell proliferation and growth by 59–73%, whereas apigenin alone potentiated the anti-proliferative effect of GEM. This effect was attributed to IKK-β-mediated NF-κB activation [14]. To improve the chemo-sensitivity of another chemotherapeutic agent, called cisplatin (CP), and to overcome the chemo-resistance of laryngeal carcinoma (Hep-2 cells), apigenin was chosen in an in vitro co-targeted therapy [15]. The results showed that CP-induced Hep-2 cell growth suppression was significantly enhanced in a time- and concentration-dependent manner with suppression of p-AKT and glucose transporter-1 (GLUT-1) involved in resistance to cancer treatments. Bao, et al. also tested this a year later against the same type of cancer [16]. In human renal proximal tubular epithelial cells, apigenin ameliorated CP-induced nephrotoxicity by promoting the PI3K/Akt pathway (Figure 3) and reducing p53 activation [18].

On the other hand, a promising combined effect was recorded with apigenin and 5-fluorouracil (5-FU), a chemotherapeutic drug belonging to the class of antimetabolite drugs [17,19]. In this context, apigenin significantly improved the treatment of hepatocellular carcinoma (HCC) by enhancing the cytotoxicity of 5-FU [17]. The combination of these two elements decreased Bcl-2 expression and mitochondrial membrane potential ($\Delta\Psi$m) while inhibiting tumor growth of HCC xenografts. This was in agreement with the results of Gaballah and collaborators [19], who also observed a reduction in tumor size and Mcl-1 expression, with an increase in Beclin-1 levels and caspase-3 and -9 activities. Furthermore, Gao, et al. [20,21] investigated the chemosensitivity of apigenin using BEL-7402/ADM cells, which are known for their resistance to DOX, a molecule belonging to the anthracycline family. Results showed that apigenin enhanced DOX sensitivity, induced apoptosis, and prevented HCC xenograft growth. Recently, treatment with apigenin was applied to ovarian cancer (OC) using ovarian cancer-sensitive cells (SKOV3) and drug-resistant cells (SKOV3/DDP) [22]. Results showed positive effects on the chemo-sensitivity of both cell types with apoptosis and reversal of drug resistance of these cancer cells through the down-regulation of the Mcl-1 gene.

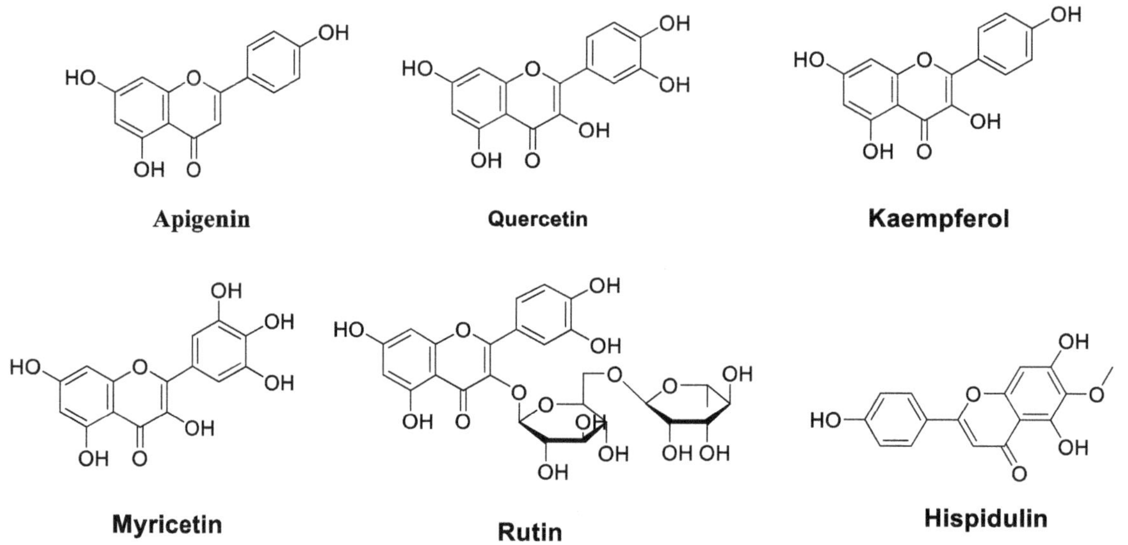

Figure 2. Chemical structures of flavonoids that improve the chemosensitivity of anticancer drugs

On the other hand, a promising combined effect was recorded with apigenin and 5-fluorouracil (5-FU), a chemotherapeutic drug belonging to the class of antimetabolite drugs [17,19]. In this context, apigenin significantly improved the treatment of hepatocellular carcinoma (HCC) by enhancing the cytotoxicity of 5-FU [17]. The combination of these two elements decreased Bcl-2 expression and mitochondrial membrane potential ($\Delta\Psi m$) while inhibiting tumor growth of HCC xenografts. This was in agreement with the results of Gaballah and collaborators [19], who also observed a reduction in tumor size and Mcl-1 expression, with an increase in Beclin-1 levels and caspase-3 and -9 activities. Furthermore, Gao, et al. [20,21] investigated the chemosensitivity of apigenin using BEL-7402/ADM cells, which are known for their resistance to DOX, a molecule belonging to the anthracycline family. Results showed that apigenin enhanced DOX sensitivity, induced apoptosis, and prevented HCC xenograft growth. Recently, treatment with apigenin was applied to ovarian cancer (OC) using ovarian cancer-sensitive cells (SKOV3) and drug-resistant cells (SKOV3/DDP) [22]. Results showed positive effects on the chemo-sensitivity of both cell types with apoptosis and reversal of drug resistance of these cancer cells through the down-regulation of the Mcl-1 gene.

2.1.2. Flavanols

Quercetin is naturally distributed in many fruits, vegetables, leaves, seeds, and grains; capers, red onions, and kale contain appreciable quantities. Regarding quercetin, several research studies have evaluated the effect of this flavonoid against multidrug resistance by several mechanisms of action in various cancer cells. Research findings indicated that a co-treatment with quercetin combined with temozolomide (TMZ), an active anticancer drug, showed positive results such as inhibition of cell viability, induction of cell apoptosis, an increase of caspase-3 activity, elimination of drug insensitivity, and improvement of TMZ inhibition [23,27]. Some of these effects, such as the decrease in colony formation, inhibition of growth, and the stimulation of apoptosis by decreasing Bcl2 gene expression and increasing p53 and caspase-9 activity in esophageal (EC9706 and Eca109) have also been observed by combining quercetin with 5-FU [24] and breast (MCF-7) [34] cancer cells.

The management of breast cancer attracted the attention of Li, et al. [25,28] who performed two experiments to evaluate the combination therapy of quercetin with DOX on MCF-7 cells. Results revealed that this treatment inhibits cell invasion and proliferation by suppressing the expression of HIF-1α and P-glycoprotein (P-gp), responsible for multidrug resistance [25]. In addition, results showed an increase in cellular apoptosis with down-regulation of p-Akt expression and up-regulation of phosphatase and tensin homolog (PTEN) expression [28]. Other effects of this combination, namely increasing cellular sensitivity to DOX and promoting DOX-induced cellular apoptosis via the mitochondrial/ROS pathway, respectively, have been noted in studies conducted by Chen, et al. [30] and by Shu, et al. [31] in the treatment of HCC (BEL-7402 cells) and prostate cancer (PC3 cells). Quercetin alone was able to down-regulate the expression of specific ABC transporters (ABCB1, ABCC1, and ABCC2) [30] with inhibition of the expression of the PI3K/AKT pathway [31].

On the other hand, the synergistic effect of quercetin was examined in vitro and in vivo with PTX, a molecule used in chemotherapy and synthesized by endophytic fungi [26]. Quercetin alone inhibited the proliferation of OC cells and increased their sensitivity to PTX [26]. Meanwhile, the combination of these two molecules showed an inhibition of the migration and proliferation of prostate cancer cells with an increase in apoptosis, and induction of G_2/M cell cycle arrest, whereas the in vivo combination showed a synergistic effect in killing cancer cells [26]. Moreover, this flavonol positively affected GEM, a drug with significant cytotoxic activity, such as the improvement of cell death associated with increased caspase-3 and -9 activities in lung cancer cells. It caused considerable suppression of HSP70 chaperone protein expression compared to treatment with GEM alone [29]. This chemo-sensitivity has also been noted in pancreatic cancer cells [32]. In a recent study, Safi, et al. [35] evaluated the synergistic effect of quercetin (95 μM) with docetaxel (7 nM), an alkaloid with anticancer properties. Results revealed a decrease in STAT3, AKT, pERK1/2, and Bcl-2 proteins in MDA-MB-231 breast cancer cells.

2.1.3. Flavonols

Kaempferol is a flavonol found in numerous fruits and vegetables such as grapes, potatoes, squash, tomatoes, broccoli, onions, brussels sprouts, green beans, green tea, peaches, spinach, blackberries, lettuce, cucumber, apples, and raspberries. It has been studied for its chemo-sensitizing activity. Its association with quercetin has shown promising results, namely growth inhibition of adriamycin-resistant K562/A cells and myeloid leukemia K562 cells, increasing their sensitivity, and induction of apoptosis [36]. Additionally, this ubiquitous flavonoid chemo-sensitized 5-FU resistant colon cancer LS174-R cells and the combination of both substances provided a synergistic effect by inhibiting cell viability and inducing cell cycle arrest [37]. This was explained recently by Wu et al. [38] who attributed these results to the inhibition of PKM2-mediated glycolysis. The combinatorial effect of 5-FU with a flavonol was further evaluated (in vitro and in vivo) with myricetin against esophageal carcinoma [39]. Several favorable outcomes such as suppression of cell proliferation, increase in cell apoptosis and caspase-3 expression, and decrease in Bcl-2 and tumor xenograft growth (in vivo) were observed. In addition, kaempferol increased the PTX cytotoxicity with modulation of anti- and pro-apoptotic markers in OC cells [40].

As previously reported in breast cancer treatment with flavonoids, these secondary metabolites reverse cancer drug resistance and sensitize tumor cells to chemotherapy via several mechanisms. In this respect, Iriti et al. studied the chemo-sensitizing potential of rutin (3′,4′,5,7-Tetrahydroxy-3-[α-L-rhamnopyranosyl-(1–6)-β-D-glucopyranosyloxy]flavone) against two breast cancer cell lines (MB-MDA-231 and MCF-7 cells) [41]. At a dose of 20 μM, these researchers found that this flavonoid acts as a chemo-sensitizing agent by improving the anti-tumor effect of two chemotherapeutic agents (methotrexate and cyclophosphamide). Furthermore, rutin improved the in vivo efficacy of another anti-cancer drug (sorafenib) in a xenograft model of human HCC [42]. As seen with quercetin and berberine, another natural flavone called hispidulin enhanced cellular chemo-sensitivity by inhibiting the expression of the transcription factor HIF-1α via AMPK signaling in gallbladder cancer [43].

2.1.4. Anthocyanidins

Anthocyanins (ACNs) are the primary color of many leaves (such as purple cabbage), fruits (such as grapes and blueberries), tubers (such as purple radishes and yams), and flowers (such as roses). In a broad sense, anthocyanidins (ACNs) present a subclass of flavonoids that have not been well investigated for their chemo-sensitizing and radio-sensitizing effects. Indeed, black raspberry ACNs improved the efficacy of two chemotherapeutic agents (5-FU and celecoxib); in vitro by inhibiting the proliferation of CRC cells and in vivo by decreasing the number of CRC tumors in animals [44]. Recently, specific molecules of this family, such as delphinidin [45] and cyanidin-3-glucoside (C3G) [46], have been studied. In radiation-exposed A549 human lung adenocarcinoma cells, delphinidin enhanced the radio-therapeutic effects (induction of autophagy and apoptosis) by activating the JNK/MAPK signaling pathway [45]. Similarly, C3G improved the sensitivity to DOX and its cytotoxicity by inhibiting the phosphorylation of Akt and increasing that of p38, mainly by reducing the expression of claudin-2 [46]. Table 2 lists anthocyanidins (Figure 4) that could improve the chemosensitivity of cancer drugs.

Table 2. Anthocyanidins that could enhance the chemosensitivity of cancer drugs.

Molecules	Origins	Experimental Approaches	Key Results	References
Delphinidin	Purchased	A549 cell line (human, lung, and carcinoma) MTT assay Immunofluorescence staining Western blot analysis qRT-PCR	Induced apoptosis in A549 cells Promoted apoptosis in the radiation-exposed A549 cells Induced autophagy in radiation-exposed A549 cellsActivated autophagic cell death and the JNK/MAPK signaling pathway in radiation-exposed A549 cells	[45]
Cyanidin-3-glucoside (C3G)	Purchased	Human lung adenocarcinoma A549 cells Immunoblotting RNA isolation and qRT-PCR Immunofluorescence measurement Luciferase reporter assay	Reduced protein level of CLDN2 in A549 cells Inhibited Akt phosphorylation Increased p38 phosphorylation Reduced CLDN2 expression at transcriptional and post-translational steps mediated by Akt inhibition and p38 activation, respectively Improved Dox accumulation and cytotoxicity in spheroid models Increased the percentages of apoptotic and necrotic cells induced by Dox	[46]
Anthocyanins (ACNs)	Black raspberry	Colon cancer cell lines, SW480 and Caco2MTT assay Colony formation assays Western blot analysis Establishment of colitis-induced colon cancer mice model	Improved the chemotherapy efficacy of 5-FU and celecoxib ACNs + (5-FU or celecoxib) inhibited CRC cell proliferation (in vitro) and decreased the number of tumors in AOM-induced CRC mice (in vivo)	[44]

2.2. *Non-Flavonoids*

2.2.1. Phenolic Acids

It has been demonstrated that phenolic acids have a chemo-sensitizing activity on several types of cancer cells to different chemotherapeutics (Table 3). Data presented in Table 3 indicate that ellagic acid was the most studied molecule. It is found in large quantities in pecans, chestnuts, raspberries, peaches, cranberries, strawberries, raw grapes, walnuts, and pomegranates. Indeed, its combination with 5-FU in treating colorectal carcinoma (CRC) gave significant effects such as inhibition of apoptotic cell death and cell proliferation. In contrast, treatment alone enhanced 5-FU chemo-sensitivity in CRC cells [47]. Indeed, ellagic acid alone potentiated CP cytotoxicity and prevented the development of CP resistance in epithelial OC cells [48]. Table 3 shows the phenolic acids (Figure 5) that improve the chemosensitivity of cancer drugs.

Caffeic acid can be derived from a variety of beverages and is relatively present at high concentrations in lingonberry, thyme, sage, and spearmint as well as in spices such as Ceylon cinnamon and star anise. Caffeic acid is moderately available in sunflower seeds, applesauce, apricots, and prunes. Caffeic acid phenethyl ester (CAPE), a central component of propolis, has also been investigated for its chemo-sensitizing [51,52] and radio-sensitizing [53] effects against various types of cancer. The radio-sensitizing effect of this substance was evaluated in 2005 by Chen, et al. [49] against CT26 colorectal adenocarcinoma cells and in vivo on BALB/c mice implanted with these cells. These authors noted, in vitro, an improvement in the destruction of CT26 cells by ionizing radiation (IR) and, in vivo, an extension of animal survival and a marked inhibition of tumor growth compared to radiotherapy alone. The mechanism of action explaining this radio-sensitivity was elucidated very recently on prostate cancer cells (DU145 and PC3) by co-treatment using gamma radiation (GR) and CAPE [53]. Results showed that this combined treatment sensitizes the cells to radiotherapy by reducing the RAD50 and RAD51 proteins and the cell migration potential, mainly by inhibiting DNA damage repair. As for the chemo-sensitivity of this phenolic compound, Lin, et al. [50] did not observe any chemo-sensitizing effect of medulloblastoma Daoy cells on the chemotherapeutics studied (DOX or CP). However, in 2018, two similar studies proved otherwise by enhancing the sensitivity of gastric and lung cancer cells to DOX and CP by decreasing proteasome function [51,52].

In contrast, Muthusamy, et al. carried out two studies on the ability of ferulic acid (FA), a phenolic acid present in seeds and leaves of certain plants and found in exceptionally high amounts in popcorn and bamboo shoots, to reverse the resistance of multiresistant cells to anticancer drugs. In the first study, FA-enhanced cell cycle arrest was exerted by PTX and decreased resistance to this drug [54]. In the second study, FA increased VCR and DOX cytotoxicity and synergistically increased DOX-induced apoptotic signaling [55]. In addition, the authors showed that the synergy between FA and DOX reduced tumor xenograft size compared to the treatment with DOX alone. They associated these results with suppressing P-gp expression by inhibiting the PI3K/Akt/NF-κB signaling pathway.

Another phenolic acid constituent, called rosmarinic acid (RA), is found in culinary herbs such as *Ocimum tenuiflorum* (holy basil), *Origanum majorana* (marjoram), *Melissa officinalis* (lemon balm), *Ocimum basilicum* (basil), *Salvia officinalis* (sage), *Salvia rosmarinus* (rosemary), peppermint, and thyme. This natural compound showed remarkable potential as an anti-leukemic agent in acute promyelocytic leukemia cells by potentiating macrophage differentiation induced by all-trans retinoic acid [56]. Furthermore, Yu, et al. [57] evaluated the impact of RA on 5-FU chemo-resistance in the treatment of gastric carcinoma. In SGC7901 gastric carcinoma cells treated with 5-FU, the application of RA increased the chemo-sensitivity of these cells to 5-FU by reducing its IC_{50} values from 208.6 to 70.43 μg/mL and the expression levels of two miRNAs (miR-642a-3p and miR-6785-5p), with increased expression of FOXO4.

2.2.2. Tannins

Although condensed tannins (also called proanthocyanidins (PCs)), found in plants, such as cranberry, blueberry, and grape seeds, are chemically polymers of flavanols, they have not been widely investigated as anticancer agents compared to flavonoids and phenolic acids. However, they have recently been studied to overcome the problems of cancer cell resistance to chemotherapy [58]. In this context, Zhang, et al. [58] showed that PCs inhibit the growth and characteristics of platinum-resistant OC cells by inducing G_1 cell cycle arrest and targeting the Wnt/β-catenin signaling pathway. On the other hand, other researchers indicated that PCs sensitize chemoresistant CC cells (HCT116 and H716) to

5-FU and oxaliplatin (OXP) [59]. In contrast, combining all these substances reduced tumor growth in chemoresistant cells and chemoresistant tumor xenografts. The mechanism suggested to overcome this chemo-resistance involves suppressing the activity of adenosine triphosphate-binding cassette transporters. Furthermore, tannic acid (TA), another plant tannin used as an anticancer agent, has been studied for its synergistic effect with chemotherapeutic drugs (5-FU, GEM, and mitomycin C) against malignant cholangiocytes [60]. Results revealed that TA exhibits a crucial synergistic effect with 5-FU and mitomycin C in modulating drug efflux pathways. The exact synergy was observed by combining TA and CP on HepG2 liver cancer cells through mitochondria-mediated apoptosis [61]. This chemotherapeutic sensitivity to CP was corroborated by co-treatment with procyanidins in TU686 laryngeal cancer cells through the apoptosis and autophagy pathway [62]. Table 4 lists condensed tannins (Figure 6) that could improve the chemosensitivity of cancer drugs.

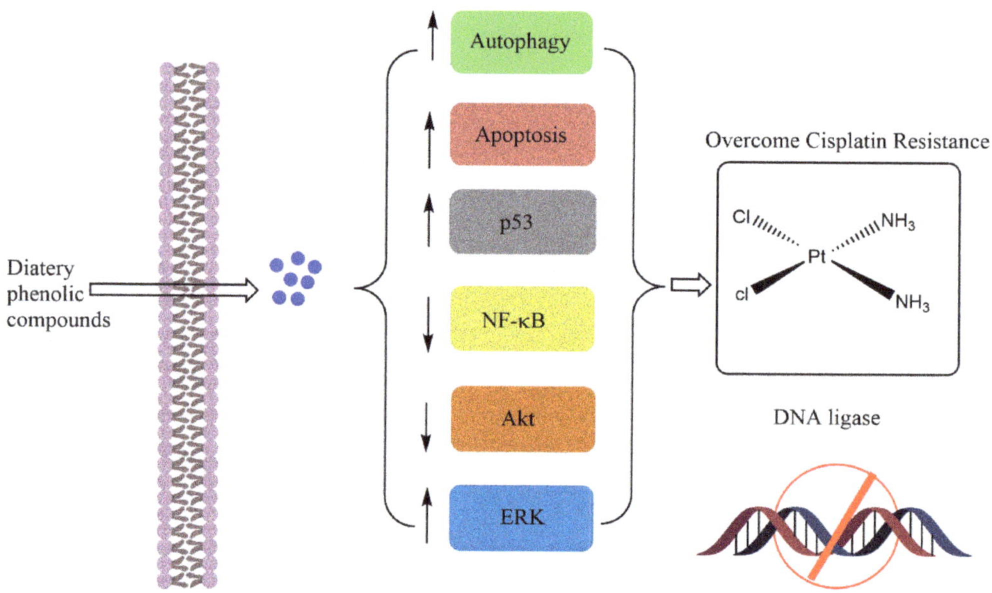

Figure 3. Mechanisms of chemosensitivity of apigenin towards sisplatin.

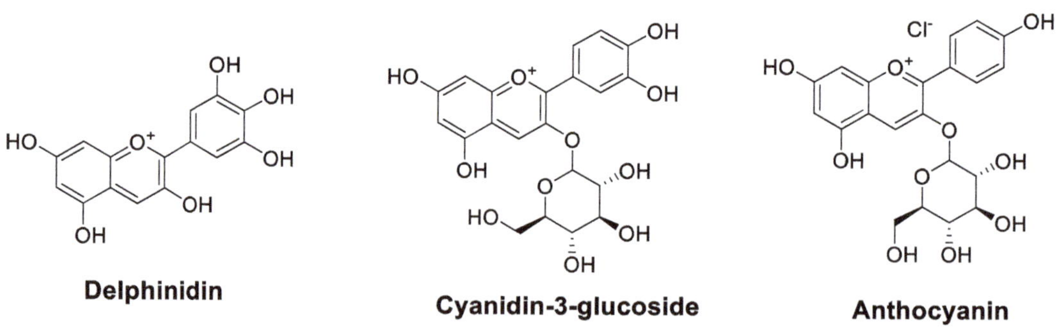

Figure 4. Chemical structures of anthocyanidins that improve chemosensitivity of anticancer drugs..

Table 3. Phenolic acids that improve the chemosensitivity of cancer drugs.

Molecules	Origins	Experimental Approaches	Key Results	References
Caffeic acid phenethyl ester (CAPE)	Not reported	Mouse CT26 colorectal adenocarcinoma cells BALB/c mouse with CT26 cells implantation Colony formation assay RT-PCR Flow cytometry	Depleted intracellular GSH in CT26 cells, but not in bone marrow cells Enhanced cell killing by IR Increased glutathione peroxidase, decreased glutathione reductase in CT26 cells Reversed radiation-activated NF-κB Induced a significant inhibition of tumor growth and prolongation of survival compared to IR alone (in vivo)	[49]
	Purchased	Human medulloblastoma Daoy cell line and Human astroglia SVGp12 MTT and trypan blue exclusion assays ELISATUNEL assay Flow cytometry Western blot analysis	Inhibited Daoy cell growth in a time- and concentration-dependent manner Decreased G_2/M fraction and increased S phase fractionDown-regulated expression of cyclin B1 protein Reduced the viability of irradiated Daoy cells No chemosensitizing effect on Dox or CP	[50]
	Purchased	Parental and the drug-resistant cells of stomach (MKN45) and colon (LoVo) cancers	Potentiated the apoptotic effects of Dox and CP against parental cells Reduced the production of Dox-induced ROS Reduced 26S proteasome-based proteolytic activities in parental MKN45 cells Up-regulated and significantly decreased chymotrypsin-like activity in Dox- or CP-resistant cells	[51]
	Not reported	Human lung adenocarcinoma A549 and RERF-LC-MS cell lines Immunoblotting RNA isolation and PCR Luciferase reporter assay Immunocytochemistry	Decreased claudin-2 protein level in a concentration-dependent manner Decreased (at 50 μM) mRNA level and promoter activity Decreased (at 50 μM) the level of p-NF−κB, and increased that of IκB Increased the expression and activity of protein phosphatase (PP) 1 and 2A Suppressed cell proliferation Enhanced Dox toxicity and accumulation in 3D spheroid cells	[52]
	Not reported	Prostate cancer (PCa) cells, DU145 and PC3 Evaluated the radiomodulatory potential of CAPE	CAPE + gamma radiation (GR) sensitized PCa cells to radiation in a concentration-dependent manner Improved the level of ionizing radiation (IR)-induced gamma H2AX foci and cell death by apoptosis CAPE + GR decreased the migration potential of PCa cells Sensitized PCa cells to radiation in vitro and induced apoptosis, increased Akt/mTOR phosphorylation and hampered cell migration CAPE + IR inhibited cell growth by decreasing RAD50 and RAD51 proteins	[53]
Ferulic acid (FA)	Purchased	Multidrug resistance (MDR) cell lines MTT assay Colony formation assay Fluorescence microscopic analysis Cell cycle analysis Tryptophan fluorescence quenching PCR array Western blot analysis	Inhibited P-glycoprotein transport function in drug-resistant KB ChR8-5 cell lines Down-regulated ABCB1 expression in a concentration-dependent manner Decreased paclitaxel resistance in KBChR8-5 and HEK293/ABCB1 cells Enhanced paclitaxel-mediated cell cycle arrest and up-regulated paclitaxel-induced apoptotic signaling in KB-resistant cells	[54]

Table 3. *Cont.*

Molecules	Origins	Experimental Approaches	Key Results	References
	Purchased	Parental KB cells and P−gp overexpressing KB Ch^{R}8-5 cell lines MTT assay γH2AX assay Western blot analysis Immunocytochemistry Animals and tumor xenograft experiments	Increased the cytotoxicity of Dox and VCR in the P-gp overexpressing KB Ch^{R}8-5 cells Enhanced the formation of Dox-induced γH2AX foci and synergistically increased Dox-induced apoptotic signaling in drug-resistant cells FA + Dox reduced KB Ch^{R}8−5 tumor xenograft size three-fold compared to the group treated with Dox alone Reversed MDR by suppressing P-gp expression via inhibition of PI3K/Akt/NF−κB signaling pathway	[55]
Rosmarinic acid (RA)	Purchased	Human acute promyelocytic leukemia NB4 cells Flow cytometry analysis Phagocytosis assay qRT-PCR	Potentiated ATRA-induced macrophage differentiation in APL cells	[56]
	Not reported	Human gastric carcinoma cell line SGC7901 Apoptosis assay CCK8 assay Apoptosis assay RNA isolation and microarray qRT-PCR Luciferase reporter assay Western blot analysis	Increased the chemosensitivity of SGC7901 cells to 5-FUReduced IC_{50} of 5-FU (70.43 ± 1.06 μg/mL) compared to untreated SGC7901/5-FU cells (208.6 ± 1.09 μg/mL) RA + 5-FU increased apoptosis rate Reduced the expression levels of two miRNAs (miR-642a−3p and miR−6785-5p) Reduced P-gp expression and increased Bax expression in SGC7901/5-FU and SGC7901/5-FU -Si cells	[57]

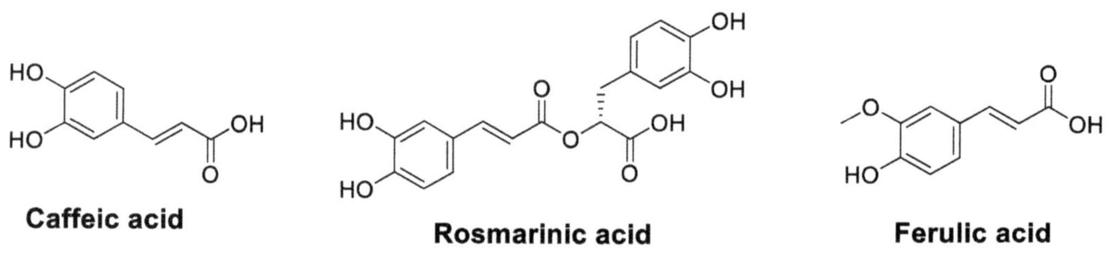

Figure 5. Chemical structures of phenolic acids that improve the chemosensitivity of anticancer drugs.

To improve the bioavailability and bioactivity of ellagic acid in vivo, Mady, et al. [63] formulated nanoparticles loaded with this acid from a biodegradable polymer [poly(ε-caprolactone)]. This encapsulation improved the oral bioavailability and the anti-tumor effect of ellagic acid. In a glioblastoma model, Cetin, et al. carried out two studies that showed an improvement in the anticancer efficacy of bevacizumab [64] and TMZ [65] by co-treatment with ellagic acid. This treatment reduced the expression of MGMT, affected caspase-3 and p53 proteins, and its combination with the chemotherapeutics reduced cell viability and the expression of MDR1.

Chemo-resistance of bladder cancer has been a serious problem in managing this type of cancer, particularly resistance to GEM. However, the underlying resistance mechanism has not been elucidated. The effect of ellagic acid or its combinatorial effect with GEM on GEM-sensitive bladder cancer cells and GEM-resistant cells was recently evaluated [66]. Results revealed that ellagic acid exerts numerous promising anticancer effects, particularly resensitization of GEM-resistant cells by inhibiting GEM transporters and the epithelial–mesenchymal transition (EMT), responsible for GEM resistance in other types of cancer. Suppression of EMT was also observed by catechol against pancreatic cancer cells, in addition to cellular chemo-sensitivity and radio-sensitivity to GEM via inhibition of the AMPK/Hippo signaling pathway [67].

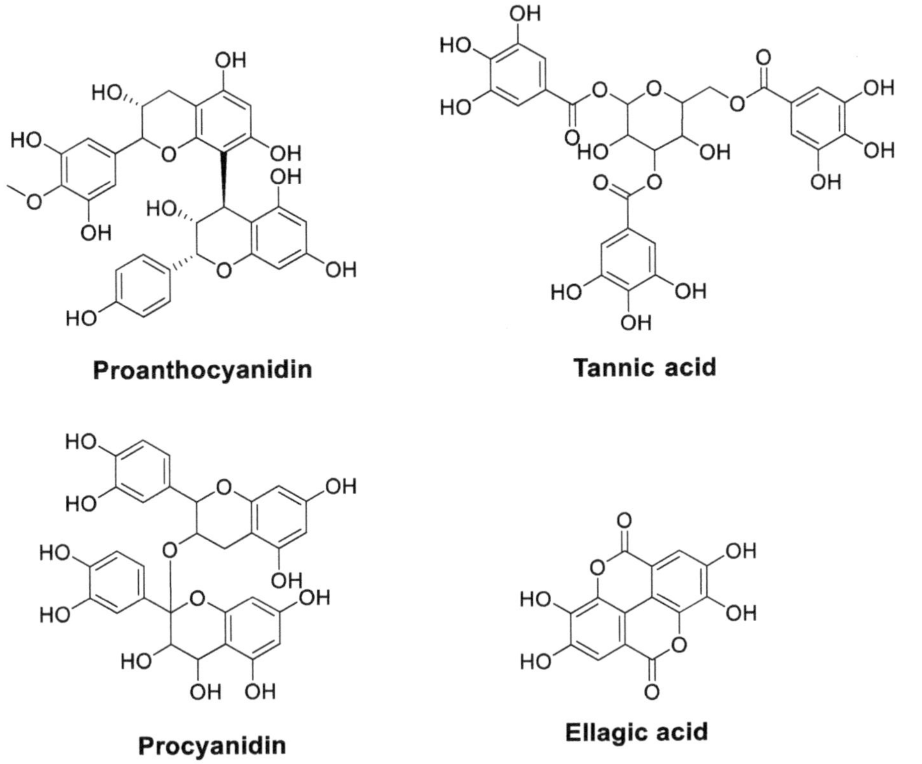

Figure 6. Chemical structures of tannins that improve chemosensitivity of anticancer drugs.

Table 4. Condensed tannins that could improve the chemosensitivity of cancer drugs.

Molecules	Origins	Experimental Approaches	Key Results	References
Proanthocyanidins	Chinese bayberry leaves	Platinum-resistant human ovarian cancer cell line OVCAR-3 Flow cytometry MTT assay Colony formation assay Western blot assay	Induced inhibitory effects on the growth and CSC characteristics of OVCAR−3 SP cells Reduced the expression of β-catenin, cyclin D1, and c-Myc and inhibited the self-renewal capacity of cells Induced G_1 cell cycle arrest in OVCAR−3 SP cells	[58]
	Grape seed extract	Colorectal cancer cell lines, HCT116 and H716 Cell cycle and apoptosis analysis Cell viability and proliferation mRNA expression analysis Genome-wide RNA-sequencing analysisXenograft animal experiments	Sensitized acquired (HCT116-FOr cells) and innately chemoresistant (H716 cells) cancer cells to 5-FU and oxaliplatin (OXP) PCs + (5-FU and OXP) inhibited the growth of chemoresistant cells and decreased the expression of several key adenosine triphosphate-binding cassette (ABC) transporters Sensitized chemoresistant cells to 5-FU and OXPPCs + (5-FU and OXP) reduced chemoresistant xenograft tumor growth in mice	[59]
Tannic acid	Purchased	Malignant human cholangiocytes Calcein retention assays Western blot analysis RT-PCR	Decreased malignant cholangiocyte growth Exhibited a synergistic effect with mitomycin C and 5-FU but not with Gem Decreased calcein efflux and expression of PGP, MRP1, and MRP2 membrane efflux pumps	[60]

Table 4. *Cont.*

Molecules	Origins	Experimental Approaches	Key Results	References
	Purchased	Liver cancer cell line HepG2 MTT assay Mitochondrial transmembrane potential qRT-PCR Western blot analysis	Inhibited HepG2 cell growth TA + CP induced mitochondria-mediated apoptosis in HepG2 cells and enhanced growth inhibitory effect compared to treatment alone	[61]
Procyanidins	Not reported	Laryngeal cancer cell line TU686 Flow cytometry Cell immunofluorescence staining Western blot analysis	Inhibited TU686 cells in a concentration-dependent manner for 24 h Induced apoptosis of TU686 cells Increased expression of LC3−II and Caspase-3	[62]
Ellagic acid	Purchased	Colorectal carcinoma HT−29, Colo 320DM, SW480, and LoVo cells Trypan blue exclusion Annexin−V labeling Mitochondrial membrane potential (Δψm) Immunoblotting	EA + 5-FU inhibited cell proliferation of HT-29, Colo 320DM and SW480 cells EA + 5-FU increased apoptotic cell death of HT−29 and Colo 320DM cells EA potentiated 5-FU chemosensitivity in at least three colorectal cancer cell lines	[47]
	Purchased	Epithelial ovarian cancer cell line A2780MTT assay Immunoblot analysis Signal pathway analysis Cell cycle analysis	Enhanced CP cytotoxicity in A2780CisR cells Prevented the development of CP resistance	[48]
	Purchased	Caco-2 and HTC-116 cells MTT assay In vitro drug release Male New Zealand white rabbits	Induced higher cell viability than EA-NP treated HCT−116 cells Oral administration of EA-NPs caused a 3.6-fold increase in the area under the curve compared to that of EA (in vivo)	[63]
	Purchased	Rat C6 glioma cells Immunohistochemistry RT-PCR	Reduced MGMT expression Affected the apoptotic proteins of p53 and caspase-3 at the protein level, but not at the gene level EA + bevacizumab (BEV) reduced cell viability EA + BEV reduced MDR1 expression only at 72 h	[64]
	Purchased	Rat C6 glioma cells Immunocytochemistry RT-PCR	EA + TMZ reduced cell viability Down-regulated MGMT expression independent of the presence of TMZ EA + TMZ reduced MDR1 expression only over 48 h compared to TMZ alone Up-regulated caspase-3 at 48 h, but up-regulated p53 at 48 and 72 h EA + TMZ enhanced immunoreactivities of p53 and caspase-3 proteins, but not of the genes	[65]
	Purchased	Four human bladder cancer cell lines, TSGH−8301, TSGH-9202, T24, and J82 MTT assay Flow cytometry Cell migration and invasion assays Western blot analysis qRT−PCR Xenograft model	Induced high cytotoxicity of Gem in GEM−resistant cells EA + Gem increased apoptosis and reduced cell motility in GCB-resistant cells Resensitized bladder cancer cells to Gem by reducing the epithelial–mesenchymal transition Reduced EMT by inhibiting the TGFβ−SMAD2/3 upward signaling pathway Inhibited the growth of bladder cancer tumors and increased the in vivo inhibitory effects of Gen on tumors	[66]

3. Conclusions and Perspectives

At present, the use of foodstuffs is attracting attention in treating and preventing diseases, including cancer. This is due to the presence of bioactive compounds such as phenolic acids, among others, in our diet. These natural compounds are gaining popularity in cancer treatment due to their lower side effects, cost, and accessibility than conventional drugs. In this review, we have shown through published research that phenolic compounds are an excellent source of natural anticancer substances providing a range of preventive and therapeutic options against several types of cancer. These compounds could be used alone or in combination with other anticancer drugs. Certain phenolic compounds such as quercetin and gallic acid have well-known mechanisms of action. These molecules act specifically on the various checkpoints of cancerous cells. Therefore, exploring these mechanisms of action could further improve the therapeutic efficacy. However, further investigations that could involve human subjects and different pharmacokinetic parameters are required to ensure the safety of these compounds before they can be used as prescription drugs. In addition, the development of a standardized extract or dosage could also be followed in clinical trials. In summary, phenolic compounds present in our food can be useful in complementary medicine for the prevention and treatment of different types of cancers due to their natural origin, safety, and low cost compared to cancer drugs.

Author Contributions: Conceptualization, A.B. (Abdelhakim Bouyahya), P.W. and M.S.M.; methodology, N.E.O., N.E.H. and S.B.; software, A.B. (Abdelaali Balahbib); validation, A.B. (Abdelhakim Bouyahya); formal analysis, A.B. (Abdelhakim Bouyahya); investigation, A.B. (Abdelhakim Bouyahya), N.E.O., N.E.H. and S.B.; writing—original draft preparation, A.B. (Abdelhakim Bouyahya); N.E.O., N.E.H. and S.B.; writing—review and editing, A.B. (Abdelhakim Bouyahya), P.W. and M.S.M.; supervision, A.B. (Abdelhakim Bouyahya) and M.S.M. All authors have read and agreed to the published version of the manuscript.

Funding: This research received no external funding.

Conflicts of Interest: The authors declare no conflict of interest.

Abbreviations

ACNs	Anthocyanidins
Akt	Protein Kinase B
APG	Apigenin
CAPE	Caffeic Acid Phenethyl Ester
CLL	Chronic Lymphocytic Leukemia
COX-2	Cyclooxygenase-2
CRC	Colorectal Carcinoma
DM	Daunomycin
DOX	Doxorubicin
ELISA	Enzyme-linked immunosorbent assay
EMT	Epithelial-Mesenchymal Transition
ERK	Extracellular Signal-Regulated Kinase
FA	Ferulic acid
GLUT-1	Glucose Transporter-1
Gem	Gemcitabine
GR	Gamma Radiation
HCC	Hepatocellular Carcinoma
HIF-1α	Hypoxia-Inducible Factor-1α
HO	Heme Oxygenase
HPD	Hispidulin
HPDE	Human pancreatic ductal epithelium
IL	Interleukin
IR	Ionizing Radiation
JNK	C-Jun N-Terminal Kinase
KAE	Kaempferol
MAPK	Mitogen-Activated Protein Kinase
MDR1	Multidrug resistance protein 1
MM	Multiple Myeloma
mTOR	mammalian Target of Rapamycin
MYR	Myricetin
NF-kB	Nuclear Factor Kappa B
Nrf2	Nuclear factor erythroid-related factor 2
NSCLC	Non-Small Cell Lung Cancer
OC	Ovarian Cancer
OXP	Oxaliplatin
P-gp	P-glycoprotein
PTEN	Phosphatase and Tensin Homolog
PTX	Paclitaxel
Que	Quercetin
ROS	Reactive Oxygen Species

RTN	Rutin
STAT3	Signal Transducer and Activator of Transcription 3
TA	Tannic acid
TNF-α	Tumor Necrosis Factor-α
TMZ	Temozolomide
VBL	Vinblastine
VCR	Vincristine
5-FU	5-Fluorouracil

References

1. Hurson, A.N.; Ahearn, T.U.; Keeman, R.; Abubakar, M.; Jung, A.Y.; Kapoor, P.M.; Koka, H.; Yang, X.R.; Chang-Claude, J.; Martínez, E. Systematic Literature Review of Risk Factor Associations with Breast Cancer Subtypes in Women of African, Asian, Hispanic, and European Descents. *Cancer Res.* **2022**, *82*, 3670. [CrossRef]
2. Stopsack, K.H.; Nandakumar, S.; Arora, K.; Nguyen, B.; Vasselman, S.E.; Nweji, B.; McBride, S.M.; Morris, M.J.; Rathkopf, D.E.; Slovin, S.F. Differences in Prostate Cancer Genomes by Self-Reported Race: Contributions of Genetic Ancestry, Modifiable Cancer Risk Factors, and Clinical FactorsRacial Differences in Prostate Cancer Genomes. *Clin. Cancer Res.* **2022**, *28*, 318–326. [CrossRef]
3. Tan, D.A.; Dayu, A.R.B. Menopausal Hormone Therapy: Why We Should No Longer Be Afraid of the Breast Cancer Risk. *Climacteric* **2022**, *25*, 362–368. [CrossRef]
4. Dobroslavić, E.; Repajić, M.; Dragović-Uzelac, V.; Elez Garofulić, I. Isolation of *Laurus Nobilis* Leaf Polyphenols: A Review on Current Techniques and Future Perspectives. *Foods* **2022**, *11*, 235. [CrossRef]
5. Mitra, S.; Tareq, A.M.; Das, R.; Emran, T.B.; Nainu, F.; Chakraborty, A.J.; Ahmad, I.; Tallei, T.E.; Idris, A.M.; Simal-Gandara, J. Polyphenols: A First Evidence in the Synergism and Bioactivities. *Food Rev. Int.* **2022**, 1–23. [CrossRef]
6. Rosero, S.; Del Pozo, F.; Simbaña, W.; Álvarez, M.; Quinteros, M.F.; Carrillo, W.; Morales, D. Polyphenols and Flavonoids Composition, Anti-Inflammatory and Antioxidant Properties of *Andean Baccharis* Macrantha Extracts. *Plants* **2022**, *11*, 1555. [CrossRef]
7. Islam, B.U.; Suhail, M.; Khan, M.K.; Zughaibi, T.A.; Alserihi, R.F.; Zaidi, S.K.; Tabrez, S. Polyphenols as Anticancer Agents: Toxicological Concern to Healthy Cells. *Phytother. Res.* **2021**, *35*, 6063–6079. [CrossRef]
8. Rauf, A.; Shariati, M.A.; Imran, M.; Bashir, K.; Khan, S.A.; Mitra, S.; Emran, T.B.; Badalova, K.; Uddin, M.; Mubarak, M.S. Comprehensive Review on Naringenin and Naringin Polyphenols as a Potent Anticancer Agent. *Environ. Sci. Pollut. Res.* **2022**, *29*, 31025–31041. [CrossRef]
9. Mottaghi, S.; Abbaszadeh, H. Natural Lignans Honokiol and Magnolol as Potential Anticarcinogenic and Anticancer Agents. A Comprehensive Mechanistic Review. *Nutr. Cancer* **2022**, *74*, 761–778. [CrossRef]
10. Yoganathan, S.; Alagaratnam, A.; Acharekar, N.; Kong, J. Ellagic Acid and Schisandrins: Natural Biaryl Polyphenols with Therapeutic Potential to Overcome Multidrug Resistance in Cancer. *Cells* **2021**, *10*, 458. [CrossRef]
11. Chan, K.-F.; Zhao, Y.; Burkett, B.A.; Wong, I.L.; Chow, L.M.; Chan, T.H. Flavonoid Dimers as Bivalent Modulators for P-Glycoprotein-Based Multidrug Resistance: Synthetic Apigenin Homodimers Linked with Defined-Length Poly (Ethylene Glycol) Spacers Increase Drug Retention and Enhance Chemosensitivity in Resistant Cancer Cells. *J. Med. Chem.* **2006**, *49*, 6742–6759. [CrossRef]
12. Gao, A.-M.; Ke, Z.-P.; Wang, J.-N.; Yang, J.-Y.; Chen, S.-Y.; Chen, H. Apigenin Sensitizes Doxorubicin-Resistant Hepatocellular Carcinoma BEL-7402/ADM Cells to Doxorubicin via Inhibiting PI3K/Akt/Nrf2 Pathway. *Carcinogenesis* **2013**, *34*, 1806–1814. [CrossRef]
13. Johnson, J.L.; de Mejia, E.G. Interactions between Dietary Flavonoids Apigenin or Luteolin and Chemotherapeutic Drugs to Potentiate Anti-Proliferative Effect on Human Pancreatic Cancer Cells, in Vitro. *Food Chem. Toxicol.* **2013**, *60*, 83–91. [CrossRef]
14. Wu, D.-G.; Yu, P.; Li, J.-W.; Jiang, P.; Sun, J.; Wang, H.-Z.; Zhang, L.-D.; Wen, M.-B.; Bie, P. Apigenin Potentiates the Growth Inhibitory Effects by IKK-β-Mediated NF-KB Activation in Pancreatic Cancer Cells. *Toxicol. Lett.* **2014**, *224*, 157–164. [CrossRef]
15. Xu, Y.-Y.; Wu, T.-T.; Zhou, S.-H.; Bao, Y.-Y.; Wang, Q.-Y.; Fan, J.; Huang, Y.-P. Apigenin Suppresses GLUT-1 and p-AKT Expression to Enhance the Chemosensitivity to Cisplatin of Laryngeal Carcinoma Hep-2 Cells: An in Vitro Study. *Int. J. Clin. Exp. Pathol.* **2014**, *7*, 3938.
16. Bao, Y.-Y.; Zhou, S.-H.; Lu, Z.-J.; Fan, J.; Huang, Y.-P. Inhibiting GLUT-1 Expression and PI3K/Akt Signaling Using Apigenin Improves the Radiosensitivity of Laryngeal Carcinoma in Vivo. *Oncol. Rep.* **2015**, *34*, 1805–1814. [CrossRef]
17. Hu, X.-Y.; Liang, J.-Y.; Guo, X.-J.; Liu, L.; Guo, Y.-B. 5-Fluorouracil Combined with Apigenin Enhances Anticancer Activity through Mitochondrial Membrane Potential (ΔΨm)-Mediated Apoptosis in Hepatocellular Carcinoma. *Clin. Exp. Pharmacol. Physiol.* **2015**, *42*, 146–153. [CrossRef]
18. Ju, S.M.; Kang, J.G.; Bae, J.S.; Pae, H.O.; Lyu, Y.S.; Jeon, B.H. The Flavonoid Apigenin Ameliorates Cisplatin-Induced Nephrotoxicity through Reduction of P53 Activation and Promotion of PI3K/Akt Pathway in Human Renal Proximal Tubular Epithelial Cells. *Evid. -Based Complementary Altern. Med.* **2015**, *2015*, 186436 . [CrossRef]
19. Gaballah, H.H.; Gaber, R.A.; Mohamed, D.A. Apigenin Potentiates the Antitumor Activity of 5-FU on Solid Ehrlich Carcinoma: Crosstalk between Apoptotic and JNK-Mediated Autophagic Cell Death Platforms. *Toxicol. Appl. Pharmacol.* **2017**, *316*, 27–35. [CrossRef]

20. Gao, A.-M.; Zhang, X.-Y.; Ke, Z.-P. Apigenin Sensitizes BEL-7402/ADM Cells to Doxorubicin through Inhibiting MiR-101/Nrf2 Pathway. *Oncotarget* **2017**, *8*, 82085. [CrossRef]
21. Gao, A.-M.; Zhang, X.-Y.; Hu, J.-N.; Ke, Z.-P. Apigenin Sensitizes Hepatocellular Carcinoma Cells to Doxorubic through Regulating MiR-520b/ATG7 Axis. *Chem.-Biol. Interact.* **2018**, *280*, 45–50. [CrossRef]
22. Li, Q.; Li, L.; Zhao, X.; Cheng, Z.; Ma, J. Apigenin Induces Apoptosis and Reverses the Drug Resistance of Ovarian Cancer Cells. *Int. J. Clin. Exp. Med.* **2020**, *13*, 1987–1994.
23. Thangasamy, T.; Sittadjody, S.; Mitchell, G.C.; Mendoza, E.E.; Radhakrishnan, V.M.; Limesand, K.H.; Burd, R. Quercetin Abrogates Chemoresistance in Melanoma Cells by Modulating ΔNp73. *BMC Cancer* **2010**, *10*, 282. [CrossRef]
24. Chuang-Xin, L.; Wen-Yu, W.; Yao, C.U.I.; Xiao-Yan, L.; Yun, Z. Quercetin Enhances the Effects of 5-Fluorouracil-Mediated Growth Inhibition and Apoptosis of Esophageal Cancer Cells by Inhibiting NF-KB. *Oncol. Lett.* **2012**, *4*, 775–778. [CrossRef]
25. Li, S.; Li, K.; Zhang, J.; Dong, Z. The Effect of Quercetin on Doxorubicin Cytotoxicity in Human Breast Cancer Cells. *Anti-Cancer Agents Med. Chem. (Former. Curr. Med. Chem. -Anti-Cancer Agents)* **2013**, *13*, 352–355. [CrossRef]
26. Maciejczyk, A.; Surowiak, P. Quercetin Inhibits Proliferation and Increases Sensitivity of Ovarian Cancer Cells to Cisplatin and Paclitaxel. *Ginekol. Pol.* **2013**, *84*, 590–595. [CrossRef]
27. Sang, D.; Li, R.; Lan, Q. Quercetin Sensitizes Human Glioblastoma Cells to Temozolomide in Vitro *via* Inhibition of Hsp27. *Acta Pharmacol. Sin.* **2014**, *35*, 832–838. [CrossRef]
28. Li, S.; Qiao, S.; Zhang, J.; Li, K. Quercetin Increase the Chemosensitivity of Breast Cancer Cells to Doxorubicin via PTEN/Akt Pathway. *Anti-Cancer Agents Med. Chem. (Former. Curr. Med. Chem. -Anti-Cancer Agents)* **2015**, *15*, 1185–1189. [CrossRef]
29. Lee, S.H.; Lee, E.J.; Min, K.H.; Hur, G.Y.; Lee, S.H.; Lee, S.Y.; Kim, J.H.; Shin, C.; Shim, J.J.; In, K.H. Quercetin Enhances Chemosensitivity to Gemcitabine in Lung Cancer Cells by Inhibiting Heat Shock Protein 70 Expression. *Clin. Lung Cancer* **2015**, *16*, e235–e243. [CrossRef]
30. Chen, Z.; Huang, C.; Ma, T.; Jiang, L.; Tang, L.; Shi, T.; Zhang, S.; Zhang, L.; Zhu, P.; Li, J. Reversal Effect of Quercetin on Multidrug Resistance *via* FZD7/β-Catenin Pathway in Hepatocellular Carcinoma Cells. *Phytomedicine* **2018**, *43*, 37–45. [CrossRef]
31. Shu, Y.; Xie, B.; Liang, Z.; Chen, J. Quercetin Reverses the Doxorubicin Resistance of Prostate Cancer Cells by Downregulating the Expression of C-Met. *Oncol. Lett.* **2018**, *15*, 2252–2258. [CrossRef]
32. Lan, C.-Y.; Chen, S.-Y.; Kuo, C.-W.; Lu, C.-C.; Yen, G.-C. Quercetin Facilitates Cell Death and Chemosensitivity through RAGE/PI3K/AKT/MTOR Axis in Human Pancreatic Cancer Cells. *J. Food Drug Anal.* **2019**, *27*, 887–896. [CrossRef]
33. Zhang, X.; Huang, J.; Yu, C.; Xiang, L.; Li, L.; Shi, D.; Lin, F. Quercetin Enhanced Paclitaxel Therapeutic Effects towards PC-3 Prostate Cancer through ER Stress Induction and ROS Production. *OncoTargets Ther.* **2020**, *13*, 513. [CrossRef]
34. Mawalizadeh, F.; Mohammadzadeh, G.; Khedri, A.; Rashidi, M. Quercetin Potentiates the Chemosensitivity of MCF-7 Breast Cancer Cells to 5-Fluorouracil. *Mol. Biol. Rep.* **2021**, *48*, 7733–7742. [CrossRef]
35. Safi, A.; Heidarian, E.; Ahmadi, R. Quercetin Synergistically Enhances the Anticancer Efficacy of Docetaxel through Induction of Apoptosis and Modulation of PI3K/AKT, MAPK/ERK, and JAK/STAT3 Signaling Pathways in MDA-MB-231 Breast Cancer Cell Line. *Int. J. Mol. Cell. Med.* **2021**, *10*, 11.
36. Yanqiu, H.; Linjuan, C.; Jin, W.; Hongjun, H.; Yongjin, S.; Guobin, X.; Hanyun, R. The Effects of Quercetin and Kaempferol on Multidrug Resistance and the Expression of Related Genes in Human Erythroleukemic K562/A Cells. *Afr. J. Biotechnol.* **2011**, *10*, 13399–13406. [CrossRef]
37. Riahi-Chebbi, I.; Souid, S.; Othman, H.; Haoues, M.; Karoui, H.; Morel, A.; Srairi-Abid, N.; Essafi, M.; Essafi-Benkhadir, K. The Phenolic Compound Kaempferol Overcomes 5-Fluorouracil Resistance in Human Resistant LS174 Colon Cancer Cells. *Sci. Rep.* **2019**, *9*, 195. [CrossRef]
38. Wu, H.; Du, J.; Li, C.; Li, H.; Guo, H.; Li, Z. Kaempferol Can Reverse the 5-Fu Resistance of Colorectal Cancer Cells by Inhibiting PKM2-Mediated Glycolysis. *Int. J. Mol. Sci.* **2022**, *23*, 3544. [CrossRef]
39. Wang, L.; Feng, J.; Chen, X.; Guo, W.; Du, Y.; Wang, Y.; Zang, W.; Zhang, S.; Zhao, G. Myricetin Enhance Chemosensitivity of 5-Fluorouracil on Esophageal Carcinoma in Vitro and in Vivo. *Cancer Cell Int.* **2014**, *14*, 71. [CrossRef]
40. Zheng, A.-W.; Chen, Y.-Q.; Zhao, L.-Q.; Feng, J.-G. Myricetin Induces Apoptosis and Enhances Chemosensitivity in Ovarian Cancer Cells. *Oncol. Lett.* **2017**, *13*, 4974–4978. [CrossRef]
41. Iriti, M.; Vitalini, S.; Arnold Apostolides, N.; El Beyrouthy, M. Chemical Composition and Antiradical Capacity of Essential Oils from Lebanese Medicinal Plants. *J. Essent. Oil Res.* **2014**, *26*, 466–472. [CrossRef]
42. Zhou, M.; Zhang, G.; Hu, J.; Zhu, Y.; Lan, H.; Shen, X.; Lv, Y.; Huang, L. Rutin Attenuates Sorafenib-Induced Chemoresistance and Autophagy in Hepatocellular Carcinoma by Regulating BANCR/MiRNA-590-5P/OLR1 Axis. *Int. J. Biol. Sci.* **2021**, *17*, 3595. [CrossRef]
43. Gao, H.; Xie, J.; Peng, J.; Han, Y.; Jiang, Q.; Han, M.; Wang, C. Hispidulin Inhibits Proliferation and Enhances Chemosensitivity of Gallbladder Cancer Cells by Targeting HIF-1α. *Exp. Cell Res.* **2015**, *332*, 236–246. [CrossRef]
44. Li, X.; Chen, L.; Gao, Y.; Zhang, Q.; Chang, A.K.; Yang, Z.; Bi, X. Black Raspberry Anthocyanins Increased the Antiproliferative Effects of 5-Fluorouracil and Celecoxib in Colorectal Cancer Cells and Mouse Model. *J. Funct. Foods* **2021**, *87*, 104801. [CrossRef]
45. Kang, S.H.; Bak, D.-H.; Chung, B.Y.; Bai, H.-W.; Kang, B.S. Delphinidin Enhances Radio-Therapeutic Effects via Autophagy Induction and JNK/MAPK Pathway Activation in Non-Small Cell Lung Cancer. *Korean J. Physiol. Pharmacol. Off. J. Korean Physiol. Soc. Korean Soc. Pharmacol.* **2020**, *24*, 413–422. [CrossRef]

46. Eguchi, H.; Matsunaga, H.; Onuma, S.; Yoshino, Y.; Matsunaga, T.; Ikari, A. Down-Regulation of Claudin-2 Expression by Cyanidin-3-Glucoside Enhances Sensitivity to Anticancer Drugs in the Spheroid of Human Lung Adenocarcinoma A549 Cells. *Int. J. Mol. Sci.* **2021**, *22*, 499. [CrossRef]
47. Kao, T.-Y.; Chung, Y.-C.; Hou, Y.-C.; Tsai, Y.-W.; Chen, C.-H.; Chang, H.-P.; Chou, J.-L.; Hsu, C.-P. Effects of Ellagic Acid on Chemosensitivity to 5-Fluorouracil in Colorectal Carcinoma Cells. *Anticancer Res.* **2012**, *32*, 4413–4418.
48. Engelke, L.H.; Hamacher, A.; Proksch, P.; Kassack, M.U. Ellagic Acid and Resveratrol Prevent the Development of Cisplatin Resistance in the Epithelial Ovarian Cancer Cell Line A2780. *J. Cancer* **2016**, *7*, 353. [CrossRef]
49. Chen, Y.-J.; Liao, H.-F.; Tsai, T.-H.; Wang, S.-Y.; Shiao, M.-S. Caffeic Acid Phenethyl Ester Preferentially Sensitizes CT26 Colorectal Adenocarcinoma to Ionizing Radiation without Affecting Bone Marrow Radioresponse. *Int. J. Radiat. Oncol. Biol. Phys.* **2005**, *63*, 1252–1261. [CrossRef]
50. Lin, Y.-H.; Chiu, J.-H.; Tseng, W.-S.; Wong, T.-T.; Chiou, S.-H.; Yen, S.-H. Antiproliferation and Radiosensitization of Caffeic Acid Phenethyl Ester on Human Medulloblastoma Cells. *Cancer Chemother. Pharmacol.* **2006**, *57*, 525–532. [CrossRef]
51. Matsunaga, T.; Tsuchimura, S.; Azuma, N.; Endo, S.; Ichihara, K.; Ikari, A. Caffeic Acid Phenethyl Ester Potentiates Gastric Cancer Cell Sensitivity to Doxorubicin and Cisplatin by Decreasing Proteasome Function. *Anti-Cancer Drugs* **2019**, *30*, 251–259. [CrossRef]
52. Sonoki, H.; Tanimae, A.; Furuta, T.; Endo, S.; Matsunaga, T.; Ichihara, K.; Ikari, A. Caffeic Acid Phenethyl Ester Down-Regulates Claudin-2 Expression at the Transcriptional and Post-Translational Levels and Enhances Chemosensitivity to Doxorubicin in Lung Adenocarcinoma A549 Cells. *J. Nutr. Biochem.* **2018**, *56*, 205–214. [CrossRef]
53. Anjaly, K.; Tiku, A.B. Caffeic Acid Phenethyl Ester Induces Radiosensitization *via* Inhibition of DNA Damage Repair in Androgen-Independent Prostate Cancer Cells. *Environ. Toxicol.* **2022**, *37*, 995–1006. [CrossRef]
54. Muthusamy, G.; Balupillai, A.; Ramasamy, K.; Shanmugam, M.; Gunaseelan, S.; Mary, B.; Prasad, N.R. Ferulic Acid Reverses ABCB1-Mediated Paclitaxel Resistance in MDR Cell Lines. *Eur. J. Pharmacol.* **2016**, *786*, 194–203. [CrossRef]
55. Muthusamy, G.; Gunaseelan, S.; Prasad, N.R. Ferulic Acid Reverses P-Glycoprotein-Mediated Multidrug Resistance *via* Inhibition of PI3K/Akt/NF-KB Signaling Pathway. *J. Nutr. Biochem.* **2019**, *63*, 62–71. [CrossRef]
56. Heo, S.-K.; Noh, E.-K.; Yoon, D.-J.; Jo, J.-C.; Koh, S.; Baek, J.H.; Park, J.-H.; Min, Y.J.; Kim, H. Rosmarinic Acid Potentiates ATRA-Induced Macrophage Differentiation in Acute Promyelocytic Leukemia NB4 Cells. *Eur. J. Pharmacol.* **2015**, *747*, 36–44. [CrossRef]
57. Yu, C.; Chen, D.; Liu, H.; Li, W.; Lu, J.; Feng, J. Rosmarinic Acid Reduces the Resistance of Gastric Carcinoma Cells to 5-Fluorouracil by Downregulating FOXO4-Targeting MiR-6785-5p. *Biomed. Pharmacother.* **2019**, *109*, 2327–2334. [CrossRef]
58. Zhang, Y.; Chen, S.; Wei, C.; Rankin, G.O.; Rojanasakul, Y.; Ren, N.; Ye, X.; Chen, Y.C. Dietary Compound Proanthocyanidins from Chinese Bayberry (*Myrica Rubra* Sieb. et Zucc.) Leaves Inhibit Angiogenesis and Regulate Cell Cycle of Cisplatin-Resistant Ovarian Cancer Cells via Targeting Akt Pathway. *J. Funct. Foods* **2018**, *40*, 573–581. [CrossRef]
59. Ravindranathan, P.; Pasham, D.; Goel, A. Oligomeric Proanthocyanidins (OPCs) from Grape Seed Extract Suppress the Activity of ABC Transporters in Overcoming Chemoresistance in Colorectal Cancer Cells. *Carcinogenesis* **2019**, *40*, 412–421. [CrossRef]
60. Naus, P.J.; Henson, R.; Bleeker, G.; Wehbe, H.; Meng, F.; Patel, T. Tannic Acid Synergizes the Cytotoxicity of Chemotherapeutic Drugs in Human Cholangiocarcinoma by Modulating Drug Efflux Pathways. *J. Hepatol.* **2007**, *46*, 222–229. [CrossRef]
61. Geng, N.; Zheng, X.; Wu, M.; Yang, L.; Li, X.; Chen, J. Tannic Acid Synergistically Enhances the Anticancer Efficacy of Cisplatin on Liver Cancer Cells through Mitochondria-Mediated Apoptosis. *Oncol. Rep.* **2019**, *42*, 2108–2116. [CrossRef]
62. Yu, F.; Liu, W.; Gong, X.R.; Zhou, Y.B.; Lin, Y. Procyanidins Enhance the Chemotherapeutic Sensitivity of Laryngeal Carcinoma Cells to Cisplatin through Autophagy Pathway. *Lin Chuang Er Bi Yan Hou Tou Jing Wai Ke Za Zhi J. Clin. Otorhinolaryngol. Head Neck Surg.* **2018**, *32*, 447–456.
63. Mady, F.M.; Shaker, M.A. Enhanced Anticancer Activity and Oral Bioavailability of Ellagic Acid through Encapsulation in Biodegradable Polymeric Nanoparticles. *Int. J. Nanomed.* **2017**, *12*, 7405. [CrossRef]
64. Cetin, A.; Biltekin, B.; Degirmencioglu, S. Ellagic Acid Enhances the Antitumor Efficacy of Bevacizumab in an in Vitro Glioblastoma Model. *World Neurosurg.* **2019**, *132*, e59–e65. [CrossRef]
65. Cetin, A.; Biltekin, B. Ellagic Acid Enhances Antitumor Efficacy of Temozolomide in an in Vitro Glioblastoma Model. *Turk Neurosurg* **2020**, *30*, 813–821. [CrossRef]
66. Wu, Y.-S.; Ho, J.-Y.; Yu, C.-P.; Cho, C.-J.; Wu, C.-L.; Huang, C.-S.; Gao, H.-W.; Yu, D.-S. Ellagic Acid Resensitizes Gemcitabine-Resistant Bladder Cancer Cells by Inhibiting Epithelial-Mesenchymal Transition and Gemcitabine Transporters. *Cancers* **2021**, *13*, 2032. [CrossRef]
67. Moon, J.Y.; Ediriweera, M.K.; Ryu, J.Y.; Kim, H.Y.; Cho, S.K. Catechol Enhances Chemo-and Radio-Sensitivity by Targeting AMPK/Hippo Signaling in Pancreatic Cancer Cells. *Oncol. Rep.* **2021**, *45*, 1133–1141. [CrossRef]

cancers

MDPI

Article

Enriched Riceberry Bran Oil Exerts Chemopreventive Properties through Anti-Inflammation and Alteration of Gut Microbiota in Carcinogen-Induced Liver and Colon Carcinogenesis in Rats

Warunyoo Phannasorn [1], Aroonrat Pharapirom [1], Parameth Thiennimitr [2], Huina Guo [1], Sunantha Ketnawa [1] and Rawiwan Wongpoomchai [1,*]

[1] Department of Biochemistry, Faculty of Medicine, Chiang Mai University, Chiang Mai 50200, Thailand
[2] Department of Microbiology, Faculty of Medicine, Chiang Mai University, Chiang Mai 50200, Thailand
* Correspondence: rawiwan.wong@cmu.ac.th; Tel.: +66-53935325; Fax: +66-53894031

Simple Summary: Rice bran oil is gaining popularity around the world due to its ability to improve lipid profiles. Recent in vitro studies have shown that the active compounds in colored rice bran oil exhibited anti-cancer properties in various cell lines. However, there has been a limited number of animal studies focusing on the anti-carcinogenic action of rice bran oil. In this study, Riceberry bran oil (RBBO) extracted from the bran of a Thai-pigmented rice variety, namely Riceberry, was investigated for its inhibitory mechanism on the early stages of liver and colorectal carcinogenesis using the dual carcinogens-induced rat model. RBBO was able to inhibit the biomarkers of rat liver cancer and colon cancer by forcing cells to undergo apoptosis, reducing inflammation, and changing the profiles of bacteria and their metabolites. These findings suggest that RBBO could be a promising source of high-value chemopreventive agents in terms of both cancer prevention and treatment.

Citation: Phannasorn, W.; Pharapirom, A.; Thiennimitr, P.; Guo, H.; Ketnawa, S.; Wongpoomchai, R. Enriched Riceberry Bran Oil Exerts Chemopreventive Properties through Anti-Inflammation and Alteration of Gut Microbiota in Carcinogen-Induced Liver and Colon Carcinogenesis in Rats. *Cancers* **2022**, *14*, 4358. https://doi.org/10.3390/cancers14184358

Academic Editor: Anupam Bishayee

Received: 29 June 2022
Accepted: 2 September 2022
Published: 7 September 2022

Abstract: Riceberry has recently been acknowledged for its beneficial pharmacological effects. Riceberry bran oil (RBBO) exhibited anti-proliferation activity in various cancer cell lines. However, animal studies of RBBO on anti-carcinogenicity and its molecular inhibitory mechanism have been limited. This study purposed to investigate the chemopreventive effects of RBBO on the carcinogen-induced liver and colorectal carcinogenesis in rats. Rats were injected with diethylnitrosamine (DEN) and 1,2-dimethylhydrazine (DMH) and further orally administered with RBBO equivalent to 100 mg/kg body weight of γ-oryzanol 5 days/week for 10 weeks. RBBO administration suppressed preneoplastic lesions including hepatic glutathione *S*-transferase placental form positive foci and colorectal aberrant crypt foci. Accordingly, RBBO induced hepatocellular and colorectal cell apoptosis and reduced pro-inflammatory cytokine expression. Interestingly, RBBO effectively promoted the alteration of gut microbiota in DEN- and DMH-induced rats, as has been shown in the elevated *Firmicutes*/*Bacteroidetes* ratio. This outcome was consistent with an increase in butyrate in the feces of carcinogen-induced rats. The increase in butyrate reflects the chemopreventive properties of RBBO through the mechanisms of its anti-inflammatory properties and cell apoptosis induction in preneoplastic cells. This would indicate that RBBO containing γ-oryzanol, phytosterols, and tocols holds significant potential in the prevention of cancer.

Keywords: anti-inflammation; anti-carcinogenicity; bioactive food components; cancer prevention; gut microbiota; Riceberry; rice bran oil; short-chain fatty acids

1. Introduction

Cancer is one of the leading causes of death worldwide with nearly 10 million deaths in 2020 reported by the World Health Organization. Colorectal and liver cancer are ranked as the second and third most common types of cancer resulting in death. Obesity, an unhealthy diet, a lack of exercise, smoking, and alcohol consumption are important risk factors for cancer. Cancer can result from interactions between an individual genetic factor and certain external agents, such as carcinogens, resulting in the transformation of normal cells into tumor cells [1]. Therefore, an intervention of the mutation and proliferation of uncommon cells is a key objective in inhibiting carcinogenesis.

At present, nutraceuticals have garnered significant attention for their nutritional value and protective capabilities against disease. They exhibit the potential to treat a variety of illnesses that include diabetes, atherosclerosis, cardiovascular disease, cancer, and neurological disorders [2]. Vegetable oil has been recommended for use in daily cooking due to its high contents of monounsaturated fatty acids (MUFAs) and polyunsaturated fatty acids (PUFAs), as well as for the positive health benefits. It has been found to exert on heart disease and cancer in clinical studies [3,4]. PUFAs and MUFAs are known to be able to reduce the risk of cardiovascular disease and lower cholesterol levels in obese patients [5]. The consumption of MUFAs that have been derived from plants, particularly olive oil, has been linked to a decreased risk of developing cancer [6]. Similarly, the substitution of plant-based MUFAs for animal-based MUFAs has been associated with a lower number of cancer deaths [7]. The effect of PUFAs on cancer risk is directly proportional to the ratio of ω-6 to ω-3 PUFAs. The 4:1 ratio of ω-6 to ω-3 has been indicated in reducing inflammation, which has been implicated as a risk factor for various chronic conditions [8]. Some documented evidence has suggested that ω-6 PUFAs could stimulate tumor development, whereas ω-3 PUFAs could protect against tumor formation. The administration of a diet rich in ω-6 given to mice resulted in increased cyclooxygenase-2 (COX-2) levels and expanded epigenetic activation of prostaglandin-endoperoxide synthase-2. These changes increased the production of prostaglandin E2 from arachidonic acid in conjunction with the gene silencing that is associated with a number of tumor protective factors. They were also observed to increase the presence of adenomatous polyposis coli and the accumulation of the factors involved in cell proliferation (*Ccnd1*). Furthermore, these changes enhanced oncogenic transformation (*c-JUN*), which may contribute to colonic inflammation and the progression of cancer [9]. On the other hand, a diet that is rich in ω-3 PUFAs inhibited the formation of MC38 colorectal cancer in mice, while the treatment of tumors with epoxydocosapentaenoic acids and ω-3 PUFAs metabolites was found to decrease proto-oncogenes expression in tumor tissues [10].

Commensal bacteria in the gastrointestinal tract serve a number of critical roles including epithelial formation, host metabolism, pathogenic defense, and immunological regulation. By contrast, dysbiosis refers to the altered composition and function of gut microbiota leading to the development of a variety of pathological diseases. This is particularly true in inflammatory bowel disease (IBD), certain IBD-associated cancers, and hepatocellular carcinoma [11]. Dietary lipids impact the microbiome that may be advantageous or detrimental to the host. Changes in the gut microbiota in mice fed a high-fat diet (HFD) enriched with saturated fat were associated with increased intestinal ROS generation and oxidative stress [12] which are known to play a crucial role in the development and progression of cancer [13]. HFD promotes colorectal carcinogenesis in both AOM-treated and $Apc^{min/+}$ mice by promoting significant changes in the composition of the gut microbiota that have been associated with increased pathogenic bacteria and reduced probiotic bacteria. Moreover, HFD has been observed to alter gut barrier functions [14]. Furthermore, a high-cholesterol diet can promote hepatocellular carcinoma in mice by increasing the hepatic retention of hydrophobic bile acids caused by dysbiosis [15]. Short-chain fatty acids (SCFA) including acetate, propionate, and butyrate, are bacterial metabolites produced from anaerobic fermentation of non-digestible dietary ingredients in the colon. They play a crucial role in the gut microbiota homeostasis and are involved in the protection of certain chronic diseases [16]. The dietary approach to modulate SCFA levels might serve as a potential chemoprevention.

Rice bran oil is considered a healthy oil due to its fatty acid profile and its unique combination of certain predominantly biologically active ingredients such as γ-oryzanol, tocopherols, tocotrienols, certain unsaponifiable substances, and many phytosterols [17]. Studies on the biological activities of rice bran oil reported effective anti-diabetic, anti-cancer, anti-inflammatory, and hypolipidemic properties [18]. Recently, various studies have reported the potential of Riceberry bran oil (RBBO) to ameliorate hyperglycemia, relevant lipid profiles, and oxidative stress in streptozotocin-induced diabetic rats fed a HFD [19]. Furthermore, it was found to be able to inhibit the proliferation of certain cancer cell lines [20,21]. However, the anti-cancer effect of RBBO in animal models has not yet been fully studied. Many forms of cancer have been linked to a range of environmental carcinogens, particularly those found in contaminated food. These carcinogens have been implicated in incidences of liver and colorectal cancer [22]. The dual organ carcinogenicity test employs both diethylnitrosamine (DEN) and 1,2-dimethylhydrazine (DMH), which are metabolized by the same cytochrome, namely P450, to initiate carcinogenesis in the liver and colorectum, respectively [23,24]. In this study, these carcinogens were administered to the same rats in order to reduce the number of animals included in the experimental procedure, according to the Three Rs principle of animal research [23–25]. Therefore, the purpose of this study was to investigate the chemopreventive effects of RBBO in cases of carcinogen-induced liver and colorectal carcinogenesis in rats, as well as to elucidate the relevant mechanisms of action at the molecular level. The important carcinogenesis-promoting factors of RBBO that were associated with its inflammatory condition, as well as those of gut microbiota and its metabolites, were also analyzed.

2. Materials and Methods

2.1. Chemicals

DEN and metaphosphoric acid were obtained from Sigma-Aldrich (St. Louis, MO, USA), while DMH was obtained from TCI (Tokyo, Japan). An ApopTag® Peroxidase in situ Apoptosis Detection Kit, hydrogen peroxide (H_2O_2), methylene blue, and skim milk were purchased from Merck (Darmstadt, Germany). Anti-rat glutathione S-transferase placental form (GST-P) was acquired from MBL (Nagoya, Japan). EnvisionTM G/2 Doublestain System Rabbit/Mouse (DAB+/Permanent Red) was bought from Agilent (Santa Clara, CA, USA). Purezol reagent was acquired from Bio-Rad (Hercules, CA, USA). A high-capacity cDNA reverse transcription kit was purchased from Applied Biosystems (Foster City, CA, USA), while a SensiFAST SYBR Lo-ROX Kit was procured from Bioline Reagent Ltd. (London, UK).

2.2. RBBO Sample

RBBO was supplied by Kurk Rice Mill (Chiang Rai, Thailand). The extraction process and major chemical constituents have been described in our previously published report [26]. Briefly, RBBO was extracted via the cold pressing method obtaining crude oil and was further purified by press filtration, and various phytochemicals were immediately analyzed by gas chromatography–mass spectrometry, high-performance liquid chromatography, and spectrophotometry. The main fatty acids of RBBO used in this study were composed of 42.61% oleic acid and 30.76% linoleic acid. One gram of RBBO contained 56.74 mg of γ-oryzanol, 6.01 mg of phytosterols, and 1.46 mg of total vitamin E with γ-tocotrienol as a major tocol [26].

2.3. Animals and Experimental Protocol

Three-week-old male Wistar rats (weighing 60–80 g) were obtained from the National Laboratory Animal Center (Nakhon Pathom, Thailand). They were housed under conventional circumstances at a temperature of 25 °C and by employing a 12-hour dark/12-h light cycle. They were given free access to drinking water and fed standard rodent food. The Animal Ethics Committee of the Faculty of Medicine, Chiang Mai University (41/2561) authorized the experimental procedure employed in this study, as presented in Figure 1. Rats were randomly separated into four groups, wherein 16 rats were placed in each group. Group 1 served as a negative control, while group 3 was representative of a positive control.

Groups 2 and 4 were fed the equivalent of 100 mg of γ-oryzanol/kg body weight of RBBO for 5 days each week throughout the entire 10 weeks of the experiment. The RBBO feeding dose was selected from the effective dose presented in our previous report [26]. Groups 3 and 4 were injected with 100 mg/kg body weight of DEN and 40 mg/kg body weight of DMH on the date stated in Figure 1 to initiate liver and colon carcinogenesis, respectively. Body weight, food consumption, and water intake were recorded twice weekly during the course of the experiment. At indicated times, rats were euthanized with anesthesia via the administration of isoflurane. This was performed to collect blood for the assessment of alanine aminotransferase (ALT) and aspartate aminotransferase (AST) levels in the serum using an automated analyzer provided by the Small Animal Hospital, Faculty of Veterinary Medicine, Chiang Mai University. Livers of the rats were then dissected and separated into two portions, one was flash frozen for molecular analysis and the other was fixed in 10% phosphate-buffered formalin for use in immunohistochemistry studies. The colons of half of the rats in each group (n = 8) were collected and placed in formalin fixative, while the colons of the remaining rats (n = 8) were washed with 0.9% normal saline solution and then longitudinally cut into segments that were placed flat on glass plates. Colonic mucosa cells were scraped off onto glass slides, collected in 1.5 mL tubes. They were then maintained at −80 °C. Moreover, feces samples were freshly collected from the anuses of the rats, placed in microcentrifuge tubes, and immediately kept at −80 °C.

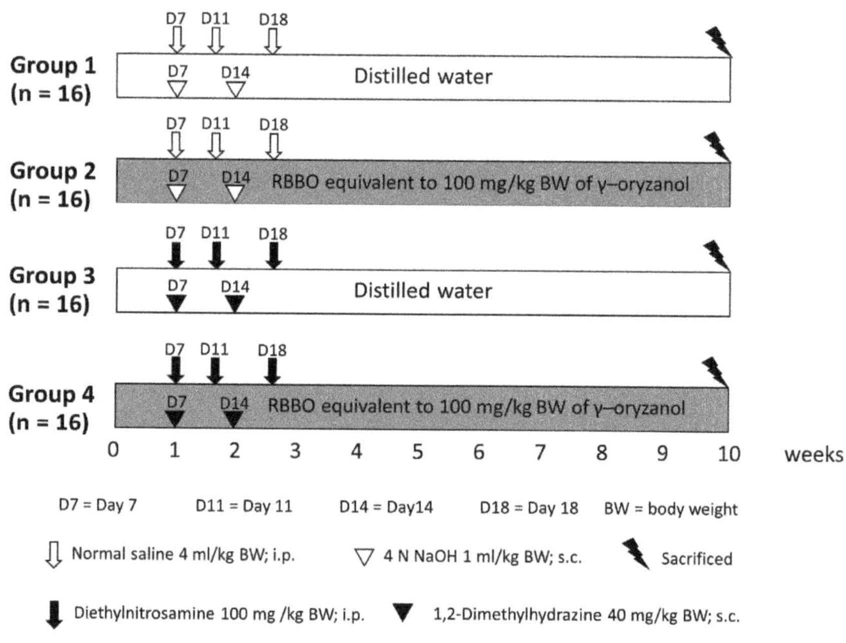

Figure 1. Experimental protocol of RBBO treatment in DEN- and DMH-induced preneoplastic lesions in livers and colons of rats.

2.4. Determination of Preneoplastic Lesions in Colon and Liver Tissues

Methylene blue staining was used to evaluate the colonic aberrant crypt foci (ACF). By filling the colon with 10% formaldehyde in phosphate-buffered saline (pH 7.4), it was enlarged and fixed. The colon was then sliced longitudinally and divided into three segments: rectum, proximal, and distal. The flattened colon was stained with 2% methylene blue for 1 min before being scored for ACF size and then examined under a light microscope at 40× magnification using Bird's criteria [27].

Liver sections of 4 μm in thickness were immunohistochemically determined for GST-P positive foci by employing the avidin–biotin complex method described by Thumvijit et al. [28]. The number and area of GST-P positive foci that were greater than 0.20 mm^2 were measured under a light microscope using the LAS Interactive Measurement program (Leica Microsystems (SEA) Pte Ltd. All Microscopy Teban Gardens Crescent Singapore, Singapore).

2.5. Immunohistochemistry of Proliferation Cell Nuclear Antigen (PCNA)

Cell proliferation biomarker in liver and colon tissue samples was examined using immunohistochemistry. The double-staining procedure for the liver tissue samples was performed using the EnVision Doublestain system. Liver slices were stained immunohistochemically with anti-PCNA antibody (Biolegend, San Diego, CA, USA) and anti-rat GST-P antibody, according to the manufacturer's instructions. Under a light microscope, the number of PCNA positive hepatocytes labeled in GST-P positive foci and its surrounding region was determined to be at least 1000 hepatocytes each.

For the colon tissue samples, sections were incubated overnight with monoclonal mouse anti-rat PCNA antibody. The steps that were then taken were similar to those presented in the manufacturer's instructions according to the liver tissue method. The number of brown-staining PCNA positive cells was determined under a light microscope and reported as the relative percentage of PCNA positive cells per total cells.

2.6. Terminal Deoxynucleotidyltransferase (TdT)–dUTP Nick End Labeling (TUNEL) Assay

TUNEL assay is a method used for the investigation of cell apoptosis by detecting 3′-OH ends from DNA fragmentations. Apoptotic cells in liver tissue samples were detected by employing the TUNEL and GST-P double-staining method using the ApopTag Peroxidase in situ kit and the EnVision Doublestain system as described by Thumvijit et al. [28]. The number of positive cells was counted both inside and throughout the surrounding area of the GST-P positive foci. Moreover, a cross-section of the colon was examined to detect cell apoptosis by TUNEL using the ApopTag Peroxidase in situ kit, according to the manufacturer's recommendations. The number of brown-staining apoptotic cells was determined under a light microscopic and reported as the relative percentage of TUNEL positive cells per total cells.

2.7. Determination of Pro-Inflammatory Cytokine Gene Expression by Quantitative Reverse Transcription Polymerase Chain Reaction (qRT-PCR)

The mRNA was extracted from defrosted liver and colonic epithelium using Purezol reagent according to the instructions presented in the user manual. Accordingly, mRNA was then synthesized to cDNA using a high-capacity cDNA reverse transcription kit, according to the manufacturer's instructions. The qPCR amplification was carried out in the QuantStudioTM 6 Flex System (Thermo Fisher Scientific, Waltham, MA, USA) using a SensiFAST SYBR Lo-ROX Kit at 95 °C for 2 min, followed by 40 cycles at 95 °C for 5 s, 60 °C for 10 s, and 72 °C for 20 s. Gene expression was standardized to β-actin levels and measured using the $2^{-\Delta\Delta ct}$ technique [29]. Table 1 presents the primer lists [29].

Table 1. Primer sequences of qRT-PCR.

Genes	Forward Primer (5′-3′)	Reverse Primer (5′-3′)
tumor necrosis factor-alpha (TNF-α)	AAATGGCCCTCTCATCAGTCC	TCTGCTTGGTGGTTTGCTACGAC
Interleukin-6 (IL-6)	TGATGGATGCTTCCAAACTG	GAGCATTGGAAGTTGGGG TA
Interleukin-1 beta (IL-1β)	CACCTCTCAAGCAGAGCACAG	GGGTTCCATGGTGAAGTCAAC
inducible nitric oxide synthase (iNOS)	CAGGTGCTATTCCCAGCCCAACA	CATTCTGTGCAGTCCCAGTGAGGAA
nuclear factor kappa B (NF-κB)	GGCATGCGTTTCCGTTACAA	TGATCTTGATGGTGGGGTGC
β-actin	ACAGGATGCAGAAGGAGATTAC	AGAGTGAGGCCAGGATAGA

2.8. Measurement of SCFA in Rat Feces

Fecal volatile acids metabolized by gut microbiota were measured using the gas chromatography (GC) technique. SCFA were extracted from the feces by employing the modified method of Calik et al. [30]. Frozen feces specimens (100 mg) were thawed and diluted 4-fold with sterile water in sterile tubes. Feces specimens were then homogenized and centrifuged for 15 min at 4 °C, 4000× *g*. The supernatant was transferred to a new tube and mixed with 200 μL ice-cold 25% metaphosphoric acid, which was then kept on ice for 30 min. The samples were centrifuged for 10 min at 4 °C at 11,000× *g* and then filtered through a 0.45-micrometer nylon filter. Samples were analyzed using a flame ionization detector and a SCION 436-GC instrument (BRUKER, Billerica, MA, USA), coupled with RestekTM RTx-1 F and Capillary columns that were 15 m in length; 0.53 mm ID, 5 μm df (Agilent Technologies, Santa Clara, CA, USA). The injector port was fixed at 250 °C. After injection, the temperature was initiated at 80 °C and increased by 15 °C/min to 200 °C where it was held for 2 min. A combination of nitrogen and helium was employed as the carrier gas. The injection volume was set at 1 μL with a total run time of 10 min and analyzed in duplicate. The amounts of acetate, propionate, butyrate, isobutyrate, valerate, and isovalerate were computed from a mixed standard curve and expressed as μ mole/g feces.

2.9. Analysis of Composition of Fecal Intestinal Microbiota in Rat

Bacterial profiles in the gut were analyzed using a next-generation sequencer. Firstly, frozen feces were thawed and bacterial DNA was extracted with the use of a QIAamp® DNA Stool Mini Kit (QIAGEN Inc, Germantown, MD, USA) by following the manufacturer's suggested protocol. Bacterial DNA was amplified by 16S ribosomal RNA gene (rDNA) amplicon PCR analysis, according to Klindworth et al. [31]. The reaction was carried out in 25-microliter volumes containing 5 ng/μL of DNA samples, 12.5 μL of KAPA HiFi HotStart ReadyMix containing 2.5 mM Mg^{2+} (Kapa Biosystems, Boston, MA, USA), and 1 μM of the forward and reverse primers. Primer pairs comprised forward 5′-TCGTCGGCAGCGTCAGATGTGTATAAGAGACAGCCTACGGGNGGCWGCAG-3′ and reverse 5′-GTCTCGTGGGCTCGGAGATGTGTATAAGAGACAGGACTACHVGGG-TATCTAATCC-3′. The following PCR steps were performed: denaturation at 95 °C for 3 min, 25 cycles of denaturation at 95 °C for 30 s, annealing at 55 °C for 30 s, and elongation at 72 °C for 30 s, with a final extension step at 72 °C for 5 min. A GeneJET PCR Purification Kit (Thermo Scientific, Waltham, MA, USA) was used to purify the PCR products. The extracted DNA was then measured and quantified using a nanodrop 800 spectrophotometer (Thermo Scientific, Waltham, MA, USA) and by administering agarose gel electrophoresis. The PCR products were stored at −20 °C for the purposes of sequencing. A minimum amount of PCR amplicon at 400 ng of each sample was then used to establish a sequencing library. The relevant PCR amplicon products were selected for next-generation sequencing using Miseq system (Illumina, San Diego, CA, USA) by Omics Sciences and Bioinformatics Center, Chulalongkorn University. Raw data were then stored in a fastq.gz file. The sequences were processed using CLC genomic workbench software version 20.0.3 to taxonomically classify the operational taxonomic unit (OTU) that was representative of sequences with a 97% similarity cutoff value in the following database: SILVA release 132 (https://www.arb-silva.de/documentation/release-132/, accessed on 1 August 2021).

2.10. Statistical Analysis

All data are presented as mean ± SEM values. The Statistical Package for the Social Sciences (SPSS) version 17.0 software was used to conduct the statistical analysis (SPSS Inc., Chicago, IL, USA). One-way analysis of variance (ANOVA) was used to determine the significant differences between groups in each experiment, followed by the least significant difference (LSD) tests. Statistical significance was defined as a value of $p < 0.05$. In terms of microbial composition, the Kruskal–Wallis *H* test was established as a non-parametric statistic in order to quantify any similarities between samples.

3. Results

3.1. Effect of RBBO on Preneoplastic Lesions of Liver and Colorectal Carcinogenesis in Rats

The inhibitory effects of RBBO on relevant biomarkers, including GST-P and the ACF of DEN- and DMH-initiated liver and colon carcinogenicity, were examined, respectively. The administration of DEN and DMH induced toxicity in rats detected by reducing body weight and increasing serum AST and ALT levels (Table 2). They did not affect the quantities of food and water ingested by the rats, as well as the relative liver, spleen, and kidney weights of those rats (data not shown). It was indicated that these carcinogens caused liver injury in rats. Feeding of RBBO did not change body and vital organ weights, and liver function enzyme levels when compared to a negative control group, suggesting non-toxicity of RBBO to the rats. However, RBBO administration could not modulate AST and ALT levels in DEN- and DMH-induced rats. Neither nodules nor tumors were observed by H&E staining in the liver and colon tissues of DEN- and DMH-induced rats in this 10-week protocol (data not shown). Furthermore, a combined DEN and DMH injection significantly induced the development of hepatic GST-P positive foci (Figure 2a) and colonic ACF (Figure 2b). The administration of 100 mg equivalent to γ-oryzanol/kg body weight of RBBO suppressed both the number and size of hepatic GST-P positive foci in DEN- and DMH-initiated rats (Figure 2c,d). In addition, RBBO administration in carcinogen-initiated rats significantly decreased the number and size of both small foci containing 1–4 crypts per focus and large foci containing more than 4 crypts per focus, as well as those of colonic ACF when compared to the carcinogen-treated alone group (Figure 2e,f). These results indicate the potential of RBBO in the inhibition of colon- and hepatocarcinogenesis. RBBO-treated alone rats did not indicate the presence of GST-P positive foci in their liver and ACF in their colons, suggesting the non-carcinogenicity of RBBO.

Table 2. Effect of RBBO on body weight and liver function test in rats.

Treatment	Final Body Weight (g)	Liver Function Test (Unit/L)	
		AST Activity	ALT Activity
Control	397.0 ± 6.6	60 ± 1.7	27 ± 1.4
RBBO	387.0 ± 3.7	67 ± 6.1	27 ± 3.5
DEN and DMH	369.4 ± 10.0 *	75 ± 2.8 *	40 ± 2.5 *
RBBO + DEN and DMH	352.5 ± 10.6	81 ± 4.8	49 ± 2.9

Values are represented as mean ± SEM values (n = 8). * Significantly different from the control group ($p < 0.05$). RBBO, Riceberry bran oil; DEN, diethylnitrosamine; DMH, dimethylhydrazine; AST, aspartate aminotransferase; ALT, alanine aminotransferase.

3.2. Inhibitory Mechanism of RBBO Involved in Cell Proliferation and Apoptosis in Liver and Colon Tissues of DEN- and DMH-Initiated Rats

To investigate whether the molecular mechanism by which RBBO inhibited preneoplastic lesions of liver and colon carcinogenicity, the biomarkers of cell proliferation and apoptosis were examined in the liver and colon tissues of DEN- and DMH-injected rats. PCNA protein representing cell proliferation was evidently verified in the liver and colon tissue samples by immunohistochemistry (Figure S1). The treatment of RBBO alone did not affect the cell proliferation of normal rat livers and colons. The number of PCNA positive cells in hepatic GST-P positive foci, those in the surrounding area, and also those in colon epithelial cells increased in the carcinogen-treated groups when compared with the negative control group. Unexpectedly, RBBO administration in carcinogen-treated rats did not alter the number of PCNA positive cells in both the liver and colon tissues when compared with those of the positive control group (Table 3). DNA fragmentation generated during apoptosis was labeled in the rat liver and colon tissues by TUNEL assay (Figure 3a,b). Rats treated with DEN and DMH revealed statistically inclined numbers of TUNEL positive hepatocytes in GST-P positive foci and in the surrounding areas, as well as in colonocytes when compared with the vehicle-injected group. Furthermore, the treatment of RBBO significantly increased the number of TUNEL positive cells in both the livers and colons of carcinogen-induced rats (Table 4). These findings indicate that RBBO could inhibit preneoplastic lesions of rat colons and hepatocarcinogenesis by the induction of cell apoptosis.

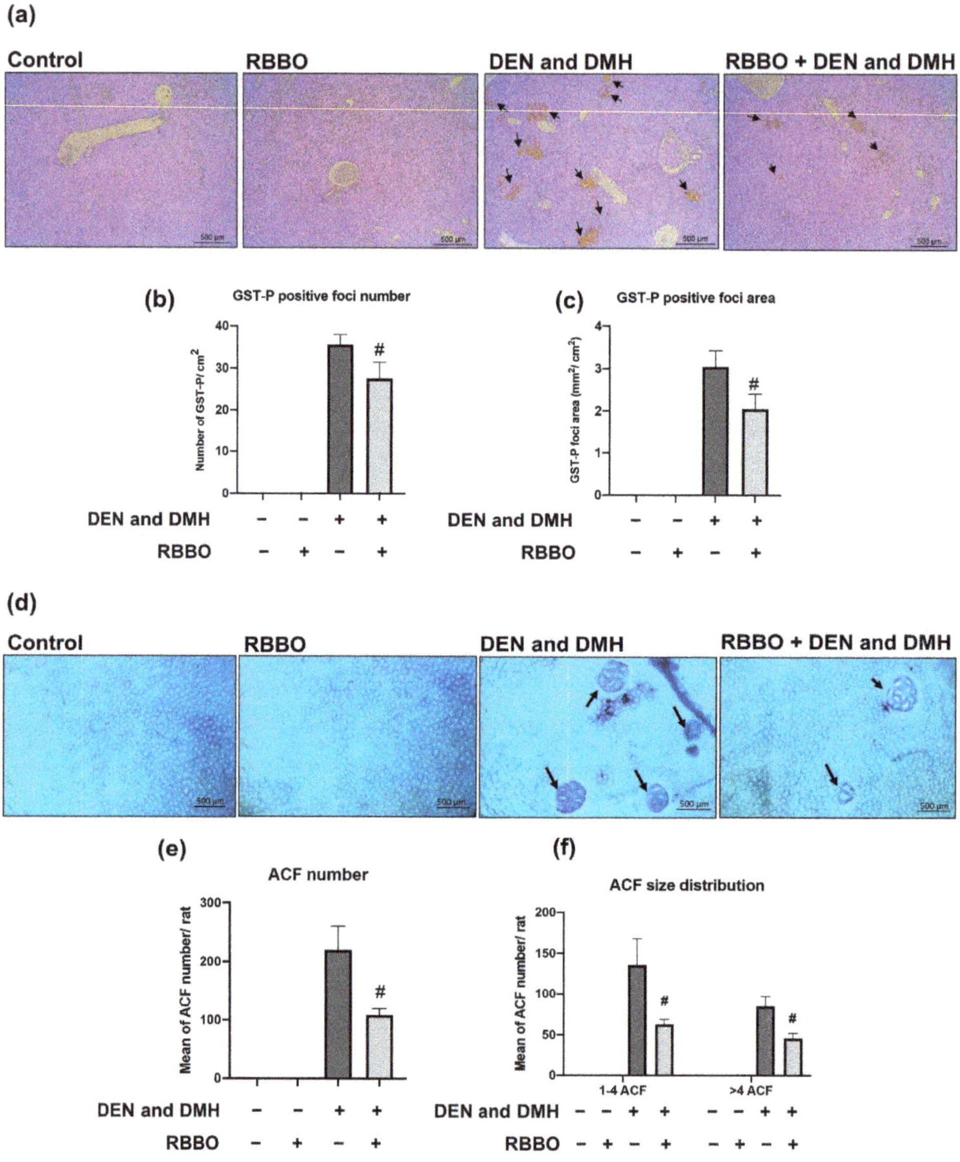

Figure 2. Effect of RBBO administration on hepatic GST-P positive foci and colonic ACF in DEN- and DMH-initiated rats. (**a**) Hepatic GST-P positive foci (100×), (**b**) number and (**c**) size of GST-P positive foci in liver tissues, (**d**) colonic ACF (100×), and (**e**) number and (**f**) size distribution of ACF in colon tissues. Arrows indicate GST-P positive foci and ACF. Results are expressed as mean ± SEM values (n = 8). # $p < 0.05$ significantly different from the DEN- and DMH-induced group. GST-P, glutathione S-transferase placental; ACF, aberrant crypt foci; RBBO, Riceberry bran oil; DEN, diethylnitrosamine; DMH, dimethylhydrazine.

Table 3. Effect of RBBO on cell proliferation in rat liver and colon tissues.

Treatment	Number of PCNA Positive Cells in Hepatocytes		% Relative (PCNA + Cells/Total Colonocytes)
	$PCNA^+$/1000GST-P^+ Cells	$PCNA^+$/1000 Surrounding Cells	
Control	ND	5.81 ± 1.39	15.31 ± 6.00
RBBO	ND	4.69 ± 2.13	15.52 ± 4.00
DEN and DMH	47.29 ± 7.98	13.58 ± 5.38 *	46.87 ± 5.38 *
RBBO + DEN and DMH	45.10 ± 8.29	12.75 ± 3.68	42.68 ± 3.68

Values are represented as mean ± SEM values (n = 8). * Significantly different from the control group ($p < 0.05$). ND, non-detectable; RBBO, Riceberry bran oil; DEN, diethylnitrosamine; DMH, dimethylhydrazine.

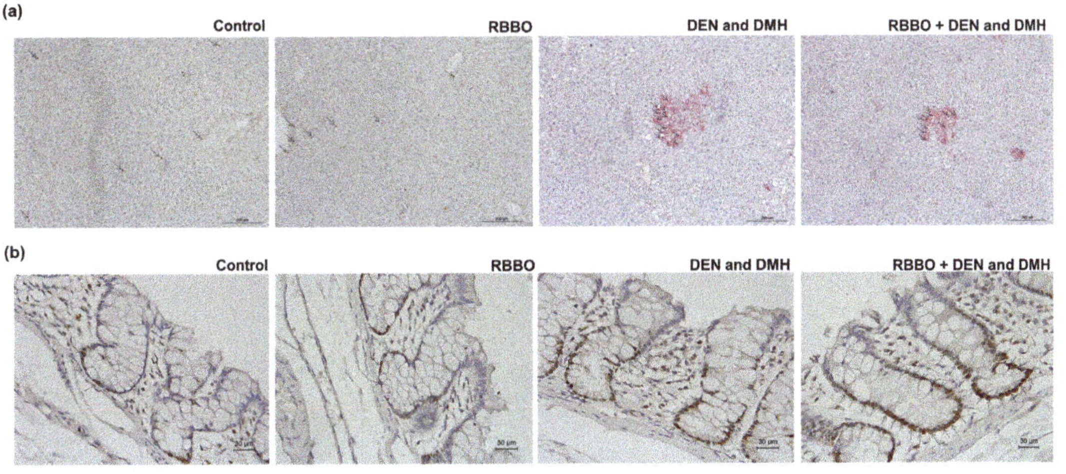

Figure 3. Effect of RBBO on cell apoptosis in liver and colon tissues of DEN- and DMH-induced rats. (**a**) Double-staining immunohistochemistry of apoptotic cells in hepatocytes (200×). Red areas demonstrate GST-P positive foci and arrows indicate TUNEL positive cells in both GST-P positive foci and normal areas. (**b**) Immunohistochemistry of apoptotic cells in colonocytes (400×). Arrows indicate TUNEL positive cells. RBBO, Riceberry bran oil; DEN, diethylnitrosamine; DMH, dimethylhydrazine.

Table 4. Effect of RBBO on cell apoptosis in rat liver and colon tissues.

Treatment	Number of TUNEL Positive Cells in Hepatocytes		% Relative (TUNEL + Cells/Total Colonocytes)
	$TUNEL^+$/1000GST-P^+ Cells	$TUNEL^+$/1000 Surrounding Cells	
Control	ND	21.47 ± 4.67	43.89 ± 8.57
RBBO	ND	26.85 ± 2.73	44.72 ± 7.48
DEN and DMH	79.86 ± 3.93	56.61 ± 5.38 *	53.92 ± 3.61 *
RBBO + DEN and DMH	91.32 ± 4.97 #	73.28 ± 6.02 #	64.84 ± 4.37 #

Values are represented as mean ± SEM values (n = 8). * Significantly different from the control group ($p < 0.05$). # Significantly different from the DEN and DMH group ($p < 0.05$). ND, non-detectable; RBBO, Riceberry bran oil; DEN, diethylnitrosamine; DMH, dimethylhydrazine.

3.3. Effect of RBBO on the Expression of Pro-Inflammatory Genes in the Livers and Colons of Rats

An injection of DEN and DMH induced the gene expression of TNF-α, IL-6, and Il-1β in hepatocytes, and also increased all genes in the colonocytes. RBBO only did not affect the inflammatory response with regard to the unchanged mRNA levels in the colons and livers of rats. Notably, the rats administrated with RBBO significantly suppressed the expression of these induced genes including the TNF-α, IL-6, and IL-1β levels in the hepatocytes of carcinogen-treated rats (Figure 4a). Furthermore, RBBO administration significantly inhibited TNF-α and IL-6 expression in the colonocytes of carcinogen-induced rats (Figure 4b). However, RBBO treatment did not alter the gene expression of NF-κB and iNOS in DEN- and DMH-induced rats (data not shown). These findings indicate that RBBO inhibited DEN- and DMH-induced liver and colorectal carcinogenesis via the inhibition of an inflammatory response through the regulation of the expression of pro-inflammatory cytokines.

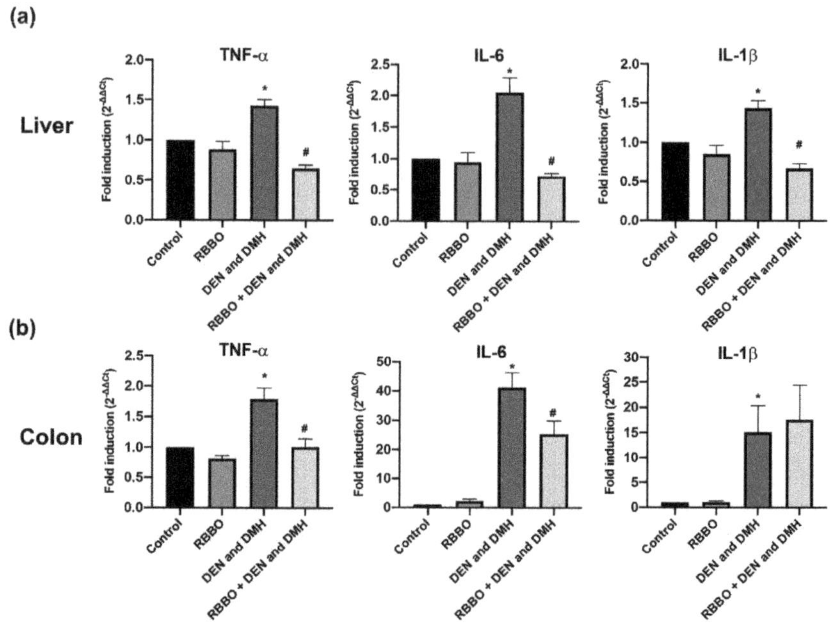

Figure 4. Effect of RBBO administration on mRNA levels of transcription factors and inflammatory response genes in liver (**a**) and colon (**b**) tissues of DEN- and DMH-induced rats measured by real-time PCR. Results are expressed as mean ± SEM values (n = 8). * $p < 0.05$ significantly different from the vehicle control. # $p < 0.05$ significantly different from the DEN- and DMH-induced alone group. TNF-α, tumor necrosis factor-alpha; IL-6, interleukin-6; IL-1β, interleukin-1beta; RBBO, Riceberry bran oil; DEN, diethylnitrosamine; DMH, 1,2-dimethylhydrazine.

3.4. *Effect of RBBO on Fecal SCFAs Production in Rats*

The SCFA produced by gut microbiota that is associated with cancer development was determined by GC-FID. The amounts of SCFA, including acetic acid, propionic acid, butyric acid, isobutyric acid, valeric acid, and isovaleric acid, are presented in Table 5. Injections of DEN and DMH significantly decreased levels of SCFA, including butyric acid, isobutyric acid, valeric acid, and isovaleric acid, in rat feces. On the other hand, RBBO treatment significantly increased the levels of butyric acid but decreased the levels of acetate in rats administrated with or without carcinogens. Furthermore, RBBO treatment statistically restored valeric acid content in carcinogen-treated rats. These findings suggest that RBBO plays a key role in the production of bacterial metabolites of gut microbiota.

Table 5. Effect of RBBO administration on the SCFA levels in the feces of DEN- and DMH-induced rats.

SCFA (μ mole/g Feces)	Treatment			
	Control	RBBO	DEN and DMH	RBBO + DEN and DMH
Acetate	46.34 ± 3.53	36.44 ± 6.20 *	42.19 ± 4.92	39.72 ± 2.37 #
Propionate	7.41 ± 1.31	6.64 ± 3.61	7.78 ± 2.29	7.36 ± 0.72
Butyrate	1.65 ± 0.11	2.15 ± 0.76 *	1.16 ± 0.22 *	2.09 ± 0.33 #
Isobutyrate	10.77 ± 2.91	6.64 ± 2.64 *	8.38 ± 1.06 *	10.63 ± 2.59
Valerate	0.84 ± 0.22	0.74 ± 0.23	0.58 ± 0.10 *	1.05 ± 0.43 #
Isovalerate	2.48 ± 0.30	2.44 ± 0.43	1.64 ± 0.37 *	1.97 ± 0.66

Results are expressed as mean ± SEM (n = 8) values. * $p < 0.05$ significantly different from the vehicle control. # $p < 0.05$ significantly different from the DEN- and DMH-induced alone group. SCFA, short-chain fatty acids; RBBO, Riceberry bran oil; DEN, diethylnitrosamine; DMH, 1,2-dimethylhydrazine.

3.5. Effect of RBBO on Bacterial Profile in Rats

The inhibition of the early stages of colon and liver carcinogenesis by RBBO was found to be involved with the bacterial metabolites that are present as a result of SCFA levels. Accordingly, the composition of fecal intestinal microbiota of the rats in each treatment was determined. Figure 5a depicts the ratio of dominant fecal microbiota between *Firmicutes* and *Bacteroidetes* phyla. The vehicle- and carcinogen-treated alone groups indicated an indifferent ratio for these two phyla suggesting that they were unaffected by carcinogen injections, as indicated by their bacterial profiles. In contrast, the administration of RBBO in both the vehicle- and carcinogen-treated rats resulted in an increase in the *Firmicutes/Bacteroidetes* (F/B) ratio by inhibiting some *Bacteroidetes* and increasing the relative abundance of *Firmicutes* when compared to the control group. This would indicate the important influence of RBBO on gut microbiota composition. The relative abundance of microbiota at the family level is demonstrated in Figure 5b. Accordingly, *Lachnospiraceae* was the predominant family of the *Firmicutes* phyla, while *Rikenellaceae*, *Prevotellaceae*, *Muribaculaceae*, and *Bacteroidaceae* represent the main families of the *Bacteroidetes* phyla in the control group, which made up 90% of the gut microbiota in normal abundance. Similar to the results of the increased *Firmicutes/Bacteroidetes* ratio, the RBBO treatment alone and the RBBO treatment in carcinogen-induced rats resulted in an increase in the *Lachnospiraceae* family as the outstanding gut microbiota in both of these groups, while also slightly reducing the abundance of *Bacteroidaceae* when compared to the negative and positive control groups. In order to demonstrate the detail in the modulation of gut microbiota by RBBO, we next compared the bacterial composition at the genus level using heatmap analysis as shown in Figure 5c. Heatmap visualization at the genus level demonstrated different bacteria levels in each group. The control group was associated with a slightly increased abundance of *Akkermansia*, *Bacteroidales bacterium*, and *Ruminococcus 2*, along with a lower abundance of various genera. The induction of rats by DEN and DMH was associated with an increased abundance of *Eubacterium coprostanoligenes*, *Ruminiclostridium 6*, and *Bacteroides* when compared with the control. The treatment of RBBO in carcinogen-induced rats was found to be related to an increase in genera in the *Ruminococcaceae UCG-013*, *Ruminococcaceae UCG-014*, *Adlercreutzia*, *Enterorhabdus*, *Papillibacter*, and *Lachnospiraceae NK4A136* groups, along with a decrease in the abundance of *Eubacterium coprostanoligenes*, *Ruminoclostridium 6*, and *Bacteroides* when compared to the carcinogen-induced group. The treatment of RBBO alone revealed an abundance of *Oscillibacter* and *Ruminococcus 1* as the main genera. Therefore, RBBO may alter the profile of gut microbiota that affect the bacterial metabolism resulting in changes in SCFA levels.

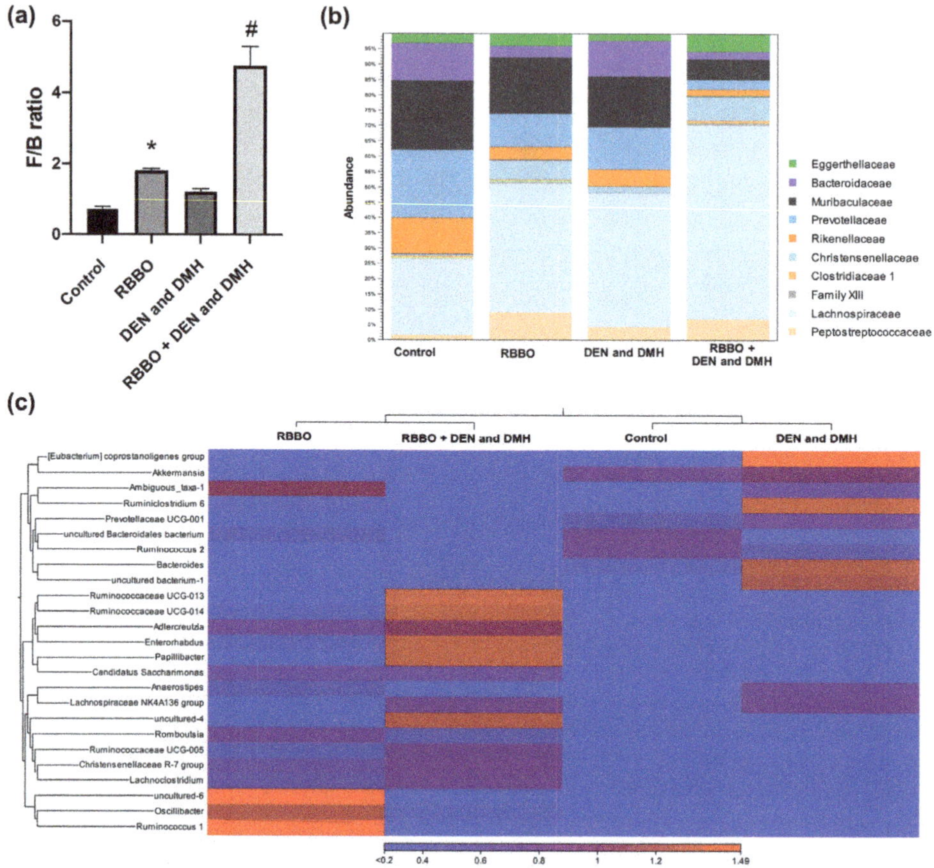

Figure 5. Effect of RBBO administration on the alteration of intestinal bacterial profiles. (**a**) *Firmicutes/Bacteroidetes* (F/B) ratio. (**b**) Relative abundance of the dominant family of each group. (**c**) Heatmap analyses of the fecal microbiota in each group. Blue-to-red shading indicates relatively lower-to-higher number of counts. Significant difference analyses were calculated using CLC Genomic workbench. * $p < 0.05$ significantly different from the vehicle control. # $p < 0.05$ significantly different from the DEN- and DMH-induced alone group. RBBO, Riceberry bran oil; DEN, diethylnitrosamine; DMH, 1,2-dimethylhydrazine.

4. Discussion

Cancer development has mainly been associated with environmental chemical carcinogens. The exposure to certain food contaminants may directly contribute to liver and colon cancers. Chemoprevention using natural or synthetic agents is an alternative way for cancer therapy to inhibit, delay, or reverse each stage of carcinogenesis [32]. Several studies have reported that a diet of vegetables, fruits, whole grains, dietary fibers, micronutrients, some fatty acids, and exercise could help to protect against various types of cancers [33]. Pigmented rice possesses a higher potency in terms of anti-oxidative activities and tumor suppression than colorless rice [34,35]. This research has determined that Riceberry bran oil (RBBO), a Thai black rice cultivar, is a rich source of oleic acid, linoleic acid, γ-oryzanol, total vitamin E, and phytosterols [26], all of which have demonstrated beneficial cancer chemopreventive properties against DEN- and DMH-induced liver and colorectal carcinogenesis in rats. However, RBBO did not injure the liver as indicated by unchanged AST and

ALT levels. In a previous study, neither significant effects on mortality nor pathological abnormalities were reported with the oral administration of γ-oryzanol obtained from rice bran extract at doses of 1000 and 2000 mg/kg body weight/day in Sprague–Dawley rats in a repeated-dose 90-day oral toxicity test that followed the Organization for Economic Co-operation and Development guidelines [36]. Consequently, RBBO was considered safe for consumption in rats. A study on the bioavailability of rice bran oil in rats by Fujiwara and his group demonstrated that γ-oryzanol is readily absorbed into the blood via the portal vein system and was subsequently raised to the highest concentration in the plasma after four hours of oral administration. Accordingly, it was then distributed to each organ in its original form. Ultimately, it was rapidly metabolized in the body as ferulic acid, triterpene alcohols, and phytosterols, but its intact form could still facilitate a range of physiological functions [37].

Gastrointestinal and hepatobiliary tracts that are routinely exposed to a variety of carcinogens via dietary contaminants lead to the most found cancer formation. The established model using DEN and DMH as the initiators to develop the early stages of liver and colon carcinogenesis was performed as a tool for exploring cancer chemopreventive agents [38]. DEN is a standard carcinogen that is routinely employed in rodent models in the study of hepatocarcinogenesis in order to induce preneoplastic lesions or liver tumors that have been implicated in incidences of liver cancer in humans [39]. DMH is a colon carcinogen that has been commonly used to study chemically induced colorectal carcinogenesis in rodent models caused by DNA methylation of colonic epithelial cells in the proliferative compartment of crypts, which can then lead to hyperproliferation and apoptosis resistance [40]. The exposure of these carcinogens caused the changes in xenobiotic-metabolizing enzymes, hepatic DNA adducts, and liver damage [38]. GST-P positive foci shaped in rat livers are recognized be preneoplastic lesions of liver cancer [41], while ACF are representative of a group of abnormal tube-like glands in the linings of the colon and rectum and can be used as a biomarker for colon carcinogenesis. These lesions are the earliest indicators of change in the development of colon cancer and have been detected in both rodents and humans [27]. However, DMH synergistically augmented DEN-induced preneoplastic lesions through the activation of xenobiotic-metabolizing enzymes in the livers of rats [25]. Therefore, the hepatocarcinogenicity of the combined administration of DEN and DMH in this study might be stronger than the single carcinogen-treated models. Our results have determined that RBBO displayed chemopreventive properties in DEN- and DMH-initiated rats indicated by the suppression of both hepatic GST-P positive foci and colonic ACF in rats. This outcome was consistent with previous studies which reported that the methanolic extract of purple rice bran containing high γ-tocotrienol could inhibit GST-P positive foci formation in the livers of DEN-induced rats [29]. Furthermore, the oral administration of δ-tocotrienol also suppressed ACF, polyps, and colon cancer in azoxymethane-induced colorectal carcinogenesis in rats [42]. Iqbal, J. and his group also suggested that the tocotrienol-rich fraction from rice bran oil could suppress hepatocarcinogenicity of DEN and 2-acetylaminofluorene in rats by modulation of hepatic GST activity [43], suggesting that the chemopreventive effect of RBBO might be mediated, at least in part, through the alteration of the carcinogen metabolism. In addition, tumor mass was decreased in transplanted BALB/c mice that had been fed a standard diet supplemented with 0.2% of γ-oryzanol [44]. However, the consumption of a diet supplemented with 0.3 to 2% of phytosterol influenced the morphology of colonic epithelial cells, which are crucial preneoplastic processes involved in colon carcinogenesis and may lead to a lower risk of cancer [45]. Hence, the prominent cancer chemopreventive ingredients in RBBO would likely be γ-oryzanol, phytosterols, and tocotrienols.

Sustaining proliferative signaling, resisting cell death, and tumor-promoting inflammation are all indicated as hallmarks of cancer [45]. RBBO administration significantly increased apoptosis cells in liver and colonic tissues. Furthermore, it also significantly suppressed the gene expression of TNF-α, IL-6, and IL-1β in the hepatocytes and colonocytes of DEN- and DMH-induced rats. Inflammation is a crucial factor that has been frequently linked to the development and progression of cancer. It can occur before cellular transformation or be directly exhibited in the tumor microenvironment leading to the promotion of tumor development [46]. An overexpression of pro-inflammatory cytokines, including TNF-α, IL-6, IL-1β, iNOS, and COX-2, in the colon tissue of rats was found after DMH injections [47]. Furthermore, DEN administration also increased liver TNF-α and IL-1β expression levels in rats [48]. Similarly, a previous study has revealed that the consumption of a diet containing rice bran oil could suppress TNF-α and IL-6 secretion in isolated bone marrow-derived macrophages of mice [49]. Recent studies have demonstrated a relationship between inflammation and apoptosis that activate signaling pathways through their mutual protein molecules. Fas/FasL has a dual function depending on engagement of the death receptors with their cognate ligands. Fas/FasL is a well-known death factor that induces apoptosis in a caspase-8-dependent manner. By contrast, it can activate transcriptional processes that result in NF-κB or AP-1-dependent pro-inflammatory cytokine expression [50]. Therefore, RBBO may drive the signal transduction associated with the Fas/FasL shift to apoptosis through the inflammatory pathway as a result of increased apoptosis and decreased pro-inflammatory expression to inhibit carcinogenesis. The results of previous studies support that the treatment of γ-tocopherol resulted in apoptosis induction for human colon cancer cell lines through the activation of caspase-3, -7, and -8 [51]. Moreover, α- and γ-tocotrienol induced the apoptosis of rat hepatoma dRLh-84 cells via DNA fragmentation, as well as the activation of caspase-3 and caspase-8 [52,53]. These findings suggest that the inhibition of preneoplastic lesions in the liver and the colorectal tissues of carcinogen-initiated rats by RBBO could be caused by the modulation of cell apoptosis and other relevant anti-inflammatory properties.

Previously published data have indicated that intestinal bacteria have been implicated in cancer development. Firmicutes and Bacteroidetes are the main phyla that are highly represented in more than 90% of a thousand different bacterial species found in the intestinal tract [54]. The alteration of gut microbiota in both composition and function has been associated with several pathological conditions such as inflammatory bowel disease, obesity, and the onset of colorectal cancer [55]. The modulation of gut microbiota may be an alternative approach for cancer prevention. Unexpectedly, the results of our experiments indicate insignificant differences in F/B ratios in comparisons between the control group and the carcinogen-induced alone group with regard to the duration of carcinogen injections and the stage of carcinogenesis. Sun and colleagues reported a decreased abundance of Firmicutes and a significant abundance of Bacteroidetes after subcutaneous injections of DMH at a dose of 20 mg/ kg body weight once a week for six consecutive weeks to establish an 'adenoma–carcinoma sequence' in mice after 26 weeks of the experiment [56]. Consequently, the frequency and number of carcinogen injections over the 10 weeks of our experiment did not result in changes in the composition of gut microbiota. Interestingly, an increase in the F/B ratio in the feces of RBBO-administrated rats was related to an increase in fecal butyrate content. Butyrate, one of the SCFA produced by the large intestinal bacteria, has been reported for its physiological function as an energy source in the growth and differentiation of human colonocytes [57]. It has also been found to be involved in numerous anti-carcinogenic actions, such as anti-inflammatory immune response, cell cycle arrest, and apoptosis induction in colon cancer, through the inhibition of histone deacetylase and by attenuating an inflammatory response in the liver [58]. The administration of RBBO in rats increased certain Firmicutes, including Lachnospiraceae, Ruminococcaceae UCG-104, and Lachnospiraceae NK4A136, which are known to be butyrate-producing bacteria [59]. These results confirm the significance of the production of butyrate by the phyla Firmicutes and their chemopreventive properties through the promotion of RBBO. Furthermore, an increase in the Eubacterium coprostanoligenes and Bacteroides families, which is evidence of colorectal cancer development [60,61], was found after DEN and DMH induction in rats. However, these levels were reduced in the RBBO-treated rats suggesting the anti-carcinogenic properties of RBBO. Moreover, conjugated linoleic acids, which were derived from the metabolism of linoleic acid in rice bran oil by probiotic bacteria, possessed anti-inflammatory and cancer preventive properties [62] while also inhibiting the growth of preneoplastic lesions of colorectal carcinogenesis in rodent models [63]. Therefore, these findings support the chemopreventive role of RBBO on the liver and in cases of colorectal carcinogenesis in rats. Because this cancer preventive activity was observed in only one dose of RBBO, the multi-dose experiment of RBBO needs to be further investigated. With regard to the advantages associated with rice bran consumption in humans, recent studies on the influence of rice bran or rice bran oil on the human gut microbiome indicate a promising potential for its application in cancer prevention. However, it is essential to highlight that increasing rice bran consumption may potentially have adverse effects. Rice bran consumption can result in a small increase in the synthesis of some bile acids, which can then result in the promotion of cancer [64]. In addition, rice bran was found to contain trace quantities of carcinogenic inorganic arsenic, which would likely be traced to the environmental contamination of the water used in the growing of rice [65]. However, the chemopreventive impact of rice bran on cancer should balance these adverse effects provided that the recommended dose of rice bran and rice bran oil is up to 30 grams per day [66].

5. Conclusions

These findings indicate the chemopreventive potential of RBBO on the liver and colorectal carcinogenesis induced by DEN and DMH along with involvement in the molecular inhibitory mechanism (Figure 6). The enriched bioactive compounds in RBBO, such as γ-oryzanol, phytosterols, and γ-tocotrienol, could inhibit an inflammatory response, delay cell cycle, and affect the alteration of gut microbiota, particularly in the SCFAs that are produced by bacteria. This is evidence of the regulation of cancer-related inflammation, as well as the induction of cell apoptosis, resulting in the inhibition of preneoplastic lesion formation in the livers and colons of rats. RBBO might be a promising source of valuable chemopreventive agents for either cancer prevention or treatment. The outcomes of this study point to the ever-increasing health benefits that can be attributed to RBBO in the prevention of carcinogenesis.

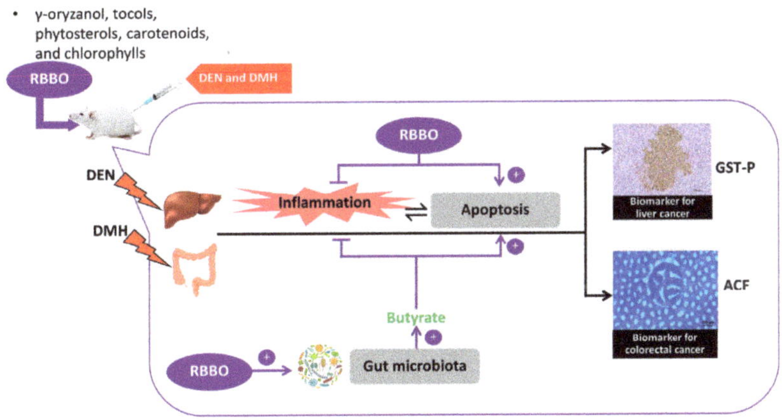

Figure 6. Summary of the mechanism of the action of RBBO as a chemopreventive agent on liver and colorectal carcinogenesis in rats.

Supplementary Materials: The following supporting information can be downloaded at: https://www.mdpi.com/article/10.3390/cancers14184358/s1, Figure S1: Effect of RBBO on cell proliferation in liver and colon tissues of DEN- and DMH-induced rats. (a) Double-staining immunohistochemistry of PCNA positive cells in hepatocytes (200×). Arrows indicate PCNA positive cells in GST-P positive foci. (b) Immunohistochemistry of PCNA positive cells in colonocytes (40×). Arrows indicate PCNA positive cells.

Author Contributions: Conceptualization, R.W.; methodology, W.P. and P.T.; software, P.T.; validation, R.W. and P.T.; formal analysis, R.W., W.P., and P.T.; investigation, W.P., A.P., H.G., and S.K.; writing—original draft preparation, W.P.; writing—review and editing, R.W.; supervision, R.W.; project administration, R.W.; funding acquisition, R.W., W.P., and S.K. All authors have read and agreed to the published version of the manuscript.

Funding: This research was funded by the Researcher and Research for industry (RRi) by Thailand Research Fund (grant number: PHD59I0088) and the Faculty of Medicine, Chiang Mai University (grant number: BIO-2562-138).

Institutional Review Board Statement: The animal study protocol was approved by the Animal Ethics Committee of the Faculty of Medicine, Chiang Mai University (41/2561).

Informed Consent Statement: Not applicable.

Data Availability Statement: All data generated or analyzed during this study are included in this published article.

Acknowledgments: We would like to thank Kurk Rice Mill, Chiang Rai for RBBO preparation. We also acknowledge the Research Center for Development of Local Lanna Rice and Rice Products, Chiang Mai University, Thailand. The authors are grateful for Chiang Mai University Presidential Scholarship on post-doctoral fellowship to S.K. This research work was partially supported by Chiang Mai University. The authors are thankful to Russell Kirk Hollis for his assistance with English editing.

Conflicts of Interest: The authors declare no conflict of interest.

Abbreviations

ACF	aberrant crypt foci
ALT	alanine aminotransferase
AP-1	activator protein 1
AST	aspartate aminotransferase
BW	body weight
Ccnd1	cyclin D1
c-JUN	Jun proto-oncogene
COX-2	cyclooxygenase-2
cDNA	complementary deoxyribonucleic acid
DAB	3,3′-diaminobenzidine
DEN	diethylnitrosamine
DMH	1,2-dimethylhydrazine
DNA	deoxyribonucleic acid
FasL	Fas ligand
F/B	*Firmicutes/Bacteroidetes*
FID	flame ionization detector
GC	gas chromatography
GST-P	glutathione *S*-transferase placental form
H&E	hematoxylin and eosin
HFD	High-fat diet
IBD	inflammatory bowel disease
IL-1β	interleukin-1 beta
IL-6	interleukin-6
iNOS	inducible nitric oxide synthase
i.p.	intraperitoneal
min	minute
mRNA	messenger ribonucleic acid
MUFAs	monounsaturated fatty acids
NF-κB	nuclear factor kappa B
PCNA	proliferation cell nuclear antigen
PCR	polymerase chain reaction
PUFAs	polyunsaturated fatty acids

qRT-PCR	quantitative reverse transcription polymerase chain reaction
RBBO	Riceberry bran oil
RNA	ribonucleic acid
s.c.	subcutaneous
SCFA	short-chain fatty acids
sec	second
TNF-α	tumor necrosis factor-alpha
TUNEL	terminal deoxynucleotidyltransferase–deoxyuridine triphosphate nick end labeling

References

1. Oliveira, P.A.; Colaço, A.; Chaves, R.; Guedes-Pinto, H.; De-La-Cruz, P.L.F.; Lopes, C. Chemical carcinogenesis. *An. Acad. Bras. Cienc.* **2007**, *79*, 593–616. [CrossRef]
2. Nasri, H.; Baradaran, A.; Shirzad, H.; Rafieian-Kopaei, M. New concepts in nutraceuticals as alternative for pharmaceuticals. *Int. J. Prev. Med.* **2014**, *5*, 1487–1499.
3. Futakuchi, M.; Cheng, J.L.; Hirose, M.; Kimoto, N.; Cho, Y.M.; Iwata, T.; Kasai, M.; Tokudome, S.; Shirai, T. Inhibition of conjugated fatty acids derived from safflower or perilla oil of induction and development of mammary tumors in rats induced by 2-amino-1-methyl-6-phenylimidazo[4,5-b]pyridine (PhIP). *Cancer Lett.* **2002**, *178*, 131–139. [CrossRef]
4. Vafa, M.; Haghighat, N.; Moslehi, N.; Eghtesadi, S.; Heydari, I. Effect of tocotrienols enriched canola oil on glycemic control and oxidative status in patients with type 2 diabetes mellitus: A randomized double-blind placebo-controlled clinical trial. *J. Res. Med. Sci.* **2015**, *20*, 540–547. [CrossRef] [PubMed]
5. Silva Figueiredo, P.; Carla Inada, A.; Marcelino, G.; Maiara Lopes Cardozo, C.; de Cássia Freitas, K.; de Cássia Avellaneda Guimarães, R.; Pereira de Castro, A.; Aragão do Nascimento, V.; Aiko Hiane, P. Fatty acids consumption: The role metabolic aspects involved in obesity and its associated disorders. *Nutrients* **2017**, *9*, 1158. [CrossRef]
6. Sellem, L.; Srour, B.; Guéraud, F.; Pierre, F.; Kesse-Guyot, E.; Fiolet, T.; Lavalette, C.; Egnell, M.; Latino-Martel, P.; Fassier, P.; et al. Saturated, mono- and polyunsaturated fatty acid intake and cancer risk: Results from the French prospective cohort NutriNet-Santé. *Eur. J. Nutr.* **2019**, *58*, 1515–1527. [CrossRef]
7. Guasch-Ferré, M.; Zong, G.; Willett, W.C.; Zock, P.L.; Wanders, A.J.; Hu, F.B.; Sun, Q. Associations of monounsaturated fatty acids from plant and animal sources with total and cause-specific mortality in two US prospective cohort studies. *Circ. Res.* **2019**, *124*, 1266–1275. [CrossRef]
8. Simopoulos, A.P. The importance of the omega-6/omega-3 fatty acid ratio in cardiovascular disease and other chronic diseases. *Exp. Biol. Med.* **2008**, *233*, 674–688. [CrossRef]
9. Romagnolo, D.F.; Donovan, M.G.; Doetschman, T.C.; Selmin, O.I. n-6 Linoleic acid induces epigenetics alterations associated with colonic inflammation and cancer. *Nutrients* **2019**, *11*, 171. [CrossRef]
10. Wang, W.; Yang, J.; Nimiya, Y.; Lee, K.S.S.; Sanidad, K.; Qi, W.; Sukamtoh, E.; Park, Y.; Liu, Z.; Zhang, G. ω-3 Polyunsaturated fatty acids and their cytochrome P450-derived metabolites suppress colorectal tumor development in mice. *J. Nutr. Biochem.* **2017**, *48*, 29–35. [CrossRef] [PubMed]
11. Thursby, E.; Juge, N. Introduction to the human gut microbiota. *Biochem. J.* **2017**, *474*, 1823–1836. [CrossRef]
12. Qiao, Y.; Sun, J.; Ding, Y.; Le, G.; Shi, Y. Alterations of the gut microbiota in high-fat diet mice is strongly linked to oxidative stress. *Appl. Microbiol. Biotechnol.* **2013**, *97*, 1689–1697. [CrossRef] [PubMed]
13. Reuter, S.; Gupta, S.C.; Chaturvedi, M.M.; Aggarwal, B.B. Oxidative stress, inflammation, and cancer: How are they linked? *Free Radic. Biol. Med.* **2010**, *49*, 1603–1616. [CrossRef] [PubMed]
14. Yang, J.; Wei, H.; Zhou, Y.; Szeto, C.H.; Li, C.; Lin, Y.; Coker, O.O.; Lau, H.C.H.; Chan, A.W.H.; Sung, J.J.Y.; et al. High-fat diet promotes colorectal tumorigenesis through modulating gut microbiota and metabolites. *Gastroenterology* **2022**, *162*, 135–149.e132. [CrossRef]
15. Zhang, X.; Coker, O.O.; Chu, E.S.; Fu, K.; Lau, H.C.H.; Wang, Y.-X.; Chan, A.W.H.; Wei, H.; Yang, X.; Sung, J.J.Y.; et al. Dietary cholesterol drives fatty liver-associated liver cancer by modulating gut microbiota and metabolites. *Gut* **2021**, *70*, 761–774. [CrossRef]
16. Flint, H.J.; Scott, K.P.; Louis, P.; Duncan, S.H. The role of the gut microbiota in nutrition and health. *Nat. Rev. Gastroenterol. Hepatol.* **2012**, *9*, 577–589. [CrossRef]
17. Wongwaiwech, D.; Weerawatanakorn, M.; Tharatha, S.; Ho, C.T. Comparative study on amount of nutraceuticals in by-products from solvent and cold pressing methods of rice bran oil processing. *J. Food Drug Anal.* **2019**, *27*, 71–82. [CrossRef]
18. Xu, Z.; Godber, J.S. Antioxidant activities of major components of γ-oryzanol from rice bran using a linoleic acid model. *J. Am. Oil Chem. Soc.* **2001**, *78*, 645. [CrossRef]
19. Posuwan, J.; Prangthip, P.; Leardkamolkarn, V.; Yamborisut, U.; Surasiang, R.; Charoensiri, R.; Kongkachuichai, R. Long-term supplementation of high pigmented rice bran oil (*Oryza sativa* L.) on amelioration of oxidative stress and histological changes in streptozotocin-induced diabetic rats fed a high fat diet; Riceberry bran oil. *Food Chem.* **2013**, *138*, 501–508. [CrossRef] [PubMed]
20. Leardkamolkarn, V.; Thongthep, W.; Suttiarporn, P.; Kongkachuichai, R.; Wongpornchai, S.; Wanavijitr, A. Chemopreventive properties of the bran extracted from a newly-developed Thai rice: The Riceberry. *Food Chem.* **2011**, *125*, 978–985. [CrossRef]

21. Suttiarporn, P.; Chumpolsri, W.; Mahatheeranont, S.; Luangkamin, S.; Teepsawang, S.; Leardkamolkarn, V. Structures of phytosterols and triterpenoids with potential anti-cancer activity in bran of black non-glutinous rice. *Nutrients* **2015**, *7*, 1672–1687. [CrossRef] [PubMed]
22. Arya, A.; Arya, S.; Arya, M. Chemical Carcinogen and Cancer Risk: An overview. *J. Chem. Pharm. Res.* **2011**, *3*, 621–631.
23. Punvittayagul, C.; Chariyakornkul, A.; Jarukamjorn, K.; Wongpoomchai, R. Protective Role of Vanillic Acid against Diethylnitrosamine- and 1,2-Dimethylhydrazine-Induced Hepatocarcinogenesis in Rats. *Molecules* **2021**, *26*, 2718. [CrossRef]
24. Chariyakornkul, A.; Inboot, N.; Taya, S.; Wongpoomchai, R. Low-polar extract from seed of Cleistocalyx nervosum var. paniala modulates initiation and promotion stages of chemically-induced carcinogenesis in rats. *Biomed. Pharmacother.* **2021**, *133*, 110963. [CrossRef] [PubMed]
25. Punvittayagul, C.; Chariyakornkul, A.; Chewonarin, T.; Jarukamjorn, K.; Wongpoomchai, R. Augmentation of diethylnitrosamine-induced early stages of rat hepatocarcinogenesis by 1,2-dimethylhydrazine. *Drug Chem. Toxicol.* **2019**, *42*, 641–648. [CrossRef]
26. Phannasorn, W.; Chariyakornkul, A.; Sookwong, P.; Wongpoomchai, R. Comparative studies on the hepatoprotective effect of white and coloured rice bran oil against acetaminophen-induced oxidative stress in mice through antioxidant- and xenobiotic-metabolizing systems. *Oxid. Med. Cell. Longev.* **2021**, *2021*, 5510230. [CrossRef] [PubMed]
27. Bird, R.P. Observation and quantification of aberrant crypts in the murine colon treated with a colon carcinogen: Preliminary findings. *Cancer Lett.* **1987**, *37*, 147–151. [CrossRef]
28. Thumvijit, T.; Taya, S.; Punvittayagul, C.; Peerapornpisal, Y.; Wongpoomchai, R. Cancer chemopreventive effect of *Spirogyra neglecta* (Hassall) Kutzing on diethylnitrosamine-induced hepatocarcinogenesis in rats. *Asian Pac. J. Cancer Prev.* **2014**, *15*, 1611–1616. [CrossRef]
29. Dokkaew, A.; Punvittayagul, C.; Insuan, O.; Limtrakul Dejkriengkraikul, P.; Wongpoomchai, R. Protective effects of defatted sticky rice bran extracts on the early stages of hepatocarcinogenesis in rats. *Molecules* **2019**, *24*, 2142. [CrossRef] [PubMed]
30. Calik, A.; Ergün, A. Effect of lactulose supplementation on growth performance, intestinal histomorphology, cecal microbial population, and short-chain fatty acid composition of broiler chickens. *Poult. Sci.* **2015**, *94*, 2173–2182. [CrossRef]
31. Klindworth, A.; Pruesse, E.; Schweer, T.; Peplies, J.; Quast, C.; Horn, M.; Glöckner, F.O. Evaluation of general 16S ribosomal RNA gene PCR primers for classical and next-generation sequencing-based diversity studies. *Nucleic Acids Res.* **2013**, *41*, e1. [CrossRef] [PubMed]
32. Benetou, V.; Lagiou, A.; Lagiou, P. Chemoprevention of cancer: Current evidence and future prospects. *F1000Res* **2015**, *4*, 916. [CrossRef] [PubMed]
33. Greenwald, P.; Clifford, C.K.; Milner, J.A. Diet and cancer prevention. *Eur. J. Cancer* **2001**, *37*, 948–965. [CrossRef]
34. Nam, S.H.; Choi, S.P.; Kang, M.Y.; Koh, H.J.; Kozukue, N.; Friedman, M. Bran extracts from pigmented rice seeds inhibit tumor promotion in lymphoblastoid B cells by phorbol ester. *Food Chem. Toxicol.* **2005**, *43*, 741–745. [CrossRef]
35. Nam, S.H.; Choi, S.P.; Kang, M.Y.; Koh, H.J.; Kozukue, N.; Friedman, M. Antioxidative activities of bran extracts from twenty one pigmented rice cultivars. *Food Chem.* **2006**, *94*, 613–620. [CrossRef]
36. Moon, S.H.; Kim, D.; Shimizu, N.; Okada, T.; Hitoe, S.; Shimoda, H. Ninety-day oral toxicity study of rice-derived γ-oryzanol in Sprague-Dawley rats. *Toxicol. Rep.* **2017**, *4*, 9–18. [CrossRef]
37. Fujiwara, S.; Sakurai, S.; Sugimoto, I.; Awata, N. Absorption and Metabolism of γ-Oryzanol in Rats. *Chem. Pharm. Bull. (Tokyo)* **1983**, *31*, 645–652. [CrossRef] [PubMed]
38. Punvittayagul, C.; Sankam, P.; Taya, S.; Wongpoomchai, R. Anticlastogenicity and anticarcinogenicity of purple rice extract in rats. *Nutr. Cancer* **2016**, *68*, 646–653. [CrossRef]
39. Chuang, S.E.; Kuo, M.L.; Hsu, C.H.; Chen, C.R.; Lin, J.K.; Lai, G.M.; Hsieh, C.Y.; Cheng, A.L. Curcumin-containing diet inhibits diethylnitrosamine-induced murine hepatocarcinogenesis. *Carcinogenesis* **2000**, *21*, 331–335. [CrossRef]
40. Grab, D.J.; Zedeck, M.S. Organ-specific Effects of the Carcinogen Methylazoxymethanol Related to Metabolism by Nicotinamide Adenine Dinucleotide-dependent Dehydrogenases. *Cancer Res.* **1977**, *37*, 4182–4189.
41. Hirose, M.; Thamavit, W.; Asamoto, M.; Osawa, T.; Ito, N. Inhibition of glutathione *S*-transferase p type-positive foci development by linolic acid hydroperoxides and their secondary oxidative products in a rat in vivo midterm test for liver carcinogens. *Toxicol. Lett.* **1986**, *32*, 51–58. [CrossRef]
42. Husain, K.; Zhang, A.; Shivers, S.; Davis-Yadley, A.; Coppola, D.; Yang, C.S.; Malafa, M.P. Chemoprevention of azoxymethane-induced colon carcinogenesis by delta-tocotrienol. *Cancer Prev. Res.* **2019**, *12*, 357–366. [CrossRef]
43. Iqbal, J.; Minhajuddin, M.; Beg, Z.H. Suppression of diethylnitrosamine and 2-acetylaminofluorene-induced hepatocarcinogenesis in rats by tocotrienol-rich fraction isolated from rice bran oil. *Eur. J. Cancer Prev.* **2004**, *13*, 515–520. [CrossRef]
44. Kim, S.P.; Kang, M.Y.; Nam, S.H.; Friedman, M. Dietary rice bran component γ-oryzanol inhibits tumor growth in tumor-bearing mice. *Mol. Nutr. Food Res.* **2012**, *56*, 935–944. [CrossRef] [PubMed]
45. Janezic, S.A.; Rao, A.V. Dose-dependent effects of dietary phytosterol on epithelial cell proliferation of the murine colon. *Food Chem. Toxicol.* **1992**, *30*, 611–616. [CrossRef]
46. Hanahan, D. Hallmarks of Cancer: New Dimensions. *Cancer Discov.* **2022**, *12*, 31. [CrossRef] [PubMed]
47. Mantovani, A.; Allavena, P.; Sica, A.; Balkwill, F. Cancer-related inflammation. *Nature* **2008**, *454*, 436–444. [CrossRef]
48. Khan, R.; Rehman, M.U.; Khan, A.Q.; Tahir, M.; Sultana, S. Glycyrrhizic acid suppresses 1,2-dimethylhydrazine-induced colon tumorigenesis in Wistar rats: Alleviation of inflammatory, proliferation, angiogenic, and apoptotic markers. *Environ. Toxicol.* **2018**, *33*, 1272–1283. [CrossRef]

49. Mansour, D.F.; Abdallah, H.M.I.; Ibrahim, B.M.M.; Hegazy, R.R.; Esmail, R.S.E.; Abdel-Salam, L.O. The carcinogenic agent diethylnitrosamine induces early oxidative stress, inflammation and proliferation in rat liver, stomach and colon: Protective effect of ginger extract. *Asian Pac. J. Cancer Prev.* **2019**, *20*, 2551–2561. [CrossRef] [PubMed]
50. Lee, S.; Yu, S.; Park, H.J.; Jung, J.; Go, G.-W.; Kim, W. Rice bran oil ameliorates inflammatory responses by enhancing mitochondrial respiration in murine macrophages. *PLoS ONE* **2019**, *14*, e0222857. [CrossRef] [PubMed]
51. Yamada, A.; Arakaki, R.; Saito, M.; Kudo, Y.; Ishimaru, N. Dual role of Fas/FasL-mediated signal in peripheral immune tolerance. *Front. Immunol.* **2017**, *8*. [CrossRef] [PubMed]
52. Campbell, S.E.; Stone, W.L.; Lee, S.; Whaley, S.; Yang, H.; Qui, M.; Goforth, P.; Sherman, D.; McHaffie, D.; Krishnan, K. Comparative effects of RRR-alpha- and RRR-gamma-tocopherol on proliferation and apoptosis in human colon cancer cell lines. *BMC Cancer* **2006**, *6*, 13. [CrossRef]
53. Sakai, M.; Okabe, M.; Yamasaki, M.; Tachibana, H.; Yamada, K. Induction of apoptosis by tocotrienol in rat hepatoma dRLh-84 cells. *Anticancer Res.* **2004**, *24*, 1683–1688. [PubMed]
54. Greenhalgh, K.; Meyer, K.M.; Aagaard, K.M.; Wilmes, P. The human gut microbiome in health: Establishment and resilience of microbiota over a lifetime. *Environ. Microbiol.* **2016**, *18*, 2103–2116. [CrossRef] [PubMed]
55. Magne, F.; Gotteland, M.; Gauthier, L.; Zazueta, A.; Pesoa, S.; Navarrete, P.; Balamurugan, R. The Firmicutes/Bacteroidetes ratio: A relevant marker of gut dysbiosis in obese patients? *Nutrients* **2020**, *12*, 1474. [CrossRef]
56. Sun, T.; Liu, S.; Zhou, Y.; Yao, Z.; Zhang, D.; Cao, S.; Wei, Z.; Tan, B.; Li, Y.; Lian, Z.; et al. Evolutionary biologic changes of gut microbiota in an 'adenoma-carcinoma sequence' mouse colorectal cancer model induced by 1, 2-Dimethylhydrazine. *Oncotarget* **2017**, *8*, 444–457. [CrossRef] [PubMed]
57. Valdes, A.M.; Walter, J.; Segal, E.; Spector, T.D. Role of the gut microbiota in nutrition and health. *BMJ* **2018**, *361*, k2179. [CrossRef]
58. McNabney, S.M.; Henagan, T.M. Short chain fatty acids in the colon and peripheral tissues: A focus on butyrate, colon cancer, obesity and insulin resistance. *Nutrients* **2017**, *9*, 1348. [CrossRef]
59. Zhang, J.; Song, L.; Wang, Y.; Liu, C.; Zhang, L.; Zhu, S.; Liu, S.; Duan, L. Beneficial effect of butyrate-producing *Lachnospiraceae* on stress-induced visceral hypersensitivity in rats. *J. Gastroenterol. Hepatol.* **2019**, *34*, 1368–1376. [CrossRef] [PubMed]
60. Cheng, W.T.; Kantilal, H.K.; Davamani, F. The mechanism of bacteroides fragilis toxin contributes to colon cancer formation. *Malays. J. Med. Sci.* **2020**, *27*, 9–21. [CrossRef]
61. Wu, Y.; Jiao, N.; Zhu, R.; Zhang, Y.; Wu, D.; Wang, A.-J.; Fang, S.; Tao, L.; Li, Y.; Cheng, S.; et al. Identification of microbial markers across populations in early detection of colorectal cancer. *Nat. Commun.* **2021**, *12*, 3063. [CrossRef] [PubMed]
62. Ewaschuk, J.B.; Walker, J.W.; Diaz, H.; Madsen, K.L. Bioproduction of conjugated linoleic acid by probiotic bacteria occurs in vitro and in vivo in mice. *J. Nutr.* **2006**, *136*, 1483–1487. [CrossRef] [PubMed]
63. Yasui, Y.; Suzuki, R.; Kohno, H.; Miyamoto, S.; Beppu, F.; Hosokawa, M.; Miyashita, K.; Tanaka, T. 9trans,11trans conjugated linoleic acid inhibits the development of azoxymethane-induced colonic aberrant crypt foci in rats. *Nutr. Cancer* **2007**, *59*, 82–91. [CrossRef] [PubMed]
64. So, W.K.; Law, B.M.; Law, P.T.; Chan, C.W.; Chair, S.Y. Current Hypothesis for the Relationship between Dietary Rice Bran Intake, the Intestinal Microbiota and Colorectal Cancer Prevention. *Nutrients* **2016**, *8*, 569. [CrossRef] [PubMed]
65. Sun, G.X.; Williams, P.N.; Carey, A.M.; Zhu, Y.G.; Deacon, C.; Raab, A.; Feldmann, J.; Islam, R.M.; Meharg, A.A. Inorganic arsenic in rice bran and its products are an order of magnitude higher than in bulk grain. *Environ. Sci. Technol.* **2008**, *42*, 7542–7546. [CrossRef] [PubMed]
66. Jariwalla, R.J. Rice-bran products: Phytonutrients with potential applications in preventive and clinical medicine. *Drugs Exp. Clin. Res.* **2001**, *27*, 17–26.

cancers

Article

Stage-Specific Effect of Inositol Hexaphosphate on Cancer Stem Cell Pool during Growth and Progression of Prostate Tumorigenesis in TRAMP Model

Komal Raina [1,2], Kushal Kandhari [1], Anil K. Jain [1], Kameswaran Ravichandran [1], Paul Maroni [3], Chapla Agarwal [1,4] and Rajesh Agarwal [1,4,*]

1 Department of Pharmaceutical Sciences, Skaggs School of Pharmacy and Pharmaceutical Sciences, University of Colorado Anschutz Medical Campus, Aurora, CO 80045, USA
2 Department of Pharmaceutical Sciences, South Dakota State University, Brookings, SD 57007, USA
3 Department of Surgery, Division of Urology, University of Colorado Anschutz Medical Campus, Aurora, CO 80045, USA
4 University of Colorado Cancer Center, University of Colorado Anschutz Medical Campus, Aurora, CO 80045, USA
* Correspondence: rajesh.agarwal@cuanschutz.edu; Tel.: +1-(303)-724-4055; Fax: +1-(303)-724-7266

Simple Summary: The stage of a tumor during cancer intervention is the most crucial factor that determines the treatment regimen. Several bioactive natural compounds have shown potential to inhibit prostate cancer growth and progression; however, there is a dearth of studies that explore their efficacy at different stages of tumorigenesis. This knowledge gap prevents researchers from fully exploiting the anti-cancer potential of these beneficial compounds. Accordingly, our present study focused on explicating the 'stage-specific' efficacy of the bioactive food component 'inositol hexaphosphate (IP6, phytic acid)' against PCa initiation, growth, and progression in the transgenic adenocarcinoma of the mouse prostate TRAMP model. Results indicated that IP6 feeding during initial stages of cancer development prevents progression of prostatic intraepithelial neoplasia lesions to adenocarcinoma, and IP6 feeding during late stage of the disease reduces tumor growth and prevents its progression to advanced stage of the disease. Thus, IP6 intervention is beneficial during all stages of prostate tumorigenesis.

Abstract: Herein, we assessed the stage-specific efficacy of inositol hexaphosphate (IP6, phytic acid), a bioactive food component, on prostate cancer (PCa) growth and progression in a transgenic mouse model of prostate cancer (TRAMP). Starting at 4, 12, 20, and 30 weeks of age, male TRAMP mice were fed either regular drinking water or 2% IP6 in water for ~8–15 weeks. Pathological assessments at study endpoint indicated that tumor grade is arrested at earlier stages by IP6 treatment; IP6 also prevented progression to more advanced forms of the disease (~55–70% decrease in moderately and poorly differentiated adenocarcinoma incidence was observed in advanced stage TRAMP cohorts). Next, we determined whether the protective effects of IP6 are mediated via its effect on the expansion of the cancer stem cells (CSCs) pool; results indicated that the anti-PCa effects of IP6 are associated with its potential to eradicate the PCa CSC pool in TRAMP prostate tumors. Furthermore, in vitro assays corroborated the above findings as IP6 decreased the % of floating PC-3 prostaspheres (self-renewal of CSCs) by ~90%. Together, these findings suggest the multifaceted chemopreventive-translational potential of IP6 intervention in suppressing the growth and progression of PCa and controlling this malignancy at an early stage.

Keywords: inositol hexaphosphate; prostate cancer; chemoprevention; cancer stem cells; TRAMP

Citation: Raina, K.; Kandhari, K.; Jain, A.K.; Ravichandran, K.; Maroni, P.; Agarwal, C.; Agarwal, R. Stage-Specific Effect of Inositol Hexaphosphate on Cancer Stem Cell Pool during Growth and Progression of Prostate Tumorigenesis in TRAMP Model. *Cancers* **2022**, *14*, 4204. https://doi.org/10.3390/cancers14174204

Academic Editor: Anupam Bishayee

Received: 1 July 2022
Accepted: 27 August 2022
Published: 30 August 2022

Publisher's Note: MDPI stays neutral with regard to jurisdictional claims in published maps and institutional affiliations.

1. Introduction

American Cancer Society data for the year 2022 estimates prostate cancer (PCa) as the most common cancer (~268,000 cases) and the second leading cause of cancer death

(~34,000 deaths) in American men [1]. On the global front, with more than 1.4 million cases, PCa is the fourth most commonly diagnosed cancer worldwide [2]. Though localized PCa has a long-term survival rate, on contrary, the metastatic PCa is still largely incurable and the principal cause of PCa related deaths [3]. Improvement in prostate-specific antigen (PSA) screening and advances in clinical practices have helped reduce PCa-associated mortality significantly in the past few decades. However, the incidence rates of localized and metastatic prostate cancer are rising and are expected to increase further in the next decade [4]. Epidemiological studies have also demonstrated significant disparities in PCa incidence worldwide. The disparity in PCa incidence has been attributed to various factors including the variations in the PSA screening, diagnostic practices, ethnicity, family/genetic history, and lifestyle [4,5]. One of the important lifestyle variables other than sedentary factor that has been suggested to be one of the possible reasons for the disparity is the dietary differences between different regions of the world [4,6].

The failure of traditionally used therapies to stem the rising incidence of PCa has compelled researchers to shift their focus to preventive intervention by dietary agents [7–10]. Inositol hexaphosphate (IP6), also known as phytic acid, is a bioactive food component present in most cereals, legumes, nuts, oilseeds, and soybean [11]. Numerous studies have identified the anti-cancer potential of IP6 against breast, colon, pancreatic, oral, and skin cancer [11,12]; also, several research groups including ours have demonstrated the anti-PCa potential of IP6 in various pre-clinical in vitro and in vivo models [11–20]. One of our previous studies reported the chemopreventive efficacy of IP6 against prostate cancer growth and progression in the transgenic adenocarcinoma of the mouse prostate TRAMP model [19]. Another study from our group elucidated the molecular mechanism of IP6-induced inhibition of PCa tumor growth, vascularity, and metabolism in TRAMP mice [20]. However, one limitation of these studies was that the chemopreventive intervention started very early and continued throughout the experiment, making it difficult to assess the clinical relevance of IP6 feeding on different tumor stages of PCa. Studies have demonstrated that the ability of dietary factors to prevent cancer is stage-dependent and thus exploring the stage-specific effects may provide insight into the uncharted potential and the associated underlying mechanisms of such dietary compounds [21]. In accordance, our present study focused on explicating the "stage-specific" efficacy of IP6 feeding against PCa initiation, growth, and progression.

2. Materials and Methods

2.1. Cell Culture and Reagents

PC-3 human prostate carcinoma cells and THP-1 monocytic cells were procured from American Type Culture Collection (ATCC) (Manassas, VA, USA). Both PC-3 and THP-1 cells were routinely cultured in RPMI-1640 medium with 10% fetal bovine serum (FBS) and 1% Penicillin-Streptomycin solution under standard culture conditions (37 °C, 95% humidified air, and 5% CO_2). THP-1 monocytes were differentiated into macrophages by 24 h exposure to 150 nM phorbol 12-myristate (PMA, #P8139 from Sigma, St. Louis, MO, USA). All cell culture reagents were procured from Gibco, Thermo Fisher Scientific (Waltham, MA, USA) unless otherwise noted. IP6 (#8810 as phytic acid sodium salt hydrate from rice, quality level M-100 from Sigma, St. Louis, MO, USA) was dissolved in water to prepare a 200 mM stock solution (for cell culture use), and pH was adjusted to 7.5. Antibody for PCNA (#M0879) was from DakoCytomation (Glostrup, Denmark). Dead End Colorimetric TUNEL System (#G7130) was purchased from Promega (Madison, WI, USA). Antibodies for VEGF (#ab46154), GLUT4 (#ab654), Sox-2 (#ab97959), and Oct-4 (#ab184665) were from Abcam (Cambridge, MA, USA). Antibody for iNOS (#NB300605) was from Novus Biologicals (Centennial, CO, USA). Antibodies for PECAM-1/CD-31 (#sc-1506) and CXCR3 (#sc-137140) were purchased from Santa Cruz Biotechnology (Dallas, TX, USA). Antibody for Shh (#ARP44235_P050) was from Aviva System Biology (San Diego, CA, USA) and antibody for cleaved Notch-1 (#4147S) was from Cell Signaling Technology (Danvers, MA, USA).

2.2. Animals, Treatment, and Necropsy

TRAMP male mice (4 weeks old) routinely obtained by breeding heterozygous TRAMP (C57BL/6) females with non-transgenic C57BL/6 breeder males were used for this study. Housing and care of the animals were as per the guidelines established by the University of Colorado, Anschutz Medical Campus animal house facility. All the animal protocols were approved by the Institutional Animal Care and Use Committee (IACUC). The mice were randomly distributed into positive control and treatment groups. Male TRAMP mice starting at 4, 12, 20, and 30 weeks of age were fed with regular drinking water (positive control group) or 2% *w/v* IP6 in regular drinking water for ~8–15 weeks as detailed previously [19,20]. Hereafter, different groups depending on their study periods are referred to as 4–12, 12–20, 20–30, and 30–45 week groups, respectively (Figure 1). Number of mice per group: [4–12 weeks: TRAMP controls (n = 11), IP6-fed (n = 13); 12–20 weeks: TRAMP controls (n = 17), IP6-fed (n = 16); 20–30 weeks: TRAMP controls (n = 14), IP6-fed (n = 14); 30–45 weeks: TRAMP controls (n = 11), IP6-fed (n = 12)] and TRAMP negative [untreated WT controls (n = 5) per study group].

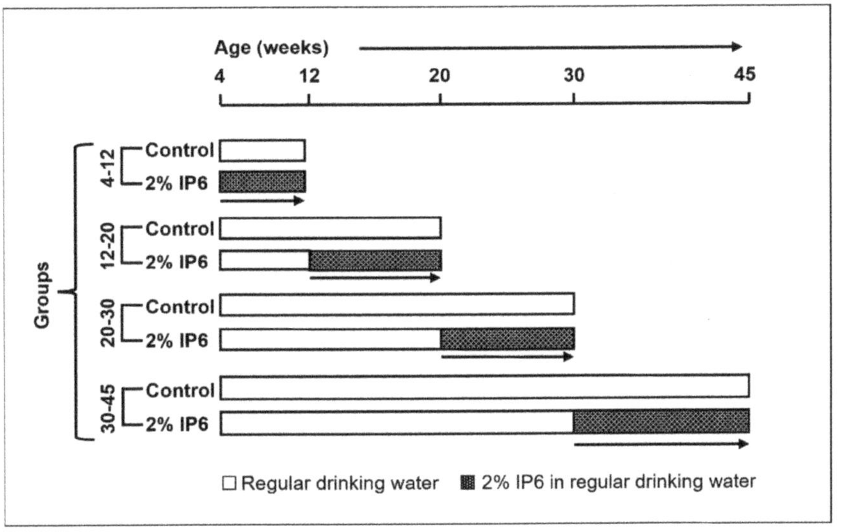

Figure 1. Study design to assess the effect of feeding IP6 during different stages of prostate cancer growth and progression in TRAMP mice. Starting at 4, 12, 20, and 30 weeks of age, male TRAMP mice were fed either regular drinking water or 2% IP6 in water, and then sacrificed at age 12, 20, 30, and 45 weeks respectively. Depending upon the feeding period, the different groups are referred to as 4–12, 12–20, 20–30, and 30–45 week groups, respectively.

At the end of each time point, mice were sacrificed by CO_2 asphyxiation followed by exsanguination. Lower urogenital tract (LUT) including bladder, seminal vesicles, and prostate were removed *en-bloc*. The prostate gland was harvested and microdissected. Gross pathology of animals, including any evidence of edema, unusual appearance, and abnormal size of any non-target organs, was also noted. All tissues were partly flash-frozen in liquid nitrogen and partly formalin-fixed for further analyses.

2.3. Histopathological and Immunohistochemical Analysis

Formalin-fixed tissues were processed as described previously [22]. Histopathological analysis of dorsolateral prostate was done using hematoxylin and eosin (H&E) stained tissues as detailed previously [22]. Given that in the TRAMP model the pathological changes associated with PCa are more evident in the dorsolateral lobes [23], our study assessments focused on these lobes only. For immunohistochemical (IHC) analysis, routine staining technique using 3, 3′-diaminobenzidine (DAB) was employed [24]. Brown-stained cells were counted as positive cells (among total number of cells) and plotted as % positive cells; these were counted in five randomly selected fields at ×400 magnification. Immunoreactivity (intensity of brown staining was represented by arbitrary values) was noted as 0 (no staining), +1 (weak intensity), +2 (moderate intensity), +3 (strong intensity), and +4 (very strong intensity) [25]. Immunopositive area was assessed as the proportion area of prostate which is positive for expression and assigned arbitrary scores as 0 (<5% positive area), +1 (5–25% positive area), +2 (26–50% positive area), +3 (51–75% positive area), and +4 (>75% positive area).

2.4. Immunofluorescence Assay

Formalin-fixed dorsolateral prostate tissues were deparaffinized and routinely processed for immunofluorescence assay as described previously [18]. Antibodies used were CD44 (#sc-9960) from Santa Cruz Biotechnology (Dallas, TX, USA) and BMI-1 (#ab38295) from Abcam (Cambridge, MA, USA). The secondary antibodies Goat anti-rabbit IgG Alexa fluor 488 (#A-11008) and Goat anti-mouse IgG Alexa fluor 647 (#A-21236) secondary antibodies were from Invitrogen, Thermo Fisher Scientific (Waltham, MA, USA). Sections were mounted using vectashield antifade mounting medium with 4′,6-diamidino-2-phenylindole (DAPI) (#H-1800) from Vector Laboratories (Burlingame, CA, USA). A Nikon D-Eclipse C1 confocal microscope (Nikon) was used for imaging. All images were taken at ×600; immunofluorescence images were evaluated using QuPath analysis software (Univ. of Edinburgh, Edinburgh, UK, Version 0.3.2).

2.5. In Vitro Prostasphere-Formation Assay

FACS sorted $CD44^{+}$ -$\alpha 2\beta 1^{high}$ subpopulation of human PCa PC-3 cell line was used for the prostaspheres formation assay in serum-free DMEM/F12 media supplemented with 20 ng/mL rhEGF, 10 ng/mL rhFGF-b, 2% B27, and 1% N2 supplement as described previously [26]. The sorted single cell suspension was plated in 6-well ultra-low attachment plates (Corning) at a density of 3000 cells/well as described previously [26]. Cells were treated with 2 mM IP6, and at the end of the experiment (after 10 days) spheres were examined for number count. To determine the impact of immune cells such as macrophages on prostasphere formation, conditioned media of human macrophage cell line [(PMA differentiated THP-1 monocytes) without or with treatment with 2 mM IP6 for 12 h (followed by drug washout and exposure to serum-free media for 48 h to collect macrophage-conditioned media)] was used in the prostasphere formation assay as above.

2.6. Statistical and Microscopic Analyses

Sigma Stat software (version 3.5, Jandel Scientific Software, San Jose, CA, USA) and GraphPad Prism (version 8.4, GraphPad Software Inc., San Diego, CA, USA) were used for statistical analyses. Incidence of PIN and adenocarcinoma lesions was compared using Fisher's Exact test and unpaired two-tailed Student's t-test was used for all other data. Quantitative data in the figures are presented as mean ± SEM; $p \leq 0.05$ was considered statistically significant. As relevant to the study, data were analyzed either intra-group (between age-matched TRAMP positive control and IP6-fed mice) or between WT controls and TRAMP positive controls. Carl Zeiss Axioscope 2 microscope (Carl Zeiss, Inc. Jena, Germany) and attached AxioCam MrC5 camera were employed for all microscopic analyses and capturing of photomicrographs.

3. Results

3.1. Stage-Specific Effect of IP6 Feeding on Pathological Changes in TRAMP Prostate

There was no significant difference in diet consumption or body weight gain between the TRAMP controls and IP6-fed mice (data not shown); though IP6-fed mice showed lower LUT weight compared to TRAMP controls, the differences were not statistically significant (Supplementary Figure S1). H&E-stained dorsolateral prostate tissue sections were microscopically evaluated and tissues were pathologically classified as described previously [10]. As shown in Figure 2A,B, there was a significant difference between the incidence of PIN and adenocarcinoma lesions between the TRAMP control and IP6-fed groups. Specifically, in the 4–12 weeks control group, ~27% of mice developed adenocarcinoma [~9% incidence each of well-differentiated (WD), moderately differentiated (MD), and poorly differentiated (PD)], whereas no mice in the IP6-fed group developed adenocarcinoma and instead showed ~30% incidence of low-grade PIN and ~70% incidence of high-grade PIN (Figure 2A, *left panel*). A similar effect was seen in the 12–20 weeks group, where ~40% of control mice developed adenocarcinoma and no mice in the IP6-fed group developed adenocarcinoma but only PIN (~19% incidence of low-grade PIN and ~81% incidence of high-grade PIN) (Figure 2A, *right panel*). In the 20–30 weeks group, the IP6-fed group did show incidence of low-grade PIN while there was no incidence of low-grade PIN lesions in control mice. On the other hand, there was a higher incidence of high-grade PIN lesions and a concomitant decrease in PD adenocarcinoma in IP6-fed mice compared to the controls (Figure 2B, *left panel*). In the 30–45 weeks group, all mice in the control group developed high-grade adenocarcinoma (~18% incidence of MD and ~81% incidence of PD), while IP6-fed mice displayed a higher incidence of PIN lesions and WD tumors; the incidence of MD and PD adenocarcinoma was also significantly decreased in the IP6-fed group (Figure 2B, *right panel*). Thus, in the 30–45 weeks cohort, there was an increase in the incidence of differentiated tumors in IP6-fed groups compared with TRAMP controls and a concomitant decrease in the incidence of more advanced tumors (Supplementary Figure S2).

Furthermore, there was a significant difference in the percentage area of dorsolateral prostate covered by PIN lesions and aggressive adenocarcinoma lesions between the TRAMP control and IP6-fed mice. As can be seen in Figure 2B, the incidence of invasive adenocarcinoma increased as a function of age in the TRAMP controls. The area of dorsolateral prostate covered by adenocarcinoma was highest in the 30–45 weeks TRAMP controls; however, in IP6-treated groups, the majority of the area was covered with non-invasive lesions (LGPIN and HGPIN). Also, in this cohort of IP6-fed mice (30–45 weeks group), there was a significant decrease in the area of MD (~79% decrease, $p \leq 0.01$) and PD lesions (~76% decrease, $p \leq 0.01$).

Next, the severity of dorsolateral prostate lesions was determined by grading the tissues for mean peak histologic score as previously described [16]. As seen in Figure 3A, TRAMP prostates had a mean peak score of ~3.8 (4–12 weeks), ~4.0 (12–20 weeks), ~5.0 (20–30 weeks), and ~5.5 (30–45 weeks) indicating a considerable increase in tumor grade as a function of age. Alternatively, IP6-treated group showed much less severe tumor grade scores in comparison to the control groups. The mean peak score of the IP6-fed group was ~2.7 (4–12 weeks), ~2.8 (12–20 weeks), ~4.0 (20–30 weeks), and ~4.3 (30–45 weeks). This corresponds to a decrease of ~15% (4–12 weeks), ~30% (12–20 weeks, $p \leq 0.01$), ~20% (20–30 weeks, $p \leq 0.05$), and ~23% (30–45 weeks, $p \leq 0.01$), indicating that IP6 feeding during different stages of tumorigenesis also decreases the severity of prostatic lesions in TRAMP mice. Altogether, these results suggest that IP6-feeding is effective in restricting the progression of both pre-malignant neoplastic lesions as well as differentiated tumors to more aggressive forms of adenocarcinoma in the TRAMP prostate.

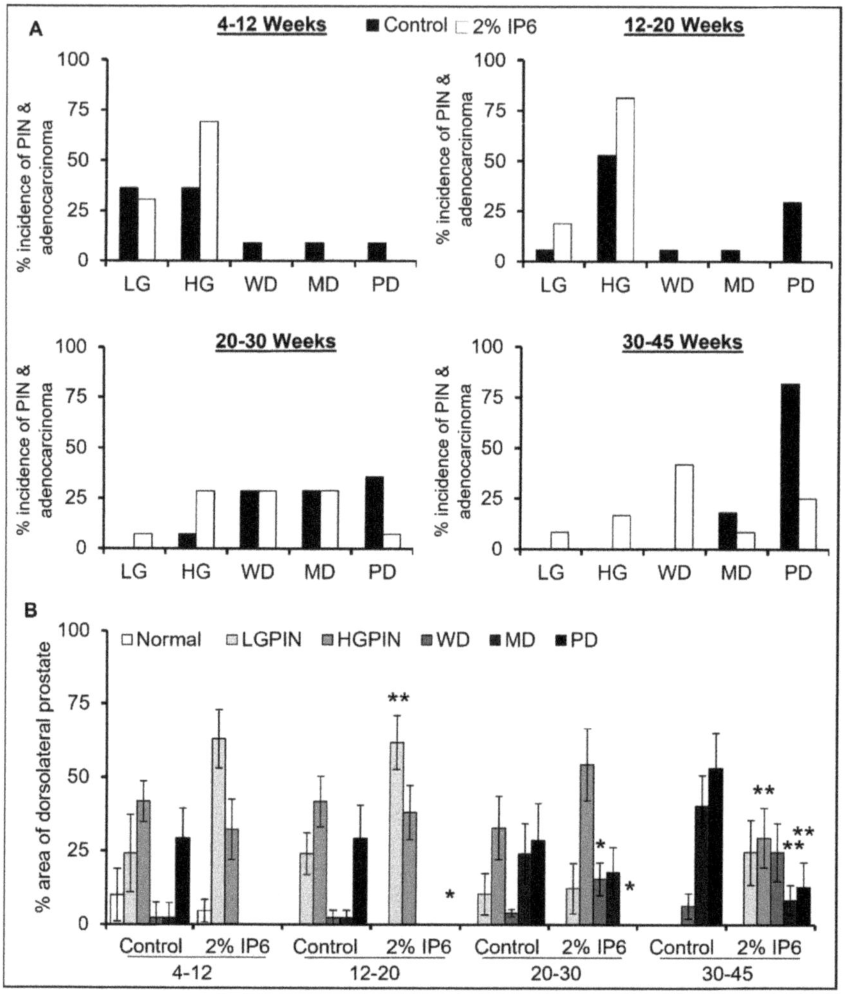

Figure 2. Stage-specific effect of IP6 feeding on pathological changes in dorsolateral prostate of TRAMP mice. (**A**) % incidence of normal, pre-neoplastic, and adenocarcinoma lesions in dorsolateral prostate tissues of TRAMP control and IP6-fed mice. (**B**) % area of dorsolateral prostate lobe displaying normal, pre-neoplastic, and adenocarcinoma lesions in TRAMP control and IP6-fed mice. LGPIN, low-grade prostatic intraepithelial neoplasia; HGPIN, high-grade prostatic intraepithelial neoplasia; WD, well-differentiated (adenocarcinoma); MD, moderately differentiated (adenocarcinoma); PD, poorly differentiated (adenocarcinoma). Quantified data are represented as columns (mean for each group); bars represent SEM. ** $p \leq 0.01$, and * $p \leq 0.05$.

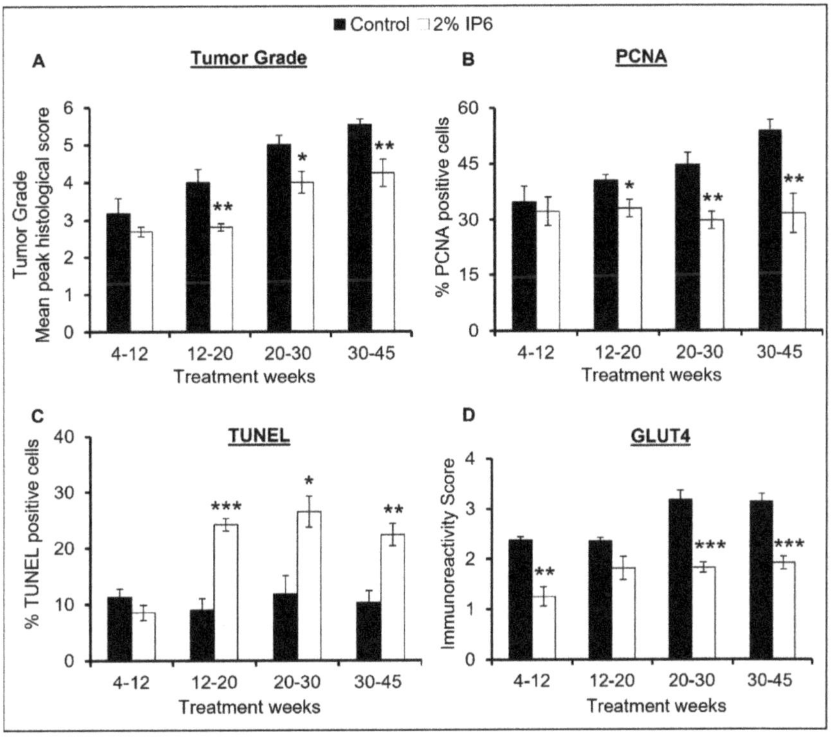

Figure 3. Stage-specific effect of IP6 feeding on tumor grade, proliferation, and apoptosis in dorsolateral prostate of TRAMP mice. Effect on (**A**) Tumor grade, (**B**) PCNA-proliferative index, (**C**) TUNEL, and (**D**) GLUT-4 (glucose transporter) in TRAMP control and IP6-fed mice. DAB, 3,3′-diaminobenzidine; PCNA, proliferating cell nuclear antigen; TUNEL, terminal deoxynucleotidyl transferase dUTP nick end labeling. Quantified data are represented as mean ± SEM. *** $p \leq 0.001$, ** $p \leq 0.01$, and * $p \leq 0.05$.

3.2. Stage-Specific Effect of IP6 Feeding on Proliferation Index and Apoptosis in TRAMP Prostate

To investigate the effect of IP6 feeding on the proliferative index in prostate tissues, immunostaining for proliferating cell nuclear antigen (PCNA) was performed on dorsolateral prostate tissues. Quantitative microscopic analyses of the stained tissues revealed that PCNA-positive cell percentage in TRAMP controls increased in an age-dependent manner. Specifically, the percentage of PCNA positive cells in the TRAMP mice was ~35% (4–12 weeks group), ~41% (12–20 weeks group), ~45% (20–30 weeks group), and ~54% (30–45 weeks group), whereas the percent PCNA positive cells in the IP6-fed group was ~32% (4–12 weeks group), ~33% (12–20 weeks group), ~30% (20–30 weeks group), and ~32% (30–45 weeks group). This corresponds to a significant decrease of ~20% (12–20 weeks group, $p \leq 0.05$), ~33% (20–30 weeks group, $p \leq 0.01$), and ~41% (30–45 weeks group, $p \leq 0.01$) in the IP6-fed mice, implying towards a more significant effect of IP6 feeding on the proliferative index in the advanced stages of PCa (Figure 3B).

Next, the apoptotic effect of IP6 feeding in dorsolateral prostate tissues of the TRAMP mice was assessed. Terminal deoxynucleotidyl transferase biotin-dUTP nick-end labeling (TUNEL) assay on the tissue samples was performed and microscopy-based examination of tissues demonstrated an increased number of apoptotic cells in the IP6-fed groups (Figure 3C). Specifically, IP6 feeding increased the number of TUNEL positive (apoptotic) cells by ~2.6 fold (12–20 weeks group, $p \leq 0.001$), ~2.3 fold (20–30 weeks group, $p \leq 0.05$), and ~2.2 fold (30–45 weeks group, $p \leq 0.01$) compared to TRAMP controls.

Thereafter, we assessed the effect of IP6 feeding on the expression of glucose transporter GLUT4 in dorsolateral prostate tissue of TRAMP mice. Studies in the past have established that PCa cells overexpress GLUT4 which plays a vital role in fulfilling the energy needs of highly proliferative PCa cells [27]. Aberrant glucose uptake in cancer cells is also known to help in PCa growth and progression [28]. IHC analysis for GLUT4 in prostate tissues revealed that the expression of GLUT4 increased as a function of age in the TRAMP controls and IP6 feeding was able to substantially decrease the expression of GLUT4 (Figure 3D). Specifically, a decrease of ~47% (4–12 weeks group, $p \leq 0.01$), ~23% (12–20 weeks group), ~43% (20–30 weeks group, $p \leq 0.001$), and ~39% (30–45 weeks group, $p \leq 0.001$) in the expression of GLUT4 was observed in the IP6-fed mice compared to TRAMP controls. Overall, these observations suggest that IP6 feeding inhibits the proliferative potential and induces apoptosis in the TRAMP mice prostate cells and that the effect is more evident in the later stages of tumorigenesis.

3.3. *Stage-Specific Effect of IP6 Feeding on Angiogenesis and Associated Regulatory Molecules in TRAMP Prostate*

CD-31: IHC analysis of the dorsolateral prostate tissues for the endothelial cell marker, platelet endothelial cell adhesion molecule-1/cluster of differentiation 31 (PECAM-1 or CD31), showed that the expression of CD-31 increased as a function of age in the TRAMP mice. However, IP6-fed mice showed an overall decrease in the expression of CD-31, especially in the later age groups, suggesting a potent efficacy of IP6 to reduce de novo angiogenesis in the TRAMP prostate. Specifically, CD-31 expression decreased by ~28% (4–12 weeks group), ~23% (12–20 weeks group), ~54% (20–30 weeks group, $p < 0.05$), and 36% (30–45 weeks group, $p \leq 0.01$) in the IP6-fed mice compared to TRAMP controls (Figure 4A).

VEGF: The effect of IP6 feeding on the expression of VEGF, an angiogenesis regulator, was also analyzed in prostate tissues. Similar to the results of CD-31, IHC analysis demonstrated that IP6 feeding substantially decreased the expression of VEGF. There was a reduction of ~65% (4–12 weeks group, $p \leq 0.05$), ~21% (12–20 weeks group), ~68% (20–30 weeks group, $p \leq 0.001$), and ~34% (30–45 weeks group) in VEGF expression in IP6-fed mice compared to controls (Figure 4B). Overall, this result in combination with the CD-31 data corroborates our histopathological analysis and suggests that IP6 feeding at different stages has the potential to impact angiogenesis in TRAMP prostate.

iNOS: Inducible nitric oxide synthase (iNOS) has been shown to play a role in PCa progression by favoring proliferation as well as angiogenesis [29,30], as such we analyzed the expression of iNOS in the prostate tissues from control and IP6-fed TRAMP mice in all age groups. IHC analysis demonstrated that IP6 treatment significantly decreased the expression of iNOS in the later stages of tumorigenesis. Specifically, iNOS expression was decreased by ~27% (12–20 weeks group, $p \leq 0.01$), ~28% (20–30 weeks group, $p \leq 0.01$), and ~37% (30–45 weeks group, $p \leq 0.05$) in the IP6-fed mice compared to the TRAMP controls (Figure 4C).

CXCR3: There is accumulating evidence that CXCR3 is a vital angiostatic receptor for various CXC chemokines such as CXCL9, CXCL10, and CXCL11 [31–33]. CXCL10-induced CXCR3 expression has been associated with reduced cell proliferation and decreased PSA levels in PCa cells [34]. Therefore, we analyzed the expression of CXCR3 in TRAMP dorsolateral prostate tissues by IHC and found that IP6 treatment was able to increase the expression of CXCR3 in all age groups. There was an increase of ~2.0 fold (4–12 weeks group), ~3.1 fold (12–20 weeks group, $p \leq 0.001$), ~1.5 fold (20–30 weeks group, $p \leq 0.01$), and ~1.3 fold (30–45 weeks group) in the IP6-fed mice compared to TRAMP controls (Figure 4D).

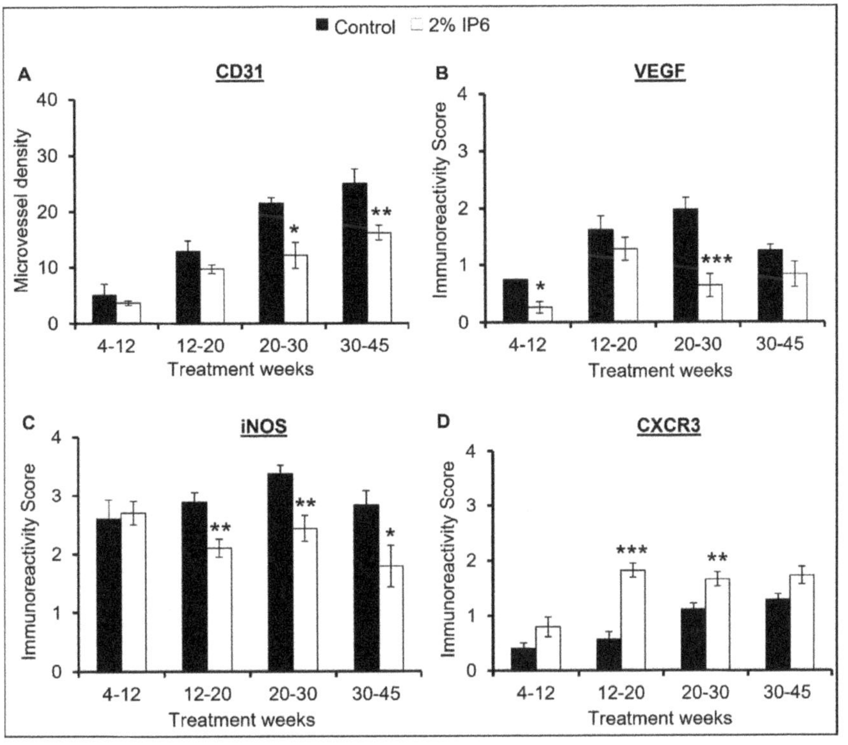

Figure 4. Stage-specific effect of IP6 feeding on angiogenic pathway in dorsolateral prostate of TRAMP mice. Effect on (**A**) microvessel density (MVD) as inferred by expression of PECAM-1/CD-31. MVD was determined by calculating the number of positive foci counted under ×400 magnifications in five selected areas in each section. Effect on (**B**) VEGF, (**C**) iNOS, (**D**) CXCR3 expression in TRAMP mice prostate and IP6-fed mice as determined by IHC. Quantified data are represented as mean ± SEM. *** $p \leq 0.001$, ** $p \leq 0.01$, and * $p \leq 0.05$.

3.4. Stage-Specific Effect of IP6 Feeding on the Expansion of Cancer Stem Cells (CSCs) Pool in TRAMP Prostate

Cancer stem cells (CSC) endowed with tumor-initiating and self-renewal capacities have been recognized as the driving force for tumor initiation and progression to advanced stages in different epithelial cancers including PCa [35–38]. CD44 is a cell-surface protein involved in cell adhesion, tumor invasion, and metastasis and its high expression is also recognized as a phenotypic marker for tumor-initiating cells (TICs) [39]. BMI-1 is responsible for cell proliferation, cell motility, self-renewal, and therapy resistance in PCa cells, and is also recognized to play a vital role in self-renewal of TICs [40]. To determine whether the protective effects of IP6 are mediated via the effect on the expansion of the TICs/CSCs pool, we analyzed the TICs pool (for dual expression of CD44 and BMI-1) as a function of tumor aggressiveness (with or without IP6 treatment).

Results revealed that both CD44 and BMI-1 had minimal expression in PIN stages and their expression increased with tumorigenesis, i.e., a strong expression was observed in MD and PD stages in TRAMP controls (Figure 5A,B). On the other hand, IP6 treatment was able to induce a significant decrease in the expression of CD44 ($p \leq 0.01$, both MD and PD stages) and BMI-1 ($p \leq 0.001$, MD stage; $p \leq 0.05$, PD stage). Notably, in the IP6-fed groups, the cells that dual stained for CD44/BMI were significantly decreased ($p \leq 0.001$, MD stage;

$p \leq 0.05$, PD stage) compared to that present in TRAMP controls (Figure 5B, *right panel*) indicating the possibility of IP6 decreasing the TICs/CSCs pool.

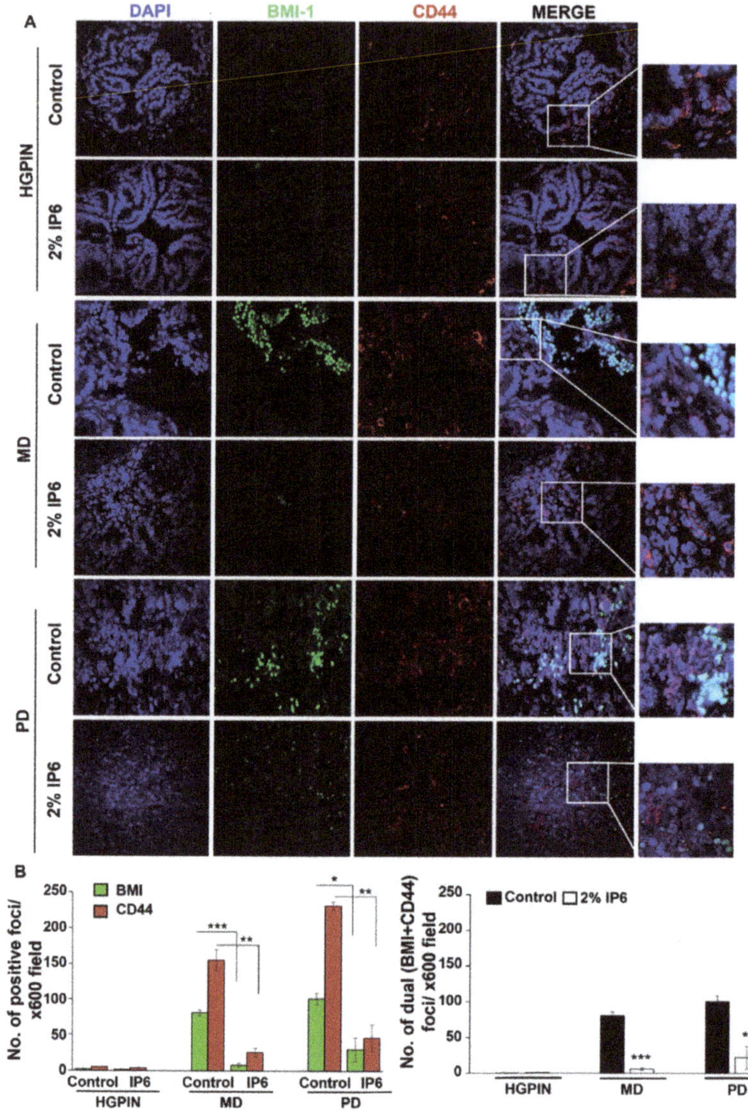

Figure 5. Stage-specific effect of IP6 feeding on the expansion of cancer stem cells (CSCs) pool in dorsolateral prostate of TRAMP mice. Immunofluorescence (IF) studies to determine the correlation and dual stained (BMI-1 and CD44 expression) tumor initiating cells (TICs/CSCs) pool in different pathological lesions of dorsolateral prostate of TRAMP controls and IP6-fed groups. Tissues were dual-stained for BMI-1 (green) and CD44 (red) expression. Nuclear staining was done with DAPI (blue). (**A**) Representative pictographs are depicted at x600 magnification and insets represent digital magnifications. (**B**) BMI-1 and CD44 positive foci was quantified using QuPATH analysis software. Quantified data are represented as mean $\pm$ SEM. *** $p \leq 0.001$, ** $p \leq 0.01$, and * $p \leq 0.05$.

3.5. *In Vitro Effect of IP6 Treatment on Prostasphere Formation*

Next, to corroborate the above findings on the potential of IP6 feeding to modulate the expansion of TICs pool and to determine the effect on the self-renewal capacity of prostate TICs/CSCs, we performed an in vitro prostasphere formation assay employing TICs/CSCs enriched ($CD44^{+}$ -$\alpha 2\beta 1^{high}$) PC-3 cells sub-population. Importantly, the % of floating spheroids (prostaspheres) generated in the presence of 2 mM IP6 was decreased by ~90% ($p \leq 0.001$) compared to control. Additionally, to account for other microenvironment triggers (such as inflammatory components) that can stimulate self-renewal capacity, the % of prostaspheres generated in the presence of macrophage THP-1 conditioned media (with and without IP6 pre-treatment) was determined. The results indicated that in vitro prostasphere assay performed with THP-1 conditioned media caused a ~1.5-fold increase ($p \leq 0.01$) in PC-3 prostaspheres formation compared to regular non-conditioned assay media. Notably, THP-1 conditioned media collected after pre-treatment of macrophages with IP6 lost its stimulating effect on self-renewal of PC-3 TICs/CSCs and was able to decrease the % prostasphere formation by ~45% ($p \leq 0.01$). Since formation of spheroids under specific in vitro conditions is a measure of stemness, it is evident that IP6 has the potential to target the self-renewal of TICs/CSCs in PCa cells (Figure 6).

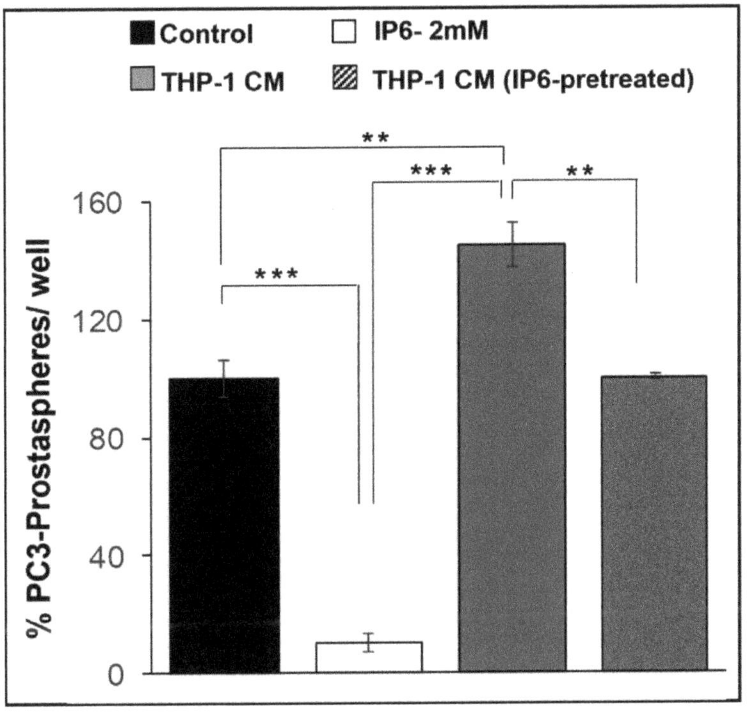

Figure 6. Effect of IP6 treatment on TICs/CSCs enriched prostaspheres in human prostate cancer PC-3 cancer cells. Effect of 2 mM IP6 treatment on TICs/CSCs ($CD44^{+}$-$\alpha 2\beta 1^{high}$) enriched prostaspheres formation, and effect on prostaspheres formation in the presence of macrophage THP-1 conditioned media and macrophage THP-1 conditioned media (pre-treated with IP6). Quantified data are represented as mean ± SEM. *** $p \leq 0.001$ and ** $p \leq 0.01$.

3.6. Stage-Specific Effect of IP6 Feeding on the Expression of CSC-Associated Signaling Molecules and Transcription Factors in TRAMP Prostate

TICs/CSCs highly express stemness-associated regulatory molecules and transcription factors such as Notch1, Shh, Sox-2, and Oct4. These molecules are associated with various signaling pathways that are recognized to be involved in tumor initiation, progression, self-renewal, stemness, neo-angiogenesis, and therapeutic resistance [41].

Cleaved Notch-1: IHC analysis for cleaved Notch-1 (activated Notch-1) expression revealed that its expression was markedly increased in all stages of PCa, especially in the more aggressive stages; however, there was no difference between low-grade and high-grade PIN stage expression, and the difference in cleaved Notch-1 expression was almost similar between WD, MD, and PD stages. Specifically, there was an increase of ~3.3 fold (LGPIN, $p \leq 0.01$), ~3.5 fold (HGPIN, $p \leq 0.001$), ~4.4 fold (WD, $p \leq 0.001$), ~4.2 fold (MD, $p \leq 0.01$), and ~4.6 fold (PD, $p \leq 0.001$) (Figure 7A, *upper left panel*) in the expression compared to WT controls. Likewise, the proportional area of dorsolateral prostate tissue having cleaved Notch-1 expression (immunopositive area) also increased compared to WT controls. Overall, there was an increase of ~2.5–3.5 fold in the average area of the prostate tissue having cleaved Notch-1 expression ($p \leq 0.01$) (Figure 7A, *upper right panel*) compared to WT controls. Next, we also assessed the effect of IP6 treatment on the expression and the area of dorsolateral positive for cleaved Notch-1 expression as a function of mice age. Results indicated that IP6-feeding had no significant effect on the cleaved Notch-1 expression nor was there any significant change in the proportion of prostate area positive for cleaved Notch-1 staining (Figure 7A, *lower panels*).

Shh: The expression of Shh increased significantly as a function of lesion stage, with a very strong expression in the adenocarcinoma stages. An increase of ~2.8 fold (LGPIN, $p \leq 0.05$), ~3.8 fold (HGPIN, $p \leq 0.05$), ~4.1 fold (WD, $p \leq 0.05$), ~5.0 fold (MD, $p \leq 0.01$), and ~5.3 fold (PD, $p \leq 0.01$) was observed for Shh expression in TRAMP prostates compared to WT controls (Figure 7B, *upper left panel*). The proportion of prostate area positive for Shh staining also increased in TRAMP controls with an increase in the aggressiveness of the tumor; specifically, there was an increase of ~1.3 fold (LGPIN), ~2.2 fold (HGPIN), ~3.6 fold (WD), and ~4.8 fold (for both MD and PD, $p \leq 0.001$) (Figure 7B, *upper right panel*) compared to WT controls. On the other hand, IP6 treatment was able to significantly decrease the expression of Shh across all the study time points. A decrease of ~38% (4–12 weeks group), ~51% (12–20 weeks group, $p \leq 0.05$), ~42% (20–30 weeks group, $p \leq 0.05$), and ~44% (30–45 weeks group, $p \leq 0.001$) in Shh expression was observed in the IP6-fed groups when compared to TRAMP controls (Figure 7B, *lower left panel*). Though a decrease in the Shh immunopositive area was also noted in the 4–12 and 30–45 weeks group by IP6 feeding, it was not statistically significant (Figure 7B, *lower right panel*).

Sox-2: Aberrant expression of Sox-2 can play a vital role in cancer progression by affecting the signaling pathways involved in tumor initiation, cell proliferation, epithelial-to-mesenchymal transition (EMT), migration, invasion, CSC regulation, and resistance to apoptosis and therapy [42]. Accordingly, we assessed the expression pattern of Sox-2 as a function of PCa aggressiveness. The expression of Sox-2 increased with aggressiveness in TRAMP prostate; however, in the PD stages, the expression was lower than in the MD stage. Specifically, Sox-2 expression increased by ~1.3 fold (LGPIN, $p \leq 0.01$), ~2.7 fold (HGPIN, $p \leq 0.001$), ~3.4 fold (WD, $p \leq 0.001$), ~3.5 fold (MD, $p \leq 0.001$), and ~2.5 fold (PD, $p \leq 0.01$) (Figure 8A, left panel) in TRAMP prostate compared to WT controls. IHC analysis in the IP6-fed groups revealed that Sox-2 expression was considerably decreased across all age groups. Specifically, the decrease in the immunoreactive score of Sox-2 in the IP6-fed group was ~93% (4–12 weeks group, $p \leq 0.05$), ~37% (12–20 weeks group), ~58% (20–30 weeks group, $p \leq 0.05$), and ~60% (30–45 weeks group, $p \leq 0.05$) (Figure 8A, *right panel*).

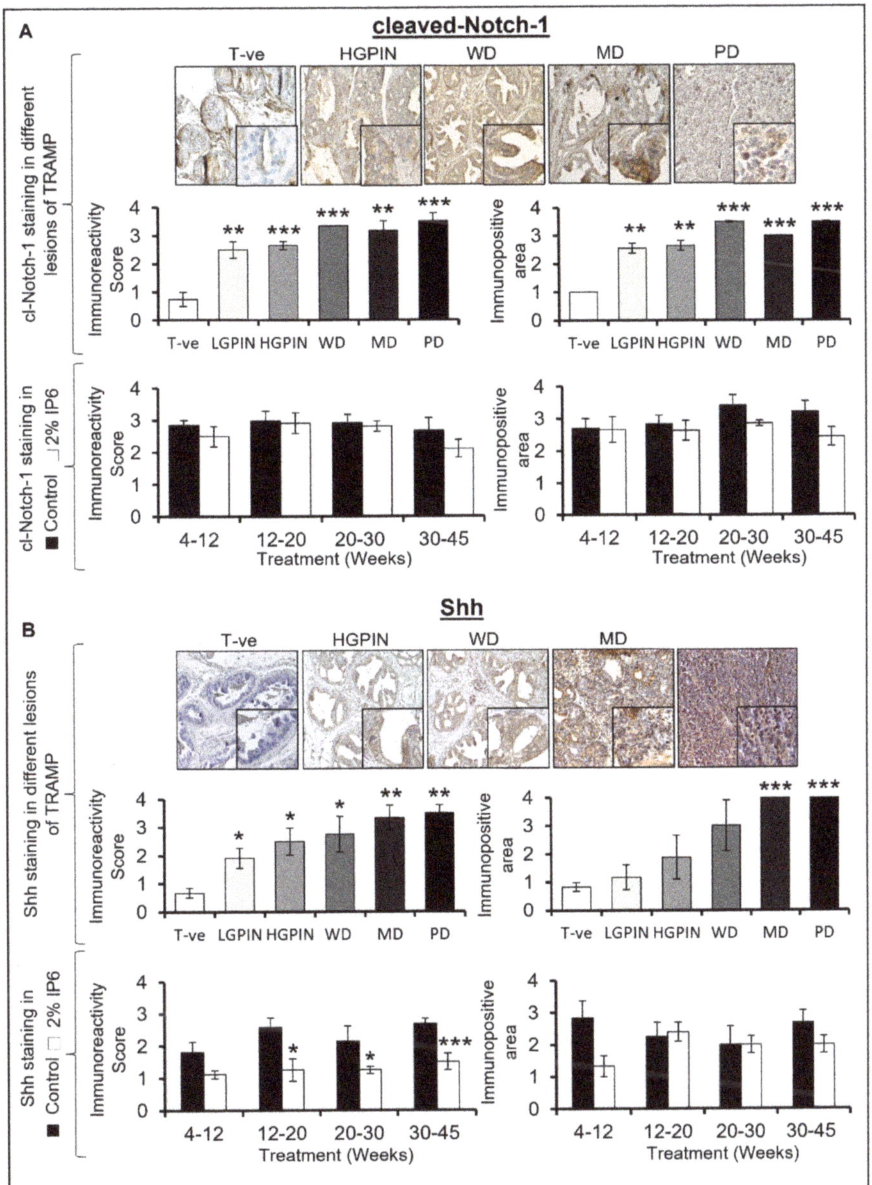

Figure 7. Stage specific effect of IP6 feeding on the expression of CSC-associated signaling molecules in the dorsolateral prostate of TRAMP mice. Pictographs and bar graphs representing the stage-specific expression of CSC-associated signaling molecules (**A**) cleaved-Notch-1, and (**B**) Shh, in WT control (T-ve), TRAMP control, and IP6-fed mice. Representative pictographs are depicted at ×100 magnification and insets represent digital magnifications. Immunoreactivity was scored as 0 (no staining), +1 (weak), +2 (moderate), +3 (strong), and +4 (very strong). The proportion area of prostate (positive for expression) was quantified as immunopositive area score and assigned arbitrary scores as 0 (<5% area), +1 (5–25% area), +2 (26–50% area), +3 (51–75% area), and +4 (>75% area). Quantified data are represented as mean ± SEM. *** $p \leq 0.001$, ** $p \leq 0.01$, and * $p \leq 0.05$.

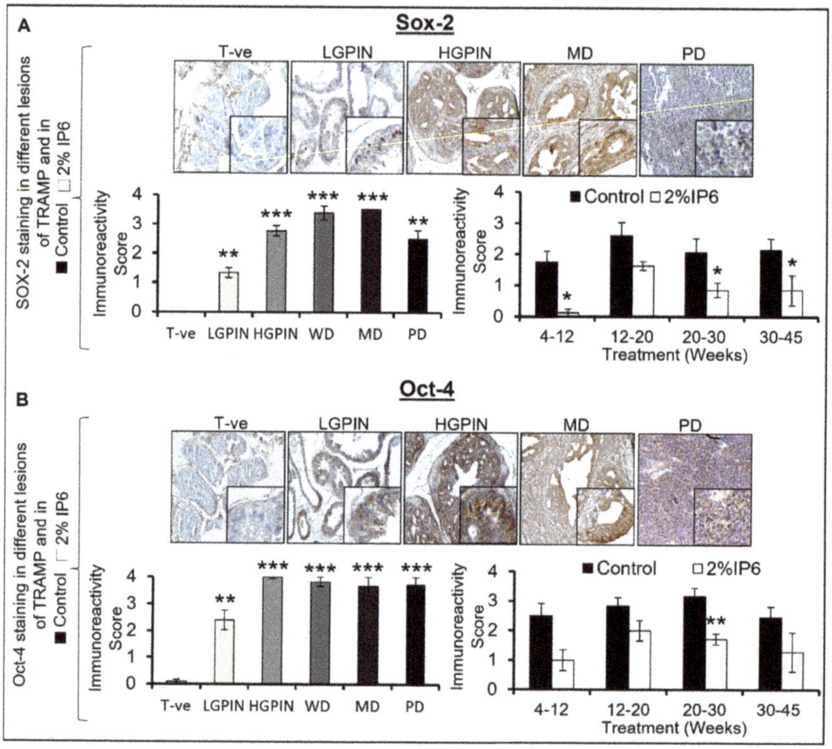

Figure 8. Stage-specific effect of IP6 feeding on the expression of CSC-associated transcription factors in the dorsolateral prostate of TRAMP mice. Pictographs and bar graphs representing the stage-specific expression of CSC-associated transcription factors (**A**) Sox-2, and (**B**) Oct-4, in WT control (Tr-ve), TRAMP control, and IP6-fed mice. Representative pictographs are depicted at ×100 magnification and insets represent digital magnifications. Immunoreactivity was scored as 0 (no staining), +1 (weak), +2 (moderate), +3 (strong), and +4 (very strong). Quantified data are represented as mean ± SEM. *** $p \leq 0.001$, ** $p \leq 0.01$, and * $p \leq 0.05$.

Oct-4: Oct-4 is a transcription factor involved in CSC maintenance and other associated oncogenic signaling pathways [43]. IHC analysis showed a marked increase in the expression of Oct-4 in PIN and adenocarcinoma stages; however, the expression in high-grade PIN and in WD, MD, and PD lesions was almost similar. Oct-4 expression increased by ~30 fold (LGPIN, $p \leq 0.01$), ~50 fold (HGPIN, $p \leq 0.001$), ~48 fold (WD, $p \leq 0.001$), ~45 fold (MD, $p \leq 0.001$), and ~47 fold (PD, $p \leq 0.001$) (Figure 8B, *left panel*) compared to WT controls. Notably, IP6 treatment decreased the expression of Oct-4 across all age groups. Specifically, IP6 treatment decreased the Oct-4 expression in the TRAMP prostates by ~60% (4–12 weeks group), ~29% (12–20 weeks group), ~46% (20–30 weeks group, $p \leq 0.01$), and ~48% (30–45 weeks group) (Figure 8B, *right panel*). Collectively, these results suggest that IP6 feeding can restrict the expansion of the TICs/CSC pool in the PCa by downregulating key molecular markers associated with the stemness and self-renewal-associated signaling pathways.

4. Discussion

Chemoprevention/intervention using natural non-toxic compounds has emerged as one of the alternate and viable therapies to control cancer prevalence [44]. This approach involves "halting or delaying" cancer at critical stages of carcinogenesis such as tumor initiation, promotion, and progression [45,46]. IP6, a naturally occurring poly-phosphorylated carbohydrate present in many dietary sources with high fiber content such as legumes, has been explored for its anti-cancer efficacy against various cancers [11,12,47]. Several studies have also demonstrated that IP6 does not cause any apparent toxicity in cell culture and animal models of different origins including the PWR-1E normal prostate epithelial cells and TRAMP mouse model [11,12,48].

In the present study, we focused on elucidating the stage-specific efficacy of IP6 against PCa growth and progression in TRAMP mice. IP6 (2% in drinking water) was fed to TRAMP mice at different stages of PCa development and then the efficacy of IP6 was evaluated on PCa growth, progression, angiogenesis, and expansion of the CSC pool. Notably, IP6 feeding to TRAMP mice at an early age restricted the onset of neoplastic characteristics and delayed the tumor growth to advanced stages. As early as 4–12 weeks of treatment regimen, in IP6-fed mice, 100% of prostate tissue was restricted to PIN stages only, whereas TRAMP prostate advanced to more aggressive adenocarcinoma lesions. This trend continued in other study time points groups with IP6-fed groups displaying much less advanced PCa lesions and TRAMP controls displaying an increased incidence of invasive adenocarcinoma lesions. For example, in the 12–20 weeks group, IP6 feeding restricted the tumor growth to PIN lesions only, while in the 20–30 and 30–45 weeks cohorts the incidence of adenocarcinoma lesions was significantly lower in IP6-fed mice compared to the TRAMP controls. This observation was also supported by the moderate decrease in the percent area covered by PIN and adenocarcinoma lesions throughout all the stages of PCa in IP6-fed TRAMP mice. IP6 feeding also reduced the mean peak tumor grades, thus suggesting that IP6 reduces the prostatic tumor lesion severity in TRAMP mice. These observations indicate the clinical potential of IP6 in restricting the growth and progression of PCa at different stages of tumorigenesis.

Aberrant cellular proliferation and evasion of apoptosis are some of the most important hallmarks of cancer [49]. Several natural compounds and dietary phytochemicals have been studied for their ability to inhibit proliferative ability and induce apoptosis in cancer cells [50]. In previous studies, IP6 was shown to inhibit cellular proliferation and induce apoptosis in PCa cells [16–18]. In the present study, IP6 considerably decreased the proliferative index and induced apoptosis in the prostatic tissues of TRAMP mice across all tumor stages.

Cancer cells exhibit high levels of aerobic glycolysis to meet the needs of aberrantly proliferating cells. In this regard, dysregulated expression of glucose transporters (GLUTs) has been observed in cancer cells [51]. GLUT4, one of the glucose transporters, is highly expressed in PCa cells [28]. Immunohistochemical staining for GLUT4 in TRAMP prostate showed a significant increase in the expression of GLUT4 as a function of mice age. On the contrary, IP6-fed groups showed a significant reduction in the expression of GLUT4 across all stages, especially in the later time points of the study. This observation suggests that IP6 exerts its anticancer efficacy by modulating glucose uptake and transport in different stages of tumorigenesis.

Activation of neo-angiogenesis is one of the early prerequisites for cancer progression to advanced stages [52]. VEGF expression has been inversely associated with survival in PCa cancer patients [53]; studies have also indicated that microvessel density increases as a function of tumor grade in prostate cancer [54]. In this regard, we observed that IP6 treatment was able to decrease the expression of both CD-31 and VEGF substantially when compared to the TRAMP controls in different stages of tumorigenesis. Additionally, IP6 treatment also modulated the expression of iNOS and CXCR3, which are recognized to play critical roles in PCa progression [30–33]. Overall, these results establish the anti-angiogenic potential of IP6 in stemming the progression of prostate cancer to advanced stages.

PCa is a highly heterogeneous cancer, genetically as well as phenotypically, which makes it difficult to treat using conventional therapies [55]. The TICs/CSCs are a subpopulation of tumor cells that are predominantly recognized as the ones imparting this heterogeneity to PCa [55]. TICs/CSCs are endowed with tumor-initiating potential and can also aid in growth and progression to advanced stages. These cells have distinct biomarkers, and they exhibit high plasticity which allows them to change their phenotypic and functional profile [56] and they can be identified based on the cell surface molecular markers such as CD44 and CD133 [57]. Genetic characterization of TICs/CSCs can be performed by investigating the expression of stemness genes, transcription factors, and associated regulatory molecules such as Oct-4, Sox-2, Shh, BMI-1, and Notch-1 [57,58]. These molecular markers collectively help maintain the TICs/CSC pool, which is vital for increased aggressiveness in cancers. Several studies have established the role of the above-mentioned markers in imparting self-renewal and therapy resistance to PCa cells [35,57,59]. A dual staining assay for CD44 and BMI-1 demonstrated that there was an elevated expression of CD44 and BMI-1 in the TRAMP prostates which was considerably downregulated by IP6 treatment across all tumor stages. Additionally, an in vitro prostasphere corroborated the above inhibitory effects of IP6 on the TICs/CSC pool (even in the presence of stimulatory signals from the immune compartment) suggesting that IP6 inhibitory effects on PCa growth could be partly attributed to its potential to target self-renewal of TICs/CSCs. Furthermore, while TICs/CSCs-associated molecular markers increased with tumorigenesis in the TRAMP prostate, IP6 feeding significantly decreased the expression of these molecules, with the most significant effect on the expression levels of Shh, Sox-2, and Oct-4. These results indicate that the molecular markers associated with the TICs/CSCs pool play a vital role in PCa progression and that IP6 exerts its inhibitory PCa effects by impacting this vital cell pool driving prostate tumorigenesis. Taken together, the efficacy outcomes from different stages of PCa and parallel molecular assessments indicated that IP6 feeding could impact tumor metabolism via interfering in glucose uptake (due to its effect on GLUT-4 expression) which in turn could slow down tumor proliferation early on. Furthermore, during the progression phase of PCa, IP6 feeding, apart from interfering with tumor metabolism, restricted angiogenesis promoting signals which arrested progression to advanced stages of PCa. In addition, the beneficial effects of IP6 against PCa could also be attributed to its negative impact on the CSC pool directly, as well as the tumor promoting signaling originating from the tumor microenvironment, which could benefit in early as well as late phases of tumorigenesis (including tumor recurrence). However, the present study did not investigate the in-depth mechanistic associations which could help establish the upstream and downstream modulators involved in cross-signaling nexus between the pathways modulated by IP6; such studies are warranted in future to delineate the anti-PCa mechanism associated with IP6 intake.

5. Conclusions

Together, these observations are highly significant and for the first time establish the stage-specific efficacy of IP6 feeding during prostate tumorigenesis in TRAMP mice. The present study, in combination with our earlier findings in pre-clinical in vitro and in vivo models including TRAMP mice, implies a strong efficacy of inositol hexaphosphate against all stages of prostate tumorigenesis with scientific rationale and it advocates for future clinical trials in patients with PIN and/or low to high-grade PCa.

Supplementary Materials: The following supporting information can be downloaded at: https://www.mdpi.com/article/10.3390/cancers14174204/s1, Figure S1: Stage-specific effect of IP6 feeding on the LUT weight of TRAMP mice; Figure S2: Representative pictographs (×100 magnification) of H&E stained dorsolateral prostate tissue from TRAMP control and IP6-fed TRAMP mice in the 30–45 week group.

Author Contributions: Concept and design: K.R. (Komal Raina) and R.A.; development of methodology: K.R. (Komal Raina) and R.A.; performed experiments: K.R. (Komal Raina), A.K.J., K.R. (Kameswaran Ravichandran) and C.A.; acquisition of data: K.R. (Komal Raina), A.K.J. and K.K.; analysis and interpretation of data: K.R. (Komal Raina), A.K.J. and K.K.; writing and revision/review of MS: K.K., K.R. (Komal Raina) and R.A.; administrative, technical, and material support: C.A., P.M. and R.A.; study supervision: K.R. (Komal Raina) and R.A. All authors have read and agreed to the published version of the manuscript.

Funding: This work was supported by NIH/National Cancer Institute grant R01-CA116636 to R.A. and generous support from the Diane D. Writer Foundation and the Barbara and Richard Gardner Fund for Prostate Cancer Research. This work was also supported by UCCSG P30CA046934 for supporting the shared resources used in this study.

Institutional Review Board Statement: All animal studies were performed under institutional guidelines using an approved Institutional Animal Care and Use Committee (IACUC) protocol [#B-57915(02)1E] in the specific pathogen-free facility at UC Denver-AMC.

Informed Consent Statement: Not applicable.

Data Availability Statement: The data presented in this study are available on request from the corresponding author.

Conflicts of Interest: The authors declare no conflict of interest.

Abbreviations

CSCs	Cancer stem cells
DAB	3, 3 -diaminobenzidine
FACS	Fluorescence-activated cell sorting
HGPIN	High-grade prostatic intraepithelial neoplasia
IHC	Immunohistochemistry
LGPIN	Low-grade prostatic intraepithelial neoplasia
LUT	Lower urogenital tract
MD	Moderately differentiated
PCa	Prostate cancer
PCNA	Proliferating cell nuclear antigen
PD	Poorly differentiated
PIN	Prostatic intraepithelial neoplasia
PMA	Phorbol 12-myristate
Shh	Sonic hedgehog
TICs	Tumor-initiating cells
TUNEL	Terminal deoxynucleotidyl transferase-mediated dUTP nick end labeling
WD	Well-differentiated

References

1. Siegel, R.L.; Miller, K.D.; Fuchs, H.E.; Jemal, A. Cancer statistics, 2022. *CA Cancer J. Clin.* **2022**, *72*, 7–33. [CrossRef] [PubMed]
2. Sung, H.; Ferlay, J.; Siegel, R.L.; Laversanne, M.; Soerjomataram, I.; Jemal, A.; Bray, F. Global Cancer Statistics 2020: GLOBOCAN Estimates of Incidence and Mortality Worldwide for 36 Cancers in 185 Countries. *CA Cancer J. Clin.* **2021**, *71*, 209–249. [CrossRef] [PubMed]
3. Dong, L.; Zieren, R.C.; Xue, W.; de Reijke, T.M.; Pienta, K.J. Metastatic prostate cancer remains incurable, why? *Asian J. Urol.* **2019**, *6*, 26–41. [CrossRef] [PubMed]
4. Rawla, P. Epidemiology of Prostate Cancer. *World J. Oncol.* **2019**, *10*, 63–89. [CrossRef]
5. Bashir, M.N. Epidemiology of Prostate Cancer. *Asian Pac. J. Cancer Prev.* **2015**, *16*, 5137–5141. [CrossRef]
6. Badal, S.; Aiken, W.; Morrison, B.; Valentine, H.; Bryan, S.; Gachii, A.; Ragin, C. Disparities in prostate cancer incidence and mortality rates: Solvable or not? *Prostate* **2020**, *80*, 3–16. [CrossRef]
7. Singla, R.K.; Sharma, P.; Dubey, A.K.; Gundamaraju, R.; Kumar, D.; Kumar, S.; Madaan, R.; Shri, R.; Tsagkaris, C.; Parisi, S.; et al. Natural Product-Based Studies for the Management of Castration-Resistant Prostate Cancer: Computational to Clinical Studies. *Front. Pharmacol.* **2021**, *12*, 732266. [CrossRef]
8. Mokbel, K.; Wazir, U.; Mokbel, K. Chemoprevention of Prostate Cancer by Natural Agents: Evidence from Molecular and Epidemiological Studies. *Anticancer Res.* **2019**, *39*, 5231–5259. [CrossRef]
9. Fontana, F.; Raimondi, M.; Marzagalli, M.; Di Domizio, A.; Limonta, P. Natural Compounds in Prostate Cancer Prevention and Treatment: Mechanisms of Action and Molecular Targets. *Cells* **2020**, *9*, 460. [CrossRef]
10. Livingstone, T.L.; Beasy, G.; Mills, R.D.; Plumb, J.; Needs, P.W.; Mithen, R.; Traka, M.H. Plant Bioactives and the Prevention of Prostate Cancer: Evidence from Human Studies. *Nutrients* **2019**, *11*, 2245. [CrossRef]
11. Vucenik, I.; Shamsuddin, A.M. Protection against cancer by dietary IP6 and inositol. *Nutr. Cancer* **2006**, *55*, 109–125. [CrossRef] [PubMed]
12. Singh, R.P.; Agarwal, R. Prostate cancer and inositol hexaphosphate: Efficacy and mechanisms. *Anticancer Res.* **2005**, *25*, 2891–2903. [PubMed]

13. Gu, M.; Raina, K.; Agarwal, C.; Agarwal, R. Inositol hexaphosphate downregulates both constitutive and ligand-induced mitogenic and cell survival signaling, and causes caspase-mediated apoptotic death of human prostate carcinoma PC-3 cells. *Mol. Carcinog.* **2010**, *49*, 1–12. [CrossRef] [PubMed]
14. Zhu, H.P.; Yun, F.; Jiu, T. Inhibitory effect of inositol hexaphosphate on proliferation of LNCaP cells and its relation to IGFBP 3 expression. *Zhejiang Da Xue Xue Bao Yi Xue Ban* **2014**, *43*, 521–527. [CrossRef]
15. Jagadeesh, S.; Banerjee, P.P. Inositol hexaphosphate represses telomerase activity and translocates TERT from the nucleus in mouse and human prostate cancer cells via the deactivation of Akt and PKC alpha. *Biochem. Biophys. Res. Commun.* **2006**, *349*, 1361–1367. [CrossRef] [PubMed]
16. Singh, R.P.; Agarwal, C.; Agarwal, R. Inositol hexaphosphate inhibits growth, and induces G1 arrest and apoptotic death of prostate carcinoma DU145 cells: Modulation of CDKI-CDK-cyclin and pRb-related protein-E2F complexes. *Carcinogenesis* **2003**, *24*, 555–563. [CrossRef]
17. Gu, M.; Roy, S.; Raina, K.; Agarwal, C.; Agarwal, R. Inositol hexaphosphate suppresses growth and induces apoptosis in prostate carcinoma cells in culture and nude mouse xenograft: PI3K-Akt pathway as potential target. *Cancer Res.* **2009**, *69*, 9465–9472. [CrossRef] [PubMed]
18. Roy, S.; Gu, M.; Ramasamy, K.; Singh, R.P.; Agarwal, C.; Siriwardana, S.; Sclafani, R.A.; Agarwal, R. p21/Cip1 and p27/Kip1 Are essential molecular targets of inositol hexaphosphate for its antitumor efficacy against prostate cancer. *Cancer Res.* **2009**, *69*, 1166–1173. [CrossRef]
19. Raina, K.; Rajamanickam, S.; Singh, R.P.; Agarwal, R. Chemopreventive efficacy of inositol hexaphosphate against prostate tumor growth and progression in TRAMP mice. *Clin. Cancer Res.* **2008**, *14*, 3177–3184. [CrossRef]
20. Raina, K.; Ravichandran, K.; Rajamanickam, S.; Huber, K.M.; Serkova, N.J.; Agarwal, R. Inositol hexaphosphate inhibits tumor growth, vascularity, and metabolism in TRAMP mice: A multiparametric magnetic resonance study. *Cancer Prev. Res.* **2013**, *6*, 40–50. [CrossRef]
21. Fenton, J.I.; Hord, N.G. Stage matters: Choosing relevant model systems to address hypotheses in diet and cancer chemoprevention research. *Carcinogenesis* **2006**, *27*, 893–902. [CrossRef] [PubMed]
22. Raina, K.; Rajamanickam, S.; Singh, R.P.; Deep, G.; Chittezhath, M.; Agarwal, R. Stage-specific inhibitory effects and associated mechanisms of silibinin on tumor progression and metastasis in transgenic adenocarcinoma of the mouse prostate model. *Cancer Res.* **2008**, *68*, 6822–6830. [CrossRef]
23. Kaplan-Lefko, P.J.; Chen, T.-M.; Ittmann, M.M.; Barrios, R.J.; Ayala, G.E.; Huss, W.J.; Maddison, L.A.; Foster, B.A.; Greenberg, N.M. Pathobiology of autochthonous prostate cancer in a pre-clinical transgenic mouse model. *Prostate* **2003**, *55*, 219–237. [CrossRef] [PubMed]
24. da Silva, R.F.; Dhar, D.; Raina, K.; Kumar, D.; Kant, R.; Cagnon, V.H.A.; Agarwal, C.; Agarwal, R. Nintedanib inhibits growth of human prostate carcinoma cells by modulating both cell cycle and angiogenesis regulators. *Sci. Rep.* **2018**, *8*, 9540. [CrossRef] [PubMed]
25. Raina, K.; Kant, R.; Prasad, R.R.; Kandhari, K.; Tomar, M.; Mishra, N.; Kumar, R.; Fox, J.T.; Sei, S.; Shoemaker, R.H.; et al. Characterization of stage-specific tumor progression in TMPRSS2-ERG (fusion)-driven and non-fusion-driven prostate cancer in GEM models. *Mol. Carcinog.* **2022**, *61*, 717–734. [CrossRef] [PubMed]
26. Tyagi, A.; Kumar, S.; Raina, K.; Wempe, M.F.; Maroni, P.D.; Agarwal, R.; Agarwal, C. Differential effect of grape seed extract and its active constituent procyanidin B2 3,3″-di-O-gallate against prostate cancer stem cells. *Mol. Carcinog.* **2019**, *58*, 1105–1117. [CrossRef]
27. Hay, N. Reprogramming glucose metabolism in cancer: Can it be exploited for cancer therapy? *Nat. Rev. Cancer* **2016**, *16*, 635–649. [CrossRef]
28. Gonzalez-Menendez, P.; Hevia, D.; Mayo, J.C.; Sainz, R.M. The dark side of glucose transporters in prostate cancer: Are they a new feature to characterize carcinomas? *Int. J. Cancer* **2018**, *142*, 2414–2424. [CrossRef]
29. Cronauer, M.V.; Ince, Y.; Engers, R.; Rinnab, L.; Weidemann, W.; Suschek, C.V.; Burchardt, M.; Kleinert, H.; Wiedenmann, J.; Sies, H.; et al. Nitric oxide-mediated inhibition of androgen receptor activity: Possible implications for prostate cancer progression. *Oncogene* **2007**, *26*, 1875–1884. [CrossRef]
30. Soni, Y.; Softness, K.; Arora, H.; Ramasamy, R. The Yin Yang Role of Nitric Oxide in Prostate Cancer. *Am. J. Mens Health* **2020**, *14*, 1557988320903191. [CrossRef]
31. Ehlert, J.E.; Addison, C.A.; Burdick, M.D.; Kunkel, S.L.; Strieter, R.M. Identification and partial characterization of a variant of human CXCR3 generated by posttranscriptional exon skipping. *J. Immunol.* **2004**, *173*, 6234–6240. [CrossRef] [PubMed]
32. Loetscher, M.; Loetscher, P.; Brass, N.; Meese, E.; Moser, B. Lymphocyte-specific chemokine receptor CXCR3: Regulation, chemokine binding and gene localization. *Eur. J. Immunol.* **1998**, *28*, 3696–3705. [CrossRef]
33. Luster, A.D.; Cardiff, R.D.; MacLean, J.A.; Crowe, K.; Granstein, R.D. Delayed wound healing and disorganized neovascularization in transgenic mice expressing the IP-10 chemokine. *Proc. Assoc. Am. Physicians* **1998**, *110*, 183–196. [PubMed]
34. Nagpal, M.L.; Davis, J.; Lin, T. Overexpression of CXCL10 in human prostate LNCaP cells activates its receptor (CXCR3) expression and inhibits cell proliferation. *Biochim. Biophys. Acta* **2006**, *1762*, 811–818. [CrossRef]
35. Mei, W.; Lin, X.; Kapoor, A.; Gu, Y.; Zhao, K.; Tang, D. The Contributions of Prostate Cancer Stem Cells in Prostate Cancer Initiation and Metastasis. *Cancers* **2019**, *11*, 434. [CrossRef]

36. Celia-Terrassa, T.; Jolly, M.K. Cancer Stem Cells and Epithelial-to-Mesenchymal Transition in Cancer Metastasis. *Cold Spring Harb. Perspect. Med.* **2020**, *10*, a036905. [CrossRef]
37. Liou, G.Y. CD133 as a regulator of cancer metastasis through the cancer stem cells. *Int. J. Biochem. Cell Biol.* **2019**, *106*, 1–7. [CrossRef]
38. Kandhari, K.; Agraval, H.; Sharma, A.; Yadav, U.C.S.; Singh, R.P. Flavonoids and Cancer Stem Cells Maintenance and Growth. In *Functional Food and Human Health*; Rani, V., Yadav, U.C.S., Eds.; Springer: Singapore, 2018; pp. 587–622.
39. Li, W.; Qian, L.; Lin, J.; Huang, G.; Hao, N.; Wei, X.; Wang, W.; Liang, J. CD44 regulates prostate cancer proliferation, invasion and migration via PDK1 and PFKFB4. *Oncotarget* **2017**, *8*, 65143–65151. [CrossRef]
40. Bansal, N.; Bartucci, M.; Yusuff, S.; Davis, S.; Flaherty, K.; Huselid, E.; Patrizii, M.; Jones, D.; Cao, L.; Sydorenko, N.; et al. BMI-1 Targeting Interferes with Patient-Derived Tumor-Initiating Cell Survival and Tumor Growth in Prostate Cancer. *Clin. Cancer Res.* **2016**, *22*, 6176–6191. [CrossRef]
41. Borovski, T.; De Sousa, E.M.F.; Vermeulen, L.; Medema, J.P. Cancer stem cell niche: The place to be. *Cancer Res.* **2011**, *71*, 634–639. [CrossRef]
42. Novak, D.; Huser, L.; Elton, J.J.; Umansky, V.; Altevogt, P.; Utikal, J. SOX2 in development and cancer biology. *Semin. Cancer Biol.* **2020**, *67*, 74–82. [CrossRef] [PubMed]
43. Zhang, Q.; Han, Z.; Zhu, Y.; Chen, J.; Li, W. The Role and Specific Mechanism of OCT4 in Cancer Stem Cells: A Review. *Int. J. Stem. Cells* **2020**, *13*, 312–325. [CrossRef] [PubMed]
44. Steward, W.P.; Brown, K. Cancer chemoprevention: A rapidly evolving field. *Br. J. Cancer* **2013**, *109*, 1–7. [CrossRef] [PubMed]
45. Ranjan, A.; Ramachandran, S.; Gupta, N.; Kaushik, I.; Wright, S.; Srivastava, S.; Das, H.; Srivastava, S.; Prasad, S.; Srivastava, S.K. Role of Phytochemicals in Cancer Prevention. *Int. J. Mol. Sci.* **2019**, *20*, 4981. [CrossRef] [PubMed]
46. Ramos, S. Cancer chemoprevention and chemotherapy: Dietary polyphenols and signalling pathways. *Mol. Nutr. Food Res.* **2008**, *52*, 507–526. [CrossRef] [PubMed]
47. Somasundar, P.; Riggs, D.R.; Jackson, B.J.; Cunningham, C.; Vona-Davis, L.; McFadden, D.W. Inositol hexaphosphate (IP6): A novel treatment for pancreatic cancer. *J. Surg. Res.* **2005**, *126*, 199–203. [CrossRef]
48. Vucenik, I.; Shamsuddin, A.M. Cancer inhibition by inositol hexaphosphate (IP6) and inositol: From laboratory to clinic. *J. Nutr.* **2003**, *133*, 3778S–3784S. [CrossRef]
49. Hanahan, D.; Weinberg, R.A. Hallmarks of cancer: The next generation. *Cell* **2011**, *144*, 646–674. [CrossRef]
50. Kotecha, R.; Takami, A.; Espinoza, J.L. Dietary phytochemicals and cancer chemoprevention: A review of the clinical evidence. *Oncotarget* **2016**, *7*, 52517–52529. [CrossRef]
51. Hamanaka, R.B.; Chandel, N.S. Targeting glucose metabolism for cancer therapy. *J. Exp. Med.* **2012**, *209*, 211–215. [CrossRef]
52. Zuazo-Gaztelu, I.; Casanovas, O. Unraveling the Role of Angiogenesis in Cancer Ecosystems. *Front. Oncol.* **2018**, *8*, 248. [CrossRef] [PubMed]
53. Zhan, P.; Ji, Y.N.; Yu, L.K. VEGF is associated with the poor survival of patients with prostate cancer: A meta-analysis. *Transl. Androl. Urol.* **2013**, *2*, 99–105. [CrossRef] [PubMed]
54. Huss, W.J.; Hanrahan, C.F.; Barrios, R.J.; Simons, J.W.; Greenberg, N.M. Angiogenesis and Prostate Cancer: Identification of A Molecular Progression Switch1. *Cancer Res.* **2001**, *61*, 2736–2743. [PubMed]
55. Haffner, M.C.; Zwart, W.; Roudier, M.P.; True, L.D.; Nelson, W.G.; Epstein, J.I.; De Marzo, A.M.; Nelson, P.S.; Yegnasubramanian, S. Genomic and phenotypic heterogeneity in prostate cancer. *Nat. Rev. Urol.* **2021**, *18*, 79–92. [CrossRef]
56. Walcher, L.; Kistenmacher, A.-K.; Suo, H.; Kitte, R.; Dluczek, S.; Strauß, A.; Blaudszun, A.-R.; Yevsa, T.; Fricke, S.; Kossatz-Boehlert, U. Cancer Stem Cells—Origins and Biomarkers: Perspectives for Targeted Personalized Therapies. *Front. Immunol.* **2020**, *11*, 1280. [CrossRef]
57. Moltzahn, F.; Thalmann, G.N. Cancer stem cells in prostate cancer. *Transl. Androl. Urol.* **2013**, *2*, 242–253. [CrossRef]
58. Thomas, E.; Thankan, R.S.; Purushottamachar, P.; Huang, W.; Kane, M.A.; Zhang, Y.; Ambulos, N.; Weber, D.J.; Njar, V.C.O. Transcriptome profiling reveals that VNPP433-3β, the lead next-generation galeterone analog inhibits prostate cancer stem cells by downregulating epithelial-mesenchymal transition and stem cell markers. *Mol. Carcinog.* **2022**, *61*, 643–654. [CrossRef]
59. Leao, R.; Domingos, C.; Figueiredo, A.; Hamilton, R.; Tabori, U.; Castelo-Branco, P. Cancer Stem Cells in Prostate Cancer: Implications for Targeted Therapy. *Urol. Int.* **2017**, *99*, 125–136. [CrossRef]

cancers

Review

Effects of Green Tea Catechins on Prostate Cancer Chemoprevention: The Role of the Gut Microbiome

Nagi B. Kumar [1,2,*], Stephanie Hogue [1], Julio Pow-Sang [2], Michael Poch [2], Brandon J. Manley [2], Roger Li [2], Jasreman Dhillon [3], Alice Yu [2] and Doratha A. Byrd [1,4]

1 Cancer Epidemiology Program, Moffitt Cancer Center and Research Institute, Tampa, FL 33612, USA
2 Genitourinary Oncology, Moffitt Cancer Center and Research Institute, Tampa, FL 33612, USA
3 Anatomic Pathology, Moffitt Cancer Center and Research Institute, Tampa, FL 33612, USA
4 Gastrointestinal Oncology, Moffitt Cancer Center and Research Institute, Tampa, FL 33612, USA
* Correspondence: nagi.kumar@moffitt.org

Simple Summary: Green tea is known for its health benefits deriving from molecules called green tea catechins (GTCs). GTCs have been demonstrated to influence molecular pathways to halt the progression of prostate cancer (PCa) and may be of particular benefit to men with low-risk PCa who are placed on active surveillance. Administering GTCs may provide patients an opportunity to be actively engaged in their treatment and help prevent cancer progression. Importantly, the trillions of microbes in the gut (the gut microbiome) metabolize GTCs, making them more accessible to the body to exert their health effects. Additionally, the gut microbiome influences multiple other processes likely involved in PCa progression, including regulating inflammation, hormones, and other known/unknown pathways. In this review, we discuss (1) the role of GTCs in preventing PCa progression; (2) current evidence for associations of the microbiome with PCa; and (3) utilizing the microbiome to identify markers that may predict improved response to GTCs to enhance clinical decision-making.

Abstract: Accumulating evidence supports green tea catechins (GTCs) in chemoprevention for prostate cancer (PCa), a leading cause of cancer morbidity and mortality among men. GTCs include (−)-epigallocatechin-3-gallate, which may modulate the molecular pathways implicated in prostate carcinogenesis. Prior studies of GTCs suggested that they are bioavailable, safe, and effective for modulating clinical and biological markers implicated in prostate carcinogenesis. GTCs may be of particular benefit to those with low-grade PCas typically managed with careful monitoring via active surveillance (AS). Though AS is recommended, it has limitations including potential under-grading, variations in eligibility, and anxiety reported by men while on AS. Secondary chemoprevention of low-grade PCas using GTCs may help address these limitations. When administrated orally, the gut microbiome enzymatically transforms GTC structure, altering its bioavailability, bioactivity, and toxicity. In addition to xenobiotic metabolism, the gut microbiome has multiple other physiological effects potentially involved in PCa progression, including regulating inflammation, hormones, and other known/unknown pathways. Therefore, it is important to consider not only the independent roles of GTCs and the gut microbiome in the context of PCa chemoprevention, but how gut microbes may relate to individual responses to GTCs, which, in turn, can enhance clinical decision-making.

Keywords: prostate cancer; green tea catechins; microbiome; chemoprevention

Citation: Kumar, N.B.; Hogue, S.; Pow-Sang, J.; Poch, M.; Manley, B.J.; Li, R.; Dhillon, J.; Yu, A.; Byrd, D.A. Effects of Green Tea Catechins on Prostate Cancer Chemoprevention: The Role of the Gut Microbiome. *Cancers* **2022**, *14*, 3988. https://doi.org/10.3390/cancers14163988

Academic Editor: Anupam Bishayee

Received: 14 July 2022
Accepted: 16 August 2022
Published: 18 August 2022

1. Introduction

The American Cancer Society estimates that there will be 268,490 and 34,500 new cases of and deaths due to prostate cancer (PCa) in the United States (US) in 2022, respectively [1]. Over the past two decades, PCa screening via serum prostate-specific antigen (PSA) led to substantial increases in detection of low-risk PCas (Gleason score ≤ 6), which pose little risk of either metastatic spread or death [2–5]. Conversely, over-treatment is a well-documented consequence of over-detection of PCa, predominantly occurring among men with low-risk PCa who may be subject to multiple treatment-related morbidities with negligible or no benefit towards cancer-specific survival [4,6]. Thus, the recommended guideline for the management of low-risk disease is active surveillance (AS). However, there are several identified challenges with AS, ranging from concerns with under-grading [7–13], patient-related factors (e.g., anxiety, depression, doubts about the possible progression of disease), and higher decisional conflict regarding the selection of AS [14–16], leading many to ultimately opt for a treatment that does not beneficially change tumor characteristics. On the other hand, men on AS are a highly motivated subgroup eager to make positive lifestyle changes to reduce their risk of PCa progression [16–21], providing an optimal opportunity to intervene during this window with promising chemopreventive agents for PCa.

Previous strategies for PCa chemoprevention included 5-alpha-reductase inhibitors, finasteride, dutasteride [22–24], trace element selenomethionine, and/or vitamin E. Collectively, these agents demonstrated greater risk for high grade disease [25] or no reduction in risk of PCa progression in large phase III trials, severely limiting their clinical adoption [23]. To date, there is minimal evidence available for the efficacy of any one agent or strategy for chemoprevention of PCa among men on AS. Therefore, the goal of our team for PCa chemoprevention is to utilize a systematic, broad-spectrum approach [26] that involves an agent shown to (a) be bioavailable; (b) have an excellent safety profile; (c) produce robust targeting of multiple relevant molecular pathways; and (d) modulate measurable intermediate endpoint biomarkers correlated with early clinical progression of PCa—an approach that collectively may be more effective than agents evaluated to date. Our team and others have evaluated several approaches (i.e., diet interventions) and agents (selenium, vitamin E, isoflavones, lycopene n-3 fatty acids, and green tea catechins, or GTCs) targeting prostate carcinogenesis.

Human PCa is a complex heterogeneous disease. The central driving forces of prostate carcinogenesis include acquisitions of diverse sets of hallmark capabilities, aberrant functioning of androgen receptor signaling, deregulation of vital cell physiological processes, inactivation of tumor-suppressive activity, and disruption of prostate gland-specific cellular homeostasis. Thus, the molecular complexity and redundancy of oncoprotein signaling in PCa demands for concurrent inhibition of multiple hallmark-associated pathways [27]. The ultimate goal for clinical cancer chemoprevention is to utilize a systematic, broad-spectrum approach that involves identifying and evaluating agents that can: (a) produce robust and concurrent inhibition of multiple hallmark-associated pathways in the target tissue/microenvironment; (b) address the underlying biology of carcinogenesis; and (c) enhance bioavailability and half-life with minimal toxicity in exceptionally high-risk populations [26,28]. GTCs comprise (−)-epigallocatechin-3-gallate (EGCG), (−)-epicatechin, (−)-epigallocatechin (EGC), and (−)-epicatechin-3-gallate. Among the agents evaluated to date, EGCG in particular has been demonstrated to affect molecular pathways implicated in prostate carcinogenesis.

The objective of this review is to summarize the current research on the safety and effectiveness of GTCs in modulating prostate carcinogenesis based on population, in vitro, pre-clinical and early clinical trials. Although previous reviews have examined the pre-clinical and early phase trials of GTCs and PCa [29–33], our review will additionally identify discrepancies in the results of previous studies and examine the early and evolving data on the role of the gut microbiome in modulating the bioavailability, safety, and anticarcinogenic properties of GTCs in prostate carcinogenesis.

2. GTCs: Promising Agent for PCa Chemoprevention

The most abundant constituents of green tea are the polyphenols, which are catechins that represent 30–40% of the dry weight of the tea leaves. The catechins in green tea belong to the flavon-3-ols of the polyphenol family [34]. Laboratory studies have identified EGCG as the most potent modulator of molecular pathways thought to be relevant to prostate carcinogenesis [35–38]. In the past two decades, research studies have shown that GTCs influence multiple biochemical and molecular cascades that inhibit several hallmarks of carcinogenesis relevant to prostate carcinogenesis. With an acceptable safety profile, GTCs are ideal candidates for PCa chemoprevention. Laboratory studies demonstrate that EGCG can affect several cancer-related proteins, including p27, Bcl-2 or Bcr-Abl oncoproteins, Bax, matrix metalloproteinases (MMP-2 and MMP-9), the androgen receptor (particularly important in PCa development and progression), epidermal growth factor receptor, activator protein 1, and some cell cycle regulators [29,35]. Using cell culture systems, Adhami et al. [39] were able to show that EGCG induces apoptosis, cyclin kinase inhibitor WAF-1/p21-mediated cell cycle-dysregulation, and cell growth inhibition. In cDNA microarrays, EGCG treatment of LNCaP cells induced genes that exhibit growth-inhibitory effects and repressed genes belonging to the G-protein signaling network [40]. The ubiquitin/proteasome pathway plays a critical role in activation of the cellular apoptotic program and the regulation of apoptosis [41]. Our work demonstrated that GTC specifically inhibits the chymotrypsin-like activity of the proteasome in several tumor and transformed cell lines, including prostate cell lines, resulting in the accumulation of two natural proteasome substrates–p27 (Kip1) and nuclear factor kappa B (NF-kB) inhibitor alpha, which inhibit transcription factor NF-kB, leading to growth arrest in the G(1) phase of the cell cycle. Synthetic analogs of EGCG were observed to be more potent as proteasome inhibitors compared to EGCG. Polyphenon E® (Poly E) and Sunphenon® 90D are standardized formulations of green tea containing 50% of the catechins from EGCG. We observed that Poly E® (>50% EGCG, 80% total catechins) preferentially inhibits the proteasomal chymotrypsin-like activities over other activities, with an IC50 value of 0.88 μM [41–44]. Standardized GTC formulations of Poly E® and Sunphenon® 90D in equal concentrations were evaluated in vitro. Pre-treatment with Sunphenon® 90D downregulated NF-kB in H_2O_2-treated C2C12 cells, while activating caspase-3 (Figure 1) [45]. Incubation of human primary osteoblasts with Sunphenon® 90D significantly reduced oxidative stress and improved cell viability [46]. EGCG has been shown to have both anti-inflammatory properties, such as through the influence of T-cell proliferation and inhibition of NF-kB, and neuroprotective properties by acting as a free radical scavenger [47,48]. More specifically, EGCG's antioxidant properties deplete reactive oxygen species, thus preventing DNA damage and inhibiting NF-kB-induced inflammation, angiogenesis, and cell survival that could otherwise propel cancer development and progression [49]. In summary, we and others have reported convincing evidence suggesting that GTCs inhibit proliferation and cell cycle events and induce apoptosis through multiple mechanisms.

The association of green tea intake with PCa risk has been investigated in several epidemiological studies. In a meta-analysis of 9 case-control studies, there was a statistically significant 57% lower risk of PCa, comparing subjects with the highest relative to lowest green tea consumption, whereas there was a null association in a meta-analysis of 4 cohort studies [50]. Similar results were observed in a more recent meta-analysis of 3 case-control and 4 cohort studies: no statistically significant associations were observed across cohort studies, while a statistically significant 55% lower odds of PCa was observed for highest versus lowest green tea intake in the case-control studies [51]. This inconsistency could be due, in part, to differences in study design, residual confounding factors such as by diet/lifestyle and biological factors, and varying formulations and subtypes of green tea studied. These studies were mostly limited to men in Asian countries, where approximately 20% of green tea is consumed globally and where mortality from PCa is the lowest compared to Western populations [36], where green tea consumption is a more recent phenomenon. Asian men who migrate to the US have a relatively increased risk of PCa compared to their counterparts in their countries of origin, potentially as a result of acculturation and adoption of Western diets [38]. Although the above study findings have been mixed—potentially due to confounding by variation in geographical location, tobacco and alcohol use, and other lifestyle factors (mainly diets) [37,52]—taken together, studies among Asian populations demonstrate a protective effect of GTCs as related to PCa [37,38,53]. Another highly plausible confounder of GTC-PCa associations is the gut microbiome, which has increasingly been implicated in the modulation of carcinogenesis. The gut microbiome comprises densely populated commensal and symbiotic microbes [54] whose composition is highly influenced by the host's dietary intake. The gut microbiome also produces metabolically active metabolites that interact with host-signaling pathways and gene expression, impacting cancer initiation and progression [55,56]. Multiple studies have observed differences in the gut microbiome between various racial and ethnic groups, even amongst those living in the same community. These differences are potentially attributed to lifestyle, dietary, social, and other uncharacterized exposures that result in variations across racial and ethnic groups [57,58]. Using fecal shotgun metagenomic data analyzed amongst 106 Japanese individuals compared with those of 11 other nations, the composition of the Japanese gut microbiome was more abundant in the phylum Actinobacteria, in particular, genus *Bifidobacterium*, compared to others [59]. In line with increased PCa rates in Asian populations living in the US, studies have shown that the gut microbiome of Southeast Asian immigrants changes after migration to the US [60], potentially indicative of an incompatibility between the incorporation of Western lifestyles with the traditionally harbored microbiome of this population [61]. These studies have provided the basis for understanding that the gut microbiome can act as an important mediating factor in investigations of diet and lifestyle differences that potentially promote cancer risk.

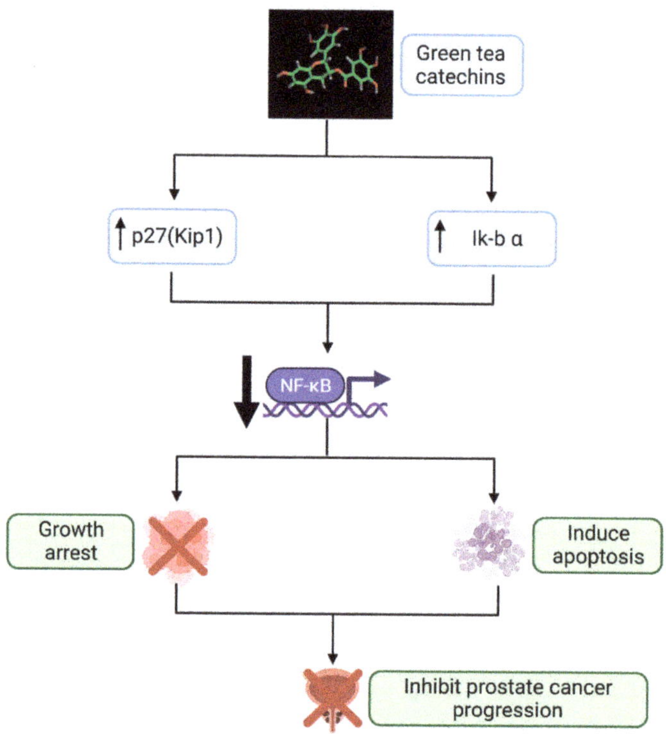

Figure 1. Mechanistic pathway by which GTCs prevent PCa progression. In vitro studies [41–44] demonstrate that GTCs block proteasomal activity in PCa cells, leading to build-up of proteasomal substrates Kip1 and Ik-b α that subsequently downregulate the activity of NF-κB. This inhibits the cell cycle and elicits apoptosis in these PCa cells. GTCs, green tea catechins; Ik-b α, NF-κB inhibitor alpha; NF-κB, nuclear factor kappa B; PCa, prostate cancer. Created with Biorender.com (accessed on 1 July 2022).

3. Pre-Clinical Evidence of the Safety and Effectiveness of GTCs in PCa Carcinogenesis

Several promising pre-clinical studies of GTC effects on prostate carcinogenesis were completed that were highly clinically relevant [39,62–66]. In studies evaluating oral GTCs (vs. pure EGCG) administered to transgenic adenocarcinoma of the mouse prostate (TRAMP) mice, greater bioavailability [29,35,62–66] of GTC was observed compared to administering EGCG alone [64]. Oral infusion of a polyphenolic fraction isolated from green tea extract at a human achievable dose (i.e., six cups of green tea per day) in a TRAMP mouse model, compared to water-fed mice [62], demonstrated significant delays in primary prostate tumor incidence and burden. Overall, they observed a decrease in prostate (64%) and genitourinary (72%) weight from baseline weight, inhibition of serum insulin-like growth factor-1 (IGF-1), and restoration of insulin-like growth factor binding protein-3 levels (IGFBP-3). Additionally, a significant reduction in the protein expression of proliferating cell nuclear antigen and apoptosis in the prostate was observed in GTC-fed mice compared to water-fed mice, resulting in reduced dissemination of cancer cells, thereby causing inhibition of development, progression, and metastasis to distant organ sites. Our team evaluated [65] the safety and efficacy of GTCs at various doses (200, 500, and 1000 mg EGCG in GTC/kg/day) in reducing the progression of PCa in a TRAMP mouse model. Significant decreases in the number and size of tumors in treated TRAMP mice were observed compared with untreated animals. We observed a dose-dependent inhibition of metastasis in GTC-treated mice ($p = 0.0003$). After 32 weeks of treatment with standardized formulation of GTC, it was found to be well-tolerated with no evidence of toxicity in C57BL/6J mice [65]. Apart from significant reductions in tumor size and multiplicity, GTCs also prevented metastatic progression of PCa in the TRAMP and other relevant mouse models. Collectively, these findings from pre-clinical studies, using doses relevant for translation to human clinical trials, provide evidence for safety and chemopreventive effects of GTCs.

4. Clinical Evidence of Bioavailability, Safety, and Effectiveness of GTCs in Modulating Prostate Carcinogenesis

Early phase I/II studies [67–76] conducted over the past decade found that doses of GTCs containing 200–1200 mg of EGCG per day (Poly E®) were tolerated by subjects, including men with precancerous lesions such as high-grade prostatic intraepithelial neoplasia, atypical small acinar proliferation, or early stage PCas.

Additionally, early phase I trials assessing standardized formulations of GTCs (Sunphenon 90D®) demonstrated increasing doses of plasma EGCG with increasing doses of the supplement [77–79]. Oral intake of GTCs in healthy subjects containing 225, 375, and 525 mg EGCG (Sunphenon® 90D) demonstrated a significant dose-dependent increase in plasma concentrations of EGCG to 657, 4300, and 4410 pmol EGCG/mL, respectively [80]. Consumption of Sunphenon® 90D containing 246 mg EGCG significantly increased plasma EGCG, which was highly correlated with attenuation of plasma phosphatidylcholine hydroperoxide levels, a marker of antioxidant capacity. Although increased bioavailability (as indicated by higher concentrations of EGCG in plasma) [81–83] occurs when GTCs are consumed in a fasting state [69] as opposed to a fed state, increased toxicity has also been reported when GTCs are taken in a fasting state. Similarly, increased bioavailability and tolerance to a multiple dosing schedule compared to a single daily dose of EGCG has been reported in phase II trials [67,75,84]. A summary of the concentration of GTCs in plasma with intervention trials targeting men at high risk for PCa is presented in Table 1. Mean plasma concentrations of EGCG varied among all these trials, potentially due to varying duration of intervention, doses, methods used in analyzing plasma EGCG, ethnicity of the target population, and nutritional and lifestyle habits. Another potential explanation may be differences in gut microbial capacity to process GTCs, as described below.

Table 1. Concentration of GTCs in plasma in interventional trials targeting men with PCa.

Author; Target Population	Dose of EGCG (mg)	Duration of Intervention	Plasma EGCG Concentration after Intervention
Nguyen et al. [84]; PCa patients prior to RP	800 (Poly E®)	3–6 weeks	146.6 pmol/mL
Kumar et al. [75]; Men with HGPIN	200 (BID) (Poly E®)	1 year	12.3 ng/mL (SD, 24.8) fed
Bettuzi et al. [67]; Men with HGPIN	200 (TID)	1 year	NA
Lane et al. [85]; Men with elevated PSA or negative prostate biopsy for PCa	GTC drink GTC capsules	6 months	24.9 nmoL/L 12.3 nmoL/L

BID, twice a day; EGCG, (−)-epigallocatechin-3-gallate; GTC, green tea catechins; HGPIN, high-grade prostatic intraepithelial neoplasia; PCa, prostate cancer; Poly E, Polyphenon E; PSA, prostate specific antigen; RP, radical prostatectomy; SD, standard deviation; TID, three times a day.

Overall, prior studies support that GTCs are generally safe for consumption in human populations. A phase II/III trial (NCT00799890) was recently completed to evaluate the effect of 200–800 mg Sunphenon® 90D on attenuating brain atrophy, targeting patients with primary or secondary chronic-progressive multiple sclerosis treated for 36 months. An additional study (NCT00951834), using a maximum dose of 800 mg EGCG for 18 months to target early Alzheimer's, has been completed with results pending. No toxicities have been reported in either of these trials. In a more recently reported phase II clinical trial that evaluated the effects of 1315 mg of total catechins, containing 843 mg of EGCG, vs. placebo in modulating mammographic density, 1075 women were evaluated in a 12-month intervention. Overall, 26 women (5.1%) in the green tea extract arm developed moderate to severe abnormalities in liver function tests during the intervention period [86,87]. In three randomized trials [84,88–90] of the effects of GTCs (800 mg EGCG), or green tea as a beverage, in men diagnosed with localized PCa prior to prostatectomy, no toxicities were observed. These trials did not collect and analyze samples to assess interactions of the gut microbiome with GTC safety and toxicity.

A summary of the changes observed in intermediate endpoint biomarkers of PCa among Phase II GTC clinical trials is presented in Table 2. The findings from our study [75] and those of Bettuzzi et al. [67,68] suggest that a daily intake of the standardized GTC formulation administered non-fasting for 12 months in divided doses: (a) accumulates in plasma; (b) reduces serum PSA; and (c) reduces the cumulative rate of progression to PCa with no toxicities [67,68,75]. In the study of the effects of green tea beverages [88], nuclear staining of NF-κB was significantly decreased in radical prostatectomy (RP) tissue of men consuming GTC ($p = 0.013$), but not black tea ($p = 0.931$), compared to water control. Further, GTCs were detected in prostate tissue from 32 of 34 men consuming green tea but not in the other groups; evidence of a systemic antioxidant effect was observed (i.e., reduced urinary 8-hyroxydeoxy-guanosine) only with green tea consumption ($p = 0.03$) [88]. In randomized trials of the effects of GTCs (800 mg EGCG) or green tea as a beverage among men diagnosed with localized PCa, prior to prostatectomy, a reduction in serum PSA was observed [88,89]. Nguyen et al. [84] observed that the proportion of subjects who had a decrease in Gleason score between biopsy and surgical specimens was greater among those randomized to GTCs, but this finding was not statistically significant for the full duration of the intervention. In an open-label, single-arm, two-stage phase II clinical trial, 26 men with positive prostate biopsies received 800 mg EGCG/day (Poly E®) for 3–6 weeks until undergoing RP. EGCG administration lowered serum concentrations of hepatocyte growth factor (HGF), vascular endothelial growth factor, IGFBP-3, IGF-1, and PSA in these patients, with no elevation of liver enzymes [89]. More recently, Lane et al. [85] completed a 6-month randomized controlled trial of green tea and lycopene among men with elevated serum PSA but negative prostate biopsies. They randomized men to consume food sources of each of these agents, to standardized formulations, or to placebo. Plasma levels of both lycopene and EGCG were higher in the treatment arms compared to the placebo arm with concentrations among the dietary source arm of these formulations being greater than the capsule group and the placebo arm. All interventions were tolerated well by the participants; however, men preferred the capsules to using food sources of lycopene and green tea. No biomarkers of disease progression were assessed in this study.

Table 2. Changes in intermediate endpoint biomarkers of PCa observed in Phase II clinical trials using GTCs.

Target Population (Ref)	Number of Subjects	Dose of GTC (EGCG)	Duration of Intervention	Biomarkers Observed
HGPIN (Betuzzi et al. [67,68])	60	200 mg TID	12 months	• Reduction in progression to PCa in treatment arm • Improvement in prostate symptom score
HGPIN (Kumar et al. [75])	97	200 mg BID Poly E®	12 months	• Cumulative rate of PCa plus ASAP among men with HGPIN without ASAP at baseline, revealed a decrease in this composite endpoint: ($p < 0.024$). • Decrease in ASAP diagnoses on the Poly E®(0/26) compared with the placebo arm (5/25). • Decrease in serum PSA was observed in the Poly E arm [−0.87 ng/mL; 95% CI, −1.66 to −0.09].
PCa patients (Henning et al. [88])	113	6 cups of green tea, black tea or water	3–8 weeks	• Nuclear staining of NF-κB was significantly decreased in RP tissue of men consuming green tea ($p = 0.013$) but not black tea ($p = 0.931$) compared to water control. • Tea polyphenols were detected in prostate tissue from 32 of 34 men consuming green tea but not in the other groups. • Evidence of a systemic antioxidant effect was observed (reduced urinary 8OHdG) only with GTC consumption ($p = 0.03$). Significant decrease in serum PSA levels ($p < 0.05$).
PCa patients (McLarty et al. [89])	26	800 mg of EGCG Poly E®	3–6 weeks	• Significant reduction in serum levels of PSA, HGF, and VEGF in men with PCa after brief treatment with EGCG (Poly E®), with no elevation of liver enzymes.

Table 2. *Cont.*

Target Population (Ref)	Number of Subjects	Dose of GTC (EGCG)	Duration of Intervention	Biomarkers Observed
PCa patients-pre-prostatectomy (Nguyen et al. [84])	52	800 mg of EGCG Poly E®	3–6 weeks	• Proportion of subjects who had a decrease in Gleason score between biopsy and surgical specimens was greater in those on Poly E®but was not statistically significant. • Favorable but not statistically significant changes in serum PSA, serum insulin-like growth factor axis, and oxidative DNA damage in blood leukocytes.

Abbreviations: 8OHdG, 8-hydroxydeoxy-guanosine; ASAP, atypical small acinar proliferation; BID, twice a day; CI, confidence interval; GTC, green tea catechins; HGF, hepatocyte growth factor; HGPIN, high-grade prostatic intraepithelial neoplasia; EGCG, epigallocatechin-3-gallate; PCa, prostate cancer; Poly E, polyphenon E; PSA, prostate specific antigen; RP, radical prostatectomy; TID, three times a day; VEGF, vascular endothelial growth factor.

In summary, evidence from epidemiological, in vitro, pre-clinical, and early phase trials completed by our team and others have shown that the standard GTC formulations (a) accumulate in plasma and tissue; (b) reduce serum PSA and cumulative rate of progression to PCa; and (c) are potent inhibitors of PCa carcinogenesis through multiple mechanisms without toxicities at these doses, establishing the evidence needed for further development of GTCs in phase II clinical trials targeting men at exceptional risk or those diagnosed with low risk PCas. Self-reported patient race/ethnicity, medical history, family history of cancer, lifestyle factors such as smoking and alcohol use, and dietary intake have been accounted for in many of these studies; however, to date, the role of the gut microbiome in the absorption, safety, and modulation of prostate carcinogenesis has not been evaluated. Although the data on the safety, effectiveness, and potential mechanism of GTCs in prostate carcinogenesis appears promising, there are gaps in knowledge pertaining the role of the gut microbiome in modulating the bioavailability and toxicity of GTCs and in prostate carcinogenesis. With significant variations observed in GTC bioavailability (Table 1) as well as in modulation of intermediate endpoint biomarkers with GTCs (Table 2) in prior clinical trials, it is imperative to evaluate the contribution of the gut microbiome to modulating the interrelationships among GTC chemoprevention and PCa progression.

5. The Gut Microbiome, PCa, and GTCs

Predictive biomarkers of responses to secondary chemoprevention are presently lacking. Identification of biomarkers, such as the gut microbiome, predictive of favorable clinical responses to secondary chemoprevention has the potential to substantially facilitate clinical decision-making. Numerous studies found that the gut microbiome directly effects drug metabolism, efficacy, and toxicity, potentially affecting disease development and progression [91]. For example, in oncology, there exists convincing evidence to support that the antitumor effects of immunotherapies can be enhanced or inhibited by the gut microbiome [92,93].

The gut microbiome likely has critical roles in regulating the bioavailability of GTCs and absorption of bioactive phenolic GTC metabolites, as demonstrated in laboratory and pre-clinical models (Figure 2). Although dietary polyphenols are absorbed by the small intestine, accumulating evidence suggests that they are metabolized to a greater extent in the colon by bacterial enzymes [94,95]. EGCG is hydrolyzed by bacteria to gallic acid or EGC and further converted to multiple metabolites, such as 5-(3,5-dihydroxyphenyl)-4-

hydroxyvaleric acid and 5-(3′,5′-dihydroxyphenyl)-g-valerolactone [95]. These metabolites are then either taken up via the portal vein and transported to the liver or excreted in the feces.

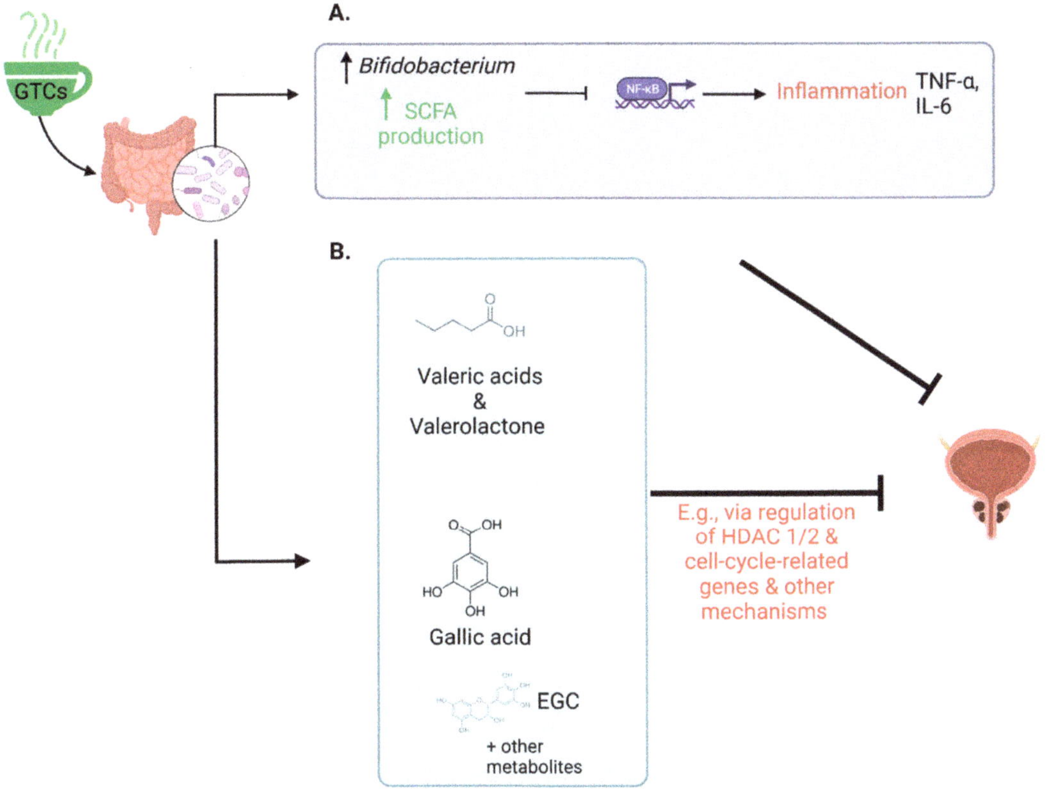

Figure 2. Examples of chemopreventive effects of GTCs in the context of PCa via gut microbiome modulation. (**A**) GTCs like EGCG have been evidenced to alter microbial composition, such as increasing abundance of Bifidobacterium [95]. This genus, for example, is known to increase production of SCFAs [95,96] which inhibit inflammatory pathways initiated by NF-κB that would otherwise propel carcinogenesis [97]. (**B**) The gut microbiome can enzymatically alter GTCs like EGCG to produce metabolites including gallic acid, EGC, valeric acid, and valerolactone, that subsequently travel to the bloodstream to exert potential chemopreventive benefits (e.g., regulating HDAC 1 and 2 and suppressing cell-cycle-related genes) [95,98–100]. EGC, epigallocatechin; EGCG, epigallocatechin gallate; GTCs, green tea catechins; HDAC, histone deacetylase; IL-6, interleukin-6; NF-κB, nuclear factor kappa B; SCFA, short chain fatty acid; TNF-α, tumor necrosis factor alpha. Created with Biorender.com (accessed on 1 July 2022).

On the other hand, several pharmacologic agents, including GTCs, were shown to influence gut microbiome composition and function. For example, in a study of 10 volunteers who drank 1000 mL of green tea daily for 10 days, Bifidobacteria abundance was increased [101]. In multiple animal studies, green tea polyphenols had similar effects on Bifidobacteria and other effects, including decreasing the Firmicutes/Bacteroidetes ratio [102,103]. In turn, gut microbiome composition and function may directly and indirectly influence PCa progression, such as through production of metabolically active metabolites or regulation of hormones and inflammation, as described below [104–106]. Given the substantial preliminary evidence for interrelationships among GTCs, the gut microbiome, and prostate carcinogenesis, it is highly likely that the gut microbiome may mediate etiological effects of GTCs, including effects on PCa progression and development of adverse events; however, little is known regarding these interrelationships among humans.

The gut microbiome has biologically plausible roles in PCa such as via its influence on hormone and inflammation regulation and production of metabolically active metabolites [104–106]. For example, gut microbes produce sex hormones, such as androgen, and, in a study by Pernigoni et al., multiple species among mice and humans produced androgens from androgen precursors, in turn promoting progression of castrate resistant PCa [107]. In a study of both mice and PCa patients, Proteobacteria was increased after antibiotic exposure, and was in turn associated with development of PCa in mice and with metastasis of PCa among humans [108]. In a study of mice on a high-fat diet, the resultant alterations to the mice fecal microbiome promoted histamine biosynthesis and increased inflammatory cancer cell growth [109]. Previous human studies of the gut microbiome and PCa included a case-control study comparing 16S rRNA sequenced fecal bacteria among 64 men with PCa and 41 without PCa, finding differences in beta diversity, higher abundances of Bacteroides and Streptococcus species, and differences in folate and arginine pathways [110]. Another case-control study compared the gut metagenome among 8 men with benign prostatic conditions and 12 men with intermediate or high risk clinically localized PCa, finding higher relative abundance of Bacteriodes massiliensis and lower relative abundances of Faecalibacterium prausnitzii and Eubacterium rectalie amongst men with intermediate/high-risk PCa [111]. In a comparison of men with and without prostate enlargement, the ratio of Firmicutes to Bacteroidetes was higher among men with enlarged prostates, potentially related to prostate inflammation [112]. Finally, evidence supports the study of the gut microbiome across the disease continuum of PCa, with evidence demonstrating that the gut microbiome may be modified by PCa treatment, including androgen deprivation therapy, among more advanced PCa patients [113].

6. Challenges and Future Directions

There is currently sufficient evidence that establishes the need to evaluate the role of the gut microbiome in modifying the response to GTCs among men diagnosed with PCa. However, there are several challenges and pitfalls pertaining to studying GTCs in the context of modification by the gut microbiome. At present, biospecimens and data available to study the role of the gut microbiome in the effects of GTCs are sparse and further research is clearly needed among diverse populations. Studying the gut microbiome itself presents several challenges, as it is a complex, dynamic ecosystem that is driven by numerous known and unknown factors, such as dietary intake, requiring comprehensive measurement of potential confounding factors. It has been well documented that methods for stool collection, DNA extraction, and sequencing can influence downstream gut microbiome metrics, potentially resulting in inconsistent study findings that hinder progress in the field. To ensure high-quality, reproducible results, it is critical to establish contemporary and validated methodologies and to optimize protocols and procedures for fecal sampling, handling, processing, and microbiome analyses [114,115].

To fill existing gaps in knowledge, detailed characterizations of the gut microbiome and its metabolites among extensively phenotyped human subjects are needed. Although sequencing of the 16S rRNA gene classifies bacteria based on conserved single marker genes, there is a lack of detailed resolution. Shotgun metagenomic sequencing, which comprises the untargeted sequencing of all DNA present in a sample, provides more detailed taxonomic information than 16S rRNA sequencing. Characterizing microbial genes, strains, and functions may provide deeper insight into GTC-gut microbiome interactions. In addition, the gut microbiome and metabolome have moderate-to-high intraindividual variability and are 'high-dimensional' in that there are typically large numbers of microbes/metabolites relative to the numbers of subjects. As a result, collecting repeat samples is particularly useful for reducing bias in estimating effects/associations and increasing statistical power [116]. Other challenges include addressing limitations of previous human studies of microbiome-PCa associations, including small sample sizes, inclusion of more advanced PCas, and cross-sectional design leading to concerns with reverse causality. Studies among large populations of men with serial microbiome and intermediate biomarker endpoint assessments are critically needed.

Future studies evaluating GTCs in prostate carcinogenesis may also include a metabolomics approach to assess EGCG- and microbiome-related metabolites from stool samples pre- and post-treatment with GTCs. In addition, these studies must include the evaluation of the correlation among specific microbial species/strains with (a) plasma levels of EGCG; (b) multiple markers of toxicity and safety; and (c) surrogate endpoint biomarkers, such as serum PSA, as an indicator for PCa progression, to provide timely evidence for a role of the gut microbiome in mediating the effects of GTCs on PCa progression. To our knowledge, studies collecting serial stool samples longitudinally to measure the microbiome in relation to these intermediate biomarkers of prostate carcinogenesis are currently unprecedented. Further, as in all biomedical research, there should be an emphasis in recruiting and studying disproportionately affected populations. In PCa, African American (AA) men are known to have the highest PCa risk. There is accumulating evidence that exposures associated with race may collectively and individually influence gut microbiome composition [57,58]. Therefore, with the inclusion of AA men in these clinical trials, we may be able to provide data to inform secondary chemoprevention efforts among this particularly at-risk population by studying a comprehensive biomarker (the gut microbiome). Finally, this review is focused and specific to the current data on the safety, effectiveness, and molecular mechanisms of GTCs in prostate carcinogenesis. Other cancers, like breast and colon cancers, may similarly be impacted by both GTCs and the gut microbiome. Collectively, these studies are critical in understanding the dynamics of the gut microbiome as we develop and evaluate promising agents such as GTCs for cancer chemoprevention.

Author Contributions: Conceptualization and writing, N.B.K. and D.A.B.; writing—original draft preparation and writing—review and editing, S.H.; Conceptualization and writing—original draft preparation, J.P.-S., M.P., B.J.M., R.L., J.D. and A.Y. All authors have read and agreed to the published version of the manuscript.

Funding: Financial support for this project was provided by funds from National Cancer Institute R01CA235032.

Conflicts of Interest: The authors declare that they have no competing financial or other interests in the results obtained within this manuscript.

Abbreviations

8OHdG	8-hydroxydeoxy-guanosine
AA	African American
AS	active surveillance
ASAP	atypical small acinar proliferation
BID	twice a day
EGC	(−)-epigallocatechin
EGCG	(−)-epigallocatechin-3-gallate
GTC(s)	green tea catechin(s)
HDAC	histone deacetylase
HGF	hepatocyte growth factor
HGPIN	high-grade prostatic intraepithelial neoplasia
IGF-1	insulin-like growth factor 1
IGFBP-3	insulin-like growth factor binding protein 3
IL-6	interleukin 6
MMP	matrix metalloproteinase
NF-kB	nuclear factor kappa b
PCa	prostate cancer

Poly E	polyphenon E®
PSA	prostate specific antigen
RP	radical prostatectomy
SCFA(s)	short-chain fatty acid(s)
SD	standard deviation
TID	three times a day
TNF-α	tumor necrosis factor alpha
TRAMP	transgenic adenocarcinoma of the mouse prostate
VEGF	vascular endothelial growth factor

References

1. American Cancer Society. Available online: http://www.cancer.org/Cancer/ProstateCancer/DetailedGuide/prostate-cancer-key-statistics (accessed on 1 July 2022).
2. Bruinsma, S.M.; Bangma, C.H.; Carroll, P.R.; Leapman, M.S.; Rannikko, A.; Petrides, N.; Weerakoon, M.; Bokhorst, L.P.; Roobol, M.J.; Movember, G.A.P.C. Active surveillance for prostate cancer: A narrative review of clinical guidelines. *Nat. Rev. Urol.* **2016**, *13*, 151–167. [CrossRef] [PubMed]
3. Ip, S.; Dahabreh, I.J.; Chung, M.; Yu, W.W.; Balk, E.M.; Iovin, R.C.; Mathew, P.; Luongo, T.; Dvorak, T.; Lau, J. An evidence review of active surveillance in men with localized prostate cancer. *Evid. Rep. Technol. Assess.* **2011**, *204*, 1–341.
4. Klotz, L. Active Surveillance for Prostate Cancer: For Whom? *J. Clin. Oncol.* **2005**, *23*, 8165–8169. [CrossRef] [PubMed]
5. Thompson, I.; Thrasher, J.B.; Aus, G.; Burnett, A.L.; Canby-Hagino, E.D.; Cookson, M.S.; D'Amico, A.V.; Dmochowski, R.R.; Eton, D.T.; Forman, J.D.; et al. Guideline for the management of clinically localized prostate cancer: 2007 update. *J. Urol.* **2007**, *177*, 2106–2131. [CrossRef] [PubMed]
6. Hamdy, F.C.; Donovan, J.L.; Neal, D.E. 10-Year Outcomes in Localized Prostate Cancer. *N. Engl. J. Med.* **2017**, *376*, 180. [CrossRef]
7. Cooperberg, M.R.; Carroll, P.R. Trends in Management for Patients With Localized Prostate Cancer, 1990–2013. *JAMA* **2015**, *314*, 80–82. [CrossRef]
8. D'Amico, A.V. Personalizing the Use of Active Surveillance As an Initial Approach for Men With Newly Diagnosed Prostate Cancer. *J. Clin. Oncol.* **2015**, *33*, 3365–3366. [CrossRef] [PubMed]
9. Klotz, L. Active surveillance for low-risk prostate cancer. *Curr. Urol. Rep.* **2015**, *16*, 24. [CrossRef]
10. Klotz, L. Active surveillance and focal therapy for low-intermediate risk prostate cancer. *Transl. Androl. Urol.* **2015**, *4*, 342–354. [CrossRef]
11. Klotz, L.; Zhang, L.; Lam, A.; Nam, R.; Mamedov, A.; Loblaw, A. Clinical results of long-term follow-up of a large, active surveillance cohort with localized prostate cancer. *J. Clin. Oncol.* **2010**, *28*, 126–131. [CrossRef]
12. Maurice, M.J.; Abouassaly, R.; Kim, S.P.; Zhu, H. Contemporary Nationwide Patterns of Active Surveillance Use for Prostate Cancer. *JAMA Intern. Med.* **2015**, *175*, 1569–1571. [CrossRef]
13. Oon, S.F.; Watson, R.W.; O'Leary, J.J.; Fitzpatrick, J.M. Epstein criteria for insignificant prostate cancer. *BJU Int.* **2011**, *108*, 518–525. [CrossRef] [PubMed]
14. NCCN. *NCCN Guidelines for Prostate Cancer*; NCCN: Bethesda, MD, USA, 2017.
15. Orom, H.; Underwood, W., 3rd; Biddle, C. Emotional Distress Increases the Likelihood of Undergoing Surgery among Men with Localized Prostate Cancer. *J. Urol.* **2017**, *197*, 350–355. [CrossRef] [PubMed]
16. Watts, S.; Leydon, G.; Eyles, C.; Moore, C.M.; Richardson, A.; Birch, B.; Prescott, P.; Powell, C.; Lewith, G. A quantitative analysis of the prevalence of clinical depression and anxiety in patients with prostate cancer undergoing active surveillance. *BMJ Open* **2015**, *5*, e006674. [CrossRef] [PubMed]
17. Avery, K.N.; Donovan, J.L.; Horwood, J.; Neal, D.E.; Hamdy, F.C.; Parker, C.; Wade, J.; Lane, A. The importance of dietary change for men diagnosed with and at risk of prostate cancer: A multi-centre interview study with men, their partners and health professionals. *BMC Fam. Pr.* **2014**, *15*, 81. [CrossRef] [PubMed]
18. Horwood, J.P.; Avery, K.N.; Metcalfe, C.; Donovan, J.L.; Hamdy, F.C.; Neal, D.E.; Lane, J.A. Men's knowledge and attitudes towards dietary prevention of a prostate cancer diagnosis: A qualitative study. *BMC Cancer* **2014**, *14*, 812. [CrossRef]
19. Kelloff, G.J.; Lieberman, R.; Steele, V.E.; Boone, C.W.; Lubet, R.A.; Kopelovitch, L.; Malone, W.A.; Crowell, J.A.; Sigman, C.C. Chemoprevention of prostate cancer: Concepts and strategies. *Eur. Urol.* **1999**, *35*, 342–350. [CrossRef] [PubMed]
20. Kumar, N.; Chornokur, G. Molecular Targeted Therapies Using Botanicals for Prostate Cancer Chemoprevention. *Transl. Med.* **2012**, *S2*, 005. [CrossRef]
21. Lieberman, R. Prostate cancer chemoprevention: Strategies for designing efficient clinical trials. *Urology* **2001**, *57*, 224–229. [CrossRef]
22. Andriole, G.L.; Bostwick, D.G.; Brawley, O.W.; Gomella, L.G.; Marberger, M.; Montorsi, F.; Pettaway, C.A.; Tammela, T.L.; Teloken, C.; Tindall, D.J.; et al. Effect of dutasteride on the risk of prostate cancer. *N. Engl. J. Med.* **2010**, *362*, 1192–1202. [CrossRef]
23. Hamilton, R.J.; Kahwati, L.C.; Kinsinger, L.S. Knowledge and use of finasteride for the prevention of prostate cancer. *Cancer Epidemiol. Biomark. Prev.* **2010**, *19*, 2164–2171. [CrossRef]
24. Thompson, I.M.; Goodman, P.J.; Tangen, C.M.; Lucia, M.S.; Miller, G.J.; Ford, L.G.; Lieber, M.M.; Cespedes, R.D.; Atkins, J.N.; Lippman, S.M.; et al. The influence of finasteride on the development of prostate cancer. *N. Engl. J. Med.* **2003**, *349*, 215–224. [CrossRef]

25. Lippman, S.M.; Klein, E.A.; Goodman, P.J.; Lucia, M.S.; Thompson, I.M.; Ford, L.G.; Parnes, H.L.; Minasian, L.M.; Gaziano, J.M.; Hartline, J.A.; et al. Effect of selenium and vitamin E on risk of prostate cancer and other cancers: The Selenium and Vitamin E Cancer Prevention Trial (SELECT). *JAMA* **2009**, *301*, 39–51. [CrossRef]
26. Block, K.I.; Gyllenhaal, C.; Lowe, L.; Amedei, A.; Amin, A.; Amin, A.; Aquilano, K.; Arbiser, J.; Arreola, A.; Arzumanyan, A.; et al. Designing a broad-spectrum integrative approach for cancer prevention and treatment. *Semin. Cancer Biol.* **2015**, *35*, S276–S304. [CrossRef]
27. Datta, D.; Aftabuddin, M.; Gupta, D.K.; Raha, S.; Sen, P. Human Prostate Cancer Hallmarks Map. *Sci. Rep.* **2016**, *6*, 30691. [CrossRef]
28. Kumar, N.B.; Pow-Sang, J.; Spiess, P.; Dickinson, S.; Schell, M.J. A phase II randomized clinical trial using aglycone isoflavones to treat patients with localized prostate cancer in the pre-surgical period prior to radical prostatectomy. *Oncotarget* **2020**, *11*, 1218–1234. [CrossRef]
29. Khan, N.; Mukhtar, H. Modulation of signaling pathways in prostate cancer by green tea polyphenols. *Biochem. Pharm.* **2013**, *85*, 667–672. [CrossRef]
30. Miyata, Y.; Shida, Y.; Hakariya, T.; Sakai, H. Anti-Cancer Effects of Green Tea Polyphenols Against Prostate Cancer. *Molecules* **2019**, *24*, 193. [CrossRef]
31. Perletti, G.; Magri, V.; Vral, A.; Stamatiou, K.; Trinchieri, A. Green tea catechins for chemoprevention of prostate cancer in patients with histologically-proven HG-PIN or ASAP. Concise review and meta-analysis. *Arch. Ital. Urol. Androl.* **2019**, *91*, 153–156. [CrossRef]
32. Rogovskii, V.S.; Popov, S.V.; Sturov, N.V.; Shimanovskii, N.L. The Possibility of Preventive and Therapeutic Use of Green Tea Catechins in Prostate Cancer. *Anticancer Agents Med. Chem.* **2019**, *19*, 1223–1231. [CrossRef]
33. Sharifi-Zahabi, E.; Hajizadeh-Sharafabad, F.; Abdollahzad, H.; Dehnad, A.; Shidfar, F. The effect of green tea on prostate specific antigen (PSA): A systematic review and meta-analysis of randomized controlled trials. *Complement. Ther. Med.* **2021**, *57*, 102659. [CrossRef]
34. Pérez-Burillo, S.; Navajas-Porras, B.; López-Maldonado, A.; Hinojosa-Nogueira, D.; Pastoriza, S.; Rufián-Henares, J. Green Tea and Its Relation to Human Gut Microbiome. *Molecules* **2021**, *26*, 3907. [CrossRef]
35. Connors, S.K.; Chornokur, G.; Kumar, N.B. New insights into the mechanisms of green tea catechins in the chemoprevention of prostate cancer. *Nutr. Cancer* **2012**, *64*, 4–22. [CrossRef]
36. Ito, K. Prostate cancer in Asian men. *Nat. Rev. Urol.* **2014**, *11*, 197–212. [CrossRef]
37. Jian, L.; Xie, L.P.; Lee, A.H.; Binns, C.W. Protective effect of green tea against prostate cancer: A case-control study in southeast China. *Int. J. Cancer* **2004**, *108*, 130–135. [CrossRef]
38. Yuan, J.M. Cancer prevention by green tea: Evidence from epidemiologic studies. *Am. J. Clin. Nutr.* **2013**, *98*, 1676S–1681S. [CrossRef]
39. Adhami, V.M.; Siddiqui, I.A.; Sarfaraz, S.; Khwaja, S.I.; Hafeez, B.B.; Ahmad, N.; Mukhtar, H. Effective Prostate Cancer Chemopreventive Intervention with Green Tea Polyphenols in the TRAMP Model Depends on the Stage of the Disease. *Clin. Cancer Res.* **2009**, *15*, 1947–1953. [CrossRef]
40. Adhami, V.M.; Ahmad, N.; Mukhtar, H. Molecular Targets for Green Tea in Prostate Cancer Prevention. *J. Nutr.* **2003**, *133*, 2417S–2424S. [CrossRef]
41. Kazi, A.; Daniel, K.G.; Smith, D.M.; Kumar, N.B.; Dou, Q.P. Inhibition of the proteasome activity, a novel mechanism associated with the tumor cell apoptosis-inducing ability of genistein. *Biochem. Pharm.* **2003**, *66*, 965–976. [CrossRef]
42. Kazi, A.; Wang, Z.; Kumar, N.; Falsetti, S.C.; Chan, T.H.; Dou, Q.P. Structure-activity relationships of synthetic analogs of (-)-epigallocatechin-3-gallate as proteasome inhibitors. *Anticancer Res.* **2004**, *24*, 943–954.
43. Nam, S.; Smith, D.M.; Dou, Q.P. Ester bond-containing tea polyphenols potently inhibit proteasome activity in vitro and in vivo. *J. Biol. Chem.* **2001**, *276*, 13322–13330. [CrossRef] [PubMed]
44. Smith, D.M.; Wang, Z.; Kazi, A.; Li, L.H.; Chan, T.H.; Dou, Q.P. Synthetic analogs of green tea polyphenols as proteasome inhibitors. *Mol. Med.* **2002**, *8*, 382–392. [CrossRef] [PubMed]
45. Sivakumar, A.S.; Hwang, I. Effects of Sunphenon and Polyphenon 60 on proteolytic pathways, inflammatory cytokines and myogenic markers in H2O2-treated C2C12 cells. *J. Biosci.* **2015**, *40*, 53–59. [CrossRef] [PubMed]
46. Vester, H.; Holzer, N.; Neumaier, M.; Lilianna, S.; Nussler, A.K.; Seeliger, C. Green Tea Extract (GTE) improves differentiation in human osteoblasts during oxidative stress. *J. Inflamm.* **2014**, *11*, 15. [CrossRef] [PubMed]
47. Aktas, O.; Prozorovski, T.; Smorodchenko, A.; Savaskan, N.E.; Lauster, R.; Kloetzel, P.M.; Infante-Duarte, C.; Brocke, S.; Zipp, F. Green tea epigallocatechin-3-gallate mediates T cellular NF-kappa B inhibition and exerts neuroprotection in autoimmune encephalomyelitis. *J. Immunol.* **2004**, *173*, 5794–5800. [CrossRef] [PubMed]
48. Sun, Q.; Zheng, Y.; Zhang, X.; Hu, X.; Wang, Y.; Zhang, S.; Zhang, D.; Nie, H. Novel immunoregulatory properties of EGCG on reducing inflammation in EAE. *Front. Biosci.* **2013**, *18*, 332–342.
49. Hayakawa, S.; Ohishi, T.; Miyoshi, N.; Oishi, Y.; Nakamura, Y.; Isemura, M. Anti-Cancer Effects of Green Tea Epigallocatchin-3-Gallate and Coffee Chlorogenic Acid. *Molecules* **2020**, *25*, 4553. [CrossRef]
50. Zheng, J.; Yang, B.; Huang, T.; Yu, Y.; Yang, J.; Li, D. Green tea and black tea consumption and prostate cancer risk: An exploratory meta-analysis of observational studies. *Nutr. Cancer* **2011**, *63*, 663–672. [CrossRef]
51. Guo, Y.; Zhi, F.; Chen, P.; Zhao, K.; Xiang, H.; Mao, Q.; Wang, X.; Zhang, X. Green tea and the risk of prostate cancer: A systematic review and meta-analysis. *Medicine* **2017**, *96*, e6426. [CrossRef]

52. Liu, J.; Li, X.; Hou, J.; Sun, J.; Guo, N.; Wang, Z. Dietary Intake of N-3 and N-6 Polyunsaturated Fatty Acids and Risk of Cancer: Meta-Analysis of Data from 32 Studies. *Nutr. Cancer* **2021**, *73*, 901–913. [CrossRef]
53. Lee, J.; Demissie, K.; Lu, S.E.; Rhoads, G.G. Cancer incidence among Korean-American immigrants in the United States and native Koreans in South Korea. *Cancer Control* **2007**, *14*, 78–85. [CrossRef] [PubMed]
54. Shen, J.; Obin, M.S.; Zhao, L. The gut microbiota, obesity and insulin resistance. *Mol. Asp. Med.* **2013**, *34*, 39–58. [CrossRef]
55. Trefflich, I.; Jabakhanji, A.; Menzel, J.; Blaut, M.; Michalsen, A.; Lampen, A.; Abraham, K.; Weikert, C. Is a vegan or a vegetarian diet associated with the microbiota composition in the gut? Results of a new cross-sectional study and systematic review. *Crit. Rev. Food Sci. Nutr.* **2020**, *60*, 2990–3004. [CrossRef] [PubMed]
56. Yang, Q.; Liang, Q.; Balakrishnan, B.; Belobrajdic, D.P.; Feng, Q.J.; Zhang, W. Role of Dietary Nutrients in the Modulation of Gut Microbiota: A Narrative Review. *Nutrients* **2020**, *12*, 381. [CrossRef] [PubMed]
57. Byrd, D.A.; Carson, T.L.; Williams, F.; Vogtmann, E. Elucidating the role of the gastrointestinal microbiota in racial and ethnic health disparities. *Genome Biol.* **2020**, *21*, 192. [CrossRef] [PubMed]
58. Dwiyanto, J.; Hussain, M.H.; Reidpath, D.; Ong, K.S.; Qasim, A.; Lee, S.W.H.; Lee, S.M.; Foo, S.C.; Chong, C.W.; Rahman, S. Ethnicity influences the gut microbiota of individuals sharing a geographical location: A cross-sectional study from a middle-income country. *Sci. Rep.* **2021**, *11*, 2618. [CrossRef]
59. Nishijima, S.; Suda, W.; Oshima, K.; Kim, S.W.; Hirose, Y.; Morita, H.; Hattori, M. The gut microbiome of healthy Japanese and its microbial and functional uniqueness. *DNA Res.* **2016**, *23*, 125–133. [CrossRef]
60. Vangay, P.; Johnson, A.J.; Ward, T.L.; Al-Ghalith, G.A.; Shields-Cutler, R.R.; Hillmann, B.M.; Lucas, S.K.; Beura, L.K.; Thompson, E.A.; Till, L.M.; et al. US Immigration Westernizes the Human Gut Microbiome. *Cell* **2018**, *175*, 962–972. [CrossRef]
61. Sankaranarayanan, R.; Ramadas, K.; Qiao, Y.L. Managing the changing burden of cancer in Asia. *BMC Med.* **2014**, *12*, 3. [CrossRef]
62. Gupta, S.; Hastak, K.; Ahmad, N.; Lewin, J.S.; Mukhtar, H. Inhibition of prostate carcinogenesis in TRAMP mice by oral infusion of green tea polyphenols. *Proc. Natl. Acad. Sci. USA* **2001**, *98*, 10350–10355. [CrossRef]
63. Harper, C.E.; Patel, B.B.; Wang, J.; Eltoum, I.A.; Lamartiniere, C.A. Epigallocatechin-3-Gallate suppresses early stage, but not late stage prostate cancer in TRAMP mice: Mechanisms of action. *Prostate* **2007**, *67*, 1576–1589. [CrossRef] [PubMed]
64. Khan, N.; Adhami, V.M.; Mukhtar, H. Review: Green tea polyphenols in chemoprevention of prostate cancer: Preclinical and clinical studies. *Nutr. Cancer* **2009**, *61*, 836–841. [CrossRef] [PubMed]
65. Kim, S.J.; Amankwah, E.; Connors, S.; Park, H.Y.; Rincon, M.; Cornnell, H.; Chornokur, G.; Hashim, A.I.; Choi, J.; Tsai, Y.Y.; et al. Safety and chemopreventive effect of polyphenon E in preventing early and metastatic progression of prostate cancer in TRAMP mice. *Cancer Prev. Res.* **2014**, *7*, 435–444. [CrossRef] [PubMed]
66. Suttie, A.; Nyska, A.; Haseman, J.K.; Moser, G.J.; Hackett, T.R.; Goldsworthy, T.L. A grading scheme for the assessment of proliferative lesions of the mouse prostate in the TRAMP model. *Toxicol. Pathol.* **2003**, *31*, 31–38. [CrossRef]
67. Bettuzzi, S.; Brausi, M.; Rizzi, F.; Castagnetti, G.; Peracchia, G.; Corti, A. Chemoprevention of human prostate cancer by oral administration of green tea catechins in volunteers with high-grade prostate intraepithelial neoplasia: A preliminary report from a one-year proof-of-principle study. *Cancer Res.* **2006**, *66*, 1234–1240. [CrossRef]
68. Brausi, M.; Rizzi, F.; Bettuzzi, S. Chemoprevention of human prostate cancer by green tea catechins: Two years later. A follow-up update. *Eur. Urol.* **2008**, *54*, 472–473. [CrossRef]
69. Chow, H.H.; Cai, Y.; Alberts, D.S.; Hakim, I.; Dorr, R.; Shahi, F.; Crowell, J.A.; Yang, C.S.; Hara, Y. Phase I pharmacokinetic study of tea polyphenols following single-dose administration of epigallocatechin gallate and polyphenon E. *Cancer Epidemiol. Biomark. Prev.* **2001**, *10*, 53–58.
70. Chow, H.H.; Cai, Y.; Hakim, I.A.; Crowell, J.A.; Shahi, F.; Brooks, C.A.; Dorr, R.T.; Hara, Y.; Alberts, D.S. Pharmacokinetics and safety of green tea polyphenols after multiple-dose administration of epigallocatechin gallate and polyphenon E in healthy individuals. *Clin. Cancer Res.* **2003**, *9*, 3312–3319.
71. Chow, H.H.; Hakim, I.A.; Vining, D.R.; Crowell, J.A.; Cordova, C.A.; Chew, W.M.; Xu, M.J.; Hsu, C.H.; Ranger-Moore, J.; Alberts, D.S. Effects of repeated green tea catechin administration on human cytochrome P450 activity. *Cancer Epidemiol. Biomark. Prev.* **2006**, *15*, 2473–2476. [CrossRef]
72. Chow, H.H.; Hakim, I.A.; Vining, D.R.; Crowell, J.A.; Ranger-Moore, J.; Chew, W.M.; Celaya, C.A.; Rodney, S.R.; Hara, Y.; Alberts, D.S. Effects of dosing condition on the oral bioavailability of green tea catechins after single-dose administration of Polyphenon E in healthy individuals. *Clin. Cancer Res.* **2005**, *11*, 4627–4633. [CrossRef]
73. Chow, H.H.; Hakim, I.A.; Vining, D.R.; Crowell, J.A.; Tome, M.E.; Ranger-Moore, J.; Cordova, C.A.; Mikhael, D.M.; Briehl, M.M.; Alberts, D.S. Modulation of human glutathione s-transferases by polyphenon e intervention. *Cancer Epidemiol. Biomark. Prev.* **2007**, *16*, 1662–1666. [CrossRef]
74. Isbrucker, R.A.; Edwards, J.A.; Wolz, E.; Davidovich, A.; Bausch, J. Safety studies on epigallocatechin gallate (EGCG) preparations. Part 2: Dermal, acute and short-term toxicity studies. *Food Chem. Toxicol.* **2006**, *44*, 636–650. [CrossRef]
75. Kumar, N.B.; Pow-Sang, J.; Egan, K.M.; Spiess, P.E.; Dickinson, S.; Salup, R.; Helal, M.; McLarty, J.; Williams, C.R.; Schreiber, F.; et al. Randomized, Placebo-Controlled Trial of Green Tea Catechins for Prostate Cancer Prevention. *Cancer Prev. Res.* **2015**, *8*, 879–887. [CrossRef]
76. Pisters, K.M.; Newman, R.A.; Coldman, B.; Shin, D.M.; Khuri, F.R.; Hong, W.K.; Glisson, B.S.; Lee, J.S. Phase I trial of oral green tea extract in adult patients with solid tumors. *J. Clin. Oncol.* **2001**, *19*, 1830–1838. [CrossRef]

77. Nakagawa, K.; Miyazawa, T. Chemiluminescence-high-performance liquid chromatographic determination of tea catechin, (−)-epigallocatechin 3-gallate, at picomole levels in rat and human plasma. *Anal. Biochem.* **1997**, *248*, 41–49. [CrossRef]
78. Nakagawa, K.; Ninomiya, M.; Okubo, T.; Aoi, N.; Juneja, L.R.; Kim, M.; Yamanaka, K.; Miyazawa, T. Tea catechin supplementation increases antioxidant capacity and prevents phospholipid hydroperoxidation in plasma of humans. *J. Agric. Food Chem.* **1999**, *47*, 3967–3973. [CrossRef]
79. Ullmann, U.; Haller, J.; Decourt, J.P.; Girault, N.; Girault, J.; Richard-Caudron, A.S.; Pineau, B.; Weber, P. A single ascending dose study of epigallocatechin gallate in healthy volunteers. *J. Int. Med. Res.* **2003**, *31*, 88–101. [CrossRef]
80. Nakagawa, K.; Okuda, S.; Miyazawa, T. Dose-dependent incorporation of tea catechins, (−)-epigallocatechin-3-gallate and (−)-epigallocatechin, into human plasma. *Biosci. Biotechnol. Biochem.* **1997**, *61*, 1981–1985. [CrossRef]
81. Kapetanovic, I.M.; Crowell, J.A.; Krishnaraj, R.; Zakharov, A.; Lindeblad, M.; Lyubimov, A. Exposure and toxicity of green tea polyphenols in fasted and non-fasted dogs. *Toxicology* **2009**, *260*, 28–36. [CrossRef]
82. Schmidt, M.; Schmitz, H.J.; Baumgart, A.; Guedon, D.; Netsch, M.I.; Kreuter, M.H.; Schmidlin, C.B.; Schrenk, D. Toxicity of green tea extracts and their constituents in rat hepatocytes in primary culture. *Food Chem. Toxicol.* **2005**, *43*, 307–314. [CrossRef]
83. Wu, K.M.; Yao, J.; Boring, D. Green tea extract-induced lethal toxicity in fasted but not in nonfasted dogs. *Int. J. Toxicol.* **2011**, *30*, 19–20. [CrossRef]
84. Nguyen, M.M.; Ahmann, F.R.; Nagle, R.B.; Hsu, C.H.; Tangrea, J.A.; Parnes, H.L.; Sokoloff, M.H.; Gretzer, M.B.; Chow, H.H. Randomized, double-blind, placebo-controlled trial of polyphenon E in prostate cancer patients before prostatectomy: Evaluation of potential chemopreventive activities. *Cancer Prev. Res.* **2012**, *5*, 290–298. [CrossRef]
85. Lane, J.A.; Er, V.; Avery, K.N.L.; Horwood, J.; Cantwell, M.; Caro, G.P.; Crozier, A.; Smith, G.D.; Donovan, J.L.; Down, L.; et al. ProDiet: A Phase II Randomized Placebo-controlled Trial of Green Tea Catechins and Lycopene in Men at Increased Risk of Prostate Cancer. *Cancer Prev. Res.* **2018**, *11*, 687–696. [CrossRef]
86. Samavat, H.; Ursin, G.; Emory, T.H.; Lee, E.; Wang, R.; Torkelson, C.J.; Dostal, A.M.; Swenson, K.; Le, C.T.; Yang, C.S.; et al. A Randomized Controlled Trial of Green Tea Extract Supplementation and Mammographic Density in Postmenopausal Women at Increased Risk of Breast Cancer. *Cancer Prev. Res.* **2017**, *10*, 710–718. [CrossRef]
87. Yu, Z.; Samavat, H.; Dostal, A.M.; Wang, R.; Torkelson, C.J.; Yang, C.S.; Butler, L.M.; Kensler, T.W.; Wu, A.H.; Kurzer, M.S.; et al. Effect of Green Tea Supplements on Liver Enzyme Elevation: Results from a Randomized Intervention Study in the United States. *Cancer Prev. Res.* **2017**, *10*, 571–579. [CrossRef]
88. Henning, S.M.; Wang, P.; Said, J.W.; Huang, M.; Grogan, T.; Elashoff, D.; Carpenter, C.L.; Heber, D.; Aronson, W.J. Randomized clinical trial of brewed green and black tea in men with prostate cancer prior to prostatectomy. *Prostate* **2015**, *75*, 550–559. [CrossRef]
89. McLarty, J.; Bigelow, R.L.; Smith, M.; Elmajian, D.; Ankem, M.; Cardelli, J.A. Tea polyphenols decrease serum levels of prostate-specific antigen, hepatocyte growth factor, and vascular endothelial growth factor in prostate cancer patients and inhibit production of hepatocyte growth factor and vascular endothelial growth factor in vitro. *Cancer Prev. Res.* **2009**, *2*, 673–682. [CrossRef]
90. Wang, P.; Aronson, W.J.; Huang, M.; Zhang, Y.; Lee, R.P.; Heber, D.; Henning, S.M. Green tea polyphenols and metabolites in prostatectomy tissue: Implications for cancer prevention. *Cancer Prev. Res.* **2010**, *3*, 985–993. [CrossRef]
91. Wilson, I.D.; Nicholson, J.K. Gut microbiome interactions with drug metabolism, efficacy, and toxicity. *Transl. Res.* **2017**, *179*, 204–222. [CrossRef]
92. Cheng, W.Y.; Wu, C.Y.; Yu, J. The role of gut microbiota in cancer treatment: Friend or foe? *Gut* **2020**, *69*, 1867–1876. [CrossRef]
93. Gopalakrishnan, V.; Spencer, C.N.; Nezi, L.; Reuben, A.; Andrews, M.C.; Karpinets, T.V.; Prieto, P.A.; Vicente, D.; Hoffman, K.; Wei, S.C.; et al. Gut microbiome modulates response to anti-PD-1 immunotherapy in melanoma patients. *Science* **2018**, *359*, 97–103. [CrossRef]
94. Gan, R.Y.; Li, H.B.; Sui, Z.Q.; Corke, H. Absorption, metabolism, anti-cancer effect and molecular targets of epigallocatechin gallate (EGCG): An updated review. *Crit. Rev. Food Sci. Nutr.* **2018**, *58*, 924–941. [CrossRef]
95. Guo, T.; Song, D.; Cheng, L.; Zhang, X. Interactions of tea catechins with intestinal microbiota and their implication for human health. *Food Sci. Biotechnol.* **2019**, *28*, 1617–1625. [CrossRef]
96. Azad, M.A.K.; Sarker, M.; Li, T.; Yin, J. Probiotic Species in the Modulation of Gut Microbiota: An Overview. *BioMed Res. Int.* **2018**, *2018*, 9478630. [CrossRef]
97. Parada Venegas, D.; De la Fuente, M.K.; Landskron, G.; González, M.J.; Quera, R.; Dijkstra, G.; Harmsen, H.J.M.; Faber, K.N.; Hermoso, M.A. Short Chain Fatty Acids (SCFAs)-Mediated Gut Epithelial and Immune Regulation and Its Relevance for Inflammatory Bowel Diseases. *Front. Immunol.* **2019**, *10*, 277. [CrossRef]
98. Chiou, Y.-S.; Wu, J.-C.; Huang, Q.; Shahidi, F.; Wang, Y.-J.; Ho, C.-T.; Pan, M.-H. Metabolic and colonic microbiota transformation may enhance the bioactivities of dietary polyphenols. *J. Funct. Foods* **2014**, *7*, 3–25. [CrossRef]
99. Jang, Y.G.; Ko, E.B.; Choi, K.C. Gallic acid, a phenolic acid, hinders the progression of prostate cancer by inhibition of histone deacetylase 1 and 2 expression. *J. Nutr. Biochem.* **2020**, *84*, 108444. [CrossRef]
100. Liu, K.C.; Huang, A.C.; Wu, P.P.; Lin, H.Y.; Chueh, F.S.; Yang, J.S.; Lu, C.C.; Chiang, J.H.; Meng, M.; Chung, J.G. Gallic acid suppresses the migration and invasion of PC-3 human prostate cancer cells via inhibition of matrix metalloproteinase-2 and -9 signaling pathways. *Oncol. Rep.* **2011**, *26*, 177–184. [CrossRef] [PubMed]
101. Jin, J.S.; Touyama, M.; Hisada, T.; Benno, Y. Effects of green tea consumption on human fecal microbiota with special reference to Bifidobacterium species. *Microbiol. Immunol.* **2012**, *56*, 729–739. [CrossRef]

102. Liao, Z.L.; Zeng, B.H.; Wang, W.; Li, G.H.; Wu, F.; Wang, L.; Zhong, Q.P.; Wei, H.; Fang, X. Impact of the Consumption of Tea Polyphenols on Early Atherosclerotic Lesion Formation and Intestinal Bifidobacteria in High-Fat-Fed ApoE$^{-/-}$ Mice. *Front. Nutr.* **2016**, *3*, 42. [CrossRef]
103. Wang, J.; Tang, L.; Zhou, H.; Zhou, J.; Glenn, T.C.; Shen, C.L.; Wang, J.S. Long-term treatment with green tea polyphenols modifies the gut microbiome of female sprague-dawley rats. *J. Nutr. Biochem.* **2018**, *56*, 55–64. [CrossRef] [PubMed]
104. Le Chatelier, E.; Nielsen, T.; Qin, J.; Prifti, E.; Hildebrand, F.; Falony, G.; Almeida, M.; Arumugam, M.; Batto, J.M.; Kennedy, S.; et al. Richness of human gut microbiome correlates with metabolic markers. *Nature* **2013**, *500*, 541–546. [CrossRef] [PubMed]
105. Schluter, J.; Peled, J.U.; Taylor, B.P.; Markey, K.A.; Smith, M.; Taur, Y.; Niehus, R.; Staffas, A.; Dai, A.; Fontana, E.; et al. The gut microbiota is associated with immune cell dynamics in humans. *Nature* **2020**, *588*, 303–307. [CrossRef]
106. Shin, J.-H.; Park, Y.-H.; Sim, M.; Kim, S.-A.; Joung, H.; Shin, D.-M. Serum level of sex steroid hormone is associated with diversity and profiles of human gut microbiome. *Res. Microbiol.* **2019**, *170*, 192–201. [CrossRef] [PubMed]
107. Pernigoni, N.; Zagato, E.; Calcinotto, A.; Troiani, M.; Mestre, R.P.; Calì, B.; Attanasio, G.; Troisi, J.; Minini, M.; Mosole, S.; et al. Commensal bacteria promote endocrine resistance in prostate cancer through androgen biosynthesis. *Science* **2021**, *374*, 216–224. [CrossRef]
108. Zhong, W.; Wu, K.; Long, Z.; Zhou, X.; Zhong, C.; Wang, S.; Lai, H.; Guo, Y.; Lv, D.; Lu, J.; et al. Gut dysbiosis promotes prostate cancer progression and docetaxel resistance via activating NF-κB-IL6-STAT3 axis. *Microbiome* **2022**, *10*, 94. [CrossRef]
109. Matsushita, M.; Fujita, K.; Hatano, K.; Hayashi, T.; Kayama, H.; Motooka, D.; Hase, H.; Yamamoto, A.; Uemura, T.; Yamamichi, G.; et al. High-fat diet promotes prostate cancer growth through histamine signaling. *Int. J. Cancer* **2022**, *151*, 623–636. [CrossRef]
110. Liss, M.A.; White, J.R.; Goros, M.; Gelfond, J.; Leach, R.; Johnson-Pais, T.; Lai, Z.; Rourke, E.; Basler, J.; Ankerst, D.; et al. Metabolic Biosynthesis Pathways Identified from Fecal Microbiome Associated with Prostate Cancer. *Eur. Urol.* **2018**, *74*, 575–582. [CrossRef]
111. Golombos, D.M.; Ayangbesan, A.; O'Malley, P.; Lewicki, P.; Barlow, L.M.; Barbieri, C.E.; Chan, C.; DuLong, C.; Abu-Ali, G.; Huttenhower, C.; et al. The Role of Gut Microbiome in the Pathogenesis of Prostate Cancer: A Prospective, Pilot Study. *Urology* **2018**, *111*, 122–128. [CrossRef]
112. Takezawa, K.; Fujita, K.; Matsushita, M.; Motooka, D.; Hatano, K.; Banno, E.; Shimizu, N.; Takao, T.; Takada, S.; Okada, K.; et al. The Firmicutes/Bacteroidetes ratio of the human gut microbiota is associated with prostate enlargement. *Prostate* **2021**, *81*, 1287–1293. [CrossRef]
113. Kure, A.; Tsukimi, T.; Ishii, C.; Aw, W.; Obana, N.; Nakato, G.; Hirayama, A.; Kawano, H.; China, T.; Shimizu, F.; et al. Gut environment changes due to androgen deprivation therapy in patients with prostate cancer. *Prostate Cancer Prostatic Dis.* **2022**. [CrossRef] [PubMed]
114. Panek, M.; Čipčić Paljetak, H.; Barešić, A.; Perić, M.; Matijašić, M.; Lojkić, I.; Vranešić Bender, D.; Krznarić, Ž.; Verbanac, D. Methodology challenges in studying human gut microbiota–effects of collection, storage, DNA extraction and next generation sequencing technologies. *Sci. Rep.* **2018**, *8*, 5143. [CrossRef] [PubMed]
115. Sanna, S.; Kurilshikov, A.; Van Der Graaf, A.; Fu, J.; Zhernakova, A. Challenges and future directions for studying effects of host genetics on the gut microbiome. *Nat. Genet.* **2022**, *54*, 100–106. [CrossRef]
116. Sinha, R.; Goedert, J.J.; Vogtmann, E.; Hua, X.; Porras, C.; Hayes, R.; Safaeian, M.; Yu, G.; Sampson, J.; Ahn, J.; et al. Quantification of Human Microbiome Stability Over 6 Months: Implications for Epidemiologic Studies. *Am. J. Epidemiol.* **2018**, *187*, 1282–1290. [CrossRef] [PubMed]

cancers

MDPI

Review

Targeting Breast Cancer-Derived Stem Cells by Dietary Phytochemicals: A Strategy for Cancer Prevention and Treatment

Kumari Sunita Prajapati [1], Sanjay Gupta [2,*] and Shashank Kumar [1,*]

1 Molecular Signaling & Drug Discovery Laboratory, Department of Biochemistry, Central University of Punjab, Guddha, Bathinda 151401, India; ksunita.prajapati@gmail.com

2 Department of Urology, Nutrition, Pharmacology and Pathology, Case Western Reserve University, Cleveland, OH 44106, USA

* Correspondence: sanjay.gupta@case.edu (S.G.); shashankbiochemau@gmail.com (S.K.)

Simple Summary: Luminal A subtype breast cancer is the most prevalent form of breast malignancy with frequent diagnosis in women. Breast cancer stem cells (BCSCs) are a rare population of cells present therein that cause cancer aggressiveness, relapse, drug-resistance, poor therapeutic outcome and a decrease in overall survival of these patients. The published literature indicates that dietary phytochemicals have the potential to target stemness and self-renewal properties in luminal A-derived BCSCs. The aim of this review is to highlight the anticancer potential of dietary phytochemicals against luminal A-derived BCSCs and their underlying mechanism(s). These findings necessitate in-depth preclinical and clinical studies on phytochemicals to explore their role in breast cancer prevention and treatment.

Abstract: Breast cancer is heterogeneous disease with variable prognosis and therapeutic response. Approximately, 70% of diagnosed breast cancer represents the luminal A subtype. This subpopulation has a fair prognosis with a lower rate of relapse than the other clinical subtypes. Acquisition of stemness in luminal A subtype modifies the phenotype plasticity to accomplish increased aggressiveness and therapeutic resistance. Therefore, targeting luminal A-derived breast cancer stem cells (BCSCs) could be a promising strategy for its prevention and treatment. Extensive studies reveal that dietary phytochemicals have the potential to target BCSCs by modulating the molecular and signal transduction pathways. Dietary phytochemicals alone or in combination with standard therapeutic modalities exert higher efficacy in targeting BCSCs through changes in stemness, self-renewal properties and hypoxia-related factors. These combinations offer achieving higher radio- and chemo- sensitization through alteration in the key signaling pathways such as AMPK, STAT3, NF-kB, Hedgehog, PI3K/Akt/mTOR, Notch, GSK3β, and Wnt related to cancer stemness and drug resistance. In this review, we highlight the concept of targeting luminal A-derived BCSCs with dietary phytochemicals by summarizing the pathways and underlying mechanism(s) involved during therapeutic resistance.

Keywords: breast cancer stem cells; dietary phytochemical; luminal A subtype; signaling pathway; cancer prevention; therapeutic resistance

Citation: Prajapati, K.S.; Gupta, S.; Kumar, S. Targeting Breast Cancer-Derived Stem Cells by Dietary Phytochemicals: A Strategy for Cancer Prevention and Treatment. *Cancers* **2022**, *14*, 2864. https://doi.org/10.3390/cancers14122864

Academic Editor: Andrea Manni

Received: 27 May 2022
Accepted: 8 June 2022
Published: 10 June 2022

1. Introduction

Breast cancer is a heterogeneous disease that generally initiates in the milk glands or in ducts, which is referred to as lobular/ductal carcinoma in situ. These neoplastic breast cancer cells migrate through the gland/duct walls and proliferate in the surrounding tissue, which ultimately transform into an invasive phenotype. Breast cancer is frequently characterized by four major molecular subtypes that includes the luminal A (HR+/HER2−), luminal B (HR+/HER2+), basal-like (HR−/HER2−), and HER2-enriched (HR−/HER2+) subpopulations. The molecular subtypes (luminal A, luminal B, basal-like, and HER2 enriched) constitute approximately 73%, 11%, 12%, and 4% of breast cancer [1]. The other less common molecular subtypes include claudin-low and molecular apocrine forms. These molecular subtypes assist patient categorization, allowing them for better management of the disease as well as therapy-type decisions. Of the four major subtypes, luminal A tumors grow at a slower rate and are less aggressive with fairly high survival and low recurrence [1]. Conventional therapies target rapidly growing malignant cells that result in extensive elimination of tumors. Nonetheless, the surviving fraction constituting the minimal residual disease expands and undergoes multi-lineage differentiation to reconstitute the tumor. The reemerged tumor is highly aggressive, drug resistant, and comprises a new phenotype exhibiting increased aggressiveness and stemness. These cells are often referred as "cancer stem-like cells". Targeting breast cancer stem cells (BCSCs) is the key to improving the efficacy of breast cancer. These cells have self-renewal properties and express stemness markers. BCSCs play an important role in the causation of drug resistance and results in a poor clinical outcome. Researchers are finding ways to target and remove the bulk of the tumor mass along with BCSCs for effective prevention and/or treatment of breast cancers. BCSCs play an important role in cancer metastasis due to the aberrant expression of some stemness-related factors, such as CD44, SOX2, OCT4, c-MYC, KLF4, Nanog, and SALL4 [2,3]. Besides the high expression of stemness and self-renewal markers, the aberrant expression of molecular signaling pathways including Wnt/β-catenin, Notch, Hedgehog, JAK-STAT, and PI3K/Akt/mTOR in BCSCs are shown to be involved in the pathophysiology of the disease [4,5]. Overall, the present literature reveals that the occurrence of BCSCs in the tumor microenvironment positively correlates with disease recurrence, low survival rate, chemo/radio therapy resistance, and low therapeutic output [6].

2. Clinical Characteristics of Breast Cancer Subtypes

Advanced molecular techniques provide a clear-cut characterization of breast cancer subtypes with better prediction and prognosis. Gene-based molecular assays, such as 70-gene and 80-gene signatures, 21-gene Recurrence Score, PAM50-ROR (50-gene Prediction Analysis of Microarrays and Risk of Recurrence), Endo-Predict, and the Breast Cancer Index (BCI) provide a precise characterization of breast cancer subtypes with better prediction and prognosis. The 21-gene recurrence score quantifies the probability of distant recurrence in patients with node-negative, ER+ breast cancer treated with tamoxifen into low, intermediate, and high-risk categories. The PAM50 classifies the intrinsic subtypes (luminal A, luminal B, HER2 enriched, basal, and normal breast) with risk of recurrence (low, intermediate, and high). The PAM50-ROR determines the probability of distant recurrence over 10 years. The 70-gene signature has the ability to divide patients into low- or high-risk corresponding to 10-year distant-metastasis-free survival (DMFS). The 80-gene signature divide patients into luminal, basal, and HER2 intrinsic subtypes. The combined 70- and 80-gene signatures are also able to classify breast cancer patients into luminal A-like (luminal subtype and low-risk), luminal B-like (luminal and high-risk), HER2, and basal subtypes [7,8].

Clinical reports suggest that at least half of the newly diagnosed breast cancer belongs to luminal A subtype. Initially, in 2011–2013, the oncologist proposed the molecular basis for the treatment of early breast cancer, which defined luminal A breast cancer patients as having a estrogen receptor (ER) positive, progesterone receptor (PR) positive (20%), HER2 negative, and Ki67 positivity of <14% [9,10]. This definition was based upon the gene profile (gene-based assay) and immunohistochemistry (IHC-based markers) of the tumor. The patients with IHC-based luminal A tumors were demonstrated to have better disease-free survival if PR expression was >20%. Especially for the luminal A breast cancer subtype, the patients and clinicians prefer surrogate IHC-based markers over gene-based biomarkers to establish the subtype. Overall, both the gene- and IHC-based biomarkers have been utilized for subtyping and treatment preference for breast cancer patients [11].

3. Relevance of Targeting Luminal A-Derived Breast Cancer Stem Cells

It has been widely accepted that the luminal cells of the mammary gland are unipotent, i.e., produce one cell type and have a self-renewal potential after evolution. Song et al. (2019) reported that during pregnancy or hormonal stimulation, the luminal cells give rise to luminal-derived basal cells (LdBCs) expressing the basal markers and ERα receptors. These cells respond to hormones and possess stem-cell renewal capability in the mammary gland [12]. Previously, it was reported that the Wnt and Notch signaling are determinants of the basal fate and luminal lineage. Recent findings align with the previous report that LdBCs demonstrated increased Wnt signaling (Figure 1). The plasticity of mammary luminal cells are associated with tumor progression in breast cancer patients [12]. The molecular subtype of breast cancer shows differential therapeutic response. Mei et al. (2020) studied the cancer stemness relationship with the molecular subtype of breast cancer in a comparative manner. The group developed MCF-7 cells (referred to as OKMS), which concomitantly overexpressed stemness-related genes (OCT4, KLF4, MYC, and SOX2) at the mRNA and protein level. These OKMS cells exhibited relatively low ER and higher HER2 expression. The cell growth and migration potential was increased up to 1.5 fold and the cancer stem cell population was increased up to 16% in OKMS cells, compared to parental MCF-7 cells. The OKMS cells demonstrated a drug response similar to HER2 positive cells after treatment with tamoxifen and trastuzumab. These results suggest a shift towards more aggressive and malignant tumors. However, luminal A cells exhibit slow growth and are less malignant but increase in stemness, transforming them to a more aggressive phenotype [13]. In another study, Yousefnia et al. (2019) reported that after a few passages, luminal A cells demonstrate a greater number of mammosphere formation in comparison to triple negative breast cancer cells [14]. Kim et al. (2012) demonstrated that tumor-derived pure luminal-like cells were capable of initiating invasive tumors, and generate larger tumors in comparison to basal-like cells in the in vivo model [15]. In addition, the stemness of cancer cells has the ability to change the tumor microenvironment in favor of supporting their aggressive natures [16]. Overall, these studies suggest that the stemness in the luminal A subtype transforms these cells to a more aggressive breast cancer phenotype. Since the luminal subtype forms the majority of breast cancer cases, targeting luminal A-derived BCSCs could provide a better therapeutic efficacy.

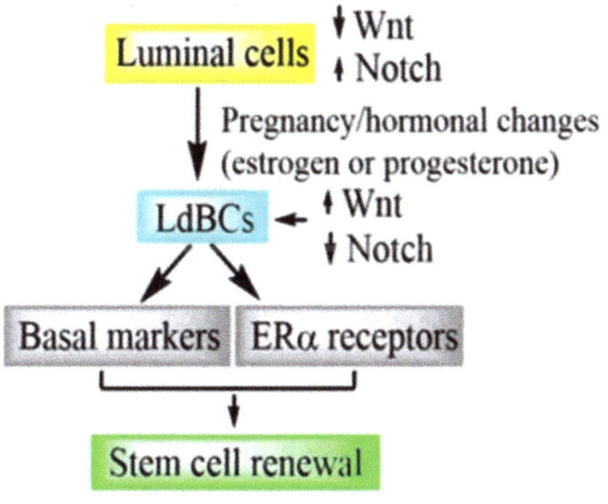

Figure 1. Sequential molecular events during self-renewal property acquisition in luminal A cells. LdBCs—Luminal-derived basal cells.

Epidemiologic and preclinical studies suggest that dietary phytochemicals possess chemopreventive properties against various cancer types. These phytochemicals possess anticancer, antioxidant, antiviral, antibacterial, and various other pharmacological activities. Dietary phytochemicals, such as curcumin, quercetin, resveratrol, silibinin, lycopene, and emodin have been found to be useful in decreasing cancer incidence. A number of studies summarize the anticancer potential of phytochemicals and their importance in drug development. Dietary phytochemicals have the ability to reduce cancer promotion by inhibiting cancer cell proliferation, survival, invasion/metastasis, angiogenesis, and eliminating toxic carcinogens from the body through targeting different cancer-related signaling pathways. Dietary compounds also regulate cell cycle progression, inflammatory cytokines, and oxidative stress response in cancer cells, and have the potential to modulate small non-coding RNAs' expression alone or in a synergistic manner. More importantly, dietary phytochemicals have a greater ability to prevent/inhibit the formation of a small population of cancer cells often referred to as cancer stem-like cells by targeting various signaling pathways [17–27]. Therefore, targeting the luminal A-derived BCSCs by dietary phytochemicals could be a better strategy in the prevention and clinical management of breast cancer. The involvement of dietary phytochemicals in the management of BCSCs may provide significant contribution in this direction due to their minimal toxicity, low-cost, and bioavailability. In this article, we have reviewed the putative role of dietary phytochemicals in targeting luminal A-derived BCSCs in order to provide a strategy to increase the therapeutic efficacy in breast cancer patients. As most studies have focused on the role of dietary and non-dietary phytochemicals in cancer stem cell pathophysiology, to date, there is no comprehensive analysis to explore the role of dietary phytochemicals related to luminal A-cell-derived BCSCs. Here, we discuss the molecular mechanism(s) and pathways through which these phytochemicals target luminal A-cell-derived BCSCs. In addition, we also provide information related to pharmacokinetics, metabolism, bioavailability, dosage, and changes in the microbiome.

4. Source of Data

The literature published (in the English language) and indexed in the PubMed database was utilized for the present review. The relevant studies were retrieved through the use of "breast cancer stem cell, luminal A, mammosphere" as keywords in searches of the database. The literature that contained the luminal A breast cell-derived cancer stem cells and phytochemicals was filtered. Various in vitro luminal A breast cancer cells (BT483, CAMA1, EFM19, HCC1428, HCC712, IBEP2, KPL1, LY2, MCF-7, MDAMB134, MDAMB134VI, MDAMB175, MDAMB175VII, MDAMB415, T47D, ZR751, and ZR75B) were taken into consideration; however, most of the studies were focused on the MCF-7 cell-derived mammosphere, which demonstrated increased stemness/self-renewal markers. Further, the literature was filtered on the basis of dietary and non-dietary phytochemicals by finding the associated published information (Table 1). Data published on the role of dietary phytochemicals on luminal A-derived breast cancer stem cells were only considered in the study. Dietary phytochemicals viz. curcumin, naringenin, resveratrol, genistein, quercetin, silibinin, and thymoquinone, comparatively cited in the literature, were used in the review. Additional phytochemicals such as ginsenoside Rg3, hisperidin, pristimerin, pterostilbene, 3-O-(E)-p-Coumaroyl betulinic acid and withaferin A, which are less studied, are discussed under a common heading, namely "other dietary phytochemicals".

Table 1. List of dietary phytochemicals and associated secondary metabolite group targeting luminal A breast cancer cells.

Phytochemical Group	Phytochemicals	Reference
Isothiocynate	Benzyl Isothiocynate	[28]
Triterpene lactone, triterpenoids, monoterpene	Brusatol, Pristimerin, Thymoquinone	[29–31]
Phenolic, isoflavones, flavonoids, flavanone glycosid	Curcumin, Eugenol, Genistein, Pterostilbene, Quercetin, Silibinin, 6-Shogoal, Hesperidin, Quercetin-3-methyl ether	[30,32–37]
Anthraquinone	Emodin	[38]
Steroidal lactone, steroidal Saponin	Withaferin-A, Ginsenoside Rg3	[35,39]
Carbazole alkaloid	Mahanine	[40]

5. Curcumin and Stemness in BCSCs

Curcumin belongs to the polyphenolic group of phytochemicals and is an important component of the spice turmeric all around the globe, especially in India. It is used for its coloring ability and taste. Moreover, curcumin has been used in various medicinal preparations of Ayurveda and Chinese Medicinal systems. Numerous studies report potent biological activity, and applications in the food, biotechnology, and cosmetics industry. Curcumin is well-known for its health promoting and disease preventive properties [41]. Yang et al. (2020) studied the effect of curcumin (alone and in combination with nanoparticles) in the radiation-treated (4Gy) MCF-7 cell-derived mammosphere. The group found that curcumin significantly increased the radio-sensitivity in the breast sphere cells alone and in combination with the gold nanoparticles. More than 60% of the sphere population was significantly damaged by curcumin treatment. Curcumin pretreatment in the radiation-exposed breast cancer MCF-7 and MDA-MB-231 cell-derived mammosphere demonstrated increased apoptosis and reactive oxygen species formation, G0/G1 phase cell cycle arrest, and decreased HIF-1α and HSP90 protein expression [42]. Sarighieh et al. (2020) tested the efficacy of curcumin in cancer stem cells isolated from MCF-7 cells. The cells were sorted in the presence of CD44+/CD24− surface markers, and the curcumin treatment was rendered both in hypoxic and normoxic conditions. The curcumin-treated MCF-7-derived cancer stem-like cells demonstrated early apoptosis and G2/M phase arrest under hypoxic conditions. Under normoxic conditions, the curcumin induced S and G2/M phase arrest in the cells [43]. The curcumin inhibits HIF1 nuclear translocation by degrading ARNT (aryl hydrocarbon receptor nuclear translocator), which is required for the transcription of hypoxia-related genes in breast cancer stem cells. The treatment also decreases HIF1 and HIF-2α expression in MCF-7 cell-derived mammospheres. In another study, Borah et al. (2020) demonstrated that curcumin in combination with GANT61 (Gli1 and 2 inhibitor of hedgehog signaling pathway) loaded PLGA (poly(lactic-co-glycolic acid) nanoparticles demonstrated self-renewal inhibitory potential in MCF-7 cell-derived mammospheres [44]. Attia et al. (2020) reported the effect of curcumin in combination with paclitaxel and vitamin D on MCF-7 cells. The study demonstrated that it improved anti-cancer activity and anti-drug resistance efficacy in MCF-7 cells by a decrease in proliferation and increased apoptosis. Further treatment significantly decreased cancer stemness markers (multidrug resistance complex and aldehyde dehrogenase-1) at the protein level [45]. Liu et al. (2019) studied the effect of a curcumin coating on a synthetic polymer (oligomeric hyaluronic acid-hydrazone bond-folic acid-biotin), which forms curcumin nano-actiniaes (Cu-NA). The Cu-NA demonstrated increased toxicity in MCF-7 cells, breast cancer stem cells, and in the in vivo anticancer experiment in comparison to free curcumin and/or other control groups [46]. Hu et al. (2019) demonstrated that curcumin has the potential to inhibit the cancer stemness property (Oct4, Nanog, and Sox2) and the epithelial to mesenchymal

(EMT) transition in luminal A cells. The group isolated the CD44+CD24−/^{low} subpopulation of MCF-7 cells, which shows breast cancer stem-like properties. The study reported that curcumin treatment resulted in a decreased cell proliferation and colony formation potential in these cells [47]. Hashemzehi et al. (2018) demonstrated the efficacy of a novel curcumin formulation (phytosomal encapsulated curcumin) on thrombin-induced cellular proliferation and metastasis in MCF-7 cells. The study demonstrated that curcumin formulation exerts its anticancer, anti-metastatic, and anti-stemness potential by activating AMPK signaling [48]. Li et al. (2018) demonstrated that curcumin treatment decreases the expression of stemness markers (ALDH1A1, CD44, Nanog, and Oct4) and inhibit Sonic hedgehog and Wnt signaling pathways in MCF-7 cell-derived mammospheres [49]. In another study, the folate decorated curcumin-loaded nanostructured lipid carriers (FA-CUR-NLCs) formulation demonstrated enhanced antitumor activity (in comparison to standard curcumin) in MCF-7 cell-inoculated animal models [50]. Yuan et al. (2018) studied the effect of the curcumin and doxorubicin combined nano-formulation (CURDOX-NPs) against drug resistance MCF-7 cell (MCF-7/ADR)-derived mammospheres. The study reported that the CURDOX-NPs significantly reduced the mammosphere formation potential in vitro and demonstrated tumor growth regression (~33%) in a mouse xenograft model [51]. Zhou et al. (2017) showed that curcumin has the potential to inhibit the drug resistance potential in breast cancer stem-like cells by improving Bcl-2-mediated apoptosis. The apoptosis inducing efficacy of curcumin was more pronounced during the combined treatment with Wnt and PI3K inhibitors. The treatment significantly decreased the anti-apoptotic proteins and increased the expression of pro-apoptotic proteins in targeted cells [52]. In a different study, Zhou et al. (2015) reported that curcumin has the potential to inhibit the cancer stem cell self-renewal potential in MCF-7 cell-derived mammospheres by lowering the expression of drug efflux transporters (ABCG2). Curcumin treatment also improved the anti-cancer efficacy of mitomycin C in the in vitro breast cancer stem cell model [53]. Further, Zhou et al. (2011) d that the co-treatment of curcumin and mitomycin C significantly reduced the mitomycin C-associated side-effects and improved its efficacy in a breast cancer xenograft model. Curcumin co-treatment altered the creatinine/blood urea nitrogen level and glutamic oxalacetic transaminase/glutamic pyruvic transaminase activity towards normal levels. The study indicated that curcumin mitigates the kidney reacted toxicity due to mitomycin C treatment in MCF-7 xenograft models. Moreover, curcumin and mitomycin C synergistically induced cell cycle arrest via the p38 MAPK pathway in the in vivo model compared to respective alone treatment(s) [54].

Other studies indicate that STAT3 (Signal Transducer and Activator of Transcription 3) and NF-κB (Nuclear factor-κB) signaling pathways play an important role in the maintenance of cancer stem-like properties in cancer cells. Chung and Vadgama, (2015) studied the effect of curcumin and EGCG co-treatment in CD44+ MCF-7-derived BCSCs. The study demonstrated a significant decrease in stem cell population, and decreased STAT3 phosphorylation and STAT3-NFkB interaction in the curcumin-treated cells [55]. Furthermore, curcumin co-treatment with interferon-β/retinoic acid (IFN-β/RA) in the MCF-7 athymic nude mouse model demonstrated synergistic anticancer potential. Curcumin increases the IFN-β/RA level with a simultaneous decrease in cyclooxygenase-2 (COX-2) activity and increases the DNA damage-inducible gene 153 (GADD153) expression, resulting in reduced tumor growth [56]. A summarization about the curcumin potential against luminal A-derived breast cancer stem cells includes (i) the decrease in self-renewal/stemness marker(s) expression, (ii) the possessed radio-sensitization and chemo-sensitization potential, (iii) targets AMPK, STAT3, and NF-kB signaling pathways and hypoxia-related markers, (iv) decreases the expression of multi-drug resistance transporters (ABCG2), and (v) the possessed synergetic anti-breast cancer stem cell potential. The overall mechanism(s) of the curcumin regulation of breast cancer stemness and associated signaling pathways is shown in Figure 2.

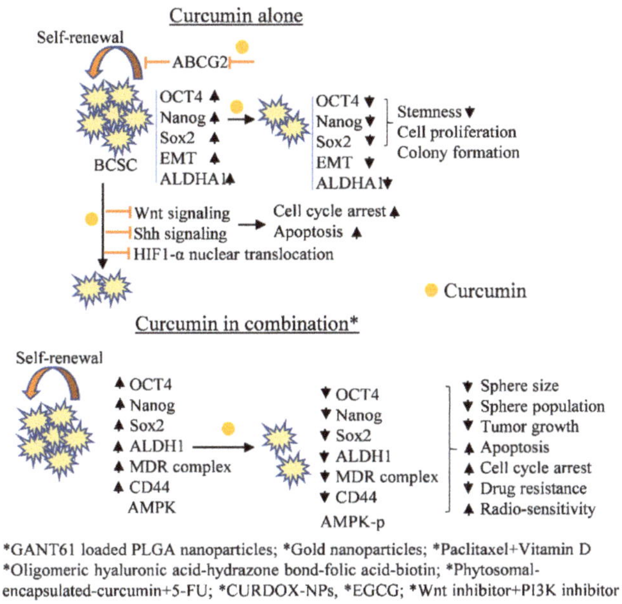

Figure 2. Effect of curcumin on luminal A-derived mammosphere. Yellow-colored circle represents curcumin. HIF-1α—Hypoxia inducing factor-1α, AMPK—AMP-activated protein kinase, EMT—Epithelial mesenchymal transition, Shh—Sonic hedgehog, ALDHA1—Aldehyde dehydrogenase A1, SRY (sex determining region Y)-box 2, and MDR—Multi-drug resistance.

6. Phytoestrogen and BCSCs

Phytoestrogens are polyphenolic naturally occurring secondary metabolites of plants. These molecules are structurally and functionally similar to the mammalian major sex hormone, 17-β-oestradiol (E2). Coumestans and isoflavones are widely researched phytoestrogens. These compounds are found in a variety of foods and possess a protective effect against hormone-related cancers and other diseases. The literature search related to the present review demonstrated that naringenin, resveratrol, genistein, apigenin, and quercetin possess the potential to target luminal A-derived BCSCs.

6.1. Genistein

Genistein is a naturally occurring isoflavone present in various dietary sources, including legumes and soybean products [57]. A hydroxyl group at carbon 7 forms a glycosidic linkage with sugar molecules and generates its dietary carbohydrate conjugates [58]. Genistein elicits several pharmacological activities, such as protein tyrosine kinase and DNA topoisomerase II inhibition, and the induction of antioxidant enzymes. The report demonstrates the role of genistein in the induction of apoptosis, cell cycle arrest, cell proliferation and metastasis inhibition in breast cancer experimental models. Genistein alters the expression of cancer-associated signaling pathways alone or in combination with standard chemotherapeutic drugs [43]. The Krüppel-like factor 4 (KLF4), an evolutionary conserved zinc finger-containing transcription factor, regulates cellular proliferation. In cancer, it functions in an organ-specific manner and displays both an oncogenic and tumor suppressive role. KLF4 is highly expressed in >70% breast cancer patients, human breast cancer cell lines, and mouse mammary cell-derived stem cells. A high KLF4 expression was positively associated with the increased self-renewal/stemness markers and side-population in experimental settings [59]. A later report demonstrates that genistein in combination with sulforaphane significantly reduces KLF4 expression at mRNA and protein levels in MCF-7 cells [60]. BCSCs undergo increased endocytosis (clathrin and caveolin independent) than analogous non-stem cancer cells. Genistein was unable to inhibit the endocytosis in the MCF-7-derived mammosphere but demonstrated a mammosphere reduction potential [61]. Genistein inhibit mammosphere formation in MCF-7 cells by downregulating the Hedgehog and PI3K/Akt pathway and inhibiting abiogenesis in mammary glands [62–64]. Further, it has been reported that genistein target adipogenesis and stem cell formation in an interleukin-6 (IL-6) independent manner [64]. In a similar study, genistein at a 25 μM dose increases the sphere formation potential in MCF-7 cell-derived tertiary spheroids. The genistein increased protease inhibitor 9 (PI-9, granzyme b inhibitor) expression and decreased estrogen receptor isoform (ERα66) [65]. It also reduced the mammosphere formation potential in MDA-MB-231 cells both in co-cultured with MCF-7 cells and in solo culture at micro and nanomolar concentrations. Although the size of the spheroids was reduced in both cultures, the morphological changes were observed only in the co-cultured experimental setup. Another study revealed that genistein inhibits the stem cell formation in MDA-MB-231 cells via induction PI3K/Akt and MEK/ERK signaling pathways in a paracrine manner through the increased expression of amphiregulin in MCF-7 cells [66]. Genistein alone or in combination with other phytoestrogens has been reported to inhibit/reduce tumor growth both in in vitro and in vivo systems. The combination of genistein (GEN) and lignan enterolactone (ENL) (100 mg/kg ENL + 100 mg/kg GEN) demonstrated that the inhibition of estradiol (E2) induced in MCF-7 cells established tumor growth and angiogenesis in mice [67]. The published literature thus far suggests the effect of genistein against luminal A-derived BCSCs through the (i) downregulation of the Hedgehog and PI3K/Akt pathway, (ii) suppression of the oncogenic transcription factors and (iii) inhibition of the mammosphere formation in ER^- breast cancer cells in a paracrine manner.

6.2. *Naringenin and Resveratrol*

Naringenin belongs to flavanones, a subclass of flavonoid. The compound is widely distributed in tomatoes, citrus, and other fruits. It is also found in glycoside form, known as naringin in various dietary sources. Naringenin is insoluble in water and soluble in organic solvents. The compound possesses antioxidant, anti-inflammatory, anti-aging, anticancer, anti-asthma, and anti-viral properties. Moreover, it has been utilized in infertility, immuno-depression, constipation, hepatic damage, pregnancy, and obesity as a therapeutic molecule [68]. Naringenin has been reported to possess anticancer activity, induce apoptosis, and cell cycle arrest at different concentrations in various human breast cancer cell lines. Naringenin has been well documented in managing the cancer cell growth and proliferation, migration, and multi-drug resistance both in in vitro and in vivo by targeting signaling pathways such as Jak/Stat3, Notch1, p38/MAPK, NF- B, PI3K/Akt, and COX2. Nanoparticle formulations of naringenin improves chemosensitization and anticancer potential [68]. Curcumin-naringenin loaded dextran-coated magnetic nanoparticles (CUR-NAR-D-MNPs) in combination with radiotherapy has been studied in the MCF-7 cell-inoculated mouse model. CUR-NAR-D-MNPs, in combination with radiotherapy, reduced tumor volume and induced cell cycle arrest and apoptosis by modulating the expression of p21, p53, TNF-α, CD44, and ROS signaling in experimental animals [69]. The group also studied the effect of phytoestrogens (naringenin, resveratrol, and quercetin) in the MCF-7 cell-derived xenograft model. The findings revealed that the phytoestrogen treatment inhibit the survival of breast tumor initiating cells, and restrict tumor growth rates and tumor initiation by increasing DAXX protein levels. Phytoestrogens demonstrated DAXX-mediated anti-breast cancer activity in the order of naringenin > resveratrol > quercetin at 20 mg/kg dose [70].

Resveratrol is a lipid soluble polyphenolic compound. The phytochemical is found in cis and trans conformations in dietary sources. The dietary source of resveratrol includes cranberry, red/white grapes, strawberry, peanuts, etc. Resveratrol has been well documented for its cardio-protective and cancer preventive properties [71]. After hormonal therapy, the tumor initiating cells in ER+ breast cancer typically demonstrate increased Notch signaling activity and resistance to therapy. These cells do not express the death domain-associated protein 6 (DAXX), resulting in the activation of notch signaling and formation of therapy-resistant tumor initiating cells (TICs) [70]. It is quite interesting that the treatment of MCF-7 cell-derived TICs with phytoestrogens (such as naringenin and resveratrol) demonstrated increased DAXX expression, which results in the inhibition of the Notch signaling-mediated TIC-cell enrichment. It should be noted that naringenin and resveratrol demonstrate this effect by selectively targeting both ERα and ERβ forms of the estrogen receptor. The findings of Peiffer et al. (2020) indicate that the selective inhibition of ER receptor isoforms by phytochemicals could be a novel therapeutic approach to target cancer stemness and tumor initiation in therapy resistant ER+ positive cells [70].

6.3. *Quercetin*

Quercetin (3,5,7,3′,4′-pentahydroxylflavone) belongs to a flavonol subclass of flavonoid. It is found in various fruits and vegetables, but at a larger quantity in apple and onion. Quercetin protects body tissues alone or in combination with other dietary antioxidants, such as vitamin C/E and carotenoids. The phytochemical is well known for its beneficial role in human health, as it is a powerful antioxidant, lowers cholesterol and erectile dysfunction, improves blood circulation, reduces inflammation, lowers the risk of neurodegenerative disease, and possesses anticancer properties [72]. Quercetin-3-methyl ether (Q3ME) is a natural analog of quercetin found in various plants. 7-O-geranylquercetin is an alkylated derivative of quercetin synthesized to overcome the poor solubility of quercetin. The compound possesses potent anti-tumor activity. It has been demonstrated that the derivative treatment in MCF-7/ADR cells inoculated in BALB/c nude mice significantly reversed drug resistance by down-regulating the expression of P-gp protein and its encoding gene MDR1 [73]. Cao et al. (2018) reported that quercetin has the potential to target MCF-7 cell-derived BCSCs alone or in combination with DAPT, a γ-secretase inhibitor. Q3ME inhibits the mammosphere formation by regulating the expression of genes involved in cancer stemness and inhibited the Notch and PI3-AKT signaling pathways [74]. The increased expression of P-glycoprotein (membrane transporter) mediated multidrug resistance (MDR) in cancer cells play a major role in decreasing the therapeutic outcome in breast cancer patients [75–77]. In this context, nuclear translocation of YB-1, a oncogenic transcription factor, is in association with the P-gp overexpressed in breast cancer cells and is associated with the stemness property [78]. Li et al. (2018) demonstrated that quercetin decreased YB-1 translocation, P-gp expression in luminal A breast cancer cells, and in the drug-resistant MCF-7 cell-derived stem-like cell population [79]. Similarly, Li et al. (2018) reported that quercetin, in combination with doxorubicin, significantly decreased the MCF-7-derived breast cancer stem-like cells [80]. Further, Li et al. (2018) demonstrated that quercetin significantly decreased the clone and sphere formation potential in MCF-7 cell-derived BCSCs [81]. Quercetin also modulated the PI3K/AkT/mTOR (phosphatidylinositol-3-kinase/Akt/mammalian target of rapamycin) signaling pathway in these cells [82]. Earlier, Imai et al. (2012) reported that the quercetin derivative (LY294002) has the capability to reduce the drug efflux in BCSCs by inhibiting the PI3K/Akt signaling pathway [83]. A summarization of the literature on the anticancer effects of quercetin against luminal A-derived breast cancer stem cells includes (i) targeting the ERα receptor, Notch and PI3/AKT/mTOR signaling pathways, (ii) lowering the expression of the multidrug resistance transporter, and (iii) inhibits the nuclear translocation of proteins involved in the breast cancer stemness and self-renewal process.

6.4. *Silibinin*

Silibinin is a natural flavonolignan compound. It is a major constituent of Silymarin, extracted from *Silybum marianum* (milk thistle), which is used for the treatment of liver diseases. Recently, silibinin has been reported to exert significant anti-neoplastic effects against breast, prostate, lung, colon, and skin cancer in the in vitro and in vivo model. It has been reported that metabolic heterogeneity plays an important role in cancer stem cell maintenance and self-renewal. Bonuccelli et al. (2017) found that MCF-7 cells possess high

PGC1α activity and reactive oxygen species production, and NADH levels in the mitochondria possess increased stem cell formation potential. Silibinin significantly reduced the mammosphere formation in this metabolic form of MCF-7 cells [84]. Studies have indicated that silibinin is a glycolytic inhibitor and also inhibits glucose uptake. Dadras et al. (2016) studied the MCF-7 cells stemness inhibition potential of silibinin-entrapped nanoparticles. The study demonstrated a significant reduction in the potential of free silibinin in MCF-7 cancer stem cell viability in the in vitro assay [85]. Published reports on the efficacy of silibinin in luminal A-derived breast cancer cells are at the preliminary levels. There is a need to explore the underlying mechanism of stemness and the self-renewal property inhibition potential of silibinin in both the in vitro and in vivo models. The literature so far has demonstrated that silibinin exerts its pharmacological effect on luminal A-derived breast cancer stem cells by targeting metabolic pathways, and reducing the viability of MCF-7 cell-derived mammospheres.

6.5. *Thymoquinone*

Nigella sativa L. (Ranunculaceae), commonly known as black cumin, is an important spice in Europe, South West Asia, and North Africa. Thymoquinone (TQ) belongs to the quinone group of phytochemicals and is the most abundant constituent of *Nigella sativa* seeds in volatile oil. Several pharmacological activities of TQ have been reported, including anti-histaminic, anti-inflammatory, anti-microbial, antioxidant, immunomodulatory, and anti-tumor effects. Various studies demonstrate that TQ possesses less toxicity and has low adverse effects on normal cells [86]. TQ demonstrated reduced self-renewal properties in the MCF-derived mammosphere. The TQ treatment decreased the number and size of spheroids in comparison to the control group. TQ, alone or in combination with the emodin, a natural anthraquinone derivative, lowered the cancer stemness-related markers viz. OCT-4, SOX-2, NANOG, and ALDH1/2 in MCF-7-derived BCSCs [87]. In another study, the TQ decreased the stem cell population by 12%; in combination with paclitaxel, the efficacy was increased up to 32%, as compared with the non-treated cells. Whereas, the paclitaxel treatment alone demonstrated an 8% reduction in stem cell population. In another study, the gemcitabine was unable to decrease the stem cell population; however, in combination with TQ, a 12% reduction was observed [88]. These studies indicate that TQ may be used in combination with standard chemotherapeutic drugs to target BCSCs effectively. However, detailed mechanisms are warranted to establish the BCSCs' reduction potential of TQ, in combination with the standard therapeutic drugs in pre-clinical models, including a reduction in mammosphere size and number alone or in combination with a phytochemical, as well as the chemosensitization potential of BCSCs. The luminal A-derived mammosphere reduction and breast cancer stemness and self-renewal regulating pathways' inhibiting potential of phytoestrogens are summarized in Figure 3.

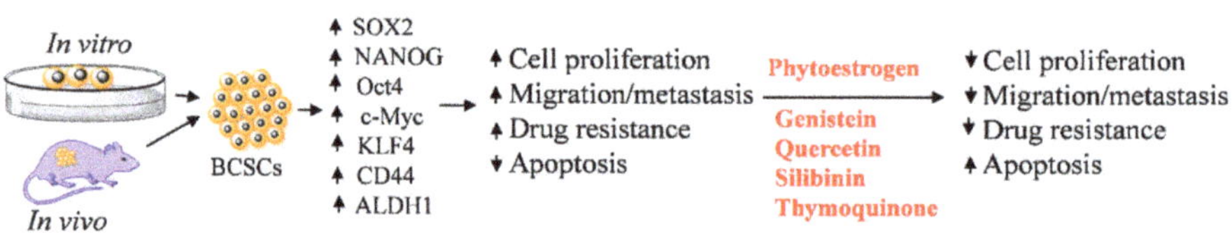

Figure 3. Effect of phytoestrogen(s) on the luminal A-derived mammosphere. ALDH1—Aldehyde dehydrogenase 1, Krüppel-like factor 4, and BCSCs—Breast cancer stem cells.

7. Other Dietary Phytochemicals

Hisperidin is a natural polyphenolic compound generally known as a citrus flavonoid. The compound is pharmacologically active and possesses significant anticancer activity. Hesperidin and its aglycone derivative (hesperitin) inhibit metastasis and tumor growth in MCF-7-inoculated experimental mice. Hesperitin (at a 1000 and 5000 ppm concentration) prevent tumor growth by reducing the plasma estrogen level and pS2 gene expression in the ovariectomized, and the aromatase overexpressing in the MCF-7 athymic xenograft mouse model. The hesperitin treatment inhibited aromatase activity and increased the cell cycle arrest and apoptosis in experimental animals [89]. Recently, Hermawan et al. (2021) reported the anticancer activity of hesperidin in luminal A-derived breast cancer spheroids using bioinformatics and an in vitro approach. A decreased sphere and colony formation potential was observed in hesperidin-treated MCF-7 cells [90].

Pristimerin is a natural occurring triterpenoid compound mainly isolated from the *Celastraceae* and *Hippocrateaceae* family. It exerts anticancer activity against different types of cancer both in in vitro and in vivo experimental models. Cevatemre et al. (2018) demonstrated that pristimerin inhibited breast tumor growth and induced apoptosis by cleaving PARP and activating caspase-3 in MCF-7-derived spheroids and in the mouse xenograft model [91]. Pristimerin demonstrated increased apoptosis, cytoplasmic vacuolation, endoplasmic reticulum stress, unfolded protein response, and autophagy flux blockage-mediated death in breast cancer spheroids. The phytochemical inhibited the Wnt signaling pathway in MCF-7-derived mammospheres by degrading the low-density lipoprotein receptor-related protein 6 (LRP6), a Wnt co-receptor [91].

Pterostilbene is a natural dimethylated analogue of resveratrol. The compound is present in blueberries in larger quantity. Pterostilbene inhibits cancer cell proliferation, invasion, and metastasis, and induced apoptosis in several experimental models. Mak et al. (2013) studied the effect of pterostilbene in M2 tumor-associated macrophages (M2TAMs) inducing stem cell generation potential in MCF-7 cells. The pterostilbene treatment significantly reduced the BCSC generation in MCF-7 cells co-cultured with the M2TAMs by decreasing the CD44+/CD24− cell population, and reduced the migratory and invasive capabilities of BCSCs. Moreover, the pterostilbene treatment reduced NF-κB, vimentin and Twist1, and elevated the E-cadherin expression in MCF-7-derived mammospheres [92]. Later, Wu et al. (2015) reported that pterostilbene produced more toxicity in MCF-7-derived cancer stem cells in comparison to MCF-7 cells. Pterostilbene significantly induced necrosis-mediated cellular membrane damage, reduced stemness markers CD44 and c-Myc, and inhibited hedgehog, Akt and GSK3β signaling pathways in MCF-7-derived spheroids [93].

Ginsenoside Rg3 (GRg3), which belongs to the *Araliaceae* family, is an important pharmacological active constituent of *Panax ginseng*. GRg3 has been known to possess potent anticancer activity by modulating several oncogenic pathways. Oh et al. (2015) comparatively studied the efficacy of low and high GRg3 containing red ginseng extract in the MCF-7 cell-derived mammosphere [94]. The high GRg3 content extract demonstrated more pronounced effect on the mammosphere by decreasing their self-renewal potential. In a different study, GRg3 decreased the stemness and self-renewal potential in MCF-7 cells' spheroids by targeting the PI3K/Akt signaling pathway, modulating Sox-2 and Bmi-1 self-renewal markers, and inhibiting the nuclear translocation of the HIFα factor [95].

Withaferin A (WA) is a major pharmacological active ingredient of Indian Ginseng (*Withania somnifera*). It belongs to the steroidal lactone group of compounds. WA inhibits luminal A-derived BCSCs by reducing the urokinase type plasminogen activator receptor (uPAR) and polycomb group protein Bmi-1 expression, which are well known factors to drive stemness and self-renewal properties in BCSCs. Inhibition of Notch4 activity reduces stem cell activity and tumor formation both in in vitro and in vivo breast cancer models [96]. Kim and Singh (2014) reported that WA has the potential to inhibit Notch4 activation and reduce KLF4 expression and ALDH1 activity in MCF-7 and SUM159 cancer stem cells [97]. The modulation of miRNAs by phytochemicals is an important strategy to modulate the expression of target mRNAs at a transcriptional level in cancer cells [13,98]. Higher expression of miR-6844 has been demonstrated in clinical specimens of invasive breast cancer patients in comparison to normal subjects. Recently, our group reported that miR-6844 is highly expressed in the luminal A-cell-derived mammosphere, compared to normal non-sphere breast cancer cells. The WA treatment significantly reversed the expression of miR-6844 and inhibited the mammosphere formation potential [99]. The aberrant expression of Notch signaling target genes has been positively correlated with the stemness and self-renewal property of BCSCs. Recently, we demonstrated that natural phytochemical 3-O-(E)-p-Coumaroylbetulinic acid possesses stemness and self-renewal inhibition potential in the MCF-7 cell-derived mammosphere by downregulating the Notch signaling pathway. The phytochemical altered the Notch target genes such as E-cadherin, Hey1, and Hes1, and breast cancer stemness markers viz. c-Myc, COX2, CD44, OCT4, NANOG, CD44, and EpCAM in MCF-7 cell-derived mammospheres [100].

Overall, the phytochemicals discussed above possess the potential to target luminal A-derived BCSCs by the selective elimination of these cells through the inhibition of Akt, Wnt, hedgehog/GSK3β signaling pathway, and nuclear translocation of the HIFα factor. These underlying mechanisms of the luminal A-derived breast cancer stemness and self-renewal inhibition potential of dietary phytochemicals is summarized in Figure 4 and Table 2.

Table 2. Stemness/self-renewal signaling regulations by dietary phytochemicals in luminal A-derived BCaSCs.

Signaling Pathway	Markers for Validation	Regulatory Outcomes	Phytochemicals	Phytochemicals Effects	References
Akt	Sox-2, Bmi-1, HIF-1α	Mammosphere formation	Ginginoside Rg3	Decrease stemness/self-renewal	[25]
p53	p21, cyclin D1, p53	Mammosphere formation	Hesperidin	Reduce sphere formation, colony formation, migration, induce cell cycle arrest, apoptosis	[90]
Wnt	LRP6, p62 and LC3-II	Spheroid formation in BCa	Pristimerin	Inhibit self-renewal, induce apoptosis, autophagy	[91]
Hedgehog, Akt, β-catenin, Wnt, NF-κB	CD44 and c-Myc, β-catenin, HIF-1α, Twist1, Vimentin, E-cadherin, miR-448	Mammosphere formation	Pterostilbene	Reduce BCa stem cell generation, stemness related markers, metastasis, induce necrosis, sensitize chemotherapy	[92,93]
Notch4	uPAR, Bmi-1, KLF4, ALDH1	Stemness and self-renewal phenotype in BCaSCs	Withaferin A	Suppress stemness and self-renewal	[96]
Hypoxia, AMPK, STAT3, NF-κB	HIF-1α, HSP90, ARNT, Oct4, Nanog, Sox2, EMT, Bcl-2, ABCG2	Mammosphere formation, mainten cancer stem-like characteristics	Curcumin	Decrease cancer stemness/self-renewal markers expression, cell proliferation and colony formation, inhibit drug efflux transporters	[42,48,49,53,55]
Notch, Hedgehog, PI3K/Akt	DAXX, KLF4, IL-6	Expression self-renewal/stemness markers and side-population	Genistein	Inhibit mammosphere formation	[59,60,62,63,70]
PI3/AKT/mTOR	P-gp, YB-1	MDR in BCa cells, Cancer stem cell viability, mammosphere formation	Quercetin	Reduces BCaSCs' proliferation, mammosphere generation, and colony formation	[74,79]
Metabolic pathway	Mitochondrial oxidative stress	Oxidative metabolism in BCaSCs	Silibinin	Reduces the sphere formation	[84]
	OCT-4, SOX-2, NANOG, ALDH1/2	Mammosphere formation	Thymoquinone	Self-renewal inhibition, mammosphere formation reduction	[87]

BCa—Breast cancer, BCaSCs—Breast cancer stem cells, Akt—Protein kinase B, SOX-2—(Sex determining region Y) box-2, Bmi-1—Polycomb protein complex, HIF-1α—Hypoxia inducing factor-1α, Wnt—Wingless/Integrated, LRP6—Low-density lipoprotein receptor-related protein 6, LC3-II—Light chain 3, NF-κB—Nuclear factor-kappa B, uPAR—Urokinase type plasminogen activator receptor, KLF4—Kruppel-like factor-4, ALDH1—Aldehyde dehydrogenase 1, AMPK-AMP—activated protein kinase, STAT3—Signal transducer and activator of transcription 3, HSP90—Heat shock protein 90, ARNT—Aryl hydrocarbon receptor nuclear transporter, Oct4—Octamer binding transcription factor, EMT—Epithelial mesenchymal transition, ABCG2—ATP-binding cassette super family G member 2, PI3K—Phosphoinositide-3-kinase, DAXX—Death-associated protein 6, IL-6—Interleukin-6, mTOR—Mammalian target of rapamycin, P-gp—P-glycoprotein, YB-1—Y-binding protein 1, and MDR—Multidrug resistance.

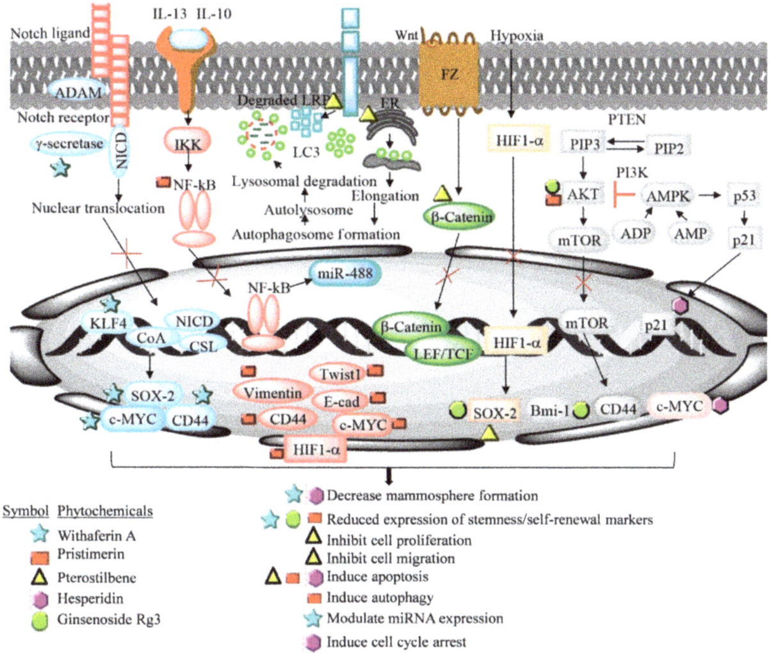

Figure 4. Luminal A-derived breast cancer stemness/self-renewal inhibiting potential of various dietary phytochemicals including *Withaferin A*, Ginsenoside Rg3 (GRg3), Pterostilbene, Hisperidin, and Pristimerin. The phytochemicals target Notch signaling, Wnt, hypoxia, NF-B, and Akt pathways involved in the maintenance of stemness and self-renewal. Withaferin A reduces the mammosphere formation in luminal A breast cancer cells by modulating the expression of Sox2, c-MYC, and CD44 via targeting Notch signaling pathway. Pterostilbene inhibits NF-κB, vimentin, and Twist1, and elevated E-cadherin expression. Ginsenoside Rg3 inhibits the nuclear translocation of HIF-1α, Sox-2, and Bmi-1 marker expression via targeting hypoxia and PI3K/Akt signaling pathway. Pristimerin mediated modulation of autophagy and degradation of LRP6, a Wnt co-receptor of Wnt signaling pathway and the expression of stemness markers. Hesperidin arrest cell progression at G0/G1 phase by targeting cyclin D1. Hesperidin modulates the expression of p21 and p53 in luminal A-derived mammosphere. [KLF4—Kruppel-like factor 4, HIF-1α—Hypoxia inducing factor-1α, VEGFA—Vascular endothelial growth factor A, Hh—Hedgehog, PTCH1—Patched1, Smo—Smoothened, GLI1—Gli family zinc finger 1, Kinesin family member 7, FZ—Frizzled, TCF/LEF—T-Cell factor/Lymphoid enhance factor, IKB—Nuclear factor of kappa light polypeptide gene enhancer in B-cells inhibitor, mTOR—Mammalian target of rapamycin, PIP3—Phosphatidylinositol (3,4,5)-trisphosphate, PIP2—Phosphatidylinositol-4, 5-bisphosphate, PTEN—Phosphatase and tensin homolog, PI3K—Phosphoinositide 3-kinases, Akt—Protein kinase B, GREB—cAMP-response element binding protein, NICD—notch intracellular domain, HAT—Histone acetyltransferases; APH-1—anterior pharynx—defective 1, *PSEN*-Presenilin-1, NCSTN—Nicastrin, MDM2-*Mouse double minute* 2 homolog, Akt—Protein kinase B, SOX-2-(Sex determining region Y) box-2, Bmi-1—Polycomb protein complex, HIF-1α—Hypoxia inducing factor-1α, Wnt—Wingless/Integrated, LRP6—Low-density lipoprotein receptor-related protein 6, LC3-II—Light chain 3, NF-κB—Nuclear factor-kappa B, KLF4—Kruppel-like factor-4, AMPK—AMP-activated protein kinase, PI3K—Phosphoinositide-3-kinase, IL-6—Interleukin-6, mTOR—Mammalian target of rapamycin, P-gp—P-glycoprotein, YB-1—Y-binding protein 1, MDR—Multidrug resistance, AMP—Adenosine monophosphate, ADP—Adenosine diphosphate, PIP3—Phosphatidylinositol (3,4,5)-trisphosphate, PIP2—Phosphatidylinositol-4, 5-bisphosphate, PTEN—Phosphatase and tensin homolog, PI3K—Phosphoinositide 3-kinases, and Akt—Protein kinase B].

8. Pharmacokinetics and Bioavailability

Liver is the primary site of metabolism for phytochemicals, together with the intestine and gut microbiota. After several metabolic reactions, phytochemical structures are modified in the hepatocytes and enterocytes, and form subsequent inactive/bioactive metabolites. Following oral ingestion, phytochemicals undergo extensive metabolism that includes chemical reactions including reduction, sulfation, and glucuronidation in the liver, kidneys, and intestinal mucosa. These metabolized products generated in the liver and intestine, as a result of their biotransformation, exhibit enhancement in their biological activity. Studies have demonstrated that the human microbiota and brush border enzymes are involved in phytoestrogen metabolism and active metabolite synthesis. Gut microbiota composition influences phytochemical bioavailability and inter-individual effects. Gut bacteria, for example, convert genistein, soy's most abundant isoflavone, into several metabolites that target and alter estrogen-dependent and non-estrogenic pathways with a variety of biological activities. As such, individual differences in the microbiome, therapeutic possibilities, and anticancer effects may be unique to each person [101–103]. Overall, these variables hinder the clinical development of dietary phytochemicals. Preclinical studies suggest that the intestinal P-glycoprotein efflux pump is responsible for the limited bioavailability of the phytochemicals. Blocking ABC transporters with quercetin increases the bioavailability and decreases their efflux. Other studies demonstrate that the combination of dietary phytochemicals such as curcumin and piperine exhibits greater bioavailability. Reports on humans suggest that the intake of nonsteroidal anti-inflammatory agents, reserpine, and blood thinners exhibit adverse effects taken together with phytochemicals [102]. Efforts are also directed to enhance the bioavailability of phytochemicals to exhibit better preventive and/or therapeutic responses. In this direction, the high-bioavailability formulation of phytochemicals is under development [104,105]. Food processing such as heating, drying, and grinding, and factors such as climate change and plant stress could impact the bioavailability of dietary phytochemicals, having an effect on their biological activity. Technological strategies such as nanoparticle synthesis, phytochemical(s) in lecithin, the phosphatidylcholine carrier, and solid lipid nanoparticles demonstrate an increase in the bioavailability of dietary phytochemicals [105–107].

In preclinical studies, phytochemicals exhibit an antitumor potential at the doses 1–200 μM and 2–100 mg/kg body weight without any apparent toxicity utilized in in vivo models [54,56,73,89]. In recent studies, it is noted that dietary phytochemicals/phytoestrogen exhibit a significant reduction in tumor volume in the MCF-7-inoculated mouse xenograft model at 2–100 mg/kg body weight [54,56,73,89]. These doses can be extrapolated in studies on humans as well. Moreover, curcumin (500 mg BID; NCT01740323), genistein (100 mg; NCT00244933), resveratrol (474 mg phenolics/day; NCT03482401), ginsenoside Rg3 (20 mg BID; NCT01717066), and thymoquinone (500 mg; NCT04852510) have been studied in various clinical trials in the range of previously reported in vivo dosages or at higher dosages. These clinical trials on dietary phytochemicals either alone or in combination with standard chemotherapy demonstrated encouraging results in breast cancer patients with less toxicity and lower side effects (NCT03072992).

9. Study Strengths and Limitations

Few studies have summarized the role of dietary phytochemicals in targeting BCSCs. Some other available reviews related to this subject are discussed under cancer stem cell physiology and related hallmarks, and their modulation by phytochemicals. The present review summarizes the role of dietary phytochemicals and their effect on luminal A-derived BCSCs' pathophysiology at the molecular level. The review emphasizes that dietary phytochemicals possess increasing potential to target breast cancer subtype (luminal A) cell-derived stem cells. This review also highlights the efficacy of dietary phytochemical-derived nanoparticles, and co-treatment with other drugs against luminal A-derived BCSCs. However, there are some limitations in the study, such as the lack of the extensive information on the effect of dietary phytochemicals in luminal A cells derived in in vivo experimental models. Because the luminal A-derived stem cell formation is an important event in the breast tumor microenvironment, further detailed studies are required to assess the stemness initiation, self-renewal, and chemotherapy resistance potential of dietary phytochemicals.

10. Conclusion and Future Prospects

Breast cancer luminal A subtype possess estrogen receptor and thus are responsive to hormone therapy. The luminal A subtype constitutes approximately 80% of the total breast cancer cases and demonstrates better prognosis and therapeutic susceptibility. Luminal A-derived T47D and MCF-7 cell culture models form tight three-dimensional cell–cell adhesion structures in comparison to luminal B breast cancer cells. As the breast tumor microenvironment constitutes nearly all subtypes of cancer cells, out of these, luminal A cells are slow growing and have the capability to transform into other breast cancer subtypes in response to changes in hormone levels and physiological states, including pregnancy status and various therapeutic modalities. Targeting luminal A cells at the initiation of breast cancer with phytochemicals could inhibit cancer progression and minimizes the casual switching to various subtypes. The dietary intake of these phytochemicals could offer prevention towards initiation and development of breast cancer, whereas cotreatment with standard chemotherapeutic drugs has the potential to increase the efficacy and therapeutic response. The present review highlights that dietary phytochemicals have the potential to target luminal A-derived BCSCs by lowering their stemness and self-renewal properties. These dietary phytochemicals demonstrate their anticancer effects by the modulation of signaling pathways, including AMPK, STAT3, NF-kB, Hedgehog, PI3K/Akt/mTOR, Notch, GSK3β, and Wnt, and other, as well as via the regulation of the mechanism(s) involved in the process of proliferation or drug resistance. These phytochemicals have the ability to target puttive molecular and biochemical events in luminal cell-derived mammospheres. The present review necessitates in-depth preclinical and clinical studies on dietary phytochemicals alone or in combination with the standard treatment to explore their cancer prevention and treatment potential.

Author Contributions: S.K. conceived and designed the study; S.K. wrote original draft of the manuscript; K.S.P. prepared figures and tables; S.G. wrote and edited the manuscript. All authors have read and agreed to the published version of the manuscript.

Funding: This research was funded by [Department of Science and Technology, India] grant number [EEQ/2016/000350].

Acknowledgments: S.K. acknowledges the Department of Science and Technology, India for providing financial support in the form of the DST-SERB Grant [EEQ/2016/000350]. S.K. also acknowledges DST-India for providing a Departmental grant to the Department of Biochemistry, Central University of Punjab, Bathinda, India in the form of the DST-FIST grant. K.S.P. acknowledges DBT, India for providing the Senior Research Fellowship.

Conflicts of Interest: The authors declare no conflict of interest.

References

1. American Cancer Society. *Breast Cancer Facts & Figure 2019 and Figure 2020*; American Cancer Society, Inc.: Atlanta, GA, USA, 2019.
2. Abraham, B.K.; Fritz, P.; McClellan, M.; Hauptvogel, P.; Athelogou, M.; Brauch, H. Prevalence of CD44+/CD24-/low cells in breast cancer may not be associated with clinical outcome but may favor distant metastasis. *Clin. Cancer Res.* **2005**, *11*, 1154–1159.
3. Charafe-Jauffret, E.; Ginestier, C.; Iovino, F.; Tarpin, C.; Diebel, M.; Esterni, B.; Houvenaeghel, G.; Extra, J.-M.; Bertucci, F.; Jacquemier, J.; et al. Aldehyde Dehydrogenase 1-Positive Cancer Stem Cells Mediate Metastasis and Poor Clinical Outcome in Inflammatory Breast Cancer. *Clin. Cancer Res.* **2009**, *16*, 45–55. [CrossRef] [PubMed]
4. Kushwaha, P.P.; Singh, A.K.; Prajapati, K.S.; Shuaib, M.; Fayez, S.; Bringmann, G.; Kumar, S. Induction of apoptosis in breast cancer cells by naphthylisoquinoline alkaloids. *Toxicol. Appl. Pharmacol.* **2020**, *409*, 115297. [CrossRef] [PubMed]
5. Gupta, S.; Singh, A.; Prajapati, K.S.; Kushwaha, P.P.; Shuaib, M.; Kumar, S. Emerging role of ZBTB7A as an oncogenic driver and transcriptional repressor. *Cancer Lett.* **2020**, *483*, 22–34. [CrossRef] [PubMed]

6. Mehraj, U.; Ganai, R.A.; Macha, M.A.; Hamid, A.; Zargar, M.A.; Bhat, A.A.; Nasser, M.W.; Haris, M.; Batra, S.K.; Alshehri, B.; et al. The tumor microenvironment as driver of stemness and therapeutic resistance in breast cancer: New challenges and therapeutic opportunities. *Cell. Oncol.* **2021**, *44*, 1209–1229. [CrossRef] [PubMed]
7. Van'T Veer, L.J.; Dai, H.; Van De Vijver, M.J.; He, Y.D.; Hart, A.A.M.; Mao, M.; Peterse, H.L.; Van Der Kooy, K.; Marton, M.J.; Witteveen, A.T.; et al. Gene expression profiling predicts clinical outcome of breast cancer. *Nature* **2002**, *415*, 530–536. [CrossRef]
8. Kittaneh, M.; Montero, A.J.; Glück, S. Molecular Profiling for Breast Cancer: A Comprehensive Review. *Biomark. Cancer* **2013**, *5*, 61–70. [CrossRef]
9. Goldhirsch, A.; Wood, W.C.; Coates, A.S.; Gelber, R.D.; Thürlimann, B.; Senn, H.-J.; Panel Members. Strategies for subtypes—dealing with the diversity of breast cancer: Highlights of the St Gallen International Expert Consensus on the Primary Therapy of Early Breast Cancer 2011. *Ann. Oncol.* **2011**, *22*, 1736–1747. [CrossRef] [PubMed]
10. Goldhirsch, A.; Winer, E.P.; Coates, A.S.; Gelber, R.D.; Piccart-Gebhart, M.; Thürlimann, B.; Senn, H.-J. Personalizing the treatment of women with early breast cancer: Highlights of the St Gallen International Expert Consensus on the Primary Therapy of Early Breast Cancer 2013. *Ann. Oncol.* **2013**, *24*, 2206–2223. [CrossRef]
11. Gao, J.J.; Swain, S.M. Luminal A Breast Cancer and Molecular Assays: A Review. *Oncologist* **2018**, *23*, 556–565. [CrossRef] [PubMed]
12. Song, W.; Wang, R.; Jiang, W.; Yin, Q.; Peng, G.; Yang, R.; Yu, Q.C.; Chen, J.; Li, J.; Cheung, T.H.; et al. Hormones induce the formation of luminal-derived basal cells in the mammary gland. *Cell Res.* **2019**, *29*, 206–220. [CrossRef] [PubMed]
13. Mei, Y.; Cai, D.; Dai, X. Modulating cancer stemness provides luminal a breast cancer cells with HER2 positive-like features. *J. Cancer* **2020**, *11*, 1162–1169. [CrossRef] [PubMed]
14. Yousefnia, S.; Ghaedi, K.; Forootan, F.S.; Esfahani, M.H.N. Characterization of the stemness potency of *mammospheres* isolated from the breast cancer cell lines. *Tumor Biol.* **2019**, *41*, 1010428319869101. [CrossRef]
15. Kim, J.; Villadsen, R.; Sørlie, T.; Fogh, L.; Grønlund, S.Z.; Fridriksdottir, A.J.; Kuhn, I.; Rank, F.; Wielenga, V.T.; Solvang, H.; et al. Tumor initiating but differentiated luminal-like breast cancer cells are highly invasive in the absence of basal-like activity. *Proc. Natl. Acad. Sci. USA* **2012**, *109*, 6124–6129. [CrossRef]
16. Bao, L.; Cardiff, R.D.; Steinbach, P.; Messer, K.S.; Ellies, L.G. Multipotent luminal mammary cancer stem cells model tumor heterogeneity. *Breast Cancer Res.* **2015**, *17*, 137. [CrossRef] [PubMed]
17. Kumar, S.; Chashoo, G.; Saxena, A.K.; Pandey, A.K. *Parthenium hysterophorus:* A Probable Source of Anticancer, Antioxidant and Anti-HIV Agents. *BioMed Res. Int.* **2013**, *2013*, 810734. [CrossRef] [PubMed]
18. Kumar, S.; Kumar, R.; Dwivedi, A.; Pandey, A.K. In Vitro Antioxidant, Antibacterial, and Cytotoxic Activity and In Vivo Effect of *Syngonium podophyllum* and *Eichhornia crassipes* Leaf Extracts on Isoniazid Induced Oxidative Stress and Hepatic Markers. *BioMed Res. Int.* **2014**, *2014*, 459452. [CrossRef] [PubMed]
19. Kumar, S.; Pandey, A.K. Medicinal attributes of Solanum xanthocarpum fruit consumed by several tribal communities as food: An in vitro antioxidant, anticancer and anti HIV perspective. *BMC Complement. Altern. Med.* **2014**, *14*, 112. [CrossRef] [PubMed]
20. Kumar, S.; Prajapati, K.S.; Shuaib, M.; Kushwaha, P.P.; Tuli, H.S.; Singh, A.K. Five-Decade Update on Chemopreventive and Other Pharmacological Potential of Kurarinone: A Natural Flavanone. *Front. Pharmacol.* **2021**, *12*, 737137. [CrossRef] [PubMed]
21. Kumar, S.; Gupta, S. Dietary phytochemicals and their role in cancer chemoprevention. *J. Cancer Metastasis Treat.* **2021**, *7*, 51. [CrossRef]
22. Kushwaha, P.P.; Kumar, R.; Neog, P.R.; Behara, M.R.; Singh, P.; Kumar, A.; Prajapati, K.S.; Singh, A.K.; Shuaib, M.; Sharma, A.K.; et al. Characterization of phytochemicals and validation of antioxidant and anticancer activity in some Indian polyherbal ayurvedic products. *Vegetos* **2021**, *34*, 286–299. [CrossRef]
23. Kushwaha, P.P.; Gupta, S.; Singh, A.K.; Prajapati, M.K.S.; Shuaib, M.; Kumar, S. MicroRNA Targeting Nicotinamide Adenine Dinucleotide Phosphate Oxidases in Cancer. *Antioxid. Redox Signal.* **2020**, *32*, 267–284. [CrossRef] [PubMed]
24. Kushwaha, P.P.; Vardhan, P.S.; Kapewangolo, P.; Shuaib, M.; Prajapati, S.K.; Singh, A.K.; Kumar, S. *Bulbine frutescens* phytochemical inhibits notch signaling pathway and induces apoptosis in triple negative and luminal breast cancer cells. *Life Sci.* **2019**, *234*, 116783. [CrossRef] [PubMed]
25. Mishra, A.; Sharma, A.K.; Kumar, S.; Saxena, A.K.; Pandey, A.K. *Bauhinia variegata*Leaf Extracts Exhibit Considerable Antibacterial, Antioxidant, and Anticancer Activities. *BioMed Res. Int.* **2013**, *2013*, 915436. [CrossRef] [PubMed]
26. Sharma, A.K.; Kumar, S.; Chashoo, G.; Saxena, A.K.; Pandey, A.K. Cell cycle inhibitory activity of Piper longum against A549 cell line and its protective effect against metal-induced toxicity in rats. *Indian J. Biochem. Biophys.* **2014**, *51*, 358–364. [PubMed]
27. Dandawate, P.; Subramaniam, D.; Jensen, R.A.; Anant, S. Targeting cancer stem cells and signaling pathways by phytochemicals: Novel approach for breast cancer therapy. *Semin. Cancer Biol.* **2016**, *40–41*, 192–208. [CrossRef]
28. Kassie, F.; Pool-Zobel, B.; Parzefall, W.; Knasmüller, S. Genotoxic effects of benzyl isothiocyanate, a natural chemopreventive agent. *Mutagenesis* **1999**, *14*, 595–604. [CrossRef] [PubMed]
29. Yang, Y.; Tian, Z.; Guo, R.; Ren, F. Nrf2 Inhibitor, Brusatol in Combination with Trastuzumab Exerts Synergistic Antitumor Activity in HER2-Positive Cancers by Inhibiting Nrf2/HO-1 and HER2-AKT/ERK1/2 Pathways. *Oxidative Med. Cell. Longev.* **2020**, *2020*, 9867595. [CrossRef] [PubMed]
30. Spagnuolo, C.; Russo, G.L.; Orhan, I.E.; Habtemariam, S.; Daglia, M.; Sureda, A.; Nabavi, S.F.; Devi, K.P.; Loizzo, M.R.; Tundis, R.; et al. Genistein and Cancer: Current Status, Challenges, and Future Directions. *Adv. Nutr.* **2015**, *6*, 408–419. [CrossRef]

31. Goyal, S.N.; Prajapati, C.P.; Gore, P.R.; Patil, C.; Mahajan, U.; Sharma, C.; Talla, S.P.; Ojha, S.K. Therapeutic Potential and Pharmaceutical Development of Thymoquinone: A Multitargeted Molecule of Natural Origin. *Front. Pharmacol.* **2017**, *8*, 656. [CrossRef] [PubMed]
32. Dei Cas, M.; Ghidoni, R. Dietary Curcumin: Correlation between Bioavailability and Health Potential. *Nutrients* **2019**, *11*, 2147. [CrossRef]
33. Khalil, A.A.; Rahman, U.U.; Khan, M.R.; Sahar, A.; Mehmood, T.; Khan, M. Essential oil eugenol: Sources, extraction techniques and nutraceutical perspectives. *RSC Adv.* **2017**, *7*, 32669–32681. [CrossRef]
34. Fenclova, M.; Novakova, A.; Viktorova, J.; Jonatova, P.; Dzuman, Z.; Ruml, T.; Kren, V.; Hajslova, J.; Vitek, L.; Stranska-Zachariasova, M. Poor chemical and microbiological quality of the commercial milk thistle-based dietary supplements may account for their reported unsatisfactory and non-reproducible clinical outcomes. *Sci. Rep.* **2019**, *9*, 11118. [CrossRef] [PubMed]
35. Dinesh, P.; Rasool, M. Herbal Formulations and Their Bioactive Components as Dietary Supplements for Treating Rheumatoid Arthritis. In *Bioactive Food as Dietary Interventions for Arthritis and Related Inflammatory Diseases*; Academic Press: Cambridge, MA, USA, 2019; pp. 385–399. [CrossRef]
36. Available online: https://foodb.ca/compounds/FDB006540 (accessed on 22 March 2022).
37. Available online: https://www.sciencedaily.com/releases/2014/10/141030102819.htm (accessed on 22 March 2022).
38. Geris, R.; Ribeiro, P.R.; Brandão, M.D.S.; Da Silva, H.H.G.; Da Silva, I.G. Bioactive Natural Products as Potential Candidates to Control Aedes aegypti, the Vector of Dengue. In *Studies in Natural Products Chemistry*; Elsevier: Amsterdam, The Netherlands, 2012; Volume 37, pp. 277–376. [CrossRef]
39. Lee, H.; Kong, G.; Tran, Q.; Kim, C.; Park, J.; Park, J. Relationship Between Ginsenoside Rg3 and Metabolic Syndrome. *Front. Pharmacol.* **2020**, *11*, 130. [CrossRef] [PubMed]
40. Das, M.; Kandimalla, R.; Gogoi, B.; Dutta, K.N.; Choudhury, P.; Devi, R.; Dutta, P.P.; Talukdar, N.C.; Samanta, S.K. Mahanine, A dietary phytochemical, represses mammary tumor burden in rat and inhibits subtype regardless breast cancer progression through suppressing self-renewal of breast cancer stem cells. *Pharmacol. Res.* **2019**, *146*, 104330. [CrossRef] [PubMed]
41. Sharifi-Rad, J.; El Rayess, Y.; Rizk, A.A.; Sadaka, C.; Zgheib, R.; Zam, W.; Sestito, S.; Rapposelli, S.; Neffe-Skocińska, K.; Zielińska, D.; et al. Turmeric and Its Major Compound Curcumin on Health: Bioactive Effects and Safety Profiles for Food, Pharmaceutical, Biotechnological and Medicinal Applications. *Front. Pharmacol.* **2020**, *11*, 01021. [CrossRef] [PubMed]
42. Yang, K.; Liao, Z.; Wu, Y.; Li, M.; Guo, T.; Lin, J.; Li, Y.; Hu, C. Curcumin and Glu-GNPs Induce Radiosensitivity against Breast Cancer Stem-Like Cells. *BioMed Res. Int.* **2020**, *2020*, 3189217. [CrossRef]
43. Sarighieh, M.A.; Montazeri, V.; Shadboorestan, A.; Ghahremani, M.H.; Ostad, S.N. The Inhibitory Effect of Curcumin on Hypoxia Inducer Factors (Hifs) as a Regulatory Factor in the Growth of Tumor Cells in Breast Cancer Stem-Like Cells. *Drug Res.* **2020**, *70*, 512–518. [CrossRef] [PubMed]
44. Borah, A.; Pillai, S.C.; Rochani, A.K.; Palaninathan, V.; Nakajima, Y.; Maekawa, T.; Kumar, D.S. GANT61 and curcumin-loaded PLGA nanoparticles for GLI1 and PI3K/Akt-mediated inhibition in breast adenocarcinoma. *Nanotechnology* **2020**, *31*, 185102. [CrossRef] [PubMed]
45. Attia, Y.M.; El-Kersh, D.M.; Ammar, R.A.; Adel, A.; Khalil, A.; Walid, H.; Eskander, K.; Hamdy, M.; Reda, N.; Mohsen, N.E.; et al. Inhibition of aldehyde dehydrogenase-1 and p-glycoprotein-mediated multidrug resistance by curcumin and vitamin D3 increases sensitivity to paclitaxel in breast cancer. *Chem. Interact.* **2019**, *315*, 108865. [CrossRef]
46. Liu, M.; Wang, B.; Guo, C.; Hou, X.; Cheng, Z.; Chen, D. Novel multifunctional triple folic acid, biotin and CD44 targeting pH-sensitive nano-actiniaes for breast cancer combinational therapy. *Drug Deliv.* **2019**, *26*, 1002–1016. [CrossRef] [PubMed]
47. Hu, C.; Li, M.; Guo, T.; Wang, S.; Huang, W.; Yang, K.; Liao, Z.; Wang, J.; Zhang, F.; Wang, H. Anti-metastasis activity of curcumin against breast cancer via the inhibition of stem cell-like properties and EMT. *Phytomedicine* **2018**, *58*, 152740. [CrossRef] [PubMed]
48. Hashemzehi, M.; Behnam-Rassouli, R.; Hassanian, S.M.; Moradi-Binabaj, M.; Moradi-Marjaneh, R.; Rahmani, F.; Fiuji, H.; Jamili, M.; Mirahmadi, M.; Boromand, N.; et al. Phytosomal-curcumin antagonizes cell growth and migration, induced by thrombin through AMP-Kinase in breast cancer. *J. Cell. Biochem.* **2018**, *119*, 5996–6007. [CrossRef]
49. Li, X.; Wang, X.; Xie, C.; Zhu, J.; Meng, Y.; Chen, Y.; Li, Y.; Jiang, Y.; Yang, X.; Wang, S.; et al. Sonic hedgehog and Wnt/β-catenin pathways mediate curcumin inhibition of breast cancer stem cells. *Anti-Cancer Drugs* **2018**, *29*, 208–215. [CrossRef]
50. Lin, M.; Teng, L.; Wang, Y.; Zhang, J.; Sun, X. Curcumin-guided nanotherapy: A lipid-based nanomedicine for targeted drug delivery in breast cancer therapy. *Drug Deliv.* **2015**, *23*, 1420–1425. [CrossRef]
51. Yuan, J.-D.; ZhuGe, D.-L.; Tong, M.-Q.; Lin, M.-T.; Xu, X.-F.; Tang, X.; Zhao, Y.-Z.; Xu, H.-L. pH-sensitive polymeric nanoparticles of mPEG-PLGA-PGlu with hybrid core for simultaneous encapsulation of curcumin and doxorubicin to kill the heterogeneous tumour cells in breast cancer. *Artif. Cells Nanomed. Biotechnol.* **2018**, *46*, 302–313. [CrossRef]
52. Zhou, Q.-M.; Sun, Y.; Lu, Y.-Y.; Zhang, H.; Chen, Q.-L.; Su, S.-B. Curcumin reduces mitomycin C resistance in breast cancer stem cells by regulating Bcl-2 family-mediated apoptosis. *Cancer Cell Int.* **2017**, *17*, 84. [CrossRef]
53. Zhou, Q.; Ye, M.; Lu, Y.; Zhang, H.; Chen, Q.; Huang, S.; Su, S. Curcumin Improves the Tumoricidal Effect of Mitomycin C by Suppressing ABCG2 Expression in Stem Cell-Like Breast Cancer Cells. *PLoS ONE* **2015**, *10*, e0136694. [CrossRef]
54. Zhou, Q.-M.; Wang, X.-F.; Liu, X.-J.; Zhang, H.; Lu, Y.-Y.; Su, S.-B. Curcumin enhanced antiproliferative effect of mitomycin C in human breast cancer MCF-7 cells in vitro and in vivo. *Acta Pharmacol. Sin.* **2011**, *32*, 1402–1410. [CrossRef]
55. Chung, S.S.; Vadgama, J.V. Curcumin and epigallocatechin gallate inhibit the cancer stem cell phenotype via down-regulation of STAT3-NFκB signaling. *Anticancer Res.* **2015**, *35*, 39–46.

56. Ren, M.; Wang, Y.; Wu, X.; Ge, S.; Wang, B. Curcumin synergistically increases effects of β-interferon and retinoic acid on breast cancer cells in vitro and in vivo by up-regulation of GRIM-19 through STAT3-dependent and STAT3-independent pathways. *J. Drug Target.* **2016**, *25*, 247–254. [CrossRef] [PubMed]
57. Liggins, J.; Bluck, L.J.C.; Runswick, S.; Atkinson, C.; Coward, W.A.; Bingham, S.A. Daidzein and genistein contents of vegetables. *Br. J. Nutr.* **2000**, *84*, 717–725. [CrossRef] [PubMed]
58. Reinli, K.; Block, G. Phytoestrogen content of foods—A compendium of literature values. *Nutr. Cancer* **1996**, *26*, 123–148. [CrossRef]
59. Yu, F.; Li, J.; Chen, H.; Fu, J.; Ray, S.; Huang, S.; Zheng, H.; Ai, W. Kruppel-like factor 4 (KLF4) is required for maintenance of breast cancer stem cells and for cell migration and invasion. *Oncogene* **2011**, *30*, 2161–2172. [CrossRef]
60. Paul, B.; Li, Y.; Tollefsbol, T.O. The Effects of Combinatorial Genistein and Sulforaphane in Breast Tumor Inhibition: Role in Epigenetic Regulation. *Int. J. Mol. Sci.* **2018**, *19*, 1754. [CrossRef]
61. Palaniy, K.; Gendler, R.J.; Palaniyandi, K.; Pockaj, B.A.; Chang, X.-B. Human Breast Cancer Stem Cells Have Significantly Higher Rate of Clathrin-Independent and Caveolin-Independent Endocytosis than the Differentiated Breast Cancer Cells. *J. Cancer Sci. Ther.* **2012**, *4*, 214–222. [CrossRef]
62. Fan, P.; Fan, S.; Wang, H.; Mao, J.; Shi, Y.; Ibrahim, M.M.; Ma, W.; Yu, X.; Hou, Z.; Wang, B.; et al. Genistein decreases the breast cancer stem-like cell population through Hedgehog pathway. *Stem Cell Res. Ther.* **2013**, *4*, 146. [CrossRef]
63. Montales, M.T.E.; Rahal, O.M.; Kang, J.; Rogers, T.J.; Prior, R.L.; Wu, X.; Simmen, R.C. Repression of mammosphere formation of human breast cancer cells by soy isoflavone genistein and blueberry polyphenolic acids suggests diet-mediated targeting of cancer stem-like/progenitor cells. *Carcinogenesis* **2012**, *33*, 652–660. [CrossRef]
64. Montales, M.T.E.; Rahal, O.M.; Nakatani, H.; Matsuda, T.; Simmen, R.C.M. Repression of mammary adipogenesis by genistein limits mammosphere formation of human MCF-7 cells. *J. Endocrinol.* **2013**, *218*, 135–149. [CrossRef]
65. Lauricella, M.; Carlisi, D.; Giuliano, M.; Calvaruso, G.; Cernigliaro, C.; Vento, R.; D'Anneo, A. The analysis of estrogen receptor-? positive breast cancer stem-like cells unveils a high expression of the serpin proteinase inhibitor PI-9: Possible regulatory mechanisms. *Int. J. Oncol.* **2016**, *49*, 352–360. [CrossRef]
66. Liu, S.; Dontu, G.; Mantle, I.D.; Patel, S.; Ahn, N.-S.; Jackson, K.W.; Suri, P.; Wicha, M.S. Hedgehog Signaling and Bmi-1 Regulate Self-renewal of Normal and Malignant Human Mammary Stem Cells. *Cancer Res.* **2006**, *66*, 6063–6071. [CrossRef]
67. Saarinen, N.M.; Abrahamsson, A.; Dabrosin, C. Estrogen-induced angiogenic factors derived from stromal and cancer cells are differently regulated by enterolactone and genistein in human breast cancer in vivo. *Int. J. Cancer* **2010**, *127*, 737–745. [CrossRef]
68. Salehi, B.; Fokou, P.V.T.; Sharifi-Rad, M.; Zucca, P.; Pezzani, R.; Martins, N.; Sharifi-Rad, J. The Therapeutic Potential of Naringenin: A Review of Clinical Trials. *Pharmaceuticals* **2019**, *12*, 11. [CrossRef] [PubMed]
69. Askar, M.A.; El Shawi, O.E.; Zaid, O.A.A.; Mansour, N.A.; Hanafy, A.M. Breast cancer suppression by curcumin-naringenin-magnetic-nano-particles: In vitro and in vivo studies. *Tumor Biol.* **2021**, *43*, 225–247. [CrossRef] [PubMed]
70. Peiffer, D.S.; Ma, E.; Wyatt, D.; Albain, K.S.; Osipo, C. DAXX-inducing phytoestrogens inhibit ER+ tumor initiating cells and delay tumor development. *Npj Breast Cancer* **2020**, *6*, 37. [CrossRef]
71. Salehi, B.; Mishra, A.P.; Nigam, M.; Sener, B.; Kilic, M.; Sharifi-Rad, M.; Fokou, P.V.T.; Martins, N.; Sharifi-Rad, J. Resveratrol: A Double-Edged Sword in Health Benefits. *Biomedicines* **2018**, *6*, 91. [CrossRef]
72. Jan, A.T.; Kamli, M.R.; Murtaza, I.; Singh, J.B.; Ali, A.; Haq, Q. Dietary Flavonoid Quercetin and Associated Health Benefits—An Overview. *Food Rev. Int.* **2010**, *26*, 302–317. [CrossRef]
73. Zhang, E.; Liu, J.; Shi, L.; Guo, X.; Liang, Z.; Zuo, J.; Xu, H.; Wang, H.; Shu, X.; Huang, S.; et al. 7-O-geranylquercetin contributes to reverse P-gp-mediated adriamycin resistance in breast cancer. *Life Sci.* **2019**, *238*, 116938. [CrossRef] [PubMed]
74. Cao, L.; Yang, Y.; Ye, Z.; Lin, B.; Zeng, J.; Li, C.; Liang, T.; Zhou, K.; Li, J. Quercetin-3-methyl ether suppresses human breast cancer stem cell formation by inhibiting the Notch1 and PI3K/Akt signaling pathways. *Int. J. Mol. Med.* **2018**, *42*, 1625–1636. [CrossRef] [PubMed]
75. Kumar, S.; Kushwaha, P.P.; Gupta, S. Emerging targets in cancer drug resistance. *Cancer Drug Resist* **2019**, *2*, 161–177. [CrossRef] [PubMed]
76. Kushwaha, P.P.; Maurya, S.K.; Singh, A.; Prajapati, K.S.; Singh, A.K.; Shuaib, M.; Kumar, S. Bulbine frutescens phytochemicals as novel ABC-transporter inhibitor: A molecular docking and molecular dynamics simulation study. *J. Cancer Metastasis Treat.* **2021**, *2021*, 1–11. [CrossRef]
77. Verma, S.; Prajapati, K.S.; Kushwaha, P.P.; Shuaib, M.; Singh, A.K.; Kumar, S.; Gupta, S. Resistance to second generation antiandrogens in prostate cancer: Pathways and mechanisms. *Cancer Drug Resist* **2020**, *3*, 7427–7461. [CrossRef] [PubMed]
78. Zhao, B.-X.; Sun, Y.-B.; Wang, S.-Q.; Duan, L.; Huo, Q.-L.; Ren, F.; Li, G.-F. Grape Seed Procyanidin Reversal of P-glycoprotein Associated Multi-Drug Resistance via Down-regulation of NF-κB and MAPK/ERK Mediated YB-1 Activity in A2780/T Cells. *PLoS ONE* **2013**, *8*, e71071. [CrossRef] [PubMed]
79. Li, S.; Zhao, Q.; Wang, B.; Yuan, S.; Wang, X.; Li, K. Quercetin reversed MDR in breast cancer cells through down-regulating P-gp expression and eliminating cancer stem cells mediated by YB-1 nuclear translocation. *Phytother. Res.* **2018**, *32*, 1530–1536. [CrossRef]
80. Li, S.; Yuan, S.; Zhao, Q.; Wang, B.; Wang, X.; Li, K. Quercetin enhances chemotherapeutic effect of doxorubicin against human breast cancer cells while reducing toxic side effects of it. *Biomed. Pharmacother.* **2018**, *100*, 441–447. [CrossRef] [PubMed]

81. Li, X.; Zhou, N.; Wang, J.; Liu, Z.; Wang, X.; Zhang, Q.; Liu, Q.; Gao, L.; Wang, R. Quercetin suppresses breast cancer stem cells (CD44+ /CD24−) by inhibiting the PI3K/Akt/mTOR-signaling pathway. *Life Sci.* **2018**, *196*, 56–62. [CrossRef]
82. Ye, X.; Wu, F.; Wu, C.; Wang, P.; Jung, K.; Gopal, K.; Ma, Y.; Li, L.; Lai, R. β-Catenin, a Sox2 binding partner, regulates the DNA binding and transcriptional activity of Sox2 in breast cancer cells. *Cell. Signal.* **2013**, *26*, 492–501. [CrossRef] [PubMed]
83. Imai, Y.; Yoshimori, M.; Fukuda, K.; Yamagishi, H.; Ueda, Y. The PI3K/Akt inhibitor LY294002 reverses BCRP-mediated drug resistance without affecting BCRP translocation. *Oncol. Rep.* **2012**, *27*, 1703–1709. [CrossRef]
84. Bonuccelli, G.; De Francesco, E.M.; De Boer, R.; Tanowitz, H.B.; Lisanti, M. NADH autofluorescence, a new metabolic biomarker for cancer stem cells: Identification of Vitamin C and CAPE as natural products targeting "stemness". *Oncotarget* **2017**, *8*, 20667–20678. [CrossRef] [PubMed]
85. Dadras, P.; Atyabi, F.; Irani, S.; Ma'Mani, L.; Foroumadi, A.; Mirzaie, Z.H.; Ebrahimi, M.; Dinarvand, R. Formulation and evaluation of targeted nanoparticles for breast cancer theranostic system. *Eur. J. Pharm. Sci.* **2016**, *97*, 47–54. [CrossRef] [PubMed]
86. Darakhshan, S.; Bidmeshki Pour, A.; Hosseinzadeh Colagar, A.H.; Sisakhtnezhad, S. Thymoquinone and its therapeutic potentials. *Pharmacol. Res.* **2015**, *95–96*, 138–158. [CrossRef] [PubMed]
87. Bhattacharjee, M.; Upadhyay, P.; Sarker, S.; Basu, A.; Das, S.; Ghosh, A.; Ghosh, S.; Adhikary, A. Combinatorial therapy of Thymoquinone and Emodin synergistically enhances apoptosis, attenuates cell migration and reduces stemness efficiently in breast cancer. *Biochim. Biophys. Acta (BBA)-Gen. Subj.* **2020**, *1864*, 129695. [CrossRef] [PubMed]
88. Bashmail, H.A.; AlAmoudi, A.A.; Noorwali, A.; Hegazy, G.; Ajabnoor, G.; Choudhry, H.; Al-Abd, A.M. Thymoquinone synergizes gemcitabine anti-breast cancer activity via modulating its apoptotic and autophagic activities. *Sci. Rep.* **2018**, *8*, 11674. [CrossRef] [PubMed]
89. Ye, L.; Chan, F.; Chen, S.; Leung, L. The citrus flavonone hesperetin inhibits growth of aromatase-expressing MCF-7 tumor in ovariectomized athymic mice. *J. Nutr. Biochem.* **2012**, *23*, 1230–1237. [CrossRef] [PubMed]
90. Hermawan, A.; Khumaira, A.; Ikawati, M.; Putri, H.; Jenie, R.I.; Angraini, S.M.; Muflikhasari, H.A. Identification of key genes of hesperidin in inhibition of breast cancer stem cells by functional network analysis. *Comput. Biol. Chem.* **2020**, *90*, 107427. [CrossRef]
91. Cevatemre, B.; Erkısa, M.; Aztopal, N.; Karakas, D.; Alper, P.; Tsimplouli, C.; Sereti, E.; Dimas, K.; Armutak, E.I.; Gurevin, E.G.; et al. A promising natural product, pristimerin, results in cytotoxicity against breast cancer stem cells in vitro and xenografts in vivo through apoptosis and an incomplete autopaghy in breast cancer. *Pharmacol. Res.* **2018**, *129*, 500–514. [CrossRef]
92. Mak, K.-K.; Wu, A.T.H.; Lee, W.-H.; Chang, T.-C.; Chiou, J.-F.; Wang, L.-S.; Wu, C.-H.; Huang, C.-Y.F.; Shieh, Y.-S.; Chao, T.-Y.; et al. Pterostilbene, a bioactive component of blueberries, suppresses the generation of breast cancer stem cells within tumor microenvironment and metastasis via modulating NF-κB/microRNA 448 circuit. *Mol. Nutr. Food Res.* **2013**, *57*, 1123–1134. [CrossRef]
93. Wu, C.-H.; Hong, B.-H.; Ho, C.-T.; Yen, G.-C. Targeting Cancer Stem Cells in Breast Cancer: Potential Anticancer Properties of 6-Shogaol and Pterostilbene. *J. Agric. Food Chem.* **2015**, *63*, 2432–2441. [CrossRef] [PubMed]
94. Oh, J.; Bin Jeon, S.; Lee, Y.; Lee, H.; Kim, J.; Kwon, B.R.; Kyung-Min, C.; Cha, J.-D.; Hwang, S.-M.; Choi, K.-M.; et al. Fermented Red Ginseng Extract Inhibits Cancer Cell Proliferation and Viability. *J. Med. Food* **2015**, *18*, 421–428. [CrossRef]
95. Oh, J.; Yoon, H.-J.; Jang, J.-H.; Kim, D.-H.; Surh, Y.-J. The standardized Korean Red Ginseng extract and its ingredient ginsenoside Rg3 inhibit manifestation of breast cancer stem cell–like properties through modulation of self-renewal signaling. *J. Ginseng Res.* **2018**, *43*, 421–430. [CrossRef] [PubMed]
96. Harrison, H.; Farnie, G.; Howell, S.J.; Rock, R.E.; Stylianou, S.; Brennan, K.R.; Bundred, N.J.; Clarke, R.B. Regulation of Breast Cancer Stem Cell Activity by Signaling through the Notch4 Receptor. *Cancer Res.* **2010**, *70*, 709–718. [CrossRef]
97. Kim, S.-H.; Singh, S.V. Mammary Cancer Chemoprevention by Withaferin a Is Accompanied by In Vivo Suppression of Self-Renewal of Cancer Stem Cells. *Cancer Prev. Res.* **2014**, *7*, 738–747. [CrossRef]
98. Shuaib, M.; Prajapati, K.S.; Singh, A.K.; Kushwaha, P.P.; Waseem, M.; Kumar, S. Identification of miRNAs and related hub genes associated with the triple negative breast cancer using integrated bioinformatics analysis and in vitro approach. *J. Biomol. Struct. Dyn.* **2021**, *39*, 1–15. [CrossRef] [PubMed]
99. Prajapati, K.S.; Shuaib, M.; Kushwaha, P.P.; Singh, A.K.; Kumar, S. Identification of cancer stemness related miRNA(s) using integrated bioinformatics analysis and in vitro validation. *3Biotech* **2021**, *11*, 446. [CrossRef]
100. Kushwaha, P.P.; Singh, A.K.; Shuaib, M.; Prajapati, K.S.; Vardhan, P.S.; Gupta, S.; Kumar, S. 3-O-(E)-p-Coumaroyl betulinic acid possess anticancer activity and inhibit Notch signaling pathway in breast cancer cells and mammosphere. *Chem. Interact.* **2020**, *328*, 109200. [CrossRef] [PubMed]
101. Jabczyk, M.; Nowak, J.; Hudzik, B.; Zubelewicz-Szkodzińska, B. Curcumin and Its Potential Impact on Microbiota. *Nutrients* **2021**, *13*, 2004. [CrossRef]
102. Cady, N.; Peterson, S.R.; Freedman, S.N.; Mangalam, A.K. Beyond Metabolism: The Complex Interplay Between Dietary Phytoestrogens, Gut Bacteria, and Cells of Nervous and Immune Systems. *Front. Neurol.* **2020**, *11*, 150. [CrossRef]
103. Ortega-Santos, C.; Al-Nakkash, L.; Whisner, C. Exercise and/or Genistein Treatment Impact Gut Microbiota and Inflammation after 12 Weeks on a High-Fat, High-Sugar Diet in C57BL/6 Mice. *Nutrients* **2020**, *12*, 3410. [CrossRef]
104. Adiwidjaja, J.; McLachlan, A.J.; Boddy, A. Curcumin as a clinically-promising anti-cancer agent: Pharmacokinetics and drug interactions. *Expert Opin. Drug Metab. Toxicol.* **2017**, *13*, 953–972. [CrossRef]

105. Aqil, F.; Munagala, R.; Jeyabalan, J.; Vadhanam, M.V. Bioavailability of phytochemicals and its enhancement by drug delivery systems. *Cancer Lett.* **2013**, *334*, 133–141. [CrossRef]
106. Xie, J.; Yang, Z.; Zhou, C.; Zhu, J.; Lee, R.J.; Teng, L. Nanotechnology for the delivery of phytochemicals in cancer therapy. *Biotechnol. Adv.* **2016**, *34*, 343–353. [CrossRef] [PubMed]
107. Ahmad, R.; Srivastava, S.; Ghosh, S.; Khare, S.K. Phytochemical delivery through nanocarriers: A review. *Colloids Surf. B Biointerfaces* **2021**, *197*, 111389. [CrossRef] [PubMed]

cancers MDPI

Correction

Correction: Bishayee et al. Lotus (*Nelumbo nucifera* Gaertn.) and Its Bioactive Phytocompounds: A Tribute to Cancer Prevention and Intervention. *Cancers* 2022, *14*, 529

Anupam Bishayee [1,*], Palak A. Patel [1], Priya Sharma [1], Shivani Thoutireddy [1] and Niranjan Das [2]

1 College of Osteopathic Medicine, Lake Erie College of Osteopathic Medicine, Bradenton, FL 34211, USA; ppatel24886@med.lecom.edu (P.A.P.); PSharma44656@med.lecom.edu (P.S.); SThoutired89922@med.lecom.edu (S.T.)

2 Department of Chemistry, Iswar Chandra Vidyasagar College, Belonia 799155, Tripura, India; ndnsmu@gmail.com

* Correspondence: abishayee@lecom.edu or abishayee@gmail.com

Table Legend

In the original article, there was a mistake in the legend for Table 2 [1]. In the table legend (page 24), "in vivo" appears incorrectly which should be replaced by "in vitro". The correct legend appears below.

Table 2. Potential anticancer effects and mechanisms of action of *N. nucifera*-derived constituents based on in vitro studies.

Error in Table

In the original article, there were mistakes in Table 3 as published. In the table legend (page 32), "in vitro" appears incorrectly which should be replaced by "in vivo". Additionally, the content of the table is same as Table 2, which should be replaced by a correct table. The corrected Table 3 along with the title appear below.

Table 3. Potential anticancer effects and mechanisms of action of *N. nucifera*-derived constituents based on in vivo studies.

Materials Tested	Animal Tumor Models	Anticancer Effects	Mechanisms	Dose (Route)	Duration	References
			Breast cancer			
Flavonoid-rich leaf extract	BALB/c athymic nude mice injected with MCF-7 cells	Reduced tumor volume and weight	↓HER2; p-HER2; ↓Fas	0.5 & 1% (diet)	28 days	Yang et al., 2011 [79]
Aqueous leaf extract	MDA-MB-231 cells injected in female C57BL/6 nude mice	Inhibited tumor growth	Not reported	0.5–2 % (s.c.)	14 days	Chang et al., 2016 [80]
Liensinine + doxorubicin	Female nude mice injected with MDA-MB-231 cells	Reduced tumor growth	↑Apoptosis; ↑cleaved caspase-3; ↓autophagy/mitophagy; ↑auto-phagosome /mitophagosome; ↑colocalization of DNM1L and TOMM20	60 mg/kg (i.p.); 2 mg/kg (i.p.)	30 days	Zhou et al., 2015 [90]

Citation: Bishayee, A.; Patel, P.A.; Sharma, P.; Thoutireddy, S.; Das, N. Correction: Bishayee et al. Lotus (*Nelumbo nucifera* Gaertn.) and Its Bioactive Phytocompounds: A Tribute to Cancer Prevention and Intervention. *Cancers* 2022, *14*, 529. *Cancers* **2022**, *14*, 2116. https://doi.org/10.3390/cancers14092116

Received: 6 April 2022
Accepted: 6 April 2022
Published: 24 April 2022

Table 3. *Cont.*

Materials Tested	Animal Tumor Models	Anticancer Effects	Mechanisms	Dose (Route)	Duration	References
			Colon cancer			
Nuciferine	CT29 cells subcutaneously implanted in nude mice	Reduced tumor weight	Not reported	9.5 mg/kg (i.p.)	3 times a week for 3 weeks	Qi et al., 2016 [96]
Liensinine	HT29 cells injected in female BALB/c nude mice	Suppressed colorectal tumorigenesis, reduced tumor size	↓Ki-67	30 mg/kg (oral)	Every other day for 15 days	Wang et al., 2018 [97]
			Eye cancer			
Neferine	WERI-Rb-1 cells injected in female athymic nude mice	Reduced tumor volume and weight	↓Ki-67; ↓VEGF; ↓SOD; ↑MDA	0.5–2 mg/kg (i.p)	Every 3 days for 30 days	Wang et al., 2020 [100]
			Gallbladder cancer			
Liensinine	NOZ cells injected in BALB/c nude mice	Reduced tumor volume and weight	↓Ki-67	2 mg/kg (i.p)	Every 2 days	Shen et al., 2019 [101]
			Gastric cancer			
Liensinine from seeds	SGC7901 cells injected in BALB/c homozygous (nu/nu) nude mice	Reduced tumor size	↓Ki-67	10 μM (i.p.)	Every 2 days for a month	Yang et al., 2019 [106]
			Head and neck cancers			
Neferine	CAL27 cells injected in male BALB/c nude mice	Reduced tumor volume	↑Apoptosis; ↑autophagy, ↑cleaved caspase-3, ↑cleaved PARP1, ↑LC3; ↑p62	10 mg/kg (i.p)	Not reported	Zhu et al., 2021 [107]
			Liver cancer			
Water-soluble polysaccharides from seeds	H22 cells injected in female Kunming mice	Reduced tumor weight	↑TNF-α; ↑IL-2; ↑SOD; ↓MDA	50–200 mg/kg (oral)	14 days	Zheng et al., 2016 [102]
Leaf extract	DEN fed male Sprague-Dawley rats	Reduced tumor size	↓AST; ↓ALT; ↓albumin; ↓total triglyceride; ↓total cholesterol; ↓lipid peroxidation; ↑GSH; ↑GSHPx; ↑SOD; ↑CAT; ↑GST; ↓Rac1; ↓PKC α; ↓TNF-α; ↓IL-6	0.5–2.0% (p.o.)	12 weeks	Horng et al., 2017 [119]
Leaf extract	2-AAF-induced male Wistar rats	Inhibited hepatic fibrosis and hepatocarcinogenesis	↓Triglycerides; ↓total cholesterol; ↓AFP; ↓IL-6; ↓TNF-α; ↓AST; ↓ALT; ↓γGT; ↓GST-Pi; ↓lipid peroxidation; ↓8-OHdG; ↑Nrf2; ↑CAT; ↑GPx; ↑SOD-1	0.5–2% in the diet (p.o.)	6 months	Yang et al., 2019 [120]
Neferine+ oxaliplatin	HepG2 and Bel-7402 cells injected in male BALB/c mice	Increased tumor volume reducing the effect of oxaliplatin	↑E-cadherin; ↓Vimentin; ↓Ki-67;	20 mg/kg/d (i.p.)	3 weeks	Deng et al., 2017 [116]
Isoliensinine	Huh-7 cells injected in male athymic nude mice and H22 cells injected in Kunming mice	Reduced tumor volume	↑caspase-3; ↓Bcl-2; ↓Bcl-xL; ↓MMP-9; ↓p65 phosphorylation	3 and 10 mg/kg/d (i.p. and gavage)	10 days; 3 weeks	Shu et al., 2015 [117]
Isoliensinine	Huh-7 cells transfectants injected in male athymic nude mice	Reduced tumor growth	↑Caspase-3 activity	10 mg/kg/d (gavage)	20 days	Shu et al., 2016 [118]

Table 3. *Cont.*

Materials Tested	Animal Tumor Models	Anticancer Effects	Mechanisms	Dose (Route)	Duration	References
			Lung cancer			
Leaf extract and leaf polyphenol extract	4T-1 metastatic tumor in the lung of BALB/c mice	Reduced metastasis and tumor weight	↓PKCα activation	0.25, 1% (p.o.)	19 days	Wu et al., 2017 [81]
Nuciferine	A549 cells injected in BALB/c mice	Reduced tumor size and weight	↑Apoptosis; ↓Bcl-2; ↑Bax; ↓Wnt/β-catenin; ↑Axin	50 mg/kg (i.p.)	3 times a week for 20 days	Liu et al., 2015 [126]
Neferine	DEN-induced lung carcinogenesis in albino male Wistar rats	Suppressed tumor growth	↓ROS; ↓lipid peroxidation; ↓protein carbonyl; ↑GSH; ↑SOD; ↑GPx; ↑GST; ↑CAT; ↓glycoprotein components; ↑ATPase; ↑p53; ↑Bax; ↑caspase-9; ↑caspase-3; ↓Bcl-2; ↓COX-2; ↓NF-κB; ↓CYP2E1; ↓VEGF; ↓PI3K; ↓Akt; ↓mTOR	10–20 mg/kg (oral)	20 alternate days	Sivalingam et al., 2019 [127]
			Neural cancer			
Nuciferine	SY5Y cells subcutaneously implanted in nude mice	Reduced tumor weight	Not reported	9.5 mg/kg (i.p.)	3 times a week for 3 weeks	Qi et al., 2016 [96]
Nuciferine	U251 cells subcutaneously inoculated in BALB/c nude mice	Suppressed tumor weight and size	↓Ki-67; ↓CDC2; ↓Bcl-2; ↓HIF1A; ↓N-cadherin; ↓VEGFA	15 mg/kg (i.p.)	Once a day for 2 weeks	Li et al., 2019 [130]
			Skin cancer			
Procyanidin extract from seedpod	B16 cells inoculated into syngeneic C57BL/6 J mice	Suppressed tumor volume and weight	↓lipid peroxidation levels; ↑SOD; ↑CAT; ↑GSPx; ↑spleen and thymus index	60–120 mg/kg (i.g.)	Every 2–3 days for 15 days	Duan et al., 2010 [137]
Leaf extract	UV-radiation exposed female guinea pigs	Reversed UVB-induced epidermal hyperplasia and hyperpigmentation	↓MITF; ↓tyrosinase; ↓TRP-1; ↓PKA; ↓ERK; ↓melanin	1–2% (topical)	2 weeks	Lai et al., 2020 [138]
7-Hydroxy-dehydronuciferine	A375.S2 cells injected in BALB/c nu/nu female mice	Reduced tumor volume	Not reported	20 mg/kg (i.p.)	Every 7 days for 28 days	Wu et al., 2015 [139]

The authors apologize for any inconvenience caused and state that the scientific conclusions are unaffected. The original article has been updated.

Reference

1. Bishayee, A.; Patel, P.A.; Sharma, P.; Thoutireddy, S.; Das, N. Lotus (*Nelumbo nucifera* Gaertn.) and Its Bioactive Phytocompounds: A Tribute to Cancer Prevention and Intervention. *Cancers* **2022**, *14*, 529. [CrossRef] [PubMed]

cancers

MDPI

Review

Lotus (*Nelumbo nucifera* Gaertn.) and Its Bioactive Phytocompounds: A Tribute to Cancer Prevention and Intervention

Anupam Bishayee [1,*], Palak A. Patel [1], Priya Sharma [1], Shivani Thoutireddy [1] and Niranjan Das [2]

1 College of Osteopathic Medicine, Lake Erie College of Osteopathic Medicine, Bradenton, FL 34211, USA; ppatel24886@med.lecom.edu (P.A.P.); PSharma44656@med.lecom.edu (P.S.); SThoutired89922@med.lecom.edu (S.T.)

2 Department of Chemistry, Iswar Chandra Vidyasagar College, Belonia 799155, Tripura, India; ndnsmu@gmail.com

* Correspondence: abishayee@lecom.edu or abishayee@gmail.com

Simple Summary: The plant *Nelumbo nucifera* (Gaertn.), commonly known as lotus, sacred lotus, Indian lotus, water lily, or Chinese water lily, is an aquatic perennial crop belonging to the family of Nelumbonaceae. *N. nucifera* has traditionally been used as an herbal medicine and functional food in many parts of Asia. It has been found that different parts of this plant consist of various bioactive phytocompounds. Within the past few decades, *N. nucifera* and its phytochemicals have been subjected to intense cancer research. In this review, we critically evaluate the potential of *N. nucifera* phytoconstituents in cancer prevention and therapy with related mechanisms of action.

Abstract: Cancer is one of the major leading causes of death worldwide. Accumulating evidence suggests a strong relationship between specific dietary habits and cancer development. In recent years, a food-based approach for cancer prevention and intervention has been gaining tremendous attention. Among diverse dietary and medicinal plants, lotus (*Nelumbo nucifera* Gaertn., family Nymphaeaceae), also known as Indian lotus, sacred lotus or Chinese water lily, has the ability to effectively combat this disease. Various parts of *N. nucifera* have been utilized as a vegetable as well as an herbal medicine for more than 2000 years in the Asian continent. The rhizome and seeds of *N. nucifera* represent the main edible parts. Different parts of *N. nucifera* have been traditionally used to manage different disorders, such as fever, inflammation, insomnia, nervous disorders, epilepsy, hypertension, cardiovascular diseases, obesity, and hyperlipidemia. It is believed that numerous bioactive components, including alkaloids, polyphenols, terpenoids, steroids, and glycosides, are responsible for its various biological and pharmacological activities, such as antioxidant, anti-inflammatory, immune-modulatory, antiviral, hepatoprotective, cardioprotective, and hypoglycemic activities. Nevertheless, there is no comprehensive review with an exclusive focus on the anticancer attributes of diverse phytochemicals from different parts of *N. nucifera*. In this review, we have analyzed the effects of *N. nucifera* extracts, fractions and pure compounds on various organ-specific cancer cells and tumor models to understand the cancer-preventive and therapeutic potential and underlying cellular and molecular mechanisms of action of this interesting medicinal and dietary plant. In addition, the bioavailability, pharmacokinetics, and possible toxicity of *N. nucifera*-derived phytochemicals, as well as current limitations, challenges and future research directions, are also presented.

Keywords: *Nelumbo nucifera*; phytochemicals; cancer; prevention; therapeutic benefits; molecular mechanisms

Citation: Bishayee, A.; Patel, P.A.; Sharma, P.; Thoutireddy, S.; Das, N. Lotus (*Nelumbo nucifera* Gaertn.) and Its Bioactive Phytocompounds: A Tribute to Cancer Prevention and Intervention. *Cancers* **2022**, *14*, 529. https://doi.org/10.3390/cancers14030529

Academic Editor: Raffaele Capasso

Received: 24 December 2021
Accepted: 17 January 2022
Published: 21 January 2022
Corrected: 24 April 2022

1. Introduction

Cancer is the second leading cause of both morbidity and mortality throughout the world, with an estimated 19.3 million new cancer cases and almost 10 million cancer deaths in the year 2020 [1]. Interestingly, it has been suggested that more than 40% of all cancer deaths could be prevented via lifestyle changes, including diet [2]. High dietary consumption of fruits and vegetables (more than 400 g/day) may prevent at least 20% of all cancers [3]. Dietary intervention may also improve the efficacy of cancer chemotherapy and lower the risk of long-term complications in cancer patients [4]. The cancer-preventive potential of various fruits, vegetables, spices, whole grains, and herbs is attributed to the presence of secondary plant metabolites, also known as phytochemicals. These naturally-occurring phytochemicals are also utilized in the discovery and development of anticancer drugs [5,6]. Emerging preclinical and clinical data shows that bioactive food components contain enormous cancer-preventive and anticancer therapeutic potential due to their unique ability to impact various cancer hallmarks, namely sustained proliferation, cell death resistance, energy metabolism, immune surveillance evasion, inflammation, invasion, angiogenesis, and metastasis, by modulating a plethora of oncogenic and oncosuppressive signaling pathways [7–17].

Nelumbo nucifera Gaertn., commonly known as lotus, sacred lotus, Indian lotus or Chinese water lily, is a well-known dietary and medicinal plant. It is a large, perennial aquatic plant that belongs to the family *Nelumbonaceae* and consists of a sole genus Nelumbo with two species, *N. nucifera* and *N. lutea*, which are called Asian lotus and American lotus, respectively [18,19]. In general, lotus refers to the Asian lotus, which is mainly distributed in India, China, Nepal, Sri Lanka, Thailand, Japan, New Guinea and Australia [20–22]. In contrast, the American lotus is predominantly found in the eastern and southern regions of North America and north of South America [18,23,24]. Since ancient times, the lotus flower (Figure 1) has been recognized as a spiritual object for Hindus, Buddhists and Egyptians, and is considered a symbol of longevity in Chinese traditional culture [25,26]. Lotus is the national flower of India and Vietnam. As a vegetable as well as a medicinal and ornamental plant, lotus has been cultivated for more than the last 7000 years [19]. Almost all parts of the lotus plant have been used as food and medicine for more than 2000 years in Asia [27]. Lotus has a significant economic value in various Asian countries, where it is emerging as a horticultural model plant [26]. China is the largest producer and consumer of lotus in the world [27]. The rhizome (modified stem), perianth (non-reproductive part of the flower) and seeds of lotus are popular food ingredients and are used in various food products due to their delicious taste and nutritional value [28,29].

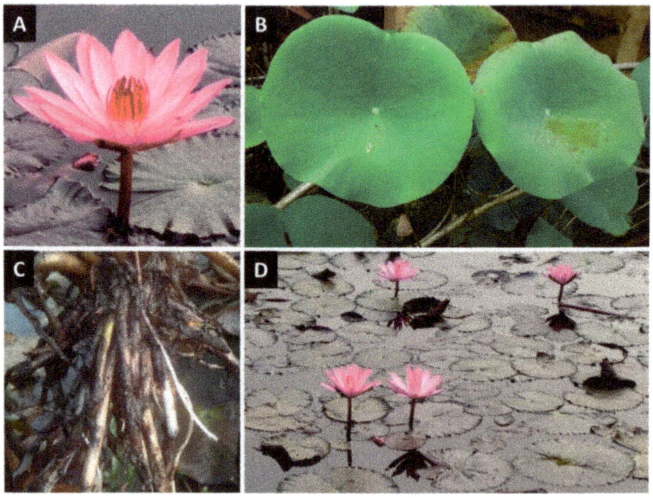

Figure 1. Photographs of lotus (*N. nucifera*). (**A**) Flower; (**B**) leaves; (**C**) rhizomes and (**D**) natural habitat.

Various parts of the lotus plant (Figure 1), from root to shoot, have documented use in different traditional systems of medicines, such as Indian traditional medicine (Ayurveda) and Chinese traditional medicine [30–32]. The whole plant, as well as crude extracts, fractions and constituents, have been found to possess numerous biological and pharmacological activities, including antioxidant, anti-inflammatory, immunomodulatory, antipyretic, antibacterial, antiviral, antifungal, antidiarrheal, diuretic, antiamnestic, antithrombotic, antiarrythmic, antidiabetic, hypocholesterolemic, antiobesity, antiaging, antiatherosclerotic, antifibrotic, sedative, antineurodegenerative, memory-improving, antifertility, hepatoprotective, skin-protective, cardiovascular-protective, and anticancer properties [24,25,29,31,33–36]. The remarkable health-promoting and disease-mitigating activities of the lotus plant have been correlated with the presence of numerous bioactive phytocompounds, including polyphenols, flavonoids, phenolic acids, alkaloids, terpenoids, steroids, fatty acids, and glycosides [25,31,33–36].

During the last several decades, *N. nucifera* has been subjected to intense research that evaluated the antineoplastic effects of various parts and active constituents of this dietary and medicinal plant. However, to the best of our knowledge, a comprehensive state-of-the-art review of all available anticancer studies has not been performed. Most of the previous reviews mainly focused on traditional and ethnopharmacological uses, biosynthesis, phytochemical analysis, industrial applications, and broad-spectrum health benefits of *N. nucifera* in which an overview of anticancer potential represents a minor representation [29,31–34,37]. Several prior publications highlighted pharmacological activities of selected phytochemicals of *N. nucifera,* and these reports did not have a sole focus on cancer [25,35,36,38,39]. Hence, the aim of this work has been to perform a systematic and critical analysis of fragmentary studies to provide an up-to-date and complete assessment of cancer-preventive and anticancer therapeutic attributes of *N. nucifera* and its bioactive phytocomponents with an understanding of the cellular and molecular mechanisms of action. Moreover, the bioavailability, pharmacokinetics and possible adverse effects of *N. nucifera*-derived phytochemicals, as well as current limitations, challenges and future research directions, are also discussed.

2. Chemical Constituents of *N. nucifera*

Several parts of *N. nucifera* are known to contain various pharmacologically active constituents and the most prominent phytochemical classes include alkaloids, flavonoids, terpenoids polysaccharides, steroids, essential oils, tannins, glycosides, proteins, fatty acids, minerals, and vitamins [29,31,34,40–43]. The main bioactive constituents of *N. nucifera* are alkaloids and flavonoids [33]. Different parts of *N. nucifera* contain several types of phytochemicals. For example, the leaves are rich in flavonoids and alkaloids, the flowers and plumules are rich in flavonoids, the seeds are rich in alkaloids, and the rhizome is rich in starch [29,40,42,44]. Procyanidins are the chief active components of *N. nucifera* receptacles [29]. A list of diverse groups of major phytochemicals present in different parts of *N. nucifera* is provided in Table 1.

Various bioactive alkaloids in different parts of *N. nucifera* include *N*-nornuciferine, nuciferine, roemerin, 2-hydroxy-1-methoxyaporphine, (6*R*,6a*R*)-roemerine-N_β-oxide, (*S*)-armepavine, (+)-1(*R*)-coclaurine, (−)-1(*S*)-norcoclaurine, lotusine, isoliensinine, liensinine, neferine, liriodenine, asimilobine, pronuciferine, oleracein E, demethyl-coclaurine, dauricine, *cis*-*N*-coumaroyltyramine, *cis*-*N*-feruloyltyramine, *trans*-*N*-coumaroyltyramine, and *trans*-*N*-feruloyltyramine (Figure 2) [31,33,34,40,44–47].

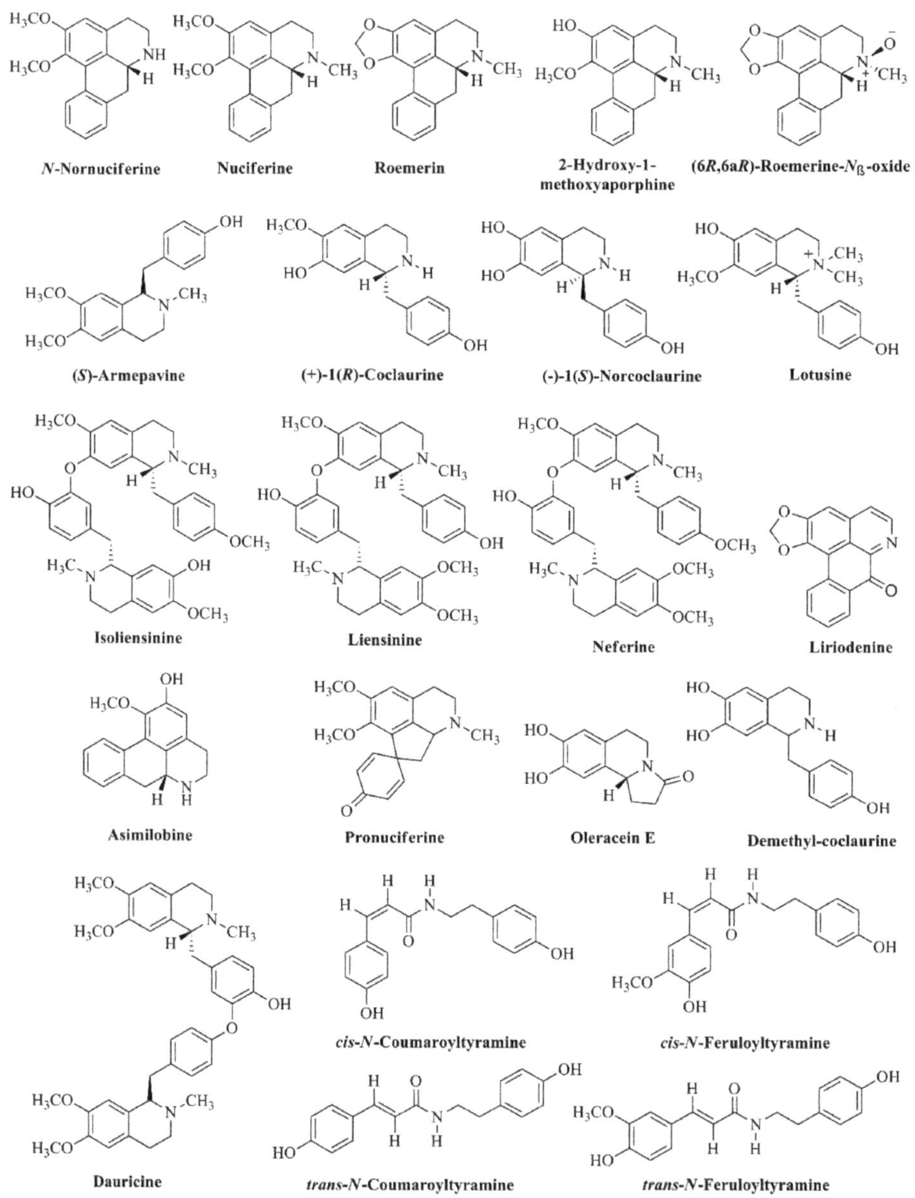

Figure 2. Chemical structures of major bioactive alkaloids isolated from different parts of *N. nucifera*.

The different parts of the *N. nucifera* plant, such as leaves, roots, seeds, and flowers, contain several bioactive flavonoid molecules, including flavonols, flavons, flavan-3-ols, flavanons, and anthocyanins [36]. The flavonols found in *N. nucifera* are myricetin, quercetin, kaempferol, and isorhamnetin, whereas the flavon molecules are diosmetin, syringetin, apigenin, luteolin, and chrysoeriol [36]. The flavan-3-ol molecules include catechin, epicatechin, catechin rhamnoside, gallocatechin gallate, and epigallocatechin gallate, along with its dimer and polymers, such as procyanidin dimer B1 and elephantorrhizol. The flavanones include naringenin and taxifolin, and the anthocyanins are cyanidin, delphinidin, malvidin, petunidin, and peonidin [36]. The major bioactive flavonoids derived from different parts of *N. nucifera* are quercetin, kaempferol, apigenin, isorhamnetin, luteolin, myricetin, syringetin, and diosmetin (Figure 3) [33,36]. A total of 16 flavonoid *C*-glycosides and 56 flavonoid *O*-glycosides have been isolated from different parts of *N. nucifera* [36]. The main flavonoid *O*-glycosides in the different parts of *N. nucifera* include myrycetin 3-*O*-galactoside, myrycetin 3-*O*-glucoside, quercetin 3-*O*-arabinopyranosyl-(1→2)-galactopyranoside, myrycetin 3-*O*-glucuronide, quercetin 3-*O*-rhamnopyranosyl-(1→6)-glucopyranoside (rutine), quercetin 3-*O*-galactoside (hyperoside), quercetin 3-*O*-glucoside (isoquercitrin), kaempferol 3-*O*-robinobioside, quercetin 3-*O*-glucuronide, kaempferol 3-*O*-galactoside, isorhamnetin 3-*O*-rutinoside, kaempferol 3-*O*-glucoside (astragalin), syringetin 3-*O*-glucoside, isorhamnetin 3-*O*-glucoside, kaempferol 3-*O*-glucuronide, kaempferol 7-*O*-glucoside, diosmetin 7-*O*-hexose, and isorhamnetin 3-*O*-glucuronide [25,42,48]. The key flavonoid *C*-glycosides in the different parts of *N. nucifera* are luteolin 8-*C*-*β*-D-glucopyranoside (orientin), luteolin 6-*C*-*β*-D-glucopyranoside (isoorientin), apigenin 8-*C*-*β*-D-glucopyranoside (vitexin), apigenin 6-*C*-*β*-D-glucopyranoside (isovitexin), apigenin 6-*C*-*β*-D-glucopyranosyl-8-*C*-*β*-D-glucopyranoside, luteolin 6-*C*-*β*-D-glucopyranosyl-8-*C*-*β*-D-pentoside, luteolin 6-*C*-*β*-D-pentosyl-8-*C*-*β*-D-glucopyranoside, apigenin 6-*C*-*β*-D-glucopyranosyl-8-*C*-*β*-D-xylopyranoside, apigenin 6-*C*-*β*-D-xylopyranosyl-8-*C*-*β*-D-glucopyranoside, apigenin 6-*C*-*β*-D-glucopyranosyl-8-*C*-*β*-D-arabionoside, apigenin 6-*C*-*β*-D-arabionosyl-8-*C*-*β*-D-glucopyranoside, apigenin 6-*C*-*β*-D-glucopyranosyl-8-*C*-*β*-D-rhamnoside, and apigenin 6-*C*-*β*-D-rhamnosyl-8-*C*-*β*-D-glucopyranoside [25]. The *N. nucifera* leaves, roots, and seed kernels contain several phenolic acids that can be classified into two categories: hydroxybenzoic acids and hydroxycinnamic acids [36]. The phenolic acids under the group of hydroxycinnamic acids include caffeic acid, protocetechuic acid, chlorogenic acid, cinnamic acid, ferulic acid, *p*-coumaric acid, and sinapic acid. The hydroxybenzoic acids include gallic acid, hydroxybenzoic acid, *p*-hydroxybenzoic acid, syringic acid, and vanillic acid [36].

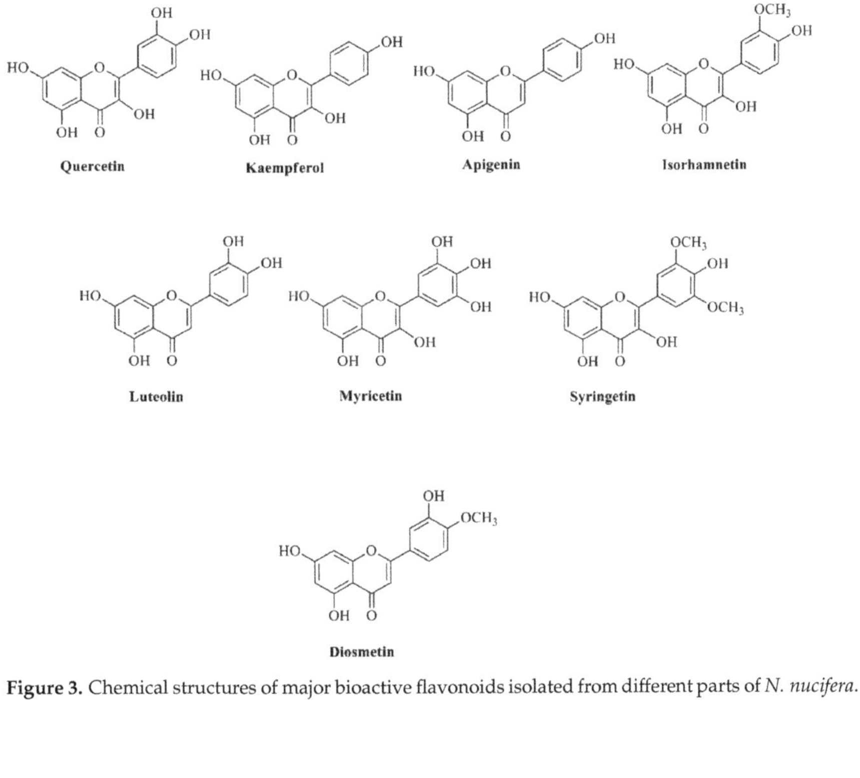

Figure 3. Chemical structures of major bioactive flavonoids isolated from different parts of *N. nucifera*.

2.1. Leaves

The leaves of *N. nucifera* are rich in alkaloids and flavonoids [29,40,44,45,47]. The phytochemical analysis of EtOAc-soluble fraction of 80% MeOH extract of leaves of *N. nucifera* revealed the presence of 33 significant bioactive constituents, including 13 megastigmanes, 1 sesquiterpene, 8 alkaloids, and 11 flavonoids [45]. The various bioactive alkaloids in *N. nucifera* have raised significant interest due to their versatile chemical and biological activities [46]. The leaves of *N. nucifera* are a rich source of various bioactive alkaloids [44–47]. The 95% EtOH extract of leaves of *N. nucifera* yielded six potent bioactive alkaloids, namely (+)-1(*R*)-coclaurine, (−)-1(*S*)-norcoclaurine, nuciferine, liensinine, neferine, and isoliensinine [40]. The high-performance liquid chromatography (HPLC) coupled with ion trap/time-of-flight mass spectrometry (LC/MS-ITTOF) analysis of *N. nucifera* leaf extract reported the existence of five isoquinoline alkaloids: dehydronuciferine, *N*-nornuciferine, *O*-nornuciferine, nuciferine, and roemerine [49]. The non-aqueous capillary electrophoresis coupled with ultraviolet and mass spectroscopy (NACE-UV-MS) analysis is a method developed by Do et al. [50] to determine the major alkaloids, such as (−)-caaverine, (+)-isoliensinine, (+)-norarmepavine, (−)-armepavine, (−)-nuciferine, (−)-nornuciferine, and (+)-pronuciferine, present in *N. nucifera* leaves. One alkaloid, *N*-methylasimilobine, has also been reported from the MeOH extract of *N. nucifera* leaves [51].

The potential bioactive flavonoids in the leaves of *N. nucifera* are quercetin, kaempferol, and luteolin [45,51]. The methanol extracts of the leaves of *N. nucifera* revealed the presence of several flavonoid compounds, including catechin, quercetin, quercetin-3-*O*-glucopyranoside, quercetin-3-*O*-glucuronide, quercetin-3-*O*-galactopyranoside, kaempferol-3-*O*-glucopyranoside, and myricetin-3-*O*-glucopyranoside [52]. The bioactive quercetin-based flavonoids and glycosides in *N. nucifera* leaves are (+)-catechin, hyperoside, isoquercitrin, and astragalin [29,40]. The in vitro lipolysis assay of the leaf extract of *N. nucifera* identified the presence of five bioactive flavonoid molecules, namely quercetin 3-*O*-α-arabinopyranosyl-(1→2)-β-galactopyranoside, (+)-catechin, hyperoside, isoquercitrin, and astragalin [53].

The gas chromatography-mass spectrometry (GC-MS) analysis of hexane extract of the leaves of *N. nucifera* revealed the presence of 38 compounds, in which 15 compounds are the essential oil composition with 9,12,15-octadecatrienoic acid, linoleic acid ethyl ester, *n*-hexadecanoic acid, hexadecanoic acid, ethyl ester, and methyl (*Z*)-5,11,14,17-eicosatetraenoate [54]. The GC-MS analysis of essential oils of *N. nucifera* leaves detected the presence of 95 constituents, in which the major constituents are *l*-(+)-ascorbic acid 2,6-dihexadecanoate, *trans*-phytol, hexahydrofarnesyl acetone, pentadecyl acrylate, β-ionone, geranyl acetone, propionic acid decyl ester, farnesyl acetone, and heneicosane [41].

The analysis of a MeOH extract of the leaves of *N. nucifera* showed the presence of five norsesquiterpenes/megastigmanes, such as (*E*)-3-hydroxymegastigm-7-en-9-one, (3*S*,5*R*,6*S*,7*E*)-megastigma-7-ene-3,5,6,9-tetrol, dendranthemoside B, icariside B2, and sedumoside F1 [51]. Two bioactive triterpenes, namely alphitolic acid and maslinic acid, have also been extracted from the MeOH extract of *N. nucifera* leaves [51].

The leaves of *N. nucifera* also contain several nonvolatile organic acids, such as alphitolic, maslinic, gallic, tartaric, malic, and anisic acids [29,51,55].

2.2. Plumules

The plumule of *N. nucifera* contains 7.8% moisture, 4.2% ash, 12.5% crude oil and 26.3% protein [56]. The *N. nucifera* plumule oil is a rich source of several fatty acids. The major fatty acids in *N. nucifera* plumule oil are linoleic acid (50.4%) and palmitic acid (18.0%), followed by oleic acid (13.5%), behenic acid (6.8%), arachidic acid (3.30%), linolenic acid (3.0%), and stearic acid (2.90%) [56]. The major triglyceride components in *N. nucifera* plumule oil include linoleic acid-linoleic acid (12.80%), β-palmitic acid-linoleic acid (11.27%), β-oleic acid-linoleic acid (9.43%), β-palmitic acid-linoleic acid-oleic acid (8.58%), β-behenic acid-linoleic acid (8.32%), β-palmitic acid-oleic acid-linoleic acid (8.28%), β-palmitic acid-linoleic acid-arachidic acid (7.99%), β-palmitic acid-linoleic acid-palmitic acid (7.71%), and β-linoleic acid-oleic acid-linoleic acid (7.13%) [56].

The unsaponifiable components in *N. nucifera* plumule oil are very high (up to 14–19%) due to the presence of several sterol compounds [56]. The major sterols present in *N. nucifera* plumule oil are β-sitosterol (31.75%), Δ5-avenasterol (19.66%), and campesterol (6.28%), followed by stigmasta-7,25-dien-3-ol (3.49%), 24-methylene-9,19-cyclolanostan-3β-ol (3.79%), α-sitosterol (3.41%), stigmasterol (2.67%) ergosta-8,24(28)-dien-3-ol (2.5%), ergosta-5,24-dien-3-ol (1.71%), lanost-7-en-3-one (1.51%), and stigmasta-7-en-3-ol (0.96%) [56].

The ultra-performance liquid chromatography coupled with quadrupole time of flight mass spectrometry analysis of *N. nucifera* plumule extracts revealed the presence of several bioactive constituents which are mainly of the alkaloid and flavonoid group of compounds [57]. The bioactive alkaloid components in *N. nucifera* plumule extracts include higenamine, lotusine, 4′-methylcoclaurine, isoliensinine, liensinine, neferine, and nuciferine [57]. Duan and Jiang [58] reported a new benzylisoquinoline alkaloid, namely nelumstemine [1-(4′-hydroxybenzoyl)-6,7-dimethoxy-3,4-dihydroisoquinoline], which was isolated from the stems of *N. nucifera*. The bioactive flavonoid constituents in *N. nucifera* plumule extracts include apigenin-6-*C*-α-L-glucopyanosyl-8-*C*-β-D-glucopyranoside and apigenin-6-*C*-α-L-arabofuranosyl-8-*C*-β-D-glucopyranoside [57].

2.3. Seeds and Rhizomes

Starch is the major ingredient (up to 70% of the dry weight) of both the rhizome and seeds of *N. nucifera* [28]. The raw and dried rhizome and seeds of *N. nucifera* are good sources of niacin and vitamin B6 [28]. The raw and dried portions of the rhizome and seeds of *N. nucifera* contain various minerals, vitamins and fatty acids [28]. The major minerals present in the seeds and dried rhizome of *N. nucifera* include potassium (16,300 µg/g), phosphorus (1715 µg/g), and magnesium (1650 µg/g), followed by aluminum (470 µg/g), calcium (445 µg/g), manganese (57 µg/g), sodium (33 µg/g), cobalt (16 µg/g), strontium (15), iron (13 µg/g), zinc (13 µg/g), copper (10 µg/g) and vanadium (7 µg/g) [24,28]. Other important nutritional agents are fat (72.17%), crude fiber (10.60%), moisture (10.50%), total ash (4.5%), proteins (2.7%), and crude carbohydrates (1.93%) [59]. The seed possesses higher energy with 348.45 cal per 100 g [59]. Vitamin C and folate are the main vitamins present in both the raw rhizome and seeds of *N. nucifera* [28]. *N. nucifera* seeds also contain several vitamins in large amounts, such as vitamin B1 (2.24 mg/kg), vitamin B2 (0.13 mg/kg), vitamin B6 (3.03 mg/kg), vitamin C (39.4 mg/kg), and vitamin E (4.6 mg/kg) [24].

Alkaloids are the key secondary metabolites in the seeds of *N. nucifera* [31]. The major alkaloids present in the seeds of *N. nucifera* are lotusine, isoliensinine, liensinine, dauricine, pronuciferine, nuciferine, procyanidin, neferine, roemerine, and armepavine [31]. The chloroform fraction of hot MeOH extract of the embryos of seeds of *N. nucifera* led to the isolation of three novel bisbenzylisoquinoline alkaloids, such as nelumboferine, nelumborines A and B, along with four previously reported alkaloids [55].

The protein, minerals, amino acids, and unsaturated fatty acids are the rich sources of the seeds of *N. nucifera* [31]. The seeds of *N. nucifera* also contain mainly four types of monosaccharide, namely D-galactose, L-arabinose, D-mannose and D-glucose [59]. The main nutrients in *N. nucifera* seeds are proteins and carbohydrates [24]. The level of polysaccharides in the rhizome of *N. nucifera* is very high [29]. Two antioxidant micromolecular constituents, such as (±)-gallocatechin and (−)-catechin, along with antioxidant macromolecular constituents as well as a polysaccharide–protein complex having α/β-pyranose and α-furanose ring of molecular mass 18.8 kDa, have been reported from the rhizome of *N. nucifera* [60]. The polysaccharide–protein complex is composed of mannose, rhamnose, glucose, galactose and xylose in the molar ratio of 2:8:7:8:1 [61]. The abundance of essential amino acids in *N. nucifera* seeds is very high [24]. The major essential amino acids present in the seeds of *N. nucifera* are methionine (1.64%), valine (1.10%), isoleucine (0.99%), lysine (0.97%), phenylalanine (0.86%), histidine (0.50%), threonine (0.45%), and leucine (0.15%) [24]). The key carbohydrates of *N. nucifera* seeds are starch, polysaccharides and oligosaccharides [24]. The main nutrients of *N. nucifera* seeds represent starch (55.77%), crude protein (16.2%), water (14.0%), sugar (8.13%), ash (4.05%) and fat (2.05%) with a total calorific value of 1432 kJ/100 g [24].

N. nucifera seeds are also rich sources of various fatty acids, such as 14-methylpentadecanoic acid, 8,11-octadecadienoic acid, anti-9-octadecenoic acid, 18-carbonate, behenic acid, 20-carbonate, 9,12,15-octadecatrienoic acid, 14-carbonate, 23-carbonate, pentadecanoate, 17-carbonate, maleic-7-hexadecene acid, anti-8-octadecenoic, and maleic-9-octadecenoic acid [24].

From the MeOH extract of *N. nucifera* rhizome, a new ursane triterpenoid ester, urs-12-*en*-3*β*-*O*-9*E*,12*E*-octadecadienoate, was isolated [62]. The fresh seed epicarps of *N. nucifera* are rich in flavonols and their glycosides. The most important flavonols in *N. nucifera* epicarps are myricetin, quercetin, kaempferol, and isorhamnetin [63]. The CC along with RP-HPLC and HPLC–ESI-MS analysis of *N. nucifera* seed epicarp at three different ripening stages, the green ripening stage, half ripening stage, and full ripening stage, revealed the presence of four bioactive polyphenolic compounds: catechin, epicatechin, hyperoside, and isoquercitrin [64]. It is reported that the levels of these four bioactive polyphenolic compounds are different during seed ripening. The levels of catechin and epicatechin decrease in the ripening stage, whereas the levels of hyperoside and isoquercitrin increase during the ripening stage [64]. The rhizome of *N. nucifera* contains considerable amounts of various phytochemicals, such as tannins, saponins, and phenolic acids [65]. The major phytochemicals present in *N. nucifera* embryo include liensinine, isoliensinine, neferine, nuciferine, lotusine, pronuciferine, rutin, hyperin, and demethylcoclaurine [33].

2.4. *Flowers*

Several classes of bioactive phytochemicals, such as polyphenols, flavonoids, tannins and terpenoids, have been isolated from the ethanolic extracts of *N. nucifera* pink flower stamens and petals [43]. Nakamura et al. [66] reported the presence of a new alkaloid, namely *N*-methylasimilobine *N*-oxide, along with 11 bioactive benzylisoquinoline alkaloids, in the methanolic extracts of flower buds and leaves of *N. nucifera*. The major phytochemicals present in the flowers of *N. nucifera* are quercetin, luteolin, luteolin glucoside, kaempferol, kaempferol-3-*O*-glucoside, and isoquercitrin [33]. The ethanolic extract of *N. nucifera* petals revealed the presence of nine potent bioactive benzylisoquinoline alkaloids: (+)-juziphine, (+)-isococlaurine, (−)-*N*-methylisococlaurine, (−)-*N*-methylcoclaurine, (+)-nor-roefractine, (+)-armepavine, (−)-caaverine, (−)-lirinidine, and (+)-glaziovine [67]. The colors of the petals of *N. nucifera* are different only due to the presence of two flavonoids, namely isorhamnetin and kaempferol [68].

Table 1. List of phytochemicals reported from the different parts of *N. nucifera*.

Phytochemicals	Plant Part	References
	Aromatic phenolic compounds	
Arbutin	Stamens	Mukherjee et al., 2009 [31]
Gallic acid	Stamens and petals	Noysang and Boonmatit, 2019 [43]
(*E*)-Ferulic acid	Seeds	Rho and Yoon, 2017 [69]
(*E*)-*p*-Coumaric acid	Seeds	Rho and Yoon, 2017 [69]
(*E*)-Sinapate-4-*O*-*β*-D-glucopyranoside	Seeds	Rho and Yoon, 2017 [69]
p-Hydroxybenzoic acid	Seeds	Rho and Yoon, 2017 [69]
Protocatechuic acid	Seeds	Rho and Yoon, 2017 [69]
Tannic acid	Stamens and petals	Noysang and Boonmatit, 2019 [43]
	Megastigmane/sesquiterpenes compounds	
(−)-Boscialin	Leaves	Ahn et al., 2013 [45]
(+)-Dehydrovomifoliol	Leaves	Ahn et al., 2013 [45]
(+)-Epiloliolide	Leaves	Ahn et al., 2013 [45]

Table 1. *Cont.*

Phytochemicals	Plant Part	References
(*E*)-3-Hydroxymegastigm-7-en-9-one	Leaves	Ahn et al., 2013 [45]
3-oxo-Retro-α-ionol I	Leaves	Ahn et al., 2013 [45]
3*S*,5*R*-Dihydroxy-6*S*,7-megastigmadien-9-one	Leaves	Ahn et al., 2013 [45]
5,6-epoxy-3-Hydroxy-7-megastigmen-9-one	Leaves	Ahn et al., 2013 [45]
Annuionone D	Leaves	Ahn et al., 2013 [45]
Byzantionoside A	Leaves	Ahn et al., 2013 [45]
Grasshopper ketone	Leaves	Ahn et al., 2013 [45]
Icariside B2	Leaves	Ahn et al., 2013 [45]
Nelumnucifoside A	Leaves	Ahn et al., 2013 [45]
Vomifoliol	Leaves	Ahn et al., 2013 [45]
Nelumnucifoside B	Leaves	Ahn et al., 2013 [45]
	Alkaloids	
(−)-1(*R*)-*N*-methylcoclaurine	Leaves	Kashiwada et al., 2005 [40]
(−)-Lirinidine (5-demethylnuciferine)	Flower buds, stamen, and leaves	Nakamura et al., 2013 [33]; Paudel & Panth, 2015 [33]
(−)-Anonaine	Leaves	Wang et al., 2011 [70]
(−)-Asimilobine	Leaves	Wang et al., 2011 [70]
(−)-Caaverine	Leaves	Wang et al., 2011 [70]
(−)-*N*-Methylasimilobine	Leaves	Wang et al., 2011 [70]
(−)-*nor*-Nuciferine	Leaves	Wang et al., 2011 [70]
(−)-Nuciferine	Leaves	Wang et al., 2011 [70]
(−)-Roemerine	Leaves	Wang et al., 2011 [70]
(6*R*,6a*R*)-Roemerine-N_{β}-oxide	Leaves	Ahn et al., 2013 [45]
(*R*)-Roemerine	Leaves	Agnihotri et al., 2008 [71]
2-Hydroxy-1-methoxy-6a,7-dehydroaporphine	Flower buds and leaves	Nakamura et al., 2013 [66]
3-Indoleacetic acid	Seeds	Rho and Yoon, 2017 [69]
4′-Methyl-*N*-methylcoclaurine	Plumule	Zhou et al., 2013 [57]
7-Hydroxydehydronuciferine	Leaves	Wang et al., 2011 [69]
Anisic acid	Seeds	Itoh et al., 2011 [55]
Anonaine	Leaves	Agnihotri et al., 2008 [71]
Anonaine	Stamen	Paudel & Panth, 2015 [33]
Armepavine	Plumule	Zhou et al., 2013 [57]
Armepavine	Stamen	Paudel & Panth, 2015 [33]
Asimilobine	Flower buds and leaves	Nakamura et al., 2013 [66]
Asimilobine	Stamen	Paudel & Panth, 2015 [33]
Cepharadione B	Leaves	Wang et al., 2011 [70]
cis-*N*-Coumaroyltyramine	Leaves	Ahn et al., 2013 [45]
cis-*N*-Feruloyltyramine	Leaves	Ahn et al., 2013 [45]
Coclaurine	Seeds	Kashiwada et al., 2005 [40]

Table 1. *Cont.*

Phytochemicals	Plant Part	References
d,l-Armepavine	Flower buds and leaves	Kashiwada et al., 2005 [40]; Nakamura et al., 2013 [65]
Dauricine	Seeds	Paudel & Panth, 2015 [33]
Dehydroanonaine	Stamen	Paudel & Panth, 2015 [33]
Dehydroemerine	Stamen	Paudel & Panth, 2015 [33]
Dehydronuciferine	Flower buds and leaves	Nakamura et al., 2013 [65]
Dehydronuciferine	Stamen	Paudel & Panth, 2015 [33]
Dehydroroemerine	Leaves	Agnihotri et al., 2008 [71]
Demethylcoclaurine	Stamen	Paudel & Panth, 2015 [33]
Higenamine	Plumule	Zhou et al., 2013 [57]
Higenamine 4′-*O*-*β*-D-glucoside	Plumule	Kato et al., 2015 [72]
Isoliensinine	Seeds, leaves, and stamen	Itoh et al., 2011 [55]; Kashiwada et al., 2005 [40]; Paudel & Panth, 2015 [33]
Liensinine	Seeds, leaves, and stamen	Itoh et al., 2011 [55]; Kashiwada et al., 2005 [40]; Paudel & Panth, 2015 [33]
Liriodenine	Leaves and stamen	Ahn et al., 2013 [45]; Wang et al., 2011 [70]; Paudel & Panth, 2015 [33]
Lotusine	Leaves and seeds	Kashiwada et al., 2005; Paudel & Panth, 2015 [33]
Lysicamine	Flower buds, leaves, and leaves	Wang et al., 2011 [70]; Nakamura et al., 2013 [66]
Neferine	Seeds and leaves	Kashiwada et al., 2005 [40]; Itoh et al., 2011 [55]; Paudel & Panth, 2015 [33]
N-methylasimilobine	Leaves	Agnihotri et al., 2008 [71]
N-Methylasimilobine	Flower buds, stamen, and leaves	Nakamura et al., 2013 [66]; Paudel & Panth, 2015 [33]
N-Methylcoclaurine	Stamen	Paudel & Panth, 2015 [33]
N-Methylisococlaurine	Stamen	Paudel & Panth, 2015 [33]
N-Norarmepavine	Stamen	Paudel & Panth, 2015 [33]
N-Nornuciferine	Flower buds and leaves	Nakamura et al., 2013 [65]
Norjuziphine	Flower	Morikawa et al., 2016 [73]
Nornuciferine	Leaves and stamen	Kashiwada et al., 2005 [40]; Paudel & Panth, 2015 [33]
Nuciferine	Flower buds, leaves, seeds, and leaves	Kashiwada et al., 2005 [40]; Agnihotri et al., 2008 [71]; Nakamura et al., 2013 [66]; Paudel & Panth, 2015 [33]
Nuciferine *N*-oxide	Flower buds and leaves	Nakamura et al., 2013 [66]
Oleracein E	Leaves	Ahn et al., 2013 [45]
O-Nornuciferine	Plumule	Zhou et al., 2013 [57]
Pronuciferine	Leaves	Ahn et al., 2013 [45]; Nakamura et al., 2013 [66]
Reserpine	Stamens and petals	Noysang and Boonmatit, 2019 [43]
Roemerin	Stamen, leaves, and plumule	Kashiwada et al., 2005 [40]; Zhou et al., 2013 [57]; Paudel & Panth, 2015 [33]
trans-*N*-Coumaroyltyramine	Leaves	Ahn et al., 2013 [45]

Table 1. *Cont.*

Phytochemicals	Plant Part	References
trans-N-Feruloyltyramine	Leaves	Ahn et al., 2013 [45]
Tryptophan	Seeds	Rho and Yoon, 2017 [69]
	Flavonoids	
(−)-Catechin	Leaves	Ahn et al., 2013 [45]
5,7,3′,5′-Tetrahydroxyflavanone	Leaves	Ahn et al., 2013 [45]
Chrysoeriol 7-*O*-*β*-D-glucopyranoside	Leaves	Wang et al., 2008 [74]; Ahn et al., 2013 [45]
Elephantorrhizol	Leaves	Ahn et al., 2013 [45]
Epitaxifolin	Leaves	Ahn et al., 2013 [45]
Hyperoside	Leaves, and plumule	Wang et al., 2008 [74]; Kashiwada et al., 2005 [40]; Zhou et al., 2013 [57]; Liu et al., 2016 [75]
Isoquercitrin (Hirsutrin)	Receptacles, Stamen, plumule, and leaves	Wang et al., 2008 [73]; Kashiwada et al., 2005 [40]; Zhou et al., 2013 [57]; Paudel & Panth, 2015 [33]; Liu et al., 2016 [75]
Isorhamnetin	Leaves	Wang et al., 2008 [74]
Isorhamnetin 3-*O*-*β*-D-glucopyranoside	Receptacles and stamens	Mukherjee et al., 2009 [31]; Liu et al., 2016 [75]
Isorhamnetin 3-*O*-rutinoside	Leaves	Kihyun et al., 2009 [51]
Isorhamnetin 3-*O*-*α*-L-rhamnopyranosyl-(1→6)-*β*-D-glucopyranoside	Stamens	Mukherjee et al., 2009 [31]
Isoschaftoside	Seeds	Rho and Yoon, 2017 [69]
Kaempferol	Leaves and stamens	Ahn et al., 2013 [45]; Wang et al., 2008 [74]; Mukherjee et al., 2009 [31]
Kaempferol 3-*O*-robinobioside	Receptacles	Liu et al., 2016 [75]
Kaempferol 3-*O*-*α*-L-rhamnopyranosyl-(1→2)-*β*-D-glucopyranoside	Stamens	Mukherjee et al., 2009 [31]
Kaempferol 3-*O*-*α*-L-rhamnopyranosyl-(1→2)-*β*-D-glucuronopyranoside	Stamens	Mukherjee et al., 2009 [31]
Kaempferol 3-*O*-*α*-L-rhamnopyranosyl-(1→6)-*β*-D-glucopyranoside	Stamens	Mukherjee et al., 2009 [31]
Kaempferol 3-*O*-*β*-D-galactopyranoside	Receptacles and stamens	Mukherjee et al., 2009 [31]; Liu et al., 2016 [75]
Kaempferol 3-*O*-*β*-D-glucopyranoside/astragalin	Receptacles, leaves, and stamens	Wang et al., 2008 [74]; Mukherjee et al., 2009 [31]; Ahn et al., 2013 [45]; Liu et al., 2016 [75]
Kaempferol 3-*O*-*β*-D-glucuronopyranoside	Stamens	Mukherjee et al., 2009 [31]; Paudel & Panth, 2015 [33]
Kaempferol 3-*O*-*β*-D-glucuronopyranosyl methylester	Stamens	Mukherjee et al., 2009 [31]
Kaempferol 7-*O*-*β*-D-glucopyranoside	Stamens	Mukherjee et al., 2009 [31]
Luteolin/luteolin glucoside	Leaves, plumule, and stamen	Ahn et al., 2013 [45]; Zhou et al., 2013 [57]; Paudel & Panth, 2015 [33]
Myricetin 3′,5′-dimethylether 3-*O*-*β*-D-glucopyranoside	Stamens	Mukherjee et al., 2009 [31]
Myricetin 3-*O*-galactoside	Receptacles	Liu et al., 2016 [75]
Myricetin 3-*O*-glucoside	Receptacles	Liu et al., 2016 [75]
Myricetin 3-*O*-glucuronide	Receptacles	Liu et al., 2016 [75]
Nelumboroside A	Stamens	Mukherjee et al., 2009 [31]

Table 1. *Cont.*

Phytochemicals	Plant Part	References
Nelumboroside B	Stamens	Mukherjee et al., 2009 [31]
Quercetin	Leaves, stamens and petals	Wang et al., 2008 [74]; Ahn et al., 2013 [45]; Paudel & Panth, 2015 [33]; Liu et al., 2016 [75]; Noysang and Boonmatit, 2019 [43]
Quercetin 3-*O*-glucuronide/Quercetin 3-*O*-β-D-glucuronide	Receptacles and leaves	Kashiwada et al., 2005 [40]; Kihyun et al., 2009 [51]; Liu et al., 2016 [75]
Quercetin 3-*O*-β-D-glucopyranoside	Leaves and stamens	Agnihotri et al., 2008 [71]; Mukherjee et al., 2009 [31]; Kihyun et al., 2009 [51]; Ahn et al., 2013 [45]
Quercetin 3-*O*-β-D-xylopyranosyl-(1$\rightarrow$2)-β-D-galactopyranoside	Leaves	Kashiwada et al., 2005 [40]
quercetin-3-*O*-β-D-xylopyranosyl-(1$\rightarrow$2)-β-D-glucopyranosyl glycoside	Leaves	Wang et al., 2008 [74]
Rutin	Leaves, stamens and petals	Kashiwada et al., 2005 [40]; Noysang and Boonmatit, 2019 [43]
Syringetin 3-*O*-glucoside	Receptacles	Liu et al., 2016 [75]
Taxifolin	Leaves	Ahn et al., 2013 [45]
	Sterols and triterpenoids	
24(*R*)-Ethylcholest-6-ene-5α-ol-3-*O*-β-D-glucopyranoside	Leaves	Agnihotri et al., 2008 [71]
Stigmasta-4,22-dien-3-one	Leaves	Wang et al., 2011 [70]
B-Sitostenone	Leaves	Wang et al., 2011 [70]
β-Sitosterol	Rhizome	Chaudhuri & Singh, 2009 [61]
β-Sitosterol-3-*O*-glucoside/β-Sitosterol-3-*O*-β-D-glucopyranoside	Rhizome, leaves, and stamens	Agnihotri et al., 2008 [71]; Chaudhuri & Singh, 2009 [62]; Mukherjee et al., 2009 [31]
Betulinic acid	Rhizome	Chaudhuri & Singh, 2009 [61]
α-Amyrin	Rhizome	Chaudhuri & Singh, 2009 [61]
	Aliphatic open chain compounds	
10-Eicosanol	Leaves	Agnihotri et al., 2008 [71]
3,7,11,15-Tetramethyl-1-hexadecen-3-ol (isophytol)	Leaves	Agnihotri et al., 2008 [71]
3,7,11,15-Tetramethyl-2-hexadecen-1-ol (*trans*-phytol)	Leaves	Agnihotri et al., 2008 [71]
7,11,15-Trimethyl-2-hexadecanone	Leaves	Agnihotri et al., 2008 [71]
Nonacosan-10-ol	Leaves	Mukherjee et al., 2009 [31]
Triacontan-7-ol	Leaves	Mukherjee et al., 2009 [31]
Nonacosane-4,10-diol	Leaves	Mukherjee et al., 2009 [31]
Nonacosane-5,10-diol	Leaves	Mukherjee et al., 2009 [31]
Nonacosane-10,13-diol	Leaves	Mukherjee et al., 2009 [31]
Hentriacontane-12,15-diol	Leaves	Mukherjee et al., 2009 [31]
Tritriacontane-9,10-diol	Leaves	Mukherjee et al., 2009 [31]
Octadecanoic acid	Leaves	Mukherjee et al., 2009 [31]
Palmitic acid	Rhizome	Chaudhuri & Singh, 2009 [62]
Linoleic acid	Rhizome	Chaudhuri & Singh, 2009 [62]

Table 1. *Cont.*

Phytochemicals	Plant Part	References
9*E*,12*E*,15*E*-Octadecatrienoic acid	Rhizome	Chaudhuri & Singh, 2009 [62]
Linalool	Stamen	Paudel & Panth, 2015 [33]
Tartaric acid	Leaves	Paudel & Panth, 2015 [33]
Gluconic acid	Leaves	Paudel & Panth, 2015 [33]
Acetic acid	Leaves	Paudel & Panth, 2015 [33]
Malic acid	Leaves	Paudel & Panth, 2015 [33]
Ginnol	Leaves	Paudel & Panth, 2015 [33]
Nonadecane	Leaves	Paudel & Panth, 2015 [33]
Succinic acid	Leaves	Paudel & Panth, 2015 [33]
	Miscellaneous compounds	
Dihydrophaseic acid	Seeds	Rho and Yoon, 2017 [69]
Dihydrophaseic acid 3′-*O*-*β*-D-glucopyranoside	Seeds	Rho and Yoon, 2017 [69]
Pheophytin-a (chlorophyll derivative)	Leaves	Wang et al., 2011 [70]
Aristophyll-C (chlorophyll derivative)	Leaves	Wang et al., 2011 [70]

3. *N. nucifera* Extracts, Fractions and Pure Compounds in Cancer Research

3.1. Literature Search Methodology

The Preferred Reporting Items for Systematic Reviews and Meta-Analysis (PRISMA) criteria [76], which is recommended for reporting systematic reviews, was followed for this work. The literature search was conducted using various databases, such as PubMed, ScienceDirect, Google Scholar, and Scopus. Publication data was not a criterion when filtering research articles. The last search was performed in December 2021. Various combinations of keywords that were used included: *Nelumbo nucifera*; lotus; cancer; in vivo, in vitro; tumor; prevention; treatment, proliferation, apoptosis, and clinical studies. Reviews, systemic reviews, meta-analyses, letters to editors, book chapters, conference abstracts, and unpublished results were not included, and only articles written in the English language were considered. Additionally, available clinical studies pertaining to *N. nucifera* and cancer were searched on clinicaltrials.gov. The quality of each animal study was evaluated according to SYRCLE's RnB tool that investigates sources of bias [77]. Reference lists from reviews and collected articles were checked for relevant publications. Articles not related to cancer or *N. nucifera* have been excluded. Upon applying these exclusion criteria, eligible full-length articles were obtained and reviewed, and a collaborative decision was made for their incorporation for further analysis. Figure 4 illustrates the overview of the literature search and study selection.

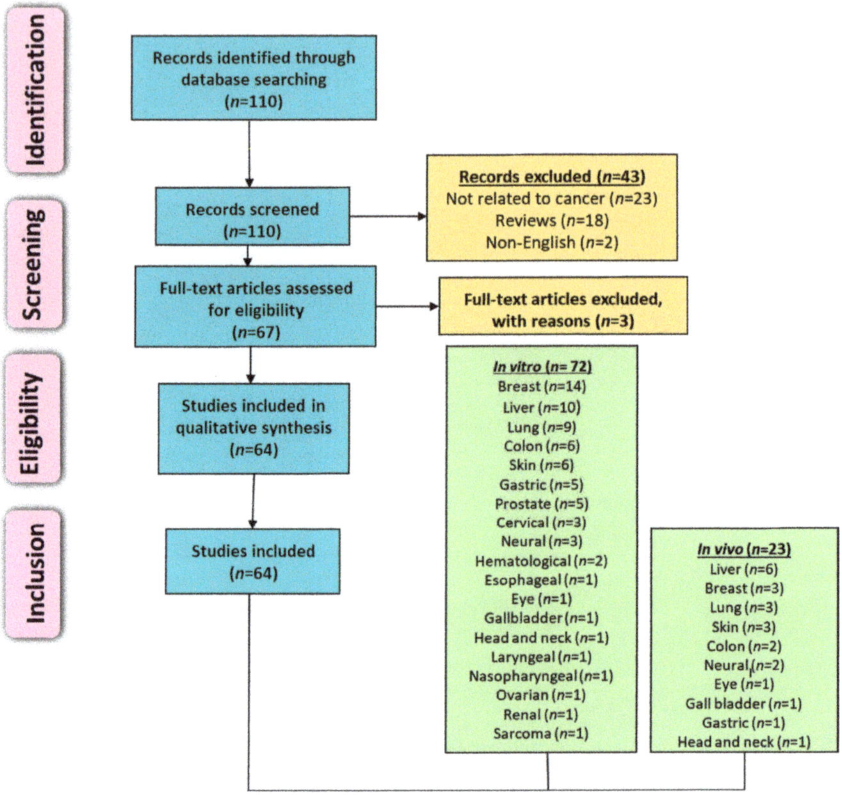

Figure 4. A PRISMA flowchart illustrating the literature search and study selection process relevant to the anticancer potential of *N. nucifera*. The total number of in vitro and in vivo studies 95 is greater than the number of studies included in this work (64) because many publications contained results based on more than one organ-specific cancer or study type (in vitro and in vivo).

3.2. Preclinical Studies (In Vitro and In Vivo)

Potential anticancer effects and mechanisms of action of *N. nucifera*-derived extracts, fractions and pure compounds have been investigated using various cancer cell lines and animal tumor models. Tables 2 and 3 summarize relevant in vitro and in vivo results, respectively.

3.2.1. Breast Cancer

The anticancer properties of various parts of the *N. nucifera* plant have been extensively investigated using different breast cancer cell lines. Karki et al. [78] explored the anticancer properties of the aqueous rhizome extract of *N. nucifera* on the MDA-MB-231 human breast cancer cell line. It was found that the extract inhibited the proliferation and migration of those cells by decreasing the levels of matrix metalloproteinase-2 (MMP-2) and MMP-9 (Table 2). Yang et al. [79] treated MCF-7 human breast cancer cells with flavonoid-rich aqueous *N. nucifera* extract (NLE) and found that it inhibited the proliferation of MCF-7 cells by arresting them in the G0/G1 phase of the cell cycle. Mechanistically, NLE induced p53 phosphorylation (p-p53), increased levels of cyclin-dependent kinase inhibitory proteins, such as p21, p27, and p16, downregulated cyclin expressions, and decreased levels of cyclin D1/cyclin-dependent kinase 4 (CDK4) and cyclin E/CDK2 complexes which led to the upregulation of Rb/E2F pathway and ultimately resulted in a G1 phase arrest. Another important observation was the NLE-mediated inactivation of fatty acid synthase (Fas). Quantitative HPLC analysis revealed gallic acid as the most abundant flavonoid within the extracts, followed by rutin. In a follow-up study, the same research group [80] treated MDA-MB-231 human breast cancer cells with the aqueous leaf extract used in the previous study (NLE) to determine its anticancer effect. NLE treatment reduced cell viability, migratory and invasive properties by decreasing the levels of phosphorylated forms of extracellular signal-regulated kinase (p-ERK), phosphoinositide-3-kinase (p-PI3K), protein kinase B (p-Akt) as well as rat sarcoma gene (RAS) and mitogen-activated extracellular signal-regulated kinase (MEK). In addition, NLE inhibited angiogenesis by downregulating the expression of connective tissue growth factor (CTGF), MMP-2, vascular endothelial growth factor (VEGF) and nuclear factor-κB (NF-κB) p65, while increasing levels of tissue inhibitor of metalloproteinase-2 (TIMP-2). In an extension of previous studies, Wu et al. [81] observed that NLE and *N. nucifera* leaf polyphenol extract (NLPE) reduced cell viability and suppressed cell proliferation in 4T-1 breast cancer cells and exhibited anti-invasive and antimigratory effects in MDA-MB-231 and 4T-1 cells. These effects occurred mechanistically through increasing apoptosis, decreasing levels of Ras homolog family member A (RhoA), Ras-related C3 botulinum toxin substrate 1 (Rac1), cyclin-dependent kinase 42 (Cdc42) and suppressing activation of ERK1/2, p38 MAPK. Additionally, NLE and NLPE reduced the expression of protein kinase Cα (PKCα) in 4T-1 cells. Arjun et al. [82] used methanol and acetone leaf extracts of *N. nucifera* to investigate their anticancer effects on MCF-7 human breast cancer cells. Although both leaf extracts inhibited proliferation and reduced viability of human breast cancer cells, the methanol extract produced the maximum inhibitory effect. However, the underlying mechanism of action of these effects has not been reported.

In addition to the leaf, other parts of the *N. nucifera* plant have also been studied for their anticancer activities. For example, *N. nucifera* flower receptacles have been investigated by Krubha and Vasan [83]. A methanolic extract from *N. nucifera* floral receptacles has shown antiproliferative and cytotoxic activities against MCF-7 human breast cancer cells by increasing antioxidant activity as demonstrated by 2,2-diphenyl-1-picrylhydrazyl radical scavenging assay.

Various researchers used pure compounds isolated from the *N. nucifera* plant to investigate their anticancer properties against breast cancer in vitro. In one study, MDA-MB-231 human breast cancer cells were treated with isoliensinine, liensinine and neferine. Although all three compounds exhibited antiproliferative effects, isoliensinine was found to be the most potent phytochemical. Isoliensinine induced cell cycle arrest at the G1 phase, which possibly occurred by downregulating cyclins and upregulating a cyclin-dependent kinase inhibitor, p21. In addition, isoliensinine also induced cell death by inducing apoptosis mediated by induction of reactive oxygen species (ROS) and alterations of Bcl-associated X protein (Bax), B cell lymphoma 2 (Bcl-2), caspase-3, and poly (ADP-ribose) polymerase-1 (PARP-1). Finally, isoliensinine activated both p38 MAPK and c-Jun N-terminal kinase (JNK) signaling, contributing to apoptosis induction [84].

The anticancer effects of neferine, another bisbenzylisoquinline alkaloid found abundantly in the *N. nucifera* plant, have been investigated by many researchers. Yang et al. [85] reported that neferine decreased MCF-7 cell viability; however, a combination treatment of neferine and dehydroepiandrosterone (DHEA), an endogenous steroid hormone, exerted a greater growth-inhibitory effect. Neferine enhanced the anticancer effect of DHEA to induce apoptosis mediated by increased levels of pro-apoptotic factors, such as caspase-3, caspase-8, caspase-9, Bax, p53, p21, transcription factor E2F1, Fas, Fas ligand (FasL), and decreased levels of antiapoptotic factors, such as Bcl-2, B-cell lymphoma-extra-large (Bcl-xL), human inhibitor of apoptosis protein-1 (HIAP-1), HIAP-2, and survivin. From the green seed embryos of *N. nucifera*, Kadioglu et al. [86] isolated neferine and compared its anticancer effect against taxol- and doxorubicin-resistant as well as sensitive MCF-7 cells. Neferine induced cytotoxicity of multidrug-resistant MCF-7 cells to a greater extent compared to the effect on sensitive cell lines by increasing rhodamine 123 (R123) uptake and inhibiting P-glycoprotein (P-gp). In a follow-up study, Law et al. [87] also reported that neferine induced cytotoxicity in drug-resistant and -sensitive MCF-7 cells. Interestingly, autophagic cell death occurred in apoptosis-resistant cells via green fluorescent protein

(GFP)-light-chain 3 (LC3) puncta formation and ryanodine receptor (Ryr) activation, which subsequently activated the calcium-dependent kinase (caMKKβ), leading to the activation of the 5′-adenosine monophosphate-activated protein kinase (AMPK)-mammalian target of rapamycin (mTOR) signaling pathway. In another study, Liu et al. [88] investigated the anticancer effects of neferine on MDA-MB-231 human breast cancer cells. Neferine significantly reduced cell proliferation, migration and invasion as well as increased apoptosis via regulation of the expression of miR-374a and fibroblast growth factor receptor 2. Neferine also suppressed the activation of PI3K, Akt, MEK, and ERK signaling pathways.

Similar to neferine, liensinine and nuciferine are two other active bisbenzylisoquinoline alkaloids found in the *N. nucifera* plant. Kang et al. [89] treated MCF-7 and MDA-MB-231 breast cancer cells with liensinine and nuciferine to investigate their anticancer properties. Liensinine and nuciferine both decreased cell viability and inhibited cell proliferation via apoptosis induction and cell cycle arrest in a concentration-dependent manner. Apoptosis was mediated by a mitochondrial-dependent pathway by decreasing Bcl-2/Bax ratio, activating caspase-3, and activating caspase-mediated PARP cleavage. Liensinine was found to be more potent in inhibiting proliferation, invasion and migration in both cell lines compared to nuciferine. In addition, both compounds inhibited osteoclast differentiation and bone resorption by blocking the receptor activator of NF-κB ligand and decreasing the secretion of cathepsin K and MMP-9. Additionally, the anticancer effects of liensinine have been studied by Zhou et al. [90], and the mechanistic results are rather unique. It was determined that treatment of MDA-MB-231 and MCF-7 human breast cancer cells with liensinine reduced the viability of these cells. Mechanistically, liensinine inhibited autophagy and induced the accumulation of autophagosomes and lysosomes by inhibiting their fusion via the recruitment of Ras-related protein Rab-7a (RAB7A) to lysosomes. This inhibition of autophagy/mitophagy by liensinine led to the sensitization of doxorubicin-induced cell death of breast cancer cells via increased dynamin-1-like protein (DNM1L) dephosphorylation and translocation to mitochondria and increased mitochondrial fission.

Very recently, Huang et al. [91] isolated three new pairs of benzyltetrahydroisoquinoline alkaloid epimers, seco-neferine A-F, from an ethanolic extract of plumula nelumbinis, a commonly used health food and traditional Chinese medicine. All six compounds were tested against MDA-MB-231 human breast cancer cells, and seco-neferine F displayed a maximum but moderate cytotoxic effect. The mechanisms behind the observed anti-breast cancer effect have not been explored.

There are at least three studies that investigated the anticancer potential of *N. nucifera* using in vivo breast cancer models. In addition to the in vitro studies presented earlier, Yang et al. [79] evaluated the effects of NLE on nude mice with an MCF-7 tumor xenograft and found that it effectively reduced tumor volume and tumor weight. Mechanistically, it was demonstrated that NLE can suppress intratumor expression of human epidermal growth factor receptor 2 (HER2), phospho-HER2 (p-HER2), and Fas (Table 3). Chang et al. [80] studied the effects of NLE in female C57BL/6 nude mice xenografted with MDA-MB-231 cells treated with various concentrations of NLE (0.5, 1, and 2%). There was a significant reduction of tumor size in animals receiving NLE-treated cells compared to control. Immunohistochemical staining of tumor tissue with CD31 antibody revealed NLE-mediated inhibition of angiogenesis as demonstrated by CD31. However, mechanisms of action of the observed antitumor and antiangiogenic effects were not studied in vivo. In addition to the in vitro experiment presented earlier, Zhou et al. [90] further performed in vivo studies to replicate the effects of liensinine on the autophagy of breast cancer cells. In this study, 5–7-week-old female nude mice were inoculated with MDA-MB-231 cells and treated with either liensinine (60 mg/kg) or doxorubicin (2 mg/kg) alone or a combination of both. It was determined that the combination treatment of liensinine and doxorubicin significantly reduced tumor growth. Mechanistically, liensinine suppressed autophagy/mitophagy, increased mitochondrial translocation of DNM1L, and increased the colocalization of DNM1L and translocase of outer mitochondrial membrane 20 (TOMM20).

All of these mechanisms led to the sensitization of doxorubicin-induced cell death via the promotion of DNM1L-mediated mitochondrial fission.

3.2.2. Cervical Cancer

N. nucifera's anticancer effect on cervical cancer has gained recent research interest. Currently, there are at least three studies that have explored this area. Maneenet et al. [67] reported a considerable cytotoxic activity of an ethanolic extract of *N. nucifera* petals against HeLa human cervical cancer cells with a preferential cytotoxicity (PC_{50}) of 10.9 μM. Phytochemical characterization of the extract revealed the presence of nine benzylisoquinoline alkaloids which exhibited significant antiausterity activity against HeLa cells. One compound, namely (−)-lirinindine, showed the greatest cytotoxicity as evidenced by cell shrinkage, plasma blebbing, and ultimately total cell death within 10 h. Mechanistically, the cytotoxic effect was achieved via induction of apoptosis, activation of caspase-3, decreased levels of Bcl-2, and downregulation of the Akt/mTOR pathway. Li et al. [92] studied the anticancer effects of liensinine on Caski, C33A, HeLa, and SiHa human cervical cancer cells. The alkaloid inhibited the proliferation of all cervical cancer cells and suppressed the colony formation of C33A and HeLa cells. A mechanistic study indicated that liensinine registered cell cycle arrest at the G0/G1 phase, increased apoptosis, elevated the levels of caspase-9 and p21 and decreased the expression of Mcl-1, CDK2, p-Akt, and GSK3α. Dasari et al. [93] focused on researching the effects of neferine on HeLa and SiHa cervical cancer cells. Treatment with various concentrations of neferine suppressed viability, induced cytotoxicity, and reduced migration in a concentration-dependent manner. Neferine induced apoptosis by promoting excess ROS formation, increasing oxidative damage, activating the expression of a DNA damage response marker (pH2AX) and upregulating the levels of pro-apoptotic markers, such as cytochrome c, Bax, cleaved caspase-3, caspase-9 and cleaved PARP1, while downregulating anti-apoptotic factors, such as Bcl-2, translational controlled tumor protein (TCTP), procaspase-3, and procaspase-9. Neferine was also shown to induce autophagy by promoting the conversion of LC3 protein from LC3-I to LC3-II and by increasing the formation of autophagosomes which was determined by an increase in autophagy factors, such as Beclin1, atg-4, atg-5, and atg-12. Migration of the cancer cells was also reduced due to cell cycle arrest at the G1/G0 phase of the cell cycle.

3.2.3. Colon Cancer

To investigate the anticancer properties of an ethanol crude extract from the stamen (a part of a flower) of Ba lotus (*N. nucifera*), Zhao et al. [94]) incubated HCT-166 human colon carcinoma cells with the extract. The test material showed an antiproliferative effect by inducing apoptosis mediated by downregulation of Bcl-2, Bcl-xL, inducible nitric oxide synthase (iNOS), cyclooxygenase-2 (COX-2), NF-κB, and upregulation of caspase-3, caspase-8, caspase-9, Fas, FasL, tumor necrosis factor-related apoptosis-inducing ligand (TRAIL), death receptor 4 (DR4), death receptor 5 (DR5), and IκBα. Additionally, the extract reduced matrix degradation and metastasis by increasing the expression of TIMP-1 and TIMP-2, which inhibited the activation of MMP-2 and MMP-9. Kadioglu et al. [86] evaluated the effect of neferine against HCT-8 human colon cancer cells. Neferine reduced cell viability by inhibiting P-gp and increasing the uptake of R123, a substrate of P-gp. Manogaran et al. [95] studied the effect of neferine and isoliensinine on HCT-15 human colon cancer cells and found that each alkaloid reduced cell viability. The underlying mechanisms for the anticancer effects of these compounds included the induction of apoptosis by increasing levels of ROS, membrane permeability, Bax, caspase-3, caspase-9, cleaved PARP, intracellular calcium, and decreasing the mitochondrial membrane potential (ΔψM) and expression of Bcl-2. In addition, Western blot analysis showed that both compounds induced the activation of the MAPK pathway and increased the protein expression of p38. Qi et al. [96] treated HT29 and HCT116 human colon cancer cells and CT26 murine undifferentiated colon carcinoma cells with nuciferine. They found that the alkaloid reduced cell viability, inhibited cell proliferation and suppressed cell invasion. In CT26 cells, nuciferine also decreased the expression of PI3K, interleukin-1β (IL-1β), and p-Akt. In another study, liensinine, extracted from the seed embryo of *N. nucifera,* suppressed cell proliferation in HT29 and DLD-1 human colorectal cancer cells. Mechanistic studies revealed that liensinine increased apoptosis, expression levels of cleaved caspase-3, cleaved PARP, cell cycle arrest in the second growth and mitosis (G2/M) phase, phosphorylated CDK1 1 (p-CDK1), cyclin A2, phosphorylated JNK (p-JNK), and Bax, and decreased Bcl-2 and Bcl-xL [97]. Guon and Chung [98] isolated two flavonol glycosides, namely hyperoside and rutin, from the roots of *N. nucifera* and determined their anticancer properties using HT29 human colorectal cancer cells. The two flavonols exhibited cytotoxicity, reduced cell viability, and inhibited cell proliferation via increased apoptosis. The observed apoptosis-inducing activity was mediated by increased Bax, caspase-3, caspase-8, and caspase-9 levels, an elevated Bax/Bcl-2 ratio, and a decreased level of Bcl-2.

Qi et al. [96] observed the anticancer properties of nuciferine through an in vivo approach in addition to the in vitro studies mentioned previously. Nude mice were subcutaneously implanted with CT29 cells and injected with 9.5 mg/kg nuciferine 3 times a week for 3 weeks immediately following tumor cell implantation or when tumor xenografts reached a size of 100 mm^3. The alkaloid resulted in reduced tumor weights in both the treatment groups compared to the control. However, the antitumor mechanisms were not explored in vivo. Wang et al. [97] also investigated the anticancer properties of liensinine in vivo by feeding it to 6–8-week-old female BALB/c nude mice injected with HT29 human colorectal cancer cells. Liensinine suppressed colorectal tumorigenesis and reduced tumor volume by decreasing cell proliferation and the expression of Ki-67.

3.2.4. Esophageal Cancer

There has been a limited amount of research investigating the anticancer properties of *N. nucifera* in esophageal cancer. An et al. [99] treated KYSE30, KYSE150, and KYSE510 human esophageal squamous cell carcinoma cells with neferine. They found that the alkaloid suppressed cell proliferation in all three cell lines and suppressed colony formation of KYSE30 and KYSE150 cells. The mechanistic studies revealed that neferine induced apoptosis, arrested cells at the G2/M, triggered the accumulation of ROS, increased the expression of cleaved PARP, cleaved caspase-3, cleaved caspase-9, p21, p-JNK, and decreased the expression of Bcl-2, cyclin B1, and Nrf2.

3.2.5. Eye Cancer

There is at least one report of the *N. nucifera* alkaloid neferine on retinoblastoma, a common primary intraocular childhood and infant malignancy. Wang et al. [100] observed that neferine inhibited the proliferation and viability of the WERI-Rb-1 human retinoblastoma cell line associated with reduced protein expression of Ki-67 and Survivin. Neferine treatment reduced microtubule-like structure formation, the number of nodes/high power field, and VEGF protein levels, demonstrating its anti-invasive capability. The results also suggested that neferine caused mitochondrial dysfunction in retinoblastoma cells through decreased SOD and GSH levels, increased MDA content, and apoptosis through down-regulation of Bcl-2 and c-Myc, upregulation of Bax expression and cleavage of caspase-3 and caspase-9.

In addition to the in vitro study, Wang et al. [100] investigated the anticancer effects of neferine using an in vivo retinoblastoma model. WERI-Rb-1 cells were subcutaneously injected in female athymic nude mice, and the tumor-bearing animals were treated with 0.5–2 mg/kg of neferine every 3 days for 30 days. Results showed a decrease in tumor volume and weight mechanistically through reduced expression of Ki-67 and VEGF, decreased SOD activity, and increased MDA content.

3.2.6. Gallbladder Cancer

The anticancer effects of *N. nucifera* have not been thoroughly investigated in regard to gallbladder cancer. There is only one study by Shen et al. [101] that explored the effects of liensinine on GBC-SD and NOZ human gallbladder carcinoma cells. Treatment with various concentrations of liensinine inhibited proliferation and suppressed cancer cell growth by inducing apoptosis and arresting the cells in the G2/M phase of the cell cycle. Western blot analysis evidenced an upregulation of cleaved caspase-3, caspase-9, PARP and Bax alongside th downregulation of Bcl-2, cyclin B1, CDK1, CDC25C, zinc finger X-chromosomal protein (ZFX), PI3K and p-Akt.

Shen et al. (2019) also performed an in vivo study on BALB/c nude mice which were injected with NOZ cells. The tumor-bearing mice were treated with 2 mg/kg of liensinine intraperitoneally. Liensinine was found to reduce tumor volume and weight with a parallel decrease in intratumor Ki-67 expression.

3.2.7. Gastric Cancer

MFC human gastric cancer cells were treated with water-soluble polysaccharides extracted from *N. nucifera* seeds, and the results showed inhibition of cell proliferation [102]. However, the underlying mechanism of action was not reported. Huang et al. [103] investigated neferine's involvement in the reversal of adriamycin (ADM) resistance in SGC7901/ADM human gastric cancer cells. It has been found that the combined treatment of hyperthermia and neferine can reverse the multidrug resistance of ADM in human gastric cancer cells by increasing cell membrane fluidity, accelerating the passive ADM permeation, and decreasing P-gp expression and the levels of multidrug resistance 1 (MDR-1) mRNA. Xue et al. [104] treated GIST-1 human gastrointestinal stromal tumor cells and SGC7901 human gastric cancer cells with neferine. In the GIST-1 cell line, neferine inhibited cell viability, proliferation, and migration. The anticancer mechanism involved the induction of apoptosis, increased expression of p15, p16, p21, Bax, cleaved caspase-3, cleaved caspase-9, microRNA-449a (miR-449a), and decreased expression of cyclin D1, Bcl-2, MMP-2, MMP-9, p-PI3K, p-Akt, Notch1, Notch2, and Notch3. In the SGC7901 cell line, neferine suppressed cell migration through increasing apoptosis and the protein expressions of Bax, cleaved caspase-3, cleaved caspase-9, and miR-449a. The alkaloid also downregulated Bcl-2, MMP-2, and MMP-9 in the SGC7901 cell line. In another study, various concentrations of 7-hydroxydehydronuciferine, a compound isolated from a methanolic extract of the leaves of *N. nucifera* Gaertn. cv. *Rosa-plena*, inhibited the proliferation of AGS human gastric cancer cells possibly by antioxidant activity [105]. Yang et al. [106] studied the effect of liensinine, an alkaloid extracted from the seeds of *N. nucifera* Gaertn., using BGC823 and SGC7901 human gastric cancer cells. Liensinine inhibited cell proliferation by increasing apoptosis, the expression of cleaved caspase-3, cleaved caspase-9, cleaved PARP, Bax, and ROS, and decreasing the expression of p-Akt and Bcl-2. The alkaloid also increased G0/G1 cell arrest and decreased levels of cyclin D1 and CDK4.

One in vivo study has been conducted regarding the anticancer effects of liensinine in gastric cancer. Yang et al. [106] tested BALB/c homozygous nude mice, xenografted with SGC7901 human gastric cancer cells, by injecting them with liensinine every two days for a month. Liensinine showed anticancer properties by reducing tumorigenesis and inhibiting cell proliferation. Mechanistic studies based on immunohistochemical analysis of tumor tissues revealed that liensinine decreased the expression of Ki-67, a marker for cell proliferation.

3.2.8. Head and Neck Cancers

Neferine's effects on mitigating head and neck cancer have been recently explored by Zhu et al. [107]. In this in vitro study, neferine reduced viability, inhibited proliferation and suppressed migration in 3 different head and neck cancer cell lines, namely HN6 and CAL27 tongue squamous cell carcinoma and HN30 pharyngeal squamous cell carcinoma. Neferine was found to trigger apoptosis and autophagy as well as increase the levels of ROS in the HN30 and Cal 20 cells. Neferine also led to the activation of the apoptosis signal-regulating kinase 1 (ASK1)/JNK pathway, leading to apoptosis. In addition, neferine induced autophagy by promoting the generation of autophagosomes, while inhibiting autophagic influx. This was observed by an increased conversion of LC3-I to LC3-II and the accumulation of p62.

In the in vivo study, CAL27 cells were injected in 5-week-old male BALB/c nude mice, which were then treated with 10 mg/kg neferine. Neferine reduced tumor volumes by increasing apoptosis and pro-apoptotic factors, such as cleaved caspase-2 and cleaved PARP. In addition, an increase in autophagy was observed, as evidenced by an increase in the conversion of LC3-I to LC3-II conversion and p62 levels [107].

3.2.9. Hematological Cancers

Limited information is available on the anticancer effect of *N. nucifera* in hematological cancers. One study used a pure compound, kaempferol, which was isolated from a methanolic extract of *N. nucifera* stamens. It has been found that kaempferol was not cytotoxic to KU812F cells, a human basophilic cell line derived from chronic myelocytic leukemia. However, kaempferol suppressed the expression of FcεR1 on the cell surface, decreased the mRNA levels of FcεR1 α- and γ-chains, reduced intracellular Ca^{2+} concentration, and diminished FcεR1-mediated histamine release in KU812F cells [108]. In a separate study, Qin and co-workers [109] experimented with neferine as a possible treatment for multi-drug resistant leukemia. They tested neferine's effect against imatinib-resistant K562/G01 human myelogenous leukemia cells. It was found that neferine, at high concentrations of 16 μM or greater, reduced cell survival rate in a concentration-dependent manner. Lower concentrations of neferine did not show any effects on cell survival. Further experimentation revealed that neferine could reverse imatinib resistance and increase its concentrations in STI571-resistant K562/G01 cells by downregulating the expression of P-gp and *MDR-1* mRNA.

3.2.10. Laryngeal Cancer

Tripartite motif-containing 44 (TRIM44) was found to be upregulated in 4 human laryngeal squamous cell carcinoma (LSCC) cell lines (AMC-HN-8, HEP-2, TU-212, and TU-686), and the knockdown of TRIM44 led to suppressed cell growth. In a recent study, 2 of these cell lines, AMC-HN-8 and TU-212, were treated with nuciferine for 24 h. Nuciferine inhibited cell survival by reducing TRIM44 expression, which led to decreased levels of Toll-like receptor 4 (TLR4) and the suppression of Akt signaling. However, with the use of a TRIM44-overexpressing plasmid transfected into LSCC cells, it was found that the overexpression of TRIM44 offset the anticancer properties of nuciferine [110].

3.2.11. Liver Cancer

Zheng et al. [102] treated HuH-7 human liver cancer and H22 mouse hepatocarcinoma cells with water-soluble polysaccharides extracted from *N. nucifera* seeds for 48 h, and the results showed inhibition of cell proliferation with no reported underlying mechanism of action. An ethanolic extract of the seedpod of *N. nucifera* showed antiproliferative and cytotoxic properties in HepG2 human liver cancer cells via antioxidant activity as demonstrated by the inhibition of the peroxidation of linoleic acid. Phytochemical analysis revealed the presence of pure compounds, such as catechin, kaempferol, quercetin, and hyperoside, in the seed extract [111]. Duan et al. [112] investigated the anticancer effects of procyanidins found in the water-acetone extract from the seed pods of *N. nucifera*. It was found that the procyanidins decreased viability, caused DNA damage and S phase cell cycle arrest, and induced autophagy of HepG2 cells by decreasing the mitochondrial membrane potential and increasing the levels of LC3, GFP-LC3, and ROS.

Multiple studies investigated the anti-liver cancer properties of neferine, an alkaloid isolated from *N. nucifera*. In one study, Xiao-Hong et al. [113] found that neferine reversed the thermotolerance of HepG2 human hepatocarcinoma cells by increasing apoptosis and downregulating the expression of Bcl-2. Yoon et al. [114] used Hep3B human liver cancer cells and reported that neferine treatment induced growth inhibition and decreased cell viability. The mechanisms associated with these anticancer effects included increased apoptosis, elevated expression of Bim, Bid, Bax, Bak, Puma, caspase-3, caspase-6, caspase-7, caspase-8, and PARP, and decreased expression of CDK4, E2F transcription factor 1 (E2F1), cyclin D1, cyclin D3, and cellular myelocytomatosis (c-Myc) oncogene. In another study, neferine reduced cell viability and induced ROS-mediated apoptosis in HepG2 human liver cancer cells. Additionally, the alkaloid increased the protein expression of Bax, Bad, cleaved caspase-3, caspase-9, PARP, tumor necrosis factor-α (TNF-α), and decreased Bcl-2. Finally, neferine increased the levels of phosphatase and tensin homolog (PTEN), p53, p38, ERK1/2, MAPK, and decreased p-Akt [115]. Deng et al. [116] also used HepG2 human liver cancer cells and found that neferine exhibited cytotoxicity and suppressed cell migration and invasion by increasing apoptosis and protein expression of E-cadherin and decreasing the expression of vimentin, snail, and N-cadherin. When both HepG2 and Hep3B human liver cancer cell lines were treated with neferine, Law et al. [87] ascertained that the alkaloid induced autophagy and displayed cytotoxicity by activating various signaling cascades, such as Unc-51-like autophagy activating kinase-1-protein kinase RNA-like ER kinase (Ulk-1-PERK) and AMPK-mTOR and increasing the amount of intracellular calcium via Ryr activation.

Two studies examined the anticancer effects of isoliensinine, an alkaloid derived from *N. nucifera* embryos, on hepatocellular cancer in vitro. Shu et al. [117] treated Hep2G, Huh-7 and H22 hepatocellular carcinoma cells with various concentrations of isoliensinine and found that it suppressed proliferation and induced apoptosis through a decrease in NF-κB activity in HCC cells, as well as through decreased phosphorylation of the NF-κB p65 subunit. The researchers also observed a decrease in NF-κB target proteins, such as Bcl-2, Bcl-xL and MMP-9, and an increase in caspase-3. In an extension of the previous study, Shu et al. [118] observed that isoliensinine suppressed NF-κB in liver cancer cells through impairing protein phosphatase 2A (PP2A)/inhibitor of PP2A (I2PP2A) interaction and stimulating PP2A-dependent p65 dephosphorylation at serine536.

Several studies have also explored the anticancer properties of *N. nucifera* using in vivo liver cancer models. In one such study, H22 human hepatocellular carcinoma cells were inoculated in 6–8-week-old female Kunming mice. After 24 h, the animals were treated with water-soluble polysaccharides from the seeds of *N. nucifera* (LSPS). After 14 days of LSPS treatment, reduced tumorigenesis was observed, as there was a significant decrease in tumor weight. Mechanistic studies revealed reduced malondialdehyde (MDA) levels in the liver, increased superoxide dismutase (SOD) activity, and an increased spleen and thymus index. In addition, there were increased levels of TNF-α and IL-2 [102]. In another study, Horng et al. [119] included 0.5–2.0% of an aqueous NLE, containing phenolic compounds such as gallic acid, catechin, peltatoside, rutin, isoquercitrin, miquelianin, and astragalin, in the diet of male Sprague-Dawley rats with hepatic carcinoma induced by diethylnitrosamine (DEN) via drinking water. By the assessment of a histopathologist, the group of rats fed DEN+2.0% NLE showed a reduction of liver carcinomas by 30% compared to the control group (DEN-fed rats). Furthermore, NLE reduced tumor size, decreased hepatocellular damage and reduced the number of glutathione S-transferase pi (GSTπ)-positive cells. Additional studies showed that NLE elicited an antioxidant effect as characterized by decreased lipid peroxidation, increased glutathione (GSH), glutathione peroxidase (GPx), SOD and catalase (CAT) as well as reduced levels of alanine aminotransferase (ALT), aspartate transaminase (AST), and albumin. Finally, NLE decreased the expression of Ras-related C3 botulinum toxin substrate 1 (Rac1), PKCα, GST, TNF-α, and IL-6. Yang et al. [120] also used dietary NLE to determine its anticancer properties in 4–5-week-old Wistar rats with 2-acetylaminofluorene (2-AAF)-induced hepatocarcinogenesis. After six months of treatment, 0.5–2% NLE was found to reduce 2-AAF-induced hepatic fibrosis (appears during the development of premalignant lesions) compared to the control (2-AAF-treatment-only rats), lower hepatic fibrosis, reduce liver weight, and enhance antioxidative potential by decreasing lipid peroxidation, levels of triglycerides, total cholesterol, α-fetoprotein (AFP), IL-6, TNF-α, AST, ALT, γ-glutamyl transferase (γGT), GSTπ, and 8-hydroxy-2′-deoxyguanosine (8-OHdG). NLE also led to increased levels of nuclear factor erythroid 2-related factor 2 (Nrf2), CAT, GPx, and SOD-1. Deng et al. [116] injected

HepG2 and Bel-7402 human hepatocellular carcinoma cells into 4-week-old male BALB/c mice and treated them with oxaliplatin (a drug used for the treatment for hepatocellular carcinoma) in the presence or absence of neferine. Neferine potentiated the tumor volume-reducing activity of oxaliplatin by depressing cell proliferation based on Ki-67 expression. The combination of oxaliplatin and neferine increased the expression of E-cadherin and decreased the expression of vimentin compared to oxaliplatin treatment alone.

There were two similarly designed studies in which the antineoplastic effects of isoliensinine were studied in vivo. H22 hepatocellular cancer cells were inoculated in male Kunming mice, and athymic male nude mice were injected with Huh-7 cells. The Kunming mice were split into 3 groups and treated with 3 or 10 mg/kg/day isoliensinine for 10 days, intraperitoneally or by gavage, or with normal saline. Athymic nude mice were also treated with isoliensinine, intraperitoneally, at a dose of 3 or 10 mg/kg/day for 3 weeks. In both models, isoliensinine showed reduced tumor growth through the apoptosis of tumor cells mediated by increased caspase-3 activity, decreased levels of Bcl-2, Bcl-xL, and MMP-9, and decreased NF-κB p65 phosphorylation [117]. In a follow-up study, the same research group [118] found that oral administration of isoliensinine at 10 mg/kg once daily for 10 days reduced tumor growth in Huh-7 xenograft model containing I2PP2A via increased caspase-3 activity.

3.2.12. Lung Cancer

There are many studies evaluating the anticancer properties of *N. nucifera* in lung cancer. One study treated A549 and H460 human non-small cell lung cancer cell lines with *N. nucifera* ethanolic seed pod extract and found it to reduce cell proliferation and colony formation. The extract also induced apoptosis through increased cleavage of PARP and increased phosphorylation of H2A histone family member X (γ-H2AX). Additionally, the extract-treated cells showed the ability to reduce the expression of mRNA and protein of Axl in both cell lines, indicating that Axl is a novel therapeutic target of the antiproliferative and proapoptotic activities of *N. nucifera* [121].

Neferine, a major bisbenzyliso-quinoline alkaloid component of *N. nucifera*, has been widely studied for its anticancer effects in lung cancer. Poornima et al. [122] investigated the effects of neferine on A549 human lung adenocarcinoma cells and found that it markedly suppressed cell proliferation in a concentration-dependent fashion. Neferine also induced autophagy as indicated by acidic vesicular accumulation and autophagosome formation measured through the expression of microtubule-associated protein-1 LC3B and conversion of LC3-I to LC3-II. Neferine decreased the expression of PI3K, Akt and mTOR, resulting in the induction of autophagy through mTOR inhibition. Finally, the investigators found that neferine-induced autophagy was mediated through ROS generation and subsequent depletion of intracellular GSH levels. In a subsequent study, the same research group [123] further investigated the effects of neferine on a panel of human lung cancer cells, such A549, H520, H661, and H441. The nontoxic nature of neferine was established in BEAS-2B normal lung cells. The cumulative findings suggested that neferine induced cytotoxicity in all lung cancer cells. In A549 cells, neferine induced apoptosis through inhibition of Bcl-2 expression and increased expression of Bax, Bad, and cytochrome c (cyt c), while the mitochondrial membrane potential was decreased. The mechanism of the observed anticancer effect of neferine was established through upregulation of p53, p27, and PTEN and downregulation of cyclin D1 and NF-κB. Increased ROS production, depletion of cellular antioxidants and activation of JNK, ERK 1/2, and p38 MAPK were also observed.

Kadioglu et al. [86] used neferine to study its cytotoxicity against paclitaxel (an anticancer drug)-resistant and -sensitive A549 cell lines. The study showed that neferine was more cytotoxic to the paclitaxel-resistant cell line. Neferine inhibited P-gp based on increased R123 uptake in the paclitaxel-resistant cell line in a comparable manner to verapamil, a known P-gp inhibitor. These results suggest that neferine has potential as a drug candidate for the treatment of multidrug-resistant cancers, since the overexpression of P-gp is linked to the efflux of chemotherapeutic drugs. Law et al. [87] confirmed the cytotoxic effect of neferine against A549 cells and also observed similar effects on other lung cancer cell lines, such as H1299 and LLC-1. Colony formation in H1299 cells was also inhibited by neferine. Neferine induced autophagy in apoptosis-resistant cell lines (A549 and LLC-1). Neferine also induced GFP-LC3 puncta formation, indicating apoptotic activity via autophagosome formation.

Kalai Selvi et al. [124] found that neferine induced cytotoxicity and enhanced the therapeutic effect of cisplatin through stimulation of non-canonical autophagy and ROS generation in A549 cells. This mechanistic study found that the neferine-cisplatin combination induced autophagy mediated through the hypergeneration of ROS, GSH depletion, and downregulation of the PI3K/Akt/mTOR pathway. In neferine- and cisplatin-treated A549 cells, autophagosome formation was measured through the expression of LC3B and increased conversion of LC3-I to LC3-II. The same research group extended the previous study and showed that neferine potentiated the cytotoxic effects of cisplatin. Combined treatment also exhibited apoptosis induction through sub-G1 cell cycle arrest and increased Bax, Bad, Bak, cyt c, caspase-3, caspase-9, PARP cleavage, and ROS generation. Additionally, the neferine and cisplatin combination downregulated the protein levels of focal adhesion kinase (FAK) and VEGF and suppressed the activity of MMP-2 [125].

Liu et al. [126] investigated the effect of nuciferine, another phytochemical present in *N. nucifera*, against nicotine (an addictive component of tobacco)-induced tumor promotion in A549 cells. Nuciferine was found to inhibit the proliferation of A549 cells in the presence of nicotine and suppressed the migration and invasion of tumor cells in the presence or absence of nicotine. Nicotine-activated Wnt/β-catenin signaling was substantially reduced after treatment with nuciferine, which was achieved by the stabilization and increased expression of Axin, while no change in adenomatous polyposis coli and glycogen synthase kinase-3β in nuciferine-treated cells was observed. Wnt/β-catenin signaling target proteins, such as c-myc, cyclin D, and VEGF-A, showed decreased expression when treated with nuciferine. Qi et al. [96] treated A549 and NCI-H1650 human lung adenocarcinoma cells with nuciferine to determine its anticancer potential. The results showed that nuciferine reduced cell viability and suppressed cell invasion via unknown mechanisms.

There are three in vivo studies that evaluated the anticancer effects of *N. nucifera* on lung cancer. Wu et al. [81] examined the anti-metastatic effects of NLE and NLPE in primary lung tumors developed following orthotopic implantation of 4T-1 cells in BALB/c mice. The researchers observed fewer lung micrometastases in the 1% NLE- and 0.25% NLPE-treated groups compared to control groups. The weight of the lungs of the treated group was also reduced compared to the control groups. Based on immunohistochemical analysis, NLE and NLPE reduced the activation of protein kinase C α in the lung tissue. Liu et al. [126] explored the antitumor effects of nuciferine (50 mg/kg 3 times a week for about 3 weeks) in BALB/c mice injected with A549 tumor cells in the presence or absence of nicotine exposure. The results indicated that nuciferine registered a significant reduction of tumor size and weight in the presence of nicotine. Mechanistic study revealed that nuciferine enhanced apoptosis of tumor cells, upregulated the expression of Bax and Axin, and downregulated the expression of Bcl-2 and β-catenin. Compared to the nicotine control group, the nuciferine-treated groups did not show any reduction in body weight or decline in liver and kidney functions. Sivalingam et al. [127] used diethylnitrosamine (DEN) to induce lung carcinogenesis in albino male Wistar rats. The rats were then treated with 10–20 mg/kg of neferine by oral intubation for 20 alternate days. The investigators found that neferine decreased lung weight and reduced pathological damage in DEN-induced rats. Neferine was shown to reduce oxidative stress in DEN-induced lung carcinogenesis through decreased ROS generation, lipid peroxidation and protein carbonyl production, as well as increased GSH, SOD, GST, and CAT. The DEN-induced increase in glycoproteins in lung tissue was significantly decreased after neferine treatment. Neferine enhanced mitochondrial-mediated apoptosis through a decreased expression of Bcl-2 and increased expression of p53, Bax, caspase-9 and caspase-3. DEN-induced animals exhibited increased inflammatory genes and proteins, such as NF-κB, COX-2, CYP2E1 and VEGF, as well as increased expression of PI3K, Akt and mTOR genes, which were all decreased with neferine treatment.

Table 2. Potential anticancer effects and mechanisms of action of *N. nucifera*-derived constituents based on in vitro studies.

Materials Tested	Cell Lines Used	Conc. (Duratdion)	Anticancer Effects	Mechanisms	References
			Breast cancer		
Aqueous rhizome extract	MDA-MB-231 (human breast cancer)	1–1000 µg/mL (24 h)	Inhibited proliferation and migration	↓MMP-2; ↓MMP-9	Karki et al., 2008 [78]
Flavonoid-rich leaf extract	MCF-7 (human breast cancer)	0.5–3 mg/mL (24 h)	Inhibited proliferation	↑p16; ↑p21; ↑p27; ↓cyclin E; ↓cyclin D1; ↓CDK2; ↓CDK4; cell cycle arrest in G0/G1 phase; ↓cyclin D1/CDK4 complex; ↓cyclin E/CDK2 complex; ↑Rb-E2Fcomplex; ↓Fas	Yang et al., 2011 [79]
Aqueous leaf extract	MDA-MB-231 (human breast cancer)	0.5–5 mg/mL (24 h)	Inhibited angiogenesis; inhibited proliferation; decreased migration rate; reduced cell invasion properties	↓MMP2; ↑TIMP; ↓VEGF, ↓CTGF; ↓VEGFR2; ↓NF-κB p65; ↓PI3K-Akt-ERK; ↓RAS; ↓MEK; ↓ERK; ↓Akt	Chang et al., 2016 [80]
Aqueous and methanol leaf extracts	4T-1 (mouse mammary carcinoma); MDA-MB-231 (human breast cancer)	2–4 mg/mL (24 h)	Reduced cell viability and attenuated migration	↑Apoptosis; ↓RhoA; ↓Rac1; ↓Cdc42; ↓ERK; ↓p38; ↓MAPK	Wu et al., 2017 [81]
Methanol and acetone leaf and flower extracts	MCF-7 (human breast cancer)	6.25–100 µg/mL (24 h)	Inhibited proliferation and reduced viability	Not reported	Arjun et al., 2012 [82]
Methanol floral receptacle extract	MCF-7 (human breast cancer)	200–600 µg/mL (24 h)	Induced cytotoxicity	Antioxidant activity	Krubha & Vasan, 2016 [83]
Isoliensinine, liensinine & neferine	MCF-10A (human breast cancer)	5–20 µM (48 h)	Induced cell death	↑Apoptosis; ↑oxidative stress; ↑p38; ↑MAPK; ↑JNK	Zhang et al., 2015 [84]
Neferine	MCF-7 (human breast cancer)	2–20 mg/mL (48 h)	Inhibited proliferation; reduced cell viability	↑Apoptosis; ↑caspase-3; ↑caspase-8; ↑caspase-9; ↑Bax; ↑p53; ↑p21; ↑E2F1; ↑Fas; ↑FasL; ↓Bcl-2; ↓Bcl-xL; ↓HIAP-1; ↓HIAP-2	Yang et al., 2016 [85]
Neferine	MCF-7 (human breast cancer)	0.039–100 µM (72 h)	Induced cytotoxicity	↑R123 uptake; ↓P-gp	Kadioglu et al., 2017 [86]
Neferine	MCF-7 (human breast cancer)	1–5 µM IC_{50} = 41.1 µM	Induced autophagy	↑Ryr; ↑cytosolic Ca^{2+}; ↑AMPk-mTOR; ↑GFP-LC3 puncta; ↑CXCR-4; ↑p-PERK; ↑PERK; ↑SQSTM; ↑Ulk-1	Law et al., 2019 [87]

Table 2. *Cont.*

Materials Tested	Cell Lines Used	Conc. (Duratdion)	Anticancer Effects	Mechanisms	References
Neferine	MDA-MB-231 (human breast cancer)	2–10 μM (24 h)	Reduced proliferation	↑Apoptosis; ↓miR-374a; ↓PI3K; ↓Akt; ↓MEK; ↓ERK	Liu et al., 2019 [88]
Liensinine and nuciferine	MCF-7; MDA-MB-231 (human breast cancer)	10–60 μM (24 h)	Inhibited proliferation	↑Apoptosis; ↑Bax/Bcl-2; ↑caspase-3	Kang et al., 2017 [89]
Liensinine	MCF-7; MDA-MB-231 (human breast cancer)	20 μM (24 h)	Reduced viability	↓Autophagy; ↓autophagosome-lysosome fusion; ↓recruitment of RAB7A to lysosomes; ↑mitochondrial fission; ↑DNM1L dephosphorylation; ↑DNM1L translocation	Zhou et al., 2015 [90]
Seco-neferine F	MDA-MB-231 (human breast cancer)	IC_{50}: 39 μM (48 h)	Induced cytotoxicity	Not reported	Huang et al., 2021 [91]
			Cervical cancer		
Ethanolic petal extract; (−)-lirinidine	HeLa (human cervical cancer)	PC_{50}: 2–11 μM (24 h)	Displayed antiausterity activities	↑Apoptosis; ↑caspase-3; ↓Bcl-2; ↓p-Akt; ↓p-mTOR	Maneenet et al., 2021 [67]
Isoliensinine	Caski, C33A, HeLa, SiHa (human cervical cancer)	5–25 μM (24 h and 48 h)	Inhibited cell proliferation and colony formation	↑Apoptosis; ↑G0/G1 phase arrest; ↑p21; ↑caspase-9; ↓Mcl-1; ↓CDK2; ↓cyclin E; ↓p-Akt; ↓GSK3α	Li et al., 2022 [92]
Neferine	HeLa, SiHa (human cervical cancer)	5–50 μM (48 h)	Suppressed viability; induced cytotoxicity; reduced migration	↑Apoptosis; ↑Bax; ↑cyt c; ↑cleaved-caspase-3; ↑cleaved-caspase-9; ↑PARP-cleavage; ↓Bcl-2; ↓procaspase-3; ↓procaspase-9; ↓TCTP; ↑beclin-1, ↑atg-4, ↑atg-5; ↑atg-12; ↑LC-3 activation; ↑P62/SQSTM1; ↑G1-G0 phase arrest; ↑ROS	Dasari et al., 2019 [93]
			Colon cancer		
Ethanolic stamen extract	HCT-116 (human colon cancer)	100–400 μg/mL (24 h)	Showed cytotoxic activity	↑Apoptosis; ↑Fas; ↑FasL; ↑TRAIL; ↑DR4; ↑DR5; ↑caspase-3, ↑caspase-8; ↑caspase-9; ↑Bax; ↓Bcl-2; ↓Bcl-xL; ↓MMP-2; ↓MMP-9; ↑TIMP-1; ↑TIMP-2; ↓iNOS; ↓COX-2; ↓NF-κB; ↑IκBα	Zhao et al., 2017 [94]

Table 2. *Cont.*

Materials Tested	Cell Lines Used	Conc. (Duratdion)	Anticancer Effects	Mechanisms	References
Neferine	HCT-8 (human colon cancer)	0.039–100 μM (72 h)	Reduced cell viability	↑R123 uptake; ↓P-gp	Kadioglu et al., 2017 [86]
Neferine; isoliensinine	HCT-15 (human colon cancer)	2–12 μM (24 h)	Showed cytotoxicity	↑Apoptosis; ↑ROS; ↑p38; ↑MAPK; ↑Bax; ↑caspase-9; ↑caspase-3; ↑cleaved PARP; ↑membrane permeability; ↓Bcl2; ↑[Ca^{2+}]; ↓ΔΨM	Manogaran et al., 2019 [95]
Nuciferine	CT26 (murine colon carcinoma); HT29 and HCT116 (human colon cancer)	0.05–1.0 mg/mL (24 h)	Reduced cell viability and inhibited cell invasion	↓PI3K; ↓IL1B; ↓p-Akt (CT26 cells only)	Qi et al., 2016 [96]
Liensinine	HT29, DLD-1 (human colorectal cancer)	5–20 μM (24–48 h)	Suppressed cell proliferation	↑Apoptosis; ↑cleaved caspase-3; ↑cleaved PARP; ↑G2/M cell arrest; ↑p-CDK1; ↑cyclin A2; ↑p-JNK; ↑Bax; ↓Bcl-2; ↓Bcl-xL	Wang et al., 2018 [97]
Hyperoxide; rutin	HT29 (human colorectal cancer)	100–200 μM (24 h)	Exhibited cytotoxicity, reduced cell viability and inhibited cell proliferation	↑Apoptosis; ↑Bax; ↓Bcl-2; ↑Bax/Bcl-2 ratio; ↑caspase-3; ↑caspase-8; ↑caspase-9	Guon and Chung, 2016 [98]
			Esophageal cancer		
Neferine	KYSE30, KYSE150 and KYSE510 (human esophageal squamous cell carcinoma)	5–30 μM (24–48 h)	Suppressed cell proliferation and colony formation	↑Apoptosis; ↑G2/M arrest; ↑cleaved PARP; ↑cleaved caspase-3; ↑cleaved caspase-9; ↑p21; ↓cyclin B1; ↓Bcl-2; ↑ROS; ↑p-JNK; ↓Nrf2	An et al., 2020 [99]
			Eye cancer		
Neferine	WERI-Rb-1 (human retinoblastoma)	0.1 to 200 μM (24 h)	Inhibited cell proliferation, migration, and viability	↓Ki-67; ↓Survivin; ↓microtubule-like structures; ↓nodes/HPF; ↓VEGF; ↓SOD; ↓GSH; ↑MDA; ↓Bcl-2; ↓c-myc; ↑Bax; ↑cleaved caspase-3; ↑cleaved caspase-9	Wang et al. 2020 [100]
			Gallbladder cancer		
Liensinine	GBC-SD and NOZ (human gallbladder carcinoma)	40–120 μM (24 and 48 h)	Inhibited proliferation and suppressed colony formation	↑Apoptosis; ↑G2/M phase arrest; ↓cyclin B1; ↓CDK1; ↓CDC25C; ↑cleaved-caspase 3; ↑cleaved-caspase 9; ↑cleaved-PARP; ↑Bax; ↓Bcl-2; ↓PI3K; ↓ZFX; ↓p-Akt	Shen et al., 2019 [101]

Table 2. *Cont.*

Materials Tested	Cell Lines Used	Conc. (Duratdion)	Anticancer Effects	Mechanisms	References
			Gastric cancer		
Water-soluble polysaccharides from seeds	MFC (human gastric cancer)	50–200 μg/mL (48 h)	Showed growth inhibition	Not reported	Zheng et al., 2016 [102]
Neferine	Adriamycin resistant SGC7901/ADM (human gastric cancer)	2.5–40 μg/mL (24 h)	Exerted cytotoxicity and reversed drug resistance	↓P-gp expression; ↓*MDR-1* mRNA	Huang et al., 2011 [103]
Neferine	GIST-1 (human gastrointestinal stromal tumor)	1–10 μM (24 h)	Inhibited cell viability, proliferation and migration	↑Apoptosis; ↑p15; ↑p16; ↑p21; ↓cyclinD1; ↑Bax; ↓Bcl-2; ↑cleaved caspase-3; ↑cleaved caspase-9; ↓MMP-2; ↓MMP-9;↑miR-449a; ↓p-PI3K; ↓p-Akt; ↓Notch1; ↓Notch2; ↓Notch3	Xue et al., 2019 [104]
7-Hydroxydehydronuciferine	AGS (human gastric cancer)	IC_{50}: 62.9 μM (duration not specified)	Inhibited cell proliferation	Antioxidant activity	Liu et al., 2014 [105]
Liensinine	BGC823 and SGC7901(human gastric cancer)	40–80 μM (48 h)	Inhibited cell proliferation	↑Apoptosis; ↑cleaved caspase-3; ↑cleaved caspase-9; ↑cleaved PARP; ↓p-Akt; ↓Bcl-2; ↑Bax; ↑ROS; ↑G0/G1 cell arrest; ↓cyclin D1; ↓CDK4	Yang et al. 2019 [106]
			Head and neck cancers		
Neferine	HN6, CAL27 (tongue squamous cell carcinoma), HN30 (pharyngeal squamous cell carcinoma)	7.5–30 μM (24 h)	Reduced cell viability and inhibited colony formation	↑Apoptosis; ↑G1 arrest; ↓Bcl-1; ↑Bax; ↑ROS; ↑autophagosome formation; ↑LC3; ↑p62; ↑p-JNK; ↑p-ASK1	Zhu et al., 2021 [107]
			Hematological cancers		
Kaempferol (from methanolic stamen extract)	KU81F (chronic myelocytic leukemia)	3.5–35 μM (24 h)	Did not display cytotoxic effect	↓FcεR1 expression; ↓FcεR1 α- and γ-chains; ↓intracellular Ca^{2+}; ↓histamine release	Shim et al., 2009 [108]
Neferine	Imatinib-resistant K562/G01 cells (human myelogenous leukemia)	4–64 μM (48 h)	Reduced cell survival rate and reversed drug resistance	↓P-gp expression; ↓*MDR-1* mRNA	Qin et al., 2011 [109]

Table 2. *Cont.*

Materials Tested	Cell Lines Used	Conc. (Duratdion)	Anticancer Effects	Mechanisms	References
			Laryngeal cancer		
Nuciferine	AMC-HN-8, TU-212 (Laryngeal squamous cell carcinoma)	25–100 µM (24 h)	Inhibited cell survival	↓TRIM44; ↓TLR4; ↓Akt signaling	Li et al., 2021 [110]
			Liver cancer		
Water-soluble polysaccharides from seeds	HuH-7 (human liver cancer); H22 (mouse hepatocarcinoma)	50–200 µg/mL (48 h)	Inhibited cell proliferation	Not reported	Zheng et al., 2016 [102]
Polyphenolic seed extract	HepG2 (human liver cancer)	6.25–50 µg/mL (24–48 h)	Showed cytotoxicity	Antioxidant activity	Shen et al., 2019 [111]
Procyanidins from seedpod extract	HepG2 (human liver cancer)	12.5–400 µg/mL (6–96 h)	Decreased viability and inhibited cell proliferation	↑Autophagy; S phase arrest; ↑LC3; ↑GFP-LC3; ↑ROS	Duan et al., 2016 [112]
Neferine	HepG2 (human hepatocarcinoma)	10–40 µM (24 h)	Reversed thermotolerance of tumor cells	↑Apoptosis; ↓Bcl-2	Xiao-Hong et al., 2007 [113]
Neferine	Hep3B (human liver cancer); Sk-hep-1 (human hepatic adenocarcinoma)	5–30 µM (24 h)	Induced growth inhibition and decreased cell viability	↑Apoptosis; ↓c-Myc; ↓cyclin D1; ↓cyclin D3; ↓CDK4; ↓E2F-1; ↑Bim; ↑Bid; ↑Bax; ↑Bak; ↑Puma; ↑caspase-3; ↑caspase-6; ↑caspase-7; caspase-8; ↑PARP	Yoon et al., 2013 [114]
Neferine	HepG2 (human liver cancer)	2–25 µM (48 h)	Reduced cell viability	↑Apoptosis; ↑Bax; ↑Bad; ↑cleaved caspase-3; ↑caspase-9; ↑PARP; ↓Bcl2; ↑p53, ↑PTEN; ↓p-Akt; ↑TNF-α; ↑p38; ↑ERK1/2 MAP kinases; ↑ROS	Poornima et al., 2013 [115]
Neferine	HepG2 (human liver cancer)	2.5–100 µM (24–48 h)	Exhibited cytotoxicity and suppressed migration and invasion	↑Apoptosis; ↑E-cadherin; ↓Vimentin; ↓Snail; ↓N-cadherin	Deng et al., 2017 [116]
Neferine	HepG2, Hep3B (human liver cancer)	1–5 µM (2 weeks)	Induced cytotoxicity	↑Autophagy; ↑Ryr; ↑cytosolic [Ca^{2+}]; ↑Ulk-1-PERK; ↑AMPK-mTOR	Law et al., 2019 [87]
Isoliensinine	HepG2, Huh-7 and H22 (human liver cancer)	3–10 µg/mL (24–48 h)	Inhibited cell proliferation	↑Apoptosis; ↑sub-G1 DNA; ↑caspase-3; ↓Bcl-2; ↓Bcl-xL; ↓MMP-9; ↓NF-κB activity; ↓p65 phosphorylation; ↑p65/PP2A binding	Shu et al., 2015 [117]; Shu et al., 2016 [118]

Table 2. *Cont.*

Materials Tested	Cell Lines Used	Conc. (Duratdion)	Anticancer Effects	Mechanisms	References
			Lung cancer		
Ethanolic seed pod extract	A549, H460 (human non-small cell lung cancer)	10–80 µM (24, 48 h)	Inhibited cell proliferation and colony formation	↑Apoptosis; ↑cleaved PARP; ↑γ-H2AX; ↓Axl	Kim et al., 2021 [121]
Neferine	A-549 (human lung carcinoma)	1–30 µM (12–72 h)	Inhibited cell proliferation	↑Autophagy; ↓PI3K; ↓Akt; ↓mTOR; ↑ROS; ↓GSH	Poornima et al., 2013 [122]
Neferine	A-549, H520, H661, H44 (human lung carcinoma)	1–30 µM (48 h)	Reduced cell viability	↑Apoptosis; G1 cell cycle arrest; ↓Bcl-2; ↑Bax; ↑Bad; ↑cyt c; ↑cleaved caspase-3; ↑cleaved caspase-9; ↓ΔΨM; ↑p53; ↑p27; ↓cyclin D1; ↓NF-κB; ↑PTEN; ↑p-JNK; ↑p-ERK1/2; ↑p-p38; ↓GSH; ↓SOD; ↓CAT; ↓GPx; ↓GST;↑[Ca^{2+}]	Poornima et al., 2014 [123]
Neferine	A549 (human lung carcinoma)	0.039–100 µM (72 h)	Reduced cell viability	↑R123 uptake; ↓P-gp	Kadioglu et al., 2017 [86]
Neferine	A549, H1299, LLC-1 (human lung cancer cells)	10 µM (4 h)	Suppressed cell growth	↑Autophagy; ↑LC3-II	Law et al., 2019 [87]
Neferine Neferine+cisplatin	A549 (human lung cancer cell)	10 µM (48 h)	Induced cytotoxicity	↑Autophagy; ↓GSH; ↑ROS; ↑LC3-II; ↓PI3K; ↓Akt; ↓mTOR	Kalai Selvi et al., 2017 [124]
Neferine Neferine + cisplatin	A549 (human lung cancer cell)	10 µM (12–72 h)	Inhibited proliferation and reduced cell viability	↑Apoptosis; ↑LDH leakage; ↑NO release; sub-G1 cell cycle arrest; ↓Bcl-2; ↑Bax; ↑Bad; ↑cyt c; ↑cleaved caspase-3; ↑cleaved caspase-9; ↑cleaved PARP; ↑p53; ↑ROS; ↓FAK; ↓VGEF; ↓MMP-2	Sivalingam et al., 2017 [125]
Nuciferine	A549 (human lung adenocarcinoma)	10–50 µM (24 h)	Exhibited antiproliferative activity and suppressed tumor cell invasion and migration	↑Apoptosis; ↓Bcl-2; ↑Bax; ↓Wnt/β-catenin signaling; ↑Axin; ↓c-myc; ↓cyclin D; ↓VEGF-A	Liu et al., 2015 [126]
Nuciferine	A549 and NCI-H1650 (human lung adenocarcinoma)	0.05–1.0 mg/mL (24 h)	Reduced cell viability and inhibited cell invasion	Not reported	Qi et al., 2016 [96]
			Nasopharyngeal cancer		

Table 2. *Cont.*

Materials Tested	Cell Lines Used	Conc. (Duratdion)	Anticancer Effects	Mechanisms	References
Alkaloids from seeds	CNE-1 (human nasopharyngeal carcinoma)	50–200 μg/mL (24 h)	Reduced cell proliferation	↑Apoptosis; ↑caspase-3; ↑caspase-8; ↑caspase-9; ↑Bax; ↑Fas;↑FasL; ↓Bcl-2; ↓Bcl-xL; ↓NF-κB; ↑IκB-α	Zhao et al., 2016 [128]
Neural cancer					
Neferine	IMR32 (human neuroblastoma)	1–30 μM (24 h)	Suppressed proliferation and migration	↑Apoptosis; G2/M phase arrest; caspase-3 cleavage; PARP cleavage; ↑autophagy; ↑LC3-II; ↑Beclin-1; ↓p-FAK; ↓p-S6K1	Pham et al., 2018 [129]
Nuciferine	SY5Y (human neuroblastoma)	0.05–1.0 mg/mL (24 h)	Reduced cell viability and suppressed cell invasion	↓PI3K; ↓IL1B; ↓p-Akt	Qi et al., 2016 [96]
Nuciferine	U87MG, U251 (human glioblastoma)	20–180 μM (24–72 h)	Inhibited cell proliferation, colony formation, mobility, invasion, migration, and epithelial-to-mesenchymal transition	↑Apoptosis; ↑Bax; ↓Bcl-2; ↓HIF1A; ↓VEGFA; ↑G2 cell cycle arrest; ↓Slug; ↓CDC2; ↑cyclin B1; ↓Vimentin; ↓N-cadherin; ↑E-cadherin; ↓SOX2; ↓p-Akt; ↓p-STAT3	Li et al., 2019 [130]
Ovarian cancer					
Neferine	A2780, HO8910; SKOV3 (human ovarian cancer)	1–10 μM (24–72 h)	Exhibited cytotoxic and growth-inhibitory effects	G1 cell cycle arrest; ↓cyclin D; ↑p27; ↑p21; ↑apoptosis; ↑autophagy; ↑LC3-II; ↑Atg7; ↓p-p70S6K; ↓p-4EBP1; ↑p-p38 MAPK; ↑p-JNK	Xu et al., 2016 [131]
Prostate cancer					
Polyphenolic seed extract	LNCaP (human prostate adenocarcinoma)	6.25–50 μg/mL (24 h & 48 h)	Exhibited antiproliferative activity	Antioxidant effects	Shen et al., 2019 [111]
Nuciferine, 7-hydroxydihydro-nuciferine, caaverine, liridodenine & anonaine	DU-145 (human prostate cancer)	IC_{50} = 80.8–218.4 μM (24 h)	Induced cytotoxicity	Not reported	Liu et al., 2014 [105]
Neferine	PC3; LNCaP (human prostate cancer); CD 44+ PC3 CSC (cancer stem cells)	3.12–100 μM (24–72 h)	Reduced cell proliferation and inhibited migration	↑Apoptosis; ↑G1 phase cell cycle arrest; ↓Bcl-2; ↓CDK4; ↑caspase-3; ↑cleaved PARP; ↑p21; ↑p27; ↑p53; ↓MMP-9; ↓Slug; ↓Snail; ↓SOD1; ↓CAT; ↓GPx	Erdogan & Turkekul, 2020 [132]

Table 2. *Cont.*

Materials Tested	Cell Lines Used	Conc. (Duratdion)	Anticancer Effects	Mechanisms	References
Neferine	DU145 and LNCaP (human prostate cancer)	5–20 µM (18 h)	Reduced cell viability	↑Apoptosis; ↑autophagy; ↓p62; ↑LC3B-II; ↑autophagosome formation; ↑p-JNK	Nazim et al., 2020 [133]
Neferine, liensinine, isoliensinine	LNCaP; PC3; DU-145 (human prostate cancer)	1–100 µM (24 and 48 h)	Induced cytotoxicity and reduced migration in PC3 and DU145 cells	↑Apoptosis; ↑autophagy; ↑Bax; ↓Bcl-2; ↑cleaved-caspase-9; ↑cleaved-PARP; ↓PARP; ↑LC3B-II; ↑AR; ↑PSA; ↑5-α reductase	Liu et al., 2021 [134]
			Renal cancer		
Neferine	Caki-1 (human renal cancer)	5–25 µM (24 h)	Inhibited cell proliferation	↑Apoptosis; ↓Bcl-2; ↑Bax; ↓XIAP; ↓sub-G1 cell population; ↓NF-κB-dependent luciferase activity; ↓p65	Kim et al., 2019 [135]
			Sarcoma		
Neferine	U2OS and Saos-2 (human osteosarcoma)	1–20 µM (24–72 h)	Inhibited cell proliferation	↑G1 arrest; ↓cyclin E; ↑p21; ↑p38 MAPK; ↑JNK	Zhang et al., 2012 [136]
			Skin cancer		
Aqueous rhizome extract	A431 (epidermoid cancer)	1–1000 µg/mL (24 h)	Inhibited proliferation and migration	↓MMP-2; ↓MMP-9	Karki et al., 2008 [78]
Methanolic extracts from flower bud and leaves	B16 melanoma 4A5 cells (murine melanoma)	3–30 µM (72 h)	Inhibited melanogenesis	↓Tyrosinase; ↓TRP-1; ↓TRP-2	Nakamura et al., 2013 [66]
Procyanidin extract from seedpod	B16 (murine melanoma)	25–100 µg/mL (1–5 days)	Displayed cytotoxicity and inhibited cell proliferation	↑Apoptosis; ↑S cell cycle arrest; ↑calcium	Duan et al., 2010 [137]
Leaf extract; gallic acid	B16F1 (murine melanoma)	NLE: 0.1–0.5 mg/mL GA: 60–100 µM (24–72 h)	Reduced melanogenesis	↓Tyrosinase; ↓MITF; TRP-1; ↓p-PKA; ↓p-CREB; ↓melanin	Lai et al., 2020 [138]
7-Hydroxydehydronuciferine	A375.S2 (human melanoma)	10–100 µM (24 h)	Inhibited cell proliferation and showed cytotoxicity	↑Apoptosis	Liu et al., 2014 [105]
7-Hydroxydehydronuciferine	A375.S2, A375 and A2058 cells (human melanoma)	10–100 µM (24 h)	Induced cytotoxicity and reduced migration	↑Apoptosis; ↑autophagy; G2/M arrest; ↑ATG-5; ↑ATG-12; ↑ATG-16; ↑AVO	Wu et al., 2015 [139]

Table 3. Potential anticancer effects and mechanisms of action of *N. nucifera*-derived constituents based on in vivo studies.

Materials Tested	Animal Tumor Models	Anticancer Effects	Mechanisms	Dose (Route)	Duration	References
			Breast cancer			
Flavonoid-rich leaf extract	BALB/c athymic nude mice injected with MCF-7 cells	Reduced tumor volume and weight	↓HER2; p-HER2; ↓Fas	0.5 & 1% (diet)	28 days	Yang et al., 2011 [79]
Aqueous leaf extract	MDA-MB-231 cells injected in female C57BL/6 nude mice	Inhibited tumor growth	Not reported	0.5–2 % (s.c.)	14 days	Chang et al., 2016 [80]
Liensinine + doxorubicin	Female nude mice injected with MDA-MB-231 cells	Reduced tumor growth	↑Apoptosis; ↑cleaved caspase-3; ↓autophagy/mitophagy; ↑auto-phagosome /mitophagosome; ↑colocalization of DNM1L and TOMM20	60 mg/kg (i.p.); 2 mg/kg (i.p.)	30 days	Zhou et al., 2015 [90]
			Colon cancer			
Nuciferine	CT29 cells subcutaneously implanted in nude mice	Reduced tumor weight	Not reported	9.5 mg/kg (i.p.)	3 times a week for 3 weeks	Qi et al., 2016 [96]
Liensinine	HT29 cells injected in female BALB/c nude mice	Suppressed colorectal tumorigenesis, reduced tumor size	↓Ki-67	30 mg/kg (oral)	Every other day for 15 days	Wang et al., 2018 [97]
			Eye cancer			
Neferine	WERI-Rb-1 cells injected in female athymic nude mice	Reduced tumor volume and weight	↓Ki-67; ↓VEGF; ↓SOD; ↑MDA	0.5–2 mg/kg (i.p)	Every 3 days for 30 days	Wang et al., 2020 [100]
			Gallbladder cancer			
Liensinine	NOZ cells injected in BALB/c nude mice	Reduced tumor volume and weight	↓Ki-67	2 mg/kg (i.p)	Every 2 days	Shen et al., 2019 [101]
			Gastric cancer			
Liensinine from seeds	SGC7901 cells injected in BALB/c homozygous (nu/nu) nude mice	Reduced tumor size	↓Ki-67	10 μM (i.p.)	Every 2 days for a month	Yang et al., 2019 [106]
			Head and neck cancers			
Neferine	CAL27 cells injected in male BALB/c nude mice	Reduced tumor volume	↑Apoptosis; ↑autophagy, ↑cleaved caspase-3, ↑cleaved PARP1, ↑LC3; ↑p62	10 mg/kg (i.p)	Not reported	Zhu et al., 2021 [107]

Table 3. *Cont.*

Materials Tested	Animal Tumor Models	Anticancer Effects	Mechanisms	Dose (Route)	Duration	References
			Liver cancer			
Water-soluble polysaccharides from seeds	H22 cells injected in female Kunming mice	Reduced tumor weight	↑TNF-α; ↑IL-2; ↑SOD; ↓MDA	50–200 mg/kg (oral)	14 days	Zheng et al., 2016 [102]
Leaf extract	DEN fed male Sprague-Dawley rats	Reduced tumor size	↓AST; ↓ALT; ↓albumin; ↓total triglyceride; ↓total cholesterol; ↓lipid peroxidation; ↑GSH; ↑GSHPx; ↑SOD; ↑CAT; ↑GST; ↓Rac1; ↓PKCα; ↓TNF-α; ↓IL-6	0.5–2.0% (p.o.)	12 weeks	Horng et al., 2017 [119]
Leaf extract	2-AAF-induced male Wistar rats	Inhibited hepatic fibrosis and hepatocarcinogenesis	↓Triglycerides; ↓total cholesterol; ↓AFP; ↓IL-6; ↓TNF-α; ↓AST; ↓ALT; ↓γGT; ↓GST-Pi; ↓lipid peroxidation; ↓8-OHdG; ↑Nrf2; ↑CAT; ↑GPx; ↑SOD-1	0.5–2% in the diet (p.o.)	6 months	Yang et al., 2019 [120]
Neferine+ oxaliplatin	HepG2 and Bel-7402 cells injected in male BALB/c mice	Increased tumor volume reducing the effect of oxaliplatin	↑E-cadherin; ↓Vimentin; ↓Ki-67;	20 mg/kg/d (i.p.)	3 weeks	Deng et al., 2017 [116]
Isoliensinine	Huh-7 cells injected in male athymic nude mice and H22 cells injected in Kunming mice	Reduced tumor volume	↑caspase-3; ↓Bcl-2; ↓Bcl-xL; ↓MMP-9; ↓p65 phosphorylation	3 and 10 mg/kg/d (i.p. and gavage)	10 days; 3 weeks	Shu et al., 2015 [117]
Isoliensinine	Huh-7 cells transfectants injected in male athymic nude mice	Reduced tumor growth	↑Caspase-3 activity	10 mg/kg/d (gavage)	20 days	Shu et al., 2016 [118]
			Lung cancer			
Leaf extract and leaf polyphenol extract	4T-1 metastatic tumor in the lung of BALB/c mice	Reduced metastasis and tumor weight	↓PKCα activation	0.25, 1% (p.o.)	19 days	Wu et al., 2017 [81]
Nuciferine	A549 cells injected in BALB/c mice	Reduced tumor size and weight	↑Apoptosis; ↓Bcl-2; ↑Bax; ↓Wnt/β-catenin; ↑Axin	50 mg/kg (i.p.)	3 times a week for 20 days	Liu et al., 2015 [126]

Table 3. *Cont.*

Materials Tested	Animal Tumor Models	Anticancer Effects	Mechanisms	Dose (Route)	Duration	References
Neferine	DEN-induced lung carcinogenesis in albino male Wistar rats	Suppressed tumor growth	↓ROS; ↓lipid peroxidation; ↓protein carbonyl; ↑GSH; ↑SOD; ↑GPx; ↑GST; ↑CAT; ↓glycoprotein components; ↑ATPase; ↑p53; ↑Bax; ↑caspase-9; ↑caspase-3; ↓Bcl-2; ↓COX-2; ↓NF-κB; ↓CYP2E1; ↓VEGF; ↓PI3K; ↓Akt; ↓mTOR	10–20 mg/kg (oral)	20 alternate days	Sivalingam et al., 2019 [127]
Neural cancer						
Nuciferine	SY5Y cells subcutaneously implanted in nude mice	Reduced tumor weight	Not reported	9.5 mg/kg (i.p.)	3 times a week for 3 weeks	Qi et al., 2016 [96]
Nuciferine	U251 cells subcutaneously inoculated in BALB/c nude mice	Suppressed tumor weight and size	↓Ki-67; ↓CDC2; ↓Bcl-2; ↓HIF1A; ↓N-cadherin; ↓VEGFA	15 mg/kg (i.p.)	Once a day for 2 weeks	Li et al., 2019 [130]
Skin cancer						
Procyanidin extract from seedpod	B16 cells inoculated into syngeneic C57BL/6 J mice	Suppressed tumor volume and weight	↓lipid peroxidation levels; ↑SOD; ↑CAT; ↑GSPx; ↑spleen and thymus index	60–120 mg/kg (i.g.)	Every 2–3 days for 15 days	Duan et al., 2010 [137]
Leaf extract	UV-radiation exposed female guinea pigs	Reversed UVB-induced epidermal hyperplasia and hyperpigmentation	↓MITF; ↓tyrosinase; ↓TRP-1; ↓PKA; ↓ERK; ↓melanin	1–2% (topical)	2 weeks	Lai et al., 2020 [138]
7-Hydroxy-dehydronuciferine	A375.S2 cells injected in BALB/c nu/nu female mice	Reduced tumor volume	Not reported	20 mg/kg (i.p.)	Every 7 days for 28 days	Wu et al., 2015 [139]

3.2.13. Nasopharyngeal Cancer

Zhao et al. [128] treated CNE-1 human nasopharyngeal carcinoma cells with alkaloids extracted from the Ba lotus (a new variety of *N. nucifera*) seeds for 24 h. The alkaloids reduced cell proliferation by increasing apoptosis and protein levels of apoptosis-associated factors, such as caspase-3, caspase-8, caspase-9, Bax, Fas, and FasL, and decreasing protein levels of antiapoptotic factors, such as Bcl-2 and Bcl-xL. The alkaloids also reduced the expression of NF-κB and increased the inhibitor of κBα (IκBα) levels to increase cell death and decrease cell growth.

3.2.14. Neural Cancer

There are at least three reports on the in vitro evaluation of *N. nucifera* pure compounds against malignant nervous system tumors. Pham et al. [129] observed that neferine disrupted the growth of IMR32 human neuroblastoma cells by the induction of G2/M phase arrest, apoptosis and autophagy, cleavage of caspase-3 and PARP, accumulation of LC3-II, overexpression of Beclin-1, and reduction in phosphorylated FAK (p-FAK) and ribosomal

S6 kinase 1 (p-S6K1). Additional results showed that neferine inhibited the migration of IMR32 cells. All these results were comparable to those of the standard anticancer drug temozolomide. Qi et al. [96] treated SY5Y human neuroblastoma cells with nuciferine and found that the alkaloid reduced cell viability and inhibited cell invasion. The mechanistic study revealed decreased expressions of PI3K, IL-1β, and p-Akt. Another research group, Li et al. [130], also investigated the anticancer properties of nuciferine in U87MG and U251 human glioblastoma cells. Nuciferine inhibited cell proliferation by increasing G2 cell cycle arrest and induced apoptosis by reducing the expression of Bcl-2 and increasing the expression of Bax. The alkaloid also reduced expression of hypoxia-inducible factor 1α (HIF-1α) and VEGFA in nuciferine-treated cells. Epithelial-to-mesenchymal transition was inhibited as nuciferine downregulated the expression of vimentin, N-cadherin, and snail family zinc finger 2 (Slug), yet upregulated E-cadherin and cyclin B1. Other proteins inhibited by nuciferine included p-Akt, phosphorylated signal transducer and activator of transcription 3 (p-STAT3), sex-determining region Y-box 2 (SOX2), and cell division control 2 (CDC2).

Qi et al. [96] also used an in vivo approach to test the anticancer potential of nuciferine against neuroblastoma. Nude mice were subcutaneously implanted with SY5Y cells and injected with nuciferine 3 times a week for 3 weeks. The alkaloid resulted in reduced tumor weights. No mechanistic study was performed. In the in vivo study conducted by Li et al. [87], U251 cells were subcutaneously inoculated into BALB/c nude mice, and the mice with tumors were intraperitoneally injected with nuciferine. Nuciferine suppressed tumor weight and size by downregulating the expression of various proteins, such as Ki-67, Bcl-2, CDC2, HIF-1α, and N-cadherin. Interestingly, ultrasonography evaluation detected reduced tumor size, angiogenesis and hardness index in the nuciferine-treated group compared to control. Magnetic resonance imaging revealed similar results with tumor growth.

3.2.15. Ovarian Cancer

The potential anticancer effects of neferine have been observed in various ovarian cancer cell lines. Xu et al. [131] studied growth-inhibitory effects of neferine on the A2780 ovarian cancer cell line and non-malignant FTE187 immortalized fallopian epithelial cell line. The results showed that neferine exhibited inhibition of the proliferation of A2780 cells, whereas less cytotoxicity was observed for FTE187 cells. Neferine substantially reduced the colony-forming abilities of various ovarian cancer cell lines, such as A2780, SKOV3, and HO8910. In A2780 cells, neferine inhibited cell cycle progression at the G1 phase via the upregulation of G1/S cell cycle proteins p21 and p27 and decreased expression of cyclin D1 in A2780 cells. Neferine also showed apoptotic potential through autophagosome formation and increased expression of GFP-LC3. The expressions of autophagy pathway biomarkers, LC-III and Atg7, were also increased in neferine-treated A2780 cells. Additionally, mTOR-dependent autophagy was observed through decreased phosphorylated levels of p70S6K and 4EBP1 in neferine-exposed A2780 cells. Finally, neferine-induced autophagy through the activation of p38 MAPK and JNK pathways was observed in A2780 and HO8910 cells.

3.2.16. Prostate Cancer

Several studies evaluated the anticancer properties of *N. nucifera* against prostate cancer. Shen et al. [111] explored the anticancer effects of the phenolic extract from the seedpods of *N. nucifera*. Phytochemicals isolated from the extract were catechin, hyperoside, kempherol, and quercetin. The phenolic seed extract induced antiproliferative activity in LNCaP human prostate adenocarcinoma cells. The seed extracts also exhibited antioxidant properties by eliciting free radical-reducing power, metal chelating capacity as well as inhibiting linoleic acid peroxidation.

In addition to extracts, the anticancer properties of several pure compounds abundantly found in *N. nucifera* were also studied. Liu et al. [105] evaluated the effects of various aporphine alkaloids extracted and purified from the leaves of *N. nucifera* against DU-145 human prostate cancer cells. The most active compound, 7-hydroxydehydronuciferine, showed significant cytotoxicity against DU-145 cells, but the underlying mechanism has not been reported. In another study, it was found that neferine inhibited the viability and reduced the proliferation of PC3 and LNCaP human prostate cancers cells and CD44+ cancer stem cells (CSC) isolated from PC3 cells by inducing apoptosis and cell cycle arrest at the G1 phase. These effects were due to the upregulation of p21, p27, p53, poly adenosine diphosphate-ribose polymerase (clePARP) and the downregulation of CDK4 and Bcl-2. In addition, neferine induced oxidative stress by significantly downregulating the mRNA expression of CAT, SOD1 and GPx. Neferine inhibited CSC migration by downregulating the expression of MMP-9 along with the transcription factors Slug and Snail. Neferine was also shown to modulate major signaling pathways by increasing phosphorylation of p38, JNK and MAPKs both in PC3 and CD44+ CSCs [132]. Nazim et al. [133] treated DU-145 and LNCap cells with various concentrations of neferine to determine its anticancer effects. The study revealed that neferine reduced cell viability significantly when combined with tumor necrosis factor-related apoptosis-inducing ligand (TRAIL). The mechanisms behind the synergistic effects of TRAIL and neferine are increased apoptosis and autophagy via increased autophagosome formation and increased levels of LC3B-II, and decreased levels of p62. Neferine was also shown to activate the JNK pathway and increase p-JNK protein expression. A recent study by Liu et al. [134] evaluated the anticancer effects of neferine, liensinine, and isoliensinine on LNCaP, PC3, and DU-145 human prostate cancer cells. These compounds induced cytotoxicity in all 3 cell lines and reduced migration, particularly in PC-3 and DU145 cells. In LNCaP cells, all 3 compounds triggered apoptosis and autophagy, downregulated the protein expression of androgen receptor (AR), prostate-specific androgen (PSA), and type II 5-α-reductase and inactivated the PI3K/Akt signaling pathway.

3.2.17. Renal Cancer

There is at least one study that evaluated the anticancer effects of *N. nucifera* in renal cancer. An investigation led by Kim et al. [135] explored the anticancer effects of neferine on Caki-1 renal cancer cells. Neferine was found to exhibit a growth-inhibitory effect in a concentration-dependent manner and caused apoptosis through the downregulation of Bcl-2 and X-linked inhibitor of apoptosis (XIAP). Further investigation revealed that the downregulation of Bcl-2 by neferine was mediated by the inhibition of the NF-κB pathway. In other renal cancer cell lines, such as ACHN and A498, neferine was also found to downregulate Bcl-2 expression, induce the cleavage of procaspase-3 and inhibit p65 expression.

3.2.18. Sarcoma

There are relatively few studies that examined the effect of neferine in sarcoma. The antiproliferative effects of neferine on U2OS and Saos-2 human osteosarcoma cell lines were demonstrated in a study by Zhang et al. [136]. This research group observed that neferine significantly reduced proliferation in the U2OS and Saos-2 cell lines with increasing concentrations of nefereine; however, normal osteoblasts, HCO, were less sensitive. The results suggested that neferine caused osteosarcoma cells to arrest in the G1 phase of the cell cycle through the increase in p21 protein level, which was independent of p53 or retinoblastoma-associated protein activation. The study went on to find that neferine treatment activated p38 MAPK and JNK through phosphorylation, leading to p21 accumulation.

3.2.19. Skin Cancer

There have been several studies evaluating the anticancer effects of *N. nucifera* on melanoma cells in vitro. Karki et al. [78] explored the anticancer effects of an aqueous rhizome extract on A431 epidermoid cancer cells. The extract was shown to inhibit cancer cell proliferation and migration by decreasing the levels of MMP-2 and MMP-9 in a concentration-dependent fashion. In another study, B16 melanoma 4A5 murine cells were treated with methanolic extracts from the flower and leaves of *N. nucifera*. These extracts inhibited cell viability by reducing the expression of tyrosinase, tyrosine-related protein-1 (TRP-1), and TRP-2. Based on phytochemical analysis, the methanolic extract yielded various constituents, such as nuciferine, N-methylasimilobine, and 2-hydroxy-1-methoxy-6a, 7-dehydroaporphine [66]. Another study investigated the anticancer effect of procyanidins extracted from the seedpod of *N. nucifera*. In this in vitro study, Duan et al. [137] treated B16 murine melanoma cells with the procyanidins, and the results showed cytotoxicity and inhibited cell proliferation via increased apoptotic activity, S phase cycle arrest, and increased intracellular calcium levels. In a recent study, NLE as well as its major component, gallic acid, induced cytotoxicity in B16F1 murine melanoma cells. Mechanistic studies using an immunoblotting assay revealed that both treatments reduced the expressions of tyrosinase, microphthalmia-associated transcription factor (MITF), TRP-1, phosphorylated protein kinase A (p-PKA), and phosphorylated cAMP response element-binding protein (p-CREB) (Lai et al., 2020). In another study, Liu et al. [138] demonstrated that 7-hydroxydehydronuciferine, a compound isolated from a methanolic extract of the leaves of *N. nucifera* Gaertn. cv. Rosa-plena, inhibited cell proliferation and showed cytotoxicity by increasing apoptosis in A375.S2 melanoma cells. Wu et al. [139] treated human melanoma cells (A375.S2, A372, and A2058) with various concentrations of 7-hydroxydehydronuciferine, isolated from the leaves of *N. nucifera*, and observed its anticancer effects. It was found that the compound induced cytotoxicity, registered G2/M phase cell cycle arrest, and reduced cellular migration in parallel with increased apoptosis, autophagy, and autophagy-related proteins (ATG-5, ATG-12, and ATG 16) as well as altered cellular acidic vesicular organelles (AVO).

In addition to their in vitro study, Duan et al. [137] also evaluated the anticancer effect of *N. nucifera* seedpod-derived procyanidins using an in vivo skin cancer model. This was performed by subcutaneously inoculating syngeneic C57BL/6 J mice with B16 melanoma cells and treating the animals with the procyanidin extract every 2–3 days for 15 days. The results showed suppressed tumor growth (reduced volume and weight) through the reduction of hepatic lipid peroxidation levels and the promotion of superoxide dismutase SOD, CAT, and GPx activity. The mice treated with the procyanidin-rich extract also displayed an increased spleen and thymus index, indicating immunomodulatory activities. Lai et al. [138] also conducted an in vivo study using ultra-violet B (UVB)-radiation exposed female guinea pigs and topically treated them with 1–2% NLE. The test agent was found to reverse UVB-induced epidermal hyperplasia and decrease melanin content, as evidenced by hematoxylin and eosin staining and Fontana-Masson staining, respectively. Western blot analysis showed that NLE downregulated the levels of MITF, tyrosinase, and TRP-1, and reduced the activity of PKA and ERK signaling. In addition to the in vitro study mentioned before, Wu et al. [139] studied the effects of 7-hydroxydehydronuciferine in vivo using BALB/c nu/nu female mice with xenotransplanted A375.S2 tumors. Intraperitoneal (i.p.) injections of the alkaloid (20 mg/kg) every 7 days for 28 days reduced tumor volume. The mechanisms behind these antitumor effects have not been reported.

4. Bioavailability and Pharmacokinetics of *N. nucifera* Constituents

Various pure compounds of *N. nucifera* have different bioavailability and pharmacokinetic characteristics. The pharmacokinetic profile of neferine, an alkaloid with significant antineoplastic activity as presented in this review, was studied by Zhao et al. [140] using canine models. Following oral administration, it was found that the plasma concentration of neferine peaked twice, first at 0.333 h and again at 0.667 h after intake. The absolute bioavailability of oral neferine was 65.36%. Another study [141] implemented rat models and also observed two absorption peaks of neferine after oral administration. The plasma concentration peaks were at 10 min and 1 h after intake. The greatest level of distribution of neferine in the liver was recorded when the rats were given 10 and 20 mg/kg of the alkaloid. However, when the rats were administered 50 mg/kg of neferine, its distribution was the greatest in the kidneys and lungs. In addition to these findings, the investigators also observed that neferine was metabolized by cytochrome P450 (CYP) 2D6 to yield metabolites, such as liensinine, isoliensinine, desmethyliensinine, and desmethylisoliensinine. A separate study evaluated the metabolism of isoliensinine identified using reversed-phase high-performance liquid chromatography and electrospray ionization tandem mass spectrometry. Using canine models, Zhou et al. [142] identified three metabolites of isoliensinine, namely 2-*N*-desmethyl-isoliensinine, 2′-*N*-desmethylisoliensinine, and 2′-*N*-6-*O*-didesmethylisoliensinine. These findings suggest that isoliensinine is primarily metabolized by *N*-demethylation and *O*-demethylation in the liver. Zhao et al. [143] also explored pharmacokinetic profiles of neferine and found it had little effect on various CYP enzymes, namely CYP1A2, CYP2D6, and CYP3A4. Kadioglu et al. [86] investigated the pharmacokinetics of neferine using an in silico absorption, distribution, metabolism, and excretion study. The values of logS for solubility, logP for the partition coefficient, and logD for the distribution coefficient were 4.302, 4.432 and 3.503, respectively, showing that neferine possessed the required druggability properties, such as aqueous solubility and lipophilicity.

Other alkaloids derived from *N. nucifera*, such as nuciferine and *N*-nuciferine, were also investigated to determine their pharmacokinetic properties. Ye et al. [47] used male rat models and found that nuciferine and N-nuciferine were rapidly absorbed in the blood and reached a maximum plasma concentration of 1.71 and 0.57 μg/mL at 0.9 and 1.65 h, respectively. The oral bioavailability for nuciferine was 58.13%, while for *N*-nuciferine, it was 79.91%. The researchers also found that the alkaloids rapidly crossed the blood-brain barrier and achieved widespread distribution in the brain. Ye et al. [144] studied the inhibitory effects of nuciferine, *N*-nuciferine, and 2-hydroxy-1-methoxyaporphine on CYP enzymes. It was found that these three alkaloids inhibited the CYP2D6-catalyzed *O*-demethylation form of metabolism. This needs to be considered when administering such *N. nucifera* compounds to patients taking anti-arrhythmia drugs (such as amiodarone and metoprolol) that are specific substrates of CYP2D6. Zou et al. [145] isolated five alkaloids (nuciferine, *O*-nornuciferin, liriodenine, armepavine, and pronuciferine) from *N. nucifera* leaf extract that were then orally administered to rats. The plasma half-lives of nunciferine, O-nornuciferin, liriodenine, armepavine, and pronuciferine were 6.18 ± 3.10, 6.67 ± 2.88, 3.77 ± 1.15, 5.22 ± 5.09, and 4.44 ± 1.88, respectively. Additionally, after giving 2.4 g/kg of the *N. nucifera* leaf extract to rats, it was found that liriodenine and pronuciferine had the slowest absorption rate. Yan et al. [146] detected an alkaloid higenamine in the green embryo of the mature seeds of *N. nucifera*, also known as plumula nelumbinis, a commonly used traditional Chinese medicine. It is interesting that higenamine is included in the Word Anti-Doping Agency (WADA) 2017 Prohibited List and is therefore checked in urine samples of athletes undergoing drug tests. Yan et al. [145] had 14 human volunteers who ingested capsules containing 0.34 g of plumula nelumbinis, and 11 human volunteers ingested capsules with 5 mg higenamine for seven days. The participants who ingested the higenamine capsules showed a maximum concentration of 2000 ng/mL in their urine, rising above the WADA reporting limit of 10 ng/mL. Within 3–7 days of ingesting the plumula nelumbinis capsules, the participants also exceeded the WADA reporting limit with a maximum concentration of 500 ng/mL of higenamine in their urine.

Overall, it has been found that multiple compounds of *N. nucifera* have high oral bioavailability, but caution needs to be taken due to their interactions with hepatic biotransformation enzymes. Further research using human models should be performed to determine the bioavailability and pharmacokinetics of *N. nucifera* compounds.

5. Toxicity Studies on *N. nucifera*

The lotus plant (*N. nucifera)* has been used in traditional medicine for many years and is consumed all around the world. Several studies have evaluated the toxicity and safety profile associated with *N. nucifera* and its constituents. There are various in vitro studies that used normal cell lines to determine the toxicity of *N. nucifera*. In one such study, a normal osteoblast cell line, HCO, was treated with neferine, and the results showed that the cell viability was not significantly affected [136]. Poornima et al. [123] treated BEAS-2B normal lung cells with neferine and found that there was no significant suppression of cell growth up to 20 μM. Xu et al. [130] used normal fallopian tube epithelial cells, FTE187, and observed that neferine did not significantly affect cell viability. In another study evaluating the toxicity of neferine, Yoon et al. [114] treated THLE-3, normal human liver cells, with 5–30 μM of the alkaloid for 24 h. The THLE-3 cells showed no cytotoxicity and change in viability even at 30 μM. Yang et al. [85] treated Hs578Bst mammary fibroblasts with neferine at concentrations up to 8 mg/mL and found that it did not affect cell growth and showed no toxicity. Liao and Lin [147] determined the safety profile of *N. nucifera* plumule polysaccharide in isolated mouse splenocytes. The results showed that the polysaccharide, even at a concentration of 125 μg/mL, did not significantly affect splenocyte viability.

There are also multiple in vivo studies that have investigated the safety profile of *N. nucifera*. Kunanusorn et al. [148] explored the acute and subchronic oral toxicity of *N. nucifera* stamens extract using a rodent model. In this experiment, 7–8-week-old male and female Sprague-Dawley rats were administered 5000 mg/kg of the extract in the acute study and 50–200 mg/kg/day for 90 days in the subchronic study. Within 14 days of the acute study and days 90–118 in the subchronic study, no signs of toxicity or significant changes in weight were noted. However, after day 118, treatment of 200 mg/kg/day in the subchronic study showed an increased number of lymphocytes, decreased number of basophils, and decreased mean corpuscular volume in the male rats. Similarly, female rats showed a decrease in red blood cells and hematocrit after 90 days and an increase in the mean corpuscular hemoglobin concentration after 118 days. In addition, after 90 days of the subchronic treatment of 200 mg/kg/day, there was a decrease in creatinine and cholesterol in male rats and a decrease in albumin in female rats. Female rats also had an increased alkaline phosphatase after 118 days. Although there were no changes in the gross appearance of the internal organs, the relative kidney, liver, and heart organ weights were lower than the control on day 90 of 200 mg/kg/day. All these results support the conclusion that the lethal oral dose of the stamen extract is more than 5000 mg/kg, and the no-observed-adverse-effect level is greater than 200 mg/kg/day for 90 days. In another in vivo study, Rajput and Khan [149] administered 10–5000 mg/kg of *N. nucifera* seed pod extract in albino mice and found that all doses up to 5000 mg/kg were tolerated for 24–48 h. No death or behavioral abnormalities were observed. Another study also utilized mice which were intragastrically administered a water extract from *N. nucifera* leaf. The median lethal dose of the extract was observed to be greater than 5000 mg/kg [150]. One study used Beagle dogs to determine the safety profile of *N. nucifera* seed extract, which was administered for over 4 weeks, and found it to be safe at 2000 mg/kg/d. The research group also used rats and found the extract at 4000 mg/kg/d to be the safe dose over a 13-week administration period [151].

Kadioglu et al. [86] evaluated the toxicity of the pure *N. nucifera* compound neferine towards normal tissues using Stardrop and Derek Nexus software. The in silico safety evaluation showed a favorable toxicity profile. No mutagenicity toxicity class was predicted. However, it has been found that neferine could cause some skin sensitization. Overall, multiple studies show that *N. nucifera* is relatively safe to use at therapeutic doses. Nevertheless, additional in vivo studies and clinical evaluations are warranted to confirm the non-toxicity and safety of *N. nucifera* for human use.

6. Conclusions, Current Challenges/Limitations and Future Directions

All parts of *N. nucifera* have been used for food and medicinal purposes across Asia for over a thousand years. More recently, *N. nucifera* constituents have been studied for their chemoprotective and antineoplastic potential. In this systematic review, we have found extensive evidence of mechanism-based cancer preventive and therapeutic effects of bioactive constituents from different parts of *N. nucifera*, as well as the bioavailability, pharmacokinetics, and toxicities of selected phytochemicals.

We analyzed a multitude of antineoplastic effects of *N. nucifera* extracts, fractions and pure compounds on various cancer types. Specific phytochemicals, including neferine, nuciferine, liensinine, 7-hydroxydehydronuciferine, cadaverine, liriodenine, anonaine, and gallic acid, have been investigated for their anticancer effects. *N. nucifera*-derived products and phytochemicals exhibit antineoplastic effects via antioxidant, anti-inflammatory, antiproliferative, cell death-inducing, cell cycle-regulatory, anti-invasive, and antiangiogenic pathways (Figure 5). *N. nucifera* phytochemicals prevented oxidative stress by altering GSH, iNOS, and CAT and modulated various proteins involved in inflammatory processes (NF-κB, COX-2, and TLR-4), proliferation (cyclins, cyclin-dependent kinases, and MAPK), apoptosis (Bax, Bad, caspase-3, caspase-6, caspase-7, caspase-8, caspase-9 and Bcl-2), invasion (MMP-2, N-cadherin, snail, and slug), and angiogenesis (VEGF and CTGF). Regarding in vitro studies, apoptosis was induced by various *N. nucifera* compounds across the majority of cancer subtypes. Various anticancer mechanisms involved activated caspase-3, caspase-6, caspase-7, caspase-8, and caspase-9, increased Bax and Bad, and decreased Bcl-2, indicating that *N. nucifera* phytochemicals induce apoptosis through extrinsic and intrinsic pathways. In vivo studies included various mechanisms without overlap between cancer subtypes.

The most-studied *N. nucifera* phytochemical has been neferine, a bis-benzylisoqunoline alkaloid, isolated from seed pod embryos. The majority of the chemotherapeutic literature on *N. nucifera* is limited to in vitro studies, as there are 72 in vitro studies and only 23 in vivo studies. The quality of each animal study was calculated using the SYRCLE's RoB tool [76]. The 17 in vivo studies had an average of 32.2% for the quality control analysis, since many protocol details were not stated. The cancer types researched include breast, colon, gastric, chronic myelocytic leukemia, laryngeal, liver, lung, nasopharyngeal, ovarian, prostate, renal and skin cancers. The most thoroughly studied cancers included gastrointestinal, breast, and lung cancers in vitro as well as in vivo studies of gastrointestinal cancers.

We have identified various limitations in the current research, including the limited bioavailability and sparse toxicology research. There are limited studies on the bioavailability of *N. nucifera*; however, some literature shows the relatively high bioavailability and distribution of *N. nucifera* constituents nuciferine, *N*-nuciferine, and neferine. *N. nucifera* compounds were also shown to interact with various hepatic CYP enzymes, which could interfere with other pharmaceuticals or chemotherapeutic drugs if used in combination with *N. nucifera*. Limited toxicity studies conclude that *N. nucifera* plumule polysaccharides and neferine are nontoxic and safe for use. Due to its limited toxicity, *N. nucifera* can pose as an alternative or in conjunction with traditional chemotherapy, which has numerous undesirable side effects.

Our group has identified many avenues of further research. Firstly, more in vivo studies should be conducted as at present, the majority of the research is limited to in vitro studies. The in vivo studies should include additional cancer subtypes and validate in vitro mechanisms of action. Currently, no clinical research has been conducted to explore the anticancer potential of *N. nucifera* constituents. Hence, randomized controlled trials are necessary to translate preclinical results into clinical practice. Another avenue of further research includes studies on synergistic effects with other anticancer drugs, as the current literature mostly examines *N. nucifera* phytochemicals individually. Along with the existing research on anticancer mechanisms of *N. nucifera*, additional research is necessary to ascertain the molecular targets of the parent compound and their metabolites in various organs. Supplementary research is needed to optimize delivery systems for *N. nucifera*'s active phytocompounds, which would increase their bioavailability and anticancer effects via efficient targeting. The quantity of *N. nucifera*-derived food items that needs to be consumed for prevention of various cancers is also yet to be determined and needs further research. Although several studies include the synergistic effects of *N. nucifera* phytochemicals and traditional chemotherapeutic drugs, such as cisplatin and oxaliplatin, additional research should be conducted to include different types of cancer as well as expansion to clinical studies. Taking into consideration the in-depth analysis of current research as presented in this review, *N. nucifera*-derived bioactive phytochemicals possess significant potential for human cancer prevention and anticancer therapy.

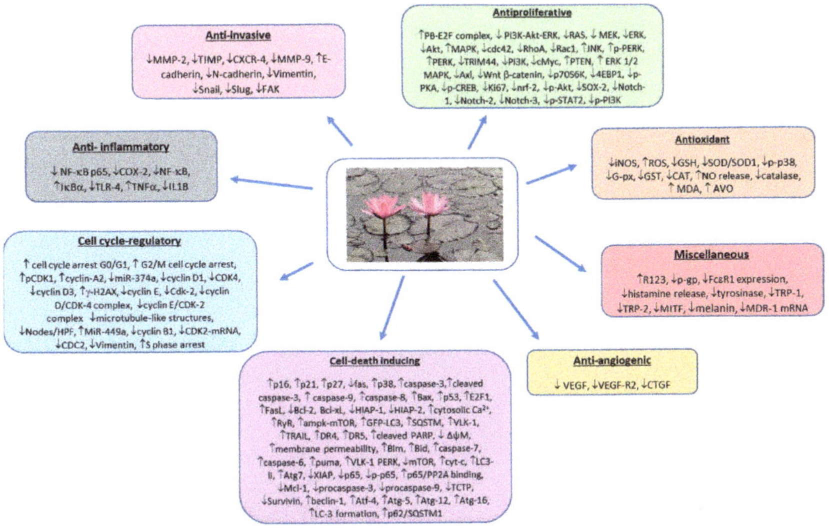

Figure 5. Overview of anticancer mechanisms, molecular targets, and signaling pathways of *N. nucifera* phytochemicals based on in vitro and studies.

Author Contributions: Conceptualization, A.B.; methodology, A.B.; investigation, A.B., P.A.P., P.S., S.T. and N.D.; writing—original draft preparation, A.B., P.A.P., P.S., S.T. and N.D.; writing—review and editing, A.B.; supervision, A.B.; project administration, A.B. All authors have read and agreed to the published version of the manuscript.

Funding: This research received no external source of funding.

Acknowledgments: We wish to convey our thanks and appreciation to investigators all over the world who have made significant contributions to our understanding of the potential of lotus in cancer prevention and therapy. We regret that we are unable to cite each and every pertinent publication due to space limitations. We also thank Sachchida Nand Rai and Vivek Chaturvedi for their assistance with literature collection and Arindam Bishayee for providing us with lotus photos.

Conflicts of Interest: The authors declare no conflict of interest.

Abbreviations

2-AAF	2-acetylaminofluorene
ADM	adriamycin
AFP	α-fetoprotein
ALT	alanine aminotransferase
AMPK	5′-adenosine monophosphate-activated protein kinase
ASK1	apoptosis signal-regulating kinase 1
AST	aspartate transaminase
AVO	acidic vesicular organelles
Bax	Bcl-associated X protein
Bcl-2	B cell lymphoma 2
Bcl-xL	B-cell lymphoma-extra-large
CAT	catalase
CDK	cyclin-dependent kinase

c-Myc	cellular myelocytomatosis
COX-2	cyclooxygenase-2
CREB	cAMP response element-binding protein
CSC	cancer stem cells
CTGF	connective tissue growth factor
cyt c	cytochrome c
CYP	cytochrome P450
DEN	diethylnitrosamine
DHEA	dehydroepiandrosterone
DNM1L	dynamin-1-like protein
DR	death receptor
E2F1	E2F transcription factor 1
ERK	extracellular signal-regulated kinase
FasL	Fas ligand
GC-MS	gas chromatography-mass spectrometry
GFP	green fluorescent protein
GPx	glutathione peroxidase
GSH	glutathione
GSTπ	glutathione S-transferase pi
γGT	γ-glutamyl transferase
γ-H2AX	H2A histone family member X
HER2	human epidermal growth factor receptor 2
HIAP	human inhibitor of apoptosis protein
HPLC	high-performance liquid chromatography
IκBα	inhibitor of κBαi
IL-1β	interleukin-1β
iNOS	inducible nitric oxide synthase
i.p.	intraperitoneal
JNK	c-Jun N-terminal kinase
LC3	light-chain 3
MAPK	mitogen activated protein kinase
MDA	malondialdehyde
MDR-1	multidrug resistance 1
MEK	mitogen-activated extracellular signal-regulated kinase
MITF	microphthalmia-associated transcription factor
MMP	matrix metalloproteinase
mTOR	mammalian target of rapamycin
NF-κB	nuclear factor-κB
NLE	*N. nucifera* leaf extract
NLPE	*N. nucifera* leaf polyphenol extract
Nrf2	nuclear factor erythroid 2-related factor 2
8-OHdG	8-hydroxy-2′-deoxyguanosine
PARP	poly (ADP-ribose) polymerase
P-gp	P-glycoprotein
PI3K	phosphoinositide-3-kinase
PKA	protein kinase A
PKCα	protein kinase Cα
PP2A	protein phosphatase 2A
PRISMA	preferred reporting items for systematic reviews and meta-analysis
PTEN	phosphatase and tensin homolog
R123	rhodamine 123
ROS	reactive oxygen species
RAB7A	Ras-related protein Rab-7a
Rac1	Ras-related C3 botulinum toxin substrate 1
Ryr	ryanodine receptor
SOD	superoxide dismutase
TIMP-2	tissue inhibitor of metalloproteinase-2
TLR4	Toll-like receptor 4

TNF-α	tumor necrosis factor-α
TOMM20	translocase of outer mitochondrial membrane 20
TRAIL	tumor necrosis factor-related apoptosis-inducing ligand
TRIM44	tripartite motif-containing 44
TRP	tyrosine related protein
Ulk-1-PERK	Unc-51-like autophagy activating kinase-1-protein kinase RNA-like ER kinase
UVB	ultra-violet B
VEGF	vascular endothelial growth factor
WADA	Word Anti-Doping Agency
XIAP	X-linked inhibitor of apoptosis
ZFX	zinc finger X-chromosomal protein

References

1. Sung, H.; Ferlay, J.; Siegel, R.L.; Laversanne, M.; Soerjomataram, I.; Jemal, A.; Bray, F. Global Cancer Statistics 2020: GLOBOCAN Estimates of Incidence and Mortality Worldwide for 36 Cancers in 185 Countries. *CA Cancer J. Clin.* **2021**, *71*, 209–249. [CrossRef]
2. Islami, F.; Goding Sauer, A.; Miller, K.D.; Siegel, R.L.; Fedewa, S.A.; Jacobs, E.J.; McCullough, M.L.; Patel, A.V.; Ma, J.; Soerjomataram, I.; et al. Proportion and number of cancer cases and deaths attributable to potentially modifiable risk factors in the United States. *CA Cancer J. Clin.* **2018**, *68*, 31–54. [CrossRef]
3. Tseng, M. Diet, cancer and public health nutrition. *Public Health Nutr.* **2009**, *12*, 737–738. [CrossRef] [PubMed]
4. Mittelman, S.D. The Role of Diet in Cancer Prevention and Chemotherapy Efficacy. *Annu. Rev. Nutr.* **2020**, *40*, 273–297. [CrossRef] [PubMed]
5. Cragg, G.M.; Pezzuto, J.M. Natural Products as a Vital Source for the Discovery of Cancer Chemotherapeutic and Chemopreventive Agents. *Med. Princ. Pract.* **2016**, *25*, 41–59. [CrossRef] [PubMed]
6. Newman, D.J.; Cragg, G.M. Natural products as sources of new drugs over the nearly four decades from 01/1981 to 09/2019. *J. Nat. Prod.* **2020**, *83*, 770–803. [CrossRef]
7. Shanmugam, M.K.; Arfuso, F.; Kumar, A.P.; Wang, L.; Goh, B.C.; Ahn, K.S.; Bishayee, A.; Sethi, G. Modulation of diverse oncogenic transcription factors by thymoquinone, an essential oil compound isolated from the seeds of Nigella sativa Linn. *Pharmacol. Res.* **2018**, *129*, 357–364. [CrossRef]
8. Tuli, H.S.; Tuorkey, M.J.; Thakral, F.; Sak, K.; Kumar, M.; Sharma, A.K.; Sharma, U.; Jain, A.; Aggarwal, V.; Bishayee, A. Molecular Mechanisms of Action of Genistein in Cancer: Recent Advances. *Front. Pharmacol.* **2019**, *10*, 1336. [CrossRef] [PubMed]
9. Aggarwal, V.; Tuli, H.S.; Tania, M.; Srivastava, S.; Ritzer, E.E.; Pandey, A.; Aggarwal, D.; Barwal, T.S.; Jain, A.; Kaur, G.; et al. Molecular mechanisms of action of epigallocatechin gallate in cancer: Recent trends and advancement. *Semin. Cancer Biol.* **2020**, *in press*. [CrossRef]
10. De Greef, D.; Barton, E.M.; Sandberg, E.N.; Croley, C.R.; Pumarol, J.; Wong, T.L.; Das, N.; Bishayee, A. Anticancer potential of garlic and its bioactive constituents: A systematic and comprehensive review. *Semin. Cancer Biol.* **2021**, *73*, 219–264. [CrossRef] [PubMed]
11. Mirza, B.; Croley, C.R.; Ahmad, M.; Pumarol, J.; Das, N.; Sethi, G.; Bishayee, A. Mango (*Mangifera indica* L.): A magnificent plant with cancer preventive and anticancer therapeutic potential. *Crit. Rev. Food Sci. Nutr.* **2021**, *61*, 2125–2151. [CrossRef]
12. Nouri, Z.; Fakhri, S.; Nouri, K.; Wallace, C.E.; Farzaei, M.H.; Bishayee, A. Targeting Multiple Signaling Pathways in Cancer: The Rutin Therapeutic Approach. *Cancers* **2020**, *12*, 2276. [CrossRef]
13. Ghanbari-Movahed, M.; Jackson, G.; Farzaei, M.H.; Bishayee, A. A Systematic Review of the Preventive and Therapeutic Effects of Naringin against Human Malignancies. *Front. Pharmacol.* **2021**, *12*, 639840. [CrossRef]
14. Jamieson, S.; E Wallace, C.; Das, N.; Bhattacharyya, P.; Bishayee, A. Guava (*Psidium guajava* L.): A glorious plant with cancer preventive and therapeutic potential. *Crit. Rev. Food Sci. Nutr.* **2021**. [CrossRef]
15. Kaiser, A.E.; Baniasadi, M.; Giansiracusa, D.; Giansiracusa, M.; Garcia, M.; Fryda, Z.; Wong, T.L.; Bishayee, A. Sulforaphane: A Broccoli Bioactive Phytocompound with Cancer Preventive Potential. *Cancers* **2021**, *13*, 4796. [CrossRef]
16. Mondal, A.; Banerjee, S.; Bose, S.; Das, P.P.; Sandberg, E.N.; Atanasov, A.G.; Bishayee, A. Cancer Preventive and Therapeutic Potential of Banana and Its Bioactive Constituents: A Systematic, Comprehensive, and Mechanistic Review. *Front. Oncol.* **2021**, *11*, 697143. [CrossRef] [PubMed]
17. Wong, T.L.; Strandberg, K.R.; Croley, C.R.; Fraser, S.E.; Venkata, K.C.N.; Fimognari, C.; Sethi, G.; Bishayee, A. Pomegranate bioactive constituents target multiple oncogenic and oncosuppressive signaling for cancer prevention and intervention. *Semin. Cancer Biol.* **2021**, *73*, 265–293. [CrossRef] [PubMed]
18. Wang, Q.; Zhang, X. *Colored Illustration of Lotus Cultivars in China*; China Forestry Publishing House: Beijing, China, 2005.
19. Ming, R.; VanBuren, R.; Liu, Y.; Yang, M.; Han, Y.; Li, L.-T.; Zhang, Q.; Kim, M.-J.; Schatz, M.C.; Campbell, M.; et al. Genome of the long-living sacred lotus (*Nelumbo nucifera* Gaertn.). *Genome Biol.* **2013**, *14*, R41. [CrossRef] [PubMed]
20. Yang, M.; Han, Y.; Xu, L.; Zhao, J.; Liu, Y. Comparative analysis of genetic diversity of lotus (Nelumbo) using SSR and SRAP markers. *Sci. Hortic.* **2012**, *142*, 185–195. [CrossRef]
21. Deng, J.; Chen, S.; Yin, X.; Wang, K.; Liu, Y.; Li, S.; Yang, P. Systematic qualitative and quantitative assessment of anthocyanins, flavones and flavonols in the petals of 108 lotus (*Nelumbo nucifera*) cultivars. *Food Chem.* **2013**, *139*, 307–312. [CrossRef] [PubMed]

22. Sheikh, S.A. Ethno-medicinal uses and pharmacological activities of lotus (*Nelumbo nucifera*). *J. Med. Plants Stud.* **2014**, *2*, 42–46.
23. Zhang, X.; Chen, L.; Wang, Q. *New Lotus Flower Cultivars in China*; China Forestry Publishing House: Beijing, China, 2011.
24. Zhang, Y.; Lu, X.; Zeng, S.; Huang, X.; Guo, Z.; Zheng, Y.; Tian, Y.; Zheng, B. Nutritional composition, physiological functions and processing of lotus (*Nelumbo nucifera* Gaertn.) seeds: A review. *Phytochem. Rev.* **2015**, *14*, 321–334. [CrossRef]
25. Tungmunnithum, D.; Pinthong, D.; Hano, C. Flavonoids from *Nelumbo nucifera* Gaertn., a Medicinal Plant: Uses in Traditional Medicine, Phytochemistry and Pharmacological Activities. *Medicines* **2018**, *5*, 127. [CrossRef]
26. Lin, Z.; Zhang, C.; Cao, D.; Damaris, R.N.; Yang, P. The Latest Studies on Lotus (*Nelumbo nucifera*)-an Emerging Horticultural Model Plant. *Int. J. Mol. Sci.* **2019**, *20*, 3680. [CrossRef]
27. Guo, H.B. Cultivation of lotus (*Nelumbo nucifera* Gaertn. ssp. nucifera) and its utilization in China. *Genet. Resour. Crop Evol.* **2009**, *56*, 323–330. [CrossRef]
28. Zhu, F. Structures, properties, and applications of lotus starches. *Food Hydrocoll.* **2017**, *63*, 332–348. [CrossRef]
29. Chen, G.; Zhu, M.; Guo, M. Research advances in traditional and modern use of *Nelumbo nucifera*: Phytochemicals, health promoting activities and beyond. *Crit. Rev. Food Sci. Nutr.* **2019**, *59*, S189–S209. [CrossRef] [PubMed]
30. Duke, J.A. *Handbook of Medicinal Herbs*, 2nd ed.; CRC Press: Boca Raton, FL, USA, 2002.
31. Mukherjee, P.K.; Mukherjee, D.; Maji, A.K.; Rai, S.; Heinrich, M. The sacred lotus (*Nelumbo nucifera*)-phytochemical and therapeutic profile. *J. Pharm. Pharmacol.* **2009**, *61*, 407–422. [CrossRef]
32. Chen, S.; Li, X.; Wu, J.; Li, J.; Xiao, M.; Yang, Y.; Liu, Z.; Cheng, Y. Plumula Nelumbinis: A review of traditional uses, phytochemistry, pharmacology, pharmacokinetics and safety. *J. Ethnopharmacol.* **2021**, *266*, 113429. [CrossRef]
33. Paudel, K.R.; Panth, N. Phytochemical Profile and Biological Activity of *Nelumbo nucifera*. *Evid.-Based Complement. Altern. Med.* **2015**, *2015*, 789124. [CrossRef] [PubMed]
34. Sharma, B.R.; Gautam, L.N.S.; Adhikari, D.; Karki, R. A Comprehensive Review on Chemical Profiling of *Nelumbo nucifera*: Potential for Drug Development. *Phytother. Res.* **2016**, *31*, 3–26. [CrossRef]
35. Asokan, S.M.; Mariappan, R.; Muthusamy, S.; Velmurugan, B.K. Pharmacological benefits of neferine—A comprehensive review. *Life Sci.* **2018**, *199*, 60–70. [CrossRef] [PubMed]
36. Limwachiranon, J.; Huang, H.; Shi, Z.; Li, L.; Luo, Z. Lotus Flavonoids and Phenolic Acids: Health Promotion and Safe Consumption Dosages. *Compr. Rev. Food Sci. Food Saf.* **2018**, *17*, 458–471. [CrossRef]
37. Wang, Z.; Li, Y.; Ma, D.; Zeng, M.; Wang, Z.; Qin, F.; Chen, J.; Christian, M.; He, Z. Alkaloids from lotus (*Nelumbo nucifera*): Recent advances in biosynthesis, pharmacokinetics, bioactivity, safety, and industrial applications. *Crit. Rev. Food Sci. Nutr.* **2021**, *30*, 1–34. [CrossRef] [PubMed]
38. Manogaran, P.; Beeraka, N.M.; Padma, V.V. The Cytoprotective and Anti-cancer Potential of Bisbenzylisoquinoline Alkaloids from *Nelumbo nucifera*. *Curr. Top. Med. Chem.* **2019**, *19*, 2940–2957. [CrossRef] [PubMed]
39. Priya, L.B.; Huang, C.; Hu, R.; Balasubramanian, B.; Baskaran, R. An updated review on pharmacological properties of neferine—A bisbenzylisoquinoline alkaloid from *Nelumbo nucifera*. *J. Food Biochem.* **2021**, *45*, e13986. [CrossRef]
40. Kashiwada, Y.; Aoshima, A.; Ikeshiro, Y.; Chen, Y.-P.; Furukawa, H.; Itoigawa, M.; Fujioka, T.; Mihashi, K.; Cosentino, L.M.; Morris-Natschke, S.L.; et al. Anti-HIV benzylisoquinoline alkaloids and flavonoids from the leaves of *Nelumbo nucifera*, and structure–activity correlations with related alkaloids. *Bioorg. Med. Chem.* **2005**, *13*, 443–448. [CrossRef]
41. Huang, B.; Ban, X.; He, J.; Tong, J.; Tian, J.; Wang, Y. Comparative Analysis of Essential Oil Components and Antioxidant Activity of Extracts of *Nelumbo nucifera* from Various Areas of China. *J. Agric. Food Chem.* **2010**, *58*, 441–448. [CrossRef]
42. Chen, S.; Wu, B.-H.; Fang, J.-B.; Liu, Y.-L.; Zhang, H.-H.; Fang, L.-C.; Guan, L.; Li, S.-H. Analysis of flavonoids from lotus (*Nelumbo nucifera*) leaves using high performance liquid chromatography/photodiode array detector tandem electrospray ionization mass spectrometry and an extraction method optimized by orthogonal design. *J. Chromatogr. A* **2012**, *1227*, 145–153. [CrossRef]
43. Noysang, C.; Boonmatit, N. Preliminary Phytochemicals and Pharmacologic Activities Assessment of White and Pink *Nelumbo nucifera* Gaertn. Flowers. *Appl. Mech. Mater.* **2019**, *891*, 41–51. [CrossRef]
44. Zhenjia, Z.; Minglin, W.; Daijie, W.; Wenjuan, D.; Xiao, W.; Chengchao, Z. Preparative separation of alkaloids from *Nelumbo nucifera* leaves by conventional and pH-zone-refining counter-current chromatography. *J. Chromatogr. B* **2010**, *878*, 1647–1651. [CrossRef]
45. Ahn, J.H.; Kim, E.S.; Lee, C.; Kim, S.; Cho, S.-H.; Hwang, B.Y.; Lee, M.K. Chemical constituents from *Nelumbo nucifera* leaves and their anti-obesity effects. *Bioorg. Med. Chem. Lett.* **2013**, *23*, 3604–3608. [CrossRef]
46. Ma, C.; Wang, J.; Chu, H.; Zhang, X.; Wang, Z.; Wang, H.; Li, G. Purification and Characterization of Aporphine Alkaloids from Leaves of *Nelumbo nucifera* Gaertn and Their Effects on Glucose Consumption in 3T3-L1 Adipocytes. *Int. J. Mol. Sci.* **2014**, *15*, 3481–3494. [CrossRef] [PubMed]
47. Ye, L.-H.; He, X.-X.; You, C.; Tao, X.; Wang, L.-S.; Zhang, M.-D.; Zhou, Y.-F.; Chang, Q. Pharmacokinetics of Nuciferine and N-Nornuciferine, Two Major Alkaloids From *Nelumbo nucifera* Leaves, in Rat Plasma and the Brain. *Front. Pharmacol.* **2018**, *9*, 902. [CrossRef]
48. Chen, S.; Fang, L.; Xi, H.; Guan, L.; Fang, J.; Liu, Y.; Wu, B.; Li, S. Simultaneous qualitative assessment and quantitative analysis of flavonoids in various tissues of lotus (*Nelumbo nucifera*) using high performance liquid chromatography coupled with triple quad mass spectrometry. *Anal. Chim. Acta* **2012**, *724*, 127–135. [CrossRef]
49. Xiao, J.; Tian, B.; Xie, B.; Yang, E.; Shi, J.; Sun, Z. Supercritical fluid extraction and identification of isoquinoline alkaloids from leaves of *Nelumbo nucifera* Gaertn. *Eur. Food Res. Technol.* **2010**, *231*, 407–414. [CrossRef]

50. Do, T.C.M.V.; Nguyen, T.D.; Tran, H.; Stuppner, H.; Ganzera, M. Analysis of alkaloids in Lotus (*Nelumbo nucifera* Gaertn.) leaves by non-aqueous capillary electrophoresis using ultraviolet and mass spectrometric detection. *J. Chromatogr. A* **2013**, *1302*, 174–180. [CrossRef] [PubMed]
51. Kihyun, K.; Chang, S.W.; Shiyong, R.; Sangun, C.; Kangro, L. Phytochemical constituents of *Nelumbo nucifera*. *Nat. Prod. Sci.* **2009**, *15*, 90–95.
52. Lin, H.-Y.; Kuo, Y.-H.; Lin, Y.-L.; Chiang, W. Antioxidative Effect and Active Components from Leaves of Lotus (*Nelumbo nucifera*). *J. Agric. Food Chem.* **2009**, *57*, 6623–6629. [CrossRef]
53. Yajima, H. Prevention of diet-induced obesity by dietary polyphenols derived from Nelumbo nucifera and black tea. In *Polyphenols in Human Health and Disease*; Academic Press: London, UK, 2014; pp. 135–142. [CrossRef]
54. Fan, X.; Zhang, Q.; Lin, X.; Chen, Y.; Qian, L.; Li, K.; Lu, X.; Zheng, B.; Chen, L. Chemical composition of essential oil from Folium nelumbinis and its antioxidant activity. *BioRxiv* **2018**, 419945. [CrossRef]
55. Itoh, A.; Saitoh, T.; Tani, K.; Uchigaki, M.; Sugimoto, Y.; Yamada, J.; Nakajima, H.; Ohshiro, H.; Sun, S.; Tanahashi, T. Bisbenzylisoquinoline Alkaloids from *Nelumbo nucifera*. *Chem. Pharm. Bull.* **2011**, *59*, 947–951. [CrossRef]
56. Bi, Y.; Yang, G.; Li, H.; Zhang, G.; Guo, Z. Characterization of the Chemical Composition of Lotus Plumule Oil. *J. Agric. Food Chem.* **2006**, *54*, 7672–7677. [CrossRef] [PubMed]
57. Zhou, M.; Jiang, M.; Ying, X.; Cui, Q.; Han, Y.; Hou, Y.; Gao, J.; Bai, G.; Luo, G. Identification and Comparison of Anti-Inflammatory Ingredients from Different Organs of Lotus Nelumbo by UPLC/Q-TOF and PCA Coupled with a NF-κB Reporter Gene Assay. *PLoS ONE* **2013**, *8*, e81971. [CrossRef]
58. Duan, X.H.; Jiang, J.Q. A new benzylisoquinoline alkaloid from stems of *Nelumbo nucifera*. *Chin. Chem. Lett.* **2008**, *19*, 308–310. [CrossRef]
59. Indrayan, A.; Sharma, S.; Durgapal, D.; Kumar, N.; Kumar, M. Determination of nutritive value and analysis of mineral el-ements for some medicinally valued plants from Uttaranchal. *Curr. Sci.* **2005**, *89*, 1252–1255.
60. Das, S.; Ray, B.; Ghosal, P.K. Structural studies of a polysaccharide from the seeds of *Nelumbo nucifera*. *Carbohydr. Res.* **1992**, *224*, 331–335. [CrossRef]
61. Jiang, Y.; Ng, T.B.; Liu, Z.; Wang, C.; Li, N.; Qiao, W.; Liua, F. Immunoregulatory and anti-HIV-1 enzyme activities of antioxidant components from lotus (*Nelumbo nucifera* Gaertn.) rhizome. *Biosci. Rep.* **2011**, *31*, 381–390. [CrossRef] [PubMed]
62. Chaudhuri, P.K.; Singh, D. A new lipid and other constituents from the rhizomes of *Nelumbo nucifera*. *J. Asian Nat. Prod. Res.* **2009**, *11*, 583–587. [CrossRef]
63. Kredy, H.M.; Huang, D.; Xie, B.; He, H.; Yang, E.; Tian, B.; Xiao, D. Flavonols of lotus (*Nelumbo nucifera*, Gaertn.) seed epicarp and their antioxidant potential. *Eur. Food Res. Technol.* **2010**, *231*, 387–394. [CrossRef]
64. Liu, Y.; Ma, S.-S.; Ibrahim, S.; Li, E.-H.; Yang, H.; Huang, W. Identification and antioxidant properties of polyphenols in lotus seed epicarp at different ripening stages. *Food Chem.* **2015**, *185*, 159–164. [CrossRef] [PubMed]
65. Shad, M.A. Phytochemical composition and antioxidant properties of rhizomes of Nilumbo nucifera. *J. Med. Plants Res.* **2012**, *6*, 972–980. [CrossRef]
66. Nakamura, S.; Nakashima, S.; Tanabe, G.; Oda, Y.; Yokota, N.; Fujimoto, K.; Matsumoto, T.; Sakuma, R.; Ohta, T.; Ogawa, K.; et al. Alkaloid constituents from flower buds and leaves of sacred lotus (*Nelumbo nucifera*, Nymphaeaceae) with melanogenesis inhibitory activity in B16 melanoma cells. *Bioorg. Med. Chem.* **2013**, *21*, 779–787. [CrossRef] [PubMed]
67. Maneenet, J.; Omar, A.M.; Sun, S.; Kim, M.J.; Daodee, S.; Monthakantirat, O.; Boonyarat, C.; Chulikhit, Y.; Awale, S. Benzylisoquinoline alkaloids from *Nelumbo nucifera* Gaertn. petals with antiausterity activities against the HeLa human cervical cancer cell line. *Z. Nat. C* **2021**, *76*, 401–406. [CrossRef] [PubMed]
68. Zhu, H.-H.; Yang, J.-X.; Xiao, C.-H.; Mao, T.-Y.; Zhang, J.; Zhang, H.-Y. Differences in flavonoid pathway metabolites and transcripts affect yellow petal colouration in the aquatic plant *Nelumbo nucifera*. *BMC Plant Biol.* **2019**, *19*, 277. [CrossRef]
69. Rho, T.; Yoon, K.D. Chemical Constituents of *Nelumbo nucifera* Seeds. *Nat. Prod. Sci.* **2017**, *23*, 253–257. [CrossRef]
70. Wang, H.M.; Yang, W.L.; Yang, S.C.; Chen, C.Y. Chemical constituents from the leaves of *Nelumbo nucifera* Gaertn. cv. Rosa-plena. *Chem. Nat. Compd.* **2011**, *47*, 316–318. [CrossRef]
71. Agnihotri, V.; ElSohly, H.N.; Khan, S.I.; Jacob, M.R.; Joshi, V.C.; Smillie, T.; Khan, I.A.; Walker, L.A. Constituents of *Nelumbo nucifera* leaves and their antimalarial and antifungal activity. *Phytochem. Lett.* **2008**, *1*, 89–93. [CrossRef]
72. Kato, E.; Inagaki, Y.; Kawabata, J. Higenamine 4′-O-β-d-glucoside in the lotus plumule induces glucose uptake of L6 cells through β2-adrenergic receptor. *Bioorg. Med. Chem.* **2015**, *23*, 3317–3321. [CrossRef]
73. Morikawa, T.; Kitagawa, N.; Tanabe, G.; Ninomiya, K.; Okugawa, S.; Motai, C.; Kamei, I.; Yoshikawa, M.; Lee, I.-J.; Muraoka, O. Quantitative Determination of Alkaloids in Lotus Flower (Flower Buds of *Nelumbo nucifera*) and Their Melanogenesis Inhibitory Activity. *Molecules* **2016**, *21*, 930. [CrossRef]
74. Wang, L.L.; Liu, B.; Shi, R.B.; Tu, G.Z. Flavonoid chemical compositions of Folium nelumbinis, Beijing Zhongyiyao Daxue Xuebao. *J. Beijing Univ. Trad. Chin. Med.* **2008**, *31*, 116–118.
75. Liu, H.; Liu, J.; Zhang, J.; Qi, Y.; Jia, X.; Zhang, B.; Xiao, P. Simultaneous Quantitative and Chemical Fingerprint Analysis of Receptaculum Nelumbinis Based on HPLC–DAD-MS Combined with Chemometrics. *J. Chromatogr. Sci.* **2016**, *54*, 618–624. [CrossRef]

76. Liberati, A.; Altman, D.G.; Tetzlaff, J.; Mulrow, C.; Gøtzsche, P.C.; Ioannidis, J.P.A.; Clarke, M.; Devereaux, P.J.; Kleijnen, J.; Moher, D. The PRISMA statement for reporting systematic reviews and meta-analyses of studies that evaluate healthcare interventions: Explanation and elaboration. *BMJ* **2009**, *339*, b2700. [CrossRef]
77. Hooijmans, C.R.; Rovers, M.M.; de Vries, R.B.M.; Leenaars, M.; Ritskes-Hoitinga, M.; Langendam, M.W. SYRCLE's risk of bias tool for animal studies. *BMC Med. Res. Methodol.* **2014**, *14*, 43. [CrossRef]
78. Karki, R.; Rhyu, D.Y.; Kim, D.W. Effect of *Nelumbo nucifera* on proliferation, migration and expression of MMP-2 and MMP-9 of rSMC, A431 and MDA-MB-231. *Korean J. Plant Res.* **2008**, *21*, 96–102.
79. Yang, M.-Y.; Chang, Y.-C.; Chan, K.-C.; Lee, Y.-J.; Wang, C.-J. Flavonoid-enriched extracts from *Nelumbo nucifera* leaves inhibits proliferation of breast cancer in vitro and in vivo. *Eur. J. Integr. Med.* **2011**, *3*, e153–e163. [CrossRef]
80. Chang, C.-H.; Ou, T.-T.; Yang, M.-Y.; Huang, C.-C.; Wang, C.-J. *Nelumbo nucifera* Gaertn leaves extract inhibits the angiogenesis and metastasis of breast cancer cells by downregulation connective tissue growth factor (CTGF) mediated PI3K/AKT/ERK signaling. *J. Ethnopharmacol.* **2016**, *188*, 111–122. [CrossRef] [PubMed]
81. Wu, C.-H.; Yang, M.-Y.; Lee, Y.-J.; Wang, C.-J. *Nelumbo nucifera* leaf polyphenol extract inhibits breast cancer cells metastasis in vitro and in vivo through PKCα targeting. *J. Funct. Foods* **2017**, *37*, 480–490. [CrossRef]
82. Arjun, P.; Priya, S.; Krishnamoorthy, M.; Balasubramanian, K. Phytochemical analysis and anticancer activity of *Nelumbo nucifera* extracts. *J. Acad. Ind. Res.* **2012**, *1*, 81–85.
83. Krubha, A.; Vasan, P.T. Phytochemical Analysis and Anticancer Activity of *Nelumbo nucifera* Floral Receptacle Extracts in MCF-7 Cell Line. *J. Acad. Ind. Res.* **2016**, *4*, 251–256. [CrossRef]
84. Zhang, X.; Wang, X.; Wu, T.; Li, B.; Liu, T.; Wang, R.; Liu, Q.; Liu, Z.; Gong, Y.; Shao, C. Isoliensinine induces apoptosis in triple-negative human breast cancer cells through ROS generation and p38 MAPK/JNK activation. *Sci. Rep.* **2015**, *5*, 12579. [CrossRef]
85. Yang, D.; Zou, X.; Yi, R.; Liu, W.; Peng, D.; Zhao, X. Neferine increase in vitro anticancer effect of dehydroepiandrosterone on MCF-7 human breast cancer cells. *Appl. Biol. Chem.* **2016**, *59*, 585–596. [CrossRef]
86. Kadioglu, O.; Law, B.Y.K.; Mok, S.W.F.; Xu, S.-W.; Efferth, T.; Wong, V.K.W. Mode of Action Analyses of Neferine, a Bisbenzylisoquinoline Alkaloid of Lotus (*Nelumbo nucifera*) against Multidrug-Resistant Tumor Cells. *Front. Pharmacol.* **2017**, *8*, 238. [CrossRef] [PubMed]
87. Law, B.Y.K.; Michelangeli, F.; Qu, Y.Q.; Xu, S.-W.; Han, Y.; Mok, S.W.F.; de Seabra Rodrigues Dias, I.R.; Javed, M.-H.; Chan, W.-K.; Xue, W.-W.; et al. Neferine induces autophagy-dependent cell death in apoptosis-resistant cancers via ryanodine receptor and Ca^{2+}-dependent mechanism. *Sci. Rep.* **2019**, *9*, 20034. [CrossRef]
88. Liu, Z.; Zhang, S.; Wang, T.; Shao, H.; Gao, J.; Wang, Y.; Ge, Y. Neferine inhibits MDA-MB-231 cells growth and metastasis by regulating miR-374a/FGFR-2. *Chem. Interact.* **2019**, *309*, 108716. [CrossRef]
89. Kang, E.J.; Lee, S.K.; Park, K.-K.; Son, S.H.; Kim, K.R.; Chung, W.-Y. Liensinine and Nuciferine, Bioactive Components of *Nelumbo nucifera*, Inhibit the Growth of Breast Cancer Cells and Breast Cancer-Associated Bone Loss. *Evid.-Based Complement. Altern. Med.* **2017**, *2017*, 1583185. [CrossRef] [PubMed]
90. Zhou, J.; Li, G.; Zheng, Y.; Shen, H.-M.; Hu, X.; Ming, Q.-L.; Huang, C.; Li, P.; Gao, N. A novel autophagy/mitophagy inhibitor liensinine sensitizes breast cancer cells to chemotherapy through DNM1L-mediated mitochondrial fission. *Autophagy* **2015**, *11*, 1259–1279. [CrossRef]
91. Huang, Z.; Xu, H.; Chen, H.; Sun, B.; Huang, H.; Fan, H.; Zheng, J. Seco-neferine A–F, three new pairs of benzyltetrahydroisoquinoline alkaloid epimers from Plumula Nelumbinis and their activity. *Fitoterapia* **2021**, *153*, 104994. [CrossRef] [PubMed]
92. Li, H.-L.; Cheng, Y.; Zhou, Z.-W.; Long, H.-Z.; Luo, H.-Y.; Wen, D.-D.; Cheng, L.; Gao, L.-C. Isoliensinine induces cervical cancer cell cycle arrest and apoptosis by inhibiting the AKT/GSK3α pathway. *Oncol. Lett.* **2022**, *23*, 8. [CrossRef]
93. Dasari, S.; Bakthavachalam, V.; Chinnapaka, S.; Venkatesan, R.; Samy, A.L.P.A.; Munirathinam, G. Neferine, an alkaloid from lotus seed embryo targets HeLa and SiHa cervical cancer cells via pro-oxidant anticancer mechanism. *Phytother. Res.* **2020**, *34*, 2366–2384. [CrossRef]
94. Zhao, X.; Feng, X.; Wang, C.; Peng, D.; Zhu, K.; Song, J.-L. Anticancer activity of *Nelumbo nucifera* stamen extract in human colon cancer HCT-116 cells in vitro. *Oncol. Lett.* **2017**, *13*, 1470–1478. [CrossRef]
95. Prasath, M.; Narasimha, M.B.; Chih-Yang, H.; Viswanadha, V.P. Neferine and isoliensinine from *Nelumbo nucifera* induced reactive oxygen species (ROS)-mediated apoptosis in colorectal cancer HCT-15 cells. *Afr. J. Pharm. Pharmacol.* **2019**, *13*, 90–99. [CrossRef]
96. Qi, Q.; Li, R.; Li, H.-Y.; Cao, Y.-B.; Bai, M.; Fan, X.-J.; Wang, S.-Y.; Zhang, B.; Li, S. Identification of the anti-tumor activity and mechanisms of nuciferine through a network pharmacology approach. *Acta Pharmacol. Sin.* **2016**, *37*, 963–972. [CrossRef] [PubMed]
97. Wang, Y.; Li, Y.-J.; Huang, X.-H.; Zheng, C.-C.; Yin, X.-F.; Li, B.; He, Q.-Y. Liensinine perchlorate inhibits colorectal cancer tumorigenesis by inducing mitochondrial dysfunction and apoptosis. *Food Funct.* **2018**, *9*, 5536–5546. [CrossRef]
98. Guon, T.E.; Chung, H.S. Hyperoside and rutin of *Nelumbo nucifera* induce mitochondrial apoptosis through a caspase-dependent mechanism in HT-29 human colon cancer cells. *Oncol. Lett.* **2016**, *11*, 2463–2470. [CrossRef]
99. An, K.; Zhang, Y.; Liu, Y.; Yan, S.; Hou, Z.; Cao, M.; Liu, G.; Dong, C.; Gao, J.; Liu, G. Neferine induces apoptosis by modulating the ROS-mediated JNK pathway in esophageal squamous cell carcinoma. *Oncol. Rep.* **2020**, *44*, 1116–1126. [CrossRef]
100. Wang, J.; Dong, Y.; Li, Q. Neferine induces mitochondrial dysfunction to exert anti-proliferative and anti-invasive activities on retinoblastoma. *Exp. Biol. Med.* **2020**, *245*, 1385–1394. [CrossRef]

101. Shen, Y.; Bian, R.; Li, Y.; Gao, Y.; Liu, Y.; Xu, Y.; Song, X.; Zhang, Y. Liensinine induces gallbladder cancer apoptosis and G2/M arrest by inhibiting ZFX-induced PI3K/AKT pathway. *Acta Biochim. Biophys. Sin.* **2019**, *51*, 607–614. [CrossRef]
102. Zheng, Y.; Wang, Q.; Zhuang, W.; Lu, X.; Miron, A.; Chai, T.-T.; Zheng, B.; Xiao, J. Cytotoxic, Antitumor and Immunomodulatory Effects of the Water-Soluble Polysaccharides from Lotus (*Nelumbo nucifera* Gaertn.) Seeds. *Molecules* **2016**, *21*, 1465. [CrossRef] [PubMed]
103. Huang, C.; Li, Y.; Cao, P.; Xie, Z.; Qin, Z. Synergistic effect of hyperthermia and neferine on reverse multidrug resistance in adriamycin-resistant SGC7901/ADM gastric cancer cells. *J. Huazhong Univ. Sci. Technol.* **2011**, *31*, 488–496. [CrossRef]
104. Xue, F.; Liu, Z.; Xu, J.; Xu, X.; Chen, X.; Tian, F. Neferine inhibits growth and migration of gastrointestinal stromal tumor cell line GIST-T1 by up-regulation of miR-449a. *Biomed. Pharmacother.* **2019**, *109*, 1951–1959. [CrossRef]
105. Liu, C.-M.; Kao, C.-L.; Wu, H.-M.; Li, W.-J.; Huang, C.-T.; Li, H.-T.; Chen, C.-Y. Antioxidant and Anticancer Aporphine Alkaloids from the Leaves of *Nelumbo nucifera* Gaertn. cv. Rosa-plena. *Molecules* **2014**, *19*, 17829–17838. [CrossRef]
106. Yang, J.-H.; Yu, K.; Si, X.-K.; Li, S.; Cao, Y.-J.; Li, W.; Zhang, J.-X. Liensinine inhibited gastric cancer cell growth through ROS generation and the PI3K/AKT pathway. *J. Cancer* **2019**, *10*, 6431–6438. [CrossRef] [PubMed]
107. Zhu, F.; Li, X.; Tang, X.; Jiang, J.; Han, Y.; Li, Y.; Ma, C.; Liu, Z.; He, Y. Neferine promotes the apoptosis of HNSCC through the accumulation of p62/SQSTM1 caused by autophagic flux inhibition. *Int. J. Mol. Med.* **2021**, *48*, 124. [CrossRef] [PubMed]
108. Byun, D.-S. Kaempferol Isolated from *Nelumbo nucifera* Stamens Negatively Regulates FcεRI Expression in Human Basophilic KU812F Cells. *J. Microbiol. Biotechnol.* **2009**, *19*, 155–160. [CrossRef]
109. Qin, Q.; Chen, X.-P.; Yang, Z.-S.; Xiao, Y.-H.; Min, H.; Li, Y.-J. Neferine increases STI571 chemosensitivity via inhibition of P-gp expression in STI571-resistant K562 cells. *Leuk. Lymphoma* **2011**, *52*, 694–700. [CrossRef]
110. Li, Q.-H.; Sui, L.-P.; Zhao, Y.-H.; Chen, B.-G.; Li, J.; Ma, Z.-H.; Hu, Z.-H.; Tang, Y.-L.; Guo, Y.-X. Tripartite Motif-Containing 44 is Involved in the Tumorigenesis of Laryngeal Squamous Cell Carcinoma, and its Expression is Downregulated by Nuciferine. *Tohoku J. Exp. Med.* **2021**, *254*, 17–23. [CrossRef] [PubMed]
111. Shen, Y.; Guan, Y.; Song, X.; He, J.; Xie, Z.; Zhang, Y.; Zhang, H.; Tang, D. Polyphenols extract from lotus seedpod (*Nelumbo nucifera* Gaertn.): Phenolic compositions, antioxidant, and antiproliferative activities. *Food Sci. Nutr.* **2019**, *7*, 3062–3070. [CrossRef]
112. Duan, Y.; Xu, H.; Luo, X.; Zhang, H.; He, Y.; Sun, G.; Sun, X. Procyanidins from *Nelumbo nucifera* Gaertn. Seedpod induce autophagy mediated by reactive oxygen species generation in human hepatoma G2 cells. *Biomed. Pharmacother.* **2016**, *79*, 135–152. [CrossRef]
113. Xiao-Hong, A.; Xiao-Qing, T.; Yan-Ping, L.; Hua-Qing, L.; Lin, D. Effect of Neferine on Adriamycin-resistance of Thermotolerant Hepatocarcinoma Cell Line HepG2/thermotolerance. *Chin. J Cancer* **2007**, *26*, 357–360.
114. Yoon, J.-S.; Kim, H.-M.; Yadunandam, A.K.; Kim, N.-H.; Jung, H.-A.; Choi, J.-S.; Kim, C.-Y.; Kim, G.-D. Neferine isolated from *Nelumbo nucifera* enhances anti-cancer activities in Hep3B cells: Molecular mechanisms of cell cycle arrest, ER stress induced apoptosis and anti-angiogenic response. *Phytomedicine* **2013**, *20*, 1013–1022. [CrossRef]
115. Poornima, P.; Quency, R.S.; Padma, V.V. Neferine induces reactive oxygen species mediated intrinsic pathway of apoptosis in HepG2 cells. *Food Chem.* **2013**, *136*, 659–667. [CrossRef] [PubMed]
116. Deng, G.; Zeng, S.; Ma, J.; Zhang, Y.; Qu, Y.; Han, Y.; Yin, L.; Cai, C.; Guo, C.; Shen, H. The anti-tumor activities of Neferine on cell invasion and oxaliplatin sensitivity regulated by EMT via Snail signaling in hepatocellular carcinoma. *Sci. Rep.* **2017**, *7*, 41616. [CrossRef] [PubMed]
117. Shu, G.; Yue, L.; Zhao, W.; Xu, C.; Yang, J.; Wang, S.; Yang, X. Isoliensinine, a Bioactive Alkaloid Derived from Embryos of *Nelumbo nucifera*, Induces Hepatocellular Carcinoma Cell Apoptosis through Suppression of NF-κB Signaling. *J. Agric. Food Chem.* **2015**, *63*, 8793–8803. [CrossRef] [PubMed]
118. Shu, G.; Zhang, L.; Jiang, S.; Cheng, Z.; Wang, G.; Huang, X.; Yang, X. Isoliensinine induces dephosphorylation of NF-κB p65 subunit at Ser536 via a PP2A-dependent mechanism in hepatocellular carcinoma cells: Roles of impairing PP2A/I2PP2A interaction. *Oncotarget* **2016**, *7*, 40285–40296. [CrossRef]
119. Horng, C.-T.; Huang, C.-W.; Yang, M.-Y.; Chen, T.-H.; Chang, Y.-C.; Wang, C.-J. *Nelumbo nucifera* leaf extract treatment attenuated preneoplastic lesions and oxidative stress in the livers of diethylnitrosamine-treated rats. *Environ. Toxicol.* **2017**, *32*, 2327–2340. [CrossRef]
120. Yang, M.-Y.; Hung, T.-W.; Wang, C.-J.; Tseng, T.-H. Inhibitory Effect of *Nelumbo nucifera* Leaf Extract on 2-Acetylaminofluorene-induced Hepatocarcinogenesis Through Enhancing Antioxidative Potential and Alleviating Inflammation in Rats. *Antioxidants* **2019**, *8*, 329. [CrossRef]
121. Kim, N.; Yang, I.; Kim, S.; Lee, C. Lotus (*Nelumbo nucifera*) seedpod extract inhibits cell proliferation and induces apoptosis in non-small cell lung cancer cells via downregulation of Axl. *J. Food Biochem.* **2021**, *45*, e13601. [CrossRef]
122. Poornima, P.; Weng, C.F.; Padma, V.V. Neferine from *Nelumbo nucifera* induces autophagy through the inhibition of PI3K/Akt/mTOR pathway and ROS hyper generation in A549 cells. *Food Chem.* **2013**, *141*, 3598–3605. [CrossRef]
123. Poornima, P.; Weng, C.F.; Padma, V.V. Neferine, an alkaloid from lotus seed embryo, inhibits human lung cancer cell growth by MAPK activation and cell cycle arrest. *BioFactors* **2014**, *40*, 121–131. [CrossRef]
124. Selvi, S.K.; Vinoth, A.; Varadharajan, T.; Weng, C.F.; Padma, V.V. Neferine augments therapeutic efficacy of cisplatin through ROS-mediated non-canonical autophagy in human lung adenocarcinoma (A549 cells). *Food Chem. Toxicol.* **2017**, *103*, 28–40. [CrossRef]
125. Sivalingam, K.S.; Paramasivan, P.; Weng, C.F.; Viswanadha, V.P. Neferine Potentiates the Antitumor Effect of Cisplatin in Human Lung Adenocarcinoma Cells via a Mitochondria-Mediated Apoptosis Pathway. *J. Cell. Biochem.* **2017**, *118*, 2865–2876. [CrossRef]

126. Liu, W.; Yi, D.-D.; Guo, J.-L.; Xiang, Z.-X.; Deng, L.-F.; He, L. Nuciferine, extracted from *Nelumbo nucifera* Gaertn, inhibits tumor-promoting effect of nicotine involving Wnt/β-catenin signaling in non-small cell lung cancer. *J. Ethnopharmacol.* **2015**, *165*, 83–93. [CrossRef] [PubMed]
127. Sivalingam, K.; Amirthalingam, V.; Ganasan, K.; Huang, C.-Y.; Viswanadha, V.P. Neferine suppresses diethylnitrosamine-induced lung carcinogenesis in Wistar rats. *Food Chem. Toxicol.* **2019**, *123*, 385–398. [CrossRef] [PubMed]
128. Zhao, X.; Feng, X.; Peng, D.; Liu, W.; Sun, P.; Li, G.; Gu, L.; Song, J.-L. Anticancer activities of alkaloids extracted from the Ba lotus seed in human nasopharyngeal carcinoma CNE-1 cells. *Exp. Ther. Med.* **2016**, *12*, 3113–3120. [CrossRef] [PubMed]
129. Pham, D.-C.; Chang, Y.-C.; Lin, S.-R.; Fuh, Y.-M.; Tsai, M.-J.; Weng, C.-F. FAK and S6K1 Inhibitor, Neferine, Dually Induces Autophagy and Apoptosis in Human Neuroblastoma Cells. *Molecules* **2018**, *23*, 3110. [CrossRef]
130. Li, Z.; Chen, Y.; An, T.; Liu, P.; Zhu, J.; Yang, H.; Zhang, W.; Dong, T.; Jiang, J.; Zhang, Y.; et al. Nuciferine inhibits the progression of glioblastoma by suppressing the SOX2-AKT/STAT3-Slug signaling pathway. *J. Exp. Clin. Cancer Res.* **2019**, *38*, 139. [CrossRef]
131. Xu, L.; Zhang, X.; Li, Y.; Lu, S.; Lu, S.; Li, J.; Wang, Y.; Tian, X.; Wei, J.-J.; Shao, C.; et al. Neferine induces autophagy of human ovarian cancer cells via p38 MAPK/JNK activation. *Tumor Biol.* **2016**, *37*, 8721–8729. [CrossRef]
132. Erdogan, S.; Turkekul, K. Neferine inhibits proliferation and migration of human prostate cancer stem cells through p38 MAPK/JNK activation. *J. Food Biochem.* **2020**, *44*, e13253. [CrossRef]
133. Nazim, U.M.; Yin, H.; Park, S. Neferine treatment enhances the TRAIL-induced apoptosis of human prostate cancer cells via autophagic flux and the JNK pathway. *Int. J. Oncol.* **2020**, *56*, 1152–1161. [CrossRef]
134. Liu, C.M.; Wu, Z.; Pan, B.; An, L.; Zhu, C.; Zhou, J.; Jiang, Y. The antiandrogenic effect of neferine, liensinine and isoliensinine by inhibiting 5-α-reductase and androgen receptor expression via PI3K/AKT signaling pathway in prostate cancer. *Pharmazie* **2021**, *76*, 225–231. [CrossRef]
135. Kim, E.; Sung, E.-G.; Song, I.-H.; Kim, J.-Y.; Sung, H.-J.; Sohn, H.-Y.; Park, J.-Y.; Lee, T.-J. Neferine-induced apoptosis is dependent on the suppression of Bcl-2 expression via downregulation of p65 in renal cancer cells. *Acta Biochim. Biophys. Sin.* **2019**, *51*, 734–742. [CrossRef]
136. Zhang, X.; Liu, Z.; Xu, B.; Sun, Z.; Gong, Y.; Shao, C. Neferine, an alkaloid ingredient in lotus seed embryo, inhibits proliferation of human osteosarcoma cells by promoting p38 MAPK-mediated p21 stabilization. *Eur. J. Pharmacol.* **2012**, *677*, 47–54. [CrossRef]
137. Duan, Y.; Zhang, H.; Xu, F.; Xie, B.; Yang, X.; Wang, Y.; Yan, Y. Inhibition effect of procyanidins from lotus seedpod on mouse B16 melanoma invivo and in vitro. *Food Chem.* **2010**, *122*, 84–91. [CrossRef]
138. Lai, P.-J.; Kao, E.-S.; Chen, S.-R.; Huang, Y.-T.; Wang, C.-J.; Huang, H.-P. *Nelumbo nucifera* Leaf Extracts Inhibit Melanogenesis in B16 Melanoma Cells and Guinea Pigs through Downregulation of CREB/MITF Activation. *J. Food Nutr. Res.* **2020**, *8*, 459–465. [CrossRef]
139. Wu, P.-F.; Chiu, C.-C.; Chen, C.-Y.; Wang, H.-M.D. 7-Hydroxydehydronuciferine induces human melanoma death via triggering autophagy and apoptosis. *Exp. Dermatol.* **2015**, *24*, 930–935. [CrossRef]
140. Zhao, L.; Wang, X.; Wu, J.; Jia, Y.; Wang, W.; Zhang, S.; Wang, J. Improved RP-HPLC method to determine neferine in dog plasma and its application to pharmacokinetics. *J. Chromatogr. B* **2007**, *857*, 341–346. [CrossRef] [PubMed]
141. Huang, Y.; Bai, Y.; Zhao, L.; Hu, T.; Hu, B.; Wang, J.; Xiang, J. Pharmacokinetics and metabolism of neferine in rats after a single oral administration. *Biopharm. Drug Dispos.* **2007**, *28*, 361–372. [CrossRef]
142. Zhou, H.; Li, L.; Jiang, H.; Zeng, S. Identification of Three New N-Demethylated and O-Demethyled Bisbenzylisoquinoline Alkaloid Metabolites of Isoliensinine from Dog Hepatic Microsomes. *Molecules* **2012**, *17*, 11712–11720. [CrossRef] [PubMed]
143. Zhao, Y.; Hellum, B.H.; Liang, A.; Nilsen, O.G. The In Vitro Inhibition of Human CYP1A2, CYP2D6 and CYP3A4 by Tetrahydropalmatine, Neferine and Berberine. *Phytother. Res.* **2011**, *26*, 277–283. [CrossRef]
144. Ye, L.-H.; He, X.-X.; Kong, L.-T.; Liao, Y.-H.; Pan, R.-L.; Xiao, B.-X.; Liu, X.-M.; Chang, Q. Identification and characterization of potent CYP2D6 inhibitors in lotus leaves. *J. Ethnopharmacol.* **2014**, *153*, 190–196. [CrossRef] [PubMed]
145. Zou, S.; Ge, Y.; Chen, X.; Li, J.; Yang, X.; Wang, H.; Gao, X.; Chang, Y.-X. Simultaneous Determination of Five Alkaloids by HPLC-MS/MS Combined With Micro-SPE in Rat Plasma and Its Application to Pharmacokinetics After Oral Administration of Lotus Leaf Extract. *Front. Pharmacol.* **2019**, *10*, 1252. [CrossRef] [PubMed]
146. Yan, K.; Wang, X.; Wang, Z.; Wang, Y.; Luan, Z.; Gao, X.; Wang, R. The risk of higenamine adverse analytical findings following oral administration of plumula nelumbinis capsules. *Drug Test. Anal.* **2019**, *11*, 1731–1736. [CrossRef] [PubMed]
147. Liao, C.-H.; Lin, J.-Y. Purified active lotus plumule (*Nelumbo nucifera* Gaertn) polysaccharides exert anti-inflammatory activity through decreasing Toll-like receptor-2 and -4 expressions using mouse primary splenocytes. *J. Ethnopharmacol.* **2013**, *147*, 164–173. [CrossRef] [PubMed]
148. Kunanusorn, P.; Panthong, A.; Pittayanurak, P.; Wanauppathamkul, S.; Nathasaen, N.; Reutrakul, V. Acute and subchronic oral toxicity studies of *Nelumbo nucifera* stamens extract in rats. *J. Ethnopharmacol.* **2011**, *134*, 789–795. [CrossRef]
149. Rajput, M.A.; Alam Khan, R. Phytochemical screening, acute toxicity, anxiolytic and antidepressant activities of the *Nelumbo nucifera* fruit. *Metab. Brain Dis.* **2017**, *32*, 743–749. [CrossRef]
150. Liu, X.; Qu, W.; Liang, J.Y. Research progress of *Nelumbo nucefera* gaertn. *Strait Pharm. J.* **2010**, *22*, 1–5.
151. Chung, H.-S.; Lee, H.J.; Shim, I.; Bae, H. Assessment of anti-depressant effect of nelumbinis semen on rats under chronic mild stress and its subchronic oral toxicity in rats and beagle dogs. *BMC Complement. Altern. Med.* **2012**, *12*, 68–82. [CrossRef]

cancers

Article

Beta-Caryophyllene Exhibits Anti-Proliferative Effects through Apoptosis Induction and Cell Cycle Modulation in Multiple Myeloma Cells

Federica Mannino [1], Giovanni Pallio [1], Roberta Corsaro [1], Letteria Minutoli [1], Domenica Altavilla [2], Giovanna Vermiglio [2], Alessandro Allegra [3], Ali H. Eid [4,5], Alessandra Bitto [1,*], Francesco Squadrito [1,*] and Natasha Irrera [1]

1 Department of Clinical and Experimental Medicine, University of Messina, Via C. Valeria Gazzi, 98125 Messina, Italy; fmannino@unime.it (F.M.); gpallio@unime.it (G.P.); robi.corsaro@libero.it (R.C.); lminutoli@unime.it (L.M.); nirrera@unime.it (N.I.)
2 Department of Biomedical, Dental, Morphological and Functional Imaging Sciences, University of Messina, Via C. Valeria Gazzi, 98125 Messina, Italy; daltavilla@unime.it (D.A.); giovanna.vermiglio1@unime.it (G.V.)
3 Department of Human Pathology in Adulthood and Childhood, University of Messina, Via C. Valeria Gazzi, 98125 Messina, Italy; alessandro.allegra@unime.it
4 Department of Basic Medical Sciences, College of Medicine, QU Health, Qatar University, 2713 Doha, Qatar; ali.eid@qu.edu.qa
5 Biomedical and Pharmaceutical Research Unit, QU Health, Qatar University, 2713 Doha, Qatar
* Correspondence: abitto@unime.it (A.B.); fsquadrito@unime.it (F.S.)

Citation: Mannino, F.; Pallio, G.; Corsaro, R.; Minutoli, L.; Altavilla, D.; Vermiglio, G.; Allegra, A.; Eid, A.H.; Bitto, A.; Squadrito, F.; et al. Beta-Caryophyllene Exhibits Anti-Proliferative Effects through Apoptosis Induction and Cell Cycle Modulation in Multiple Myeloma Cells. *Cancers* **2021**, *13*, 5741. https://doi.org/10.3390/cancers13225741

Academic Editors: Sikander Ailawadhi and Anupam Bishayee

Received: 12 October 2021
Accepted: 15 November 2021
Published: 16 November 2021

Simple Summary: Multiple myeloma (MM) is a malignant B-cell neoplasm characterized by the uncontrolled proliferation of plasma cells. MM cells highly express cannabinoid type 2 receptors (CB2Rs), and previous studies have already demonstrated that the Cannabis plant and its derivatives may have anti-emetic as well as anti-neoplastic effects. In the present study, β-caryophyllene (BCP), a natural CB2R agonist, was evaluated for its anti-proliferative and anti-cancer effects. BCP was able to induce the apoptotic mechanism by activating the molecules involved in triggering apoptosis, such as Bax and caspase 3, and it reduced the anti-apoptotic protein Bcl-2; BCP also regulated cell proliferation through sophisticated crosstalk between Akt, β-catenin, and cyclin D1/CDK 4-6 in a concentration-dependent manner. These effects were counteracted by AM630, a CB2R antagonist, thus showing that BCP acts through CB2R. The data obtained so far demonstrate that BCP, thanks to its anti-proliferative effects, might represent an interesting additional therapeutic approach to improve anti-myeloma therapy.

Abstract: Cannabinoid receptors, which are widely distributed in the body, have been considered as possible pharmacological targets for the management of several tumors. Cannabinoid type 2 receptors (CB2Rs) belong to the G protein-coupled receptor family and are mainly expressed in hematopoietic and immune cells, such as B-cells, T-cells, and macrophages; thus, CB2R activation might be useful for treating cancers affecting plasma cells, such as multiple myeloma (MM). Previous studies have shown that CB2R stimulation may have anti-proliferative effects; therefore, the purpose of the present study was to explore the antitumor effect of beta-caryophyllene (BCP), a CB2R agonist, in an in vitro model of MM. Dexamethasone-resistant (MM.1R) and sensitive (MM.1S) human multiple myeloma cell lines were used in this study. Cells were treated with different concentrations of BCP for 24 h, and a group of cells was pre-incubated with AM630, a specific CB2R antagonist. BCP treatment reduced cell proliferation through CB2R stimulation; notably, BCP considerably increased the pro-apoptotic protein Bax and decreased the anti-apoptotic molecule Bcl-2. Furthermore, an increase in caspase 3 protein levels was detected following BCP incubation, thus demonstrating its anti-proliferative effect through apoptosis activation. In addition, BCP regulated AKT, Wnt1, and beta-catenin expression, showing that CB2R stimulation may decrease cancer cell proliferation by modulating Wnt/β-catenin signaling. These effects were counteracted by AM630 co-incubation, thus confirming that BCP's mechanism of action is mainly related to CB2R modulation. A decrease in β-catenin regulated the impaired cell cycle and especially promoted cyclin D1 and CDK 4/6 reduction.

Taken together, these data revealed that BCP might have significant and effective anti-cancer and anti-proliferative effects in MM cells by activating apoptosis, modulating different molecular pathways, and downregulating the cell cycle.

Keywords: beta-caryophyllene; cannabinoid receptor 2; multiple myeloma; apoptosis; Wnt/β-catenin

1. Introduction

Multiple myeloma (MM) is a malignant B-cell neoplasm characterized by monoclonal plasma cell proliferation in the bone marrow. Among the hematologic tumors, MM is the second-most frequent malignancy worldwide, with over 30,000 cases of MM reported in the United States in 2019 [1]. One of the main hallmarks of MM is the uncontrolled proliferation of clonal plasma cells, which is responsible for its malignancy and possible invasion [2]. This uncontrolled proliferation is mainly due to the dysregulation of the cell cycle, which contributes to the progression of the disease and worsens the prognosis. Some patients may become refractory to the current therapies, which are mainly based on the use of proteasome inhibitors, bisphosphonates, corticosteroids, immunosuppressant drugs, and peripheral blood stem cell transplantation; for this reason, MM is still an incurable cancer [3], and various efforts are devoted to discovering new therapeutic approaches. In this context, previous studies have shown that cannabinoid type 2 receptors (CB2Rs) are highly expressed in B-cells, which are plasma cell (PCs) precursors, and in hematopoietic cells [4,5]. In addition, MM cell lines and primary MM cells highly express CB2Rs, suggesting significant expression of CB2Rs in B PCs as well [6]. Interestingly, some studies have indicated that immune cells are able to secrete 2-arachidonoyl glycerol (2-AG), an endocannabinoid that acts as an agonist of cannabinoid receptors [7–9]. Several studies have demonstrated the anti-cancer activity of cannabinoids [10–13], which is mainly ascribed to cell proliferation arrest, selective apoptosis induction, cell cycle modulation, and tumor growth inhibition [14,15]. In particular, a previous study demonstrated that cannabinoid derivatives are able to reduce the cell viability of the MM cell line and primary MPCs collected from high-risk MM patients; interestingly, this anti-proliferative effect was selective toward cancer cells and not normal healthy cells [10].

The high selectivity of cannabinoid derivatives assumes an important translational significance since the available chemotherapeutic agents are not specific to cancer cells and are responsible for a great number of adverse events.

Beta-caryophyllene (β-caryophyllene, BCP) is a non-psychoactive sesquiterpene extracted from Copaifera spp and Cannabis spp with significant antioxidant, anti-inflammatory, chemo-preventive, neuroprotective, and anti-proliferative effects [16–18]. BCP has been approved by the Food and Drug Administration (FDA) as a food additive, taste enhancer, and flavoring agent, and it could be used as a nutraceutical and a dietary supplement [16,19]. However, BCP is poorly aqueous-soluble and is sensitive to light, oxygen, humidity, and high temperatures; for this reason, its bioavailability may be affected, thus reducing its pharmacologic activity [20]. In fact, several delivery systems have been developed to overcome this significant limitation and improve both BCP stability and bioavailability [21–23] so that this promising compound could be used in future clinical practice.

BCP selectively binds CB2R [24,25], and as a result, it does not induce any psychoactive effects related to CB1 receptor binding. This mechanism of action is responsible for the pharmacological effects of BCP, and its anti-cancer activity is mainly based on cell survival protein inhibition, cell cycle modulation, and apoptosis activation [13].

In the light of the cannabinoid's anti-cancer effects, evidenced by high CB2R expression in myeloma cells, the aim of this study was to evaluate the effects of BCP, a CB2R agonist, in dexamethasone-resistant (MM.1R) and sensitive (MM.1S) human MM cell lines.

2. Materials and Methods

2.1. Cell Cultures

MM.1S (steroid-based therapy-resistant) and MM.1R (dexamethasone-resistant), human B lymphoblasts obtained from the peripheral blood of a patient affected by MM, were provided by ATCC® CRL-2974™ and ATCC® CRL-2975™ (ATCC Manassas, Manassas, VA, USA), respectively. Both cell cultures were plated in RPMI-1640 media (ATCC Manassas, Manassas, VA, USA) with 2 mM L-glutamine, 1 mM sodium pyruvate, 1% antibiotic mixture (Sigma-Aldrich, St. Louis, MO, USA), and 10% fetal bovine serum (FBS) (ATCC Manassas, Manassas, VA, USA) in a humidified incubator at 37 °C with a percentage of 5% CO_2. In addition, RPMI 1788 cells (ATCC® CCL-156™; ATCC Manassas, Manassas, VA, USA), which are human B lymphoblasts obtained from the peripheral blood of a healthy donor, were cultured in RPMI-1640 medium supplemented with 20% FBS (ATCC Manassas, Manassas, VA, USA) and a 1% antibiotic mixture (Sigma-Aldrich, St. Louis, MO, USA) in a humidified incubator at 37 °C with a percentage of 5% CO_2.

2.2. Cell Treatment

MM.1S and MM.1R were placed in culture using 6-well plates with a density of 2.5×10^5 cells/well; cells were treated with BCP (Sigma-Aldrich, St. Louis, MO, USA; purity >80%) at concentrations of 50 and 100 μM for 24 h. At the end of BCP treatment, cells were collected to perform fluorescein diacetate/propidium iodide (FDA/PI) staining, molecular evaluations, and immunofluorescence. In addition, a group of MM.1S and MM.1R cells were treated with AM630 (Tocris Bioscience, Oxford, UK), a CB2 receptor antagonist, at a concentration of 100 nM 2 h before BCP treatment.

2.3. FDA/PI Staining

FDA/PI staining (Sigma-Aldrich, St. Louis, MO, USA) was used to evaluate MM.1S and MM.1R cell viability. FDA stock solution was prepared by dissolving 5 mg of FDA in 1 mL of acetone, and a PI stock solution was prepared by dissolving 2 mg of PI in 1 mL of phosphate-buffered saline (PBS). The FDA/PI staining solution was prepared by adding 8 μL of FDA (5mg/mL) and 50 μL of PI (2 mg/mL) in 5 mL of culture medium without FBS. Cells were seeded at a density of 5×10^5 cells/well in a 24-well plate and treated with 50 and 100 μM BCP. The culture medium was removed after 24 h, and cells were stained with the FDA/PI staining solution for 5 min at room temperature in the dark. Viable cells were observed with a fluorescence microscope. The quantification of positive cells was performed with ImageJ software for Windows (Softonic, Barcelona, Spain).

2.4. MTT Assay

An MTT assay was carried out to evaluate cancer cell viability following BCP treatment. MM.1S, MM.1R, and RPMI 1788 were seeded in a 96-well plate at a density of 2×10^5 cells/well for 24 h. The day after, cells were treated with doubling concentrations of BCP (6.25, 12.5, 25, 50, 100, and 200 μM) for 24 h in order to evaluate the cytotoxic effect, as previously described [25].

2.5. Trypan Blue Assay

Trypan blue dye was used to quantify the comparative number of live and dead cells. Cells were collected and centrifuged at 1200 rpm for 5 min. The obtained cell pellets were resuspended in 1 mL of fresh medium. The suspension and a 0.4% trypan blue/PBS solution were mixed in a 1:1 ratio. Ten microliters of this mixture was loaded on a hemocytometer and visualized with an optical microscope. The percent viability was determined using the following formula:

$$\% \text{ viable cells} = [1.00 - (\text{Number of blue cells} \div \text{Number of total cells})] \times 100$$

2.6. Measurements of Proteins by Enzyme-Linked Immunosorbent Assay (ELISA)

CDK4, CDK6, and Wnt1 levels were evaluated in the cell lysates, using the respective enzyme-linked immunosorbent assay (ELISA) kits (LSBio, Seattle, WA, USA, or MyBioSource, San Diego, CA, USA), following the instructions reported by the manufacturer [26].

2.7. Western Blot Analysis

After 24 h of BCP treatment, cells were collected, and the protein expressions of phospho-β-catenin, phospho-Akt, Bax, caspase-3 (Cell Signaling, Danvers, MA, USA), cyclin D1 (Gentex, Irvine, CA, USA), and Bcl-2 (Abcam, Cambridge, UK) were evaluated, as previously described in detail [27,28].

2.8. Immunofluorescence Staining

MM.1S and MM.1R were seeded onto glass coverslips, processed for immunofluorescence following 24 h of BCP treatment, and photographed according to the techniques previously described in detail [29].

2.9. Statistical Analysis

All results are expressed as means ± standard error of the mean (SEM). The reported results are the means of three experiments. In order to guarantee reproducibility, all assays were performed in duplicate. Statistical analysis was conducted using one-way ANOVA with Tukey's post hoc test for intergroup comparisons. A p-value less than 0.05 was considered significant. Graphs were prepared using GraphPad Prism software (Version 8.0 for macOS, San Diego, CA, USA).

3. Results

3.1. BCP Reduces Cancer Cells Viability

Cell viability was evaluated by incubating MM.1S, MM.1R, and RPMI 1788 cell lines with increasing concentrations of BCP, ranging from 6.25 μM to 200 μM. The results of the MTT assay showed that MM.1R cell viability was reduced when cells were treated with BCP at concentrations of 25 μM to 200 μM; in particular, cell viability was reduced to about 80% when BCP was used at a concentration of 50 μM and to 50% with 100 μM BCP following 24 h of treatment (Figure 1A). As shown in Figure 1B, reductions in cell viability of about 70% and 50% were observed when MM.1S cells were treated with 50 and 100 μM BCP, respectively. Moreover, BCP treatment did not affect the cell viability of RPMI1788 cells, demonstrating its selective antiproliferative effect on MM cells (Figure 1C).

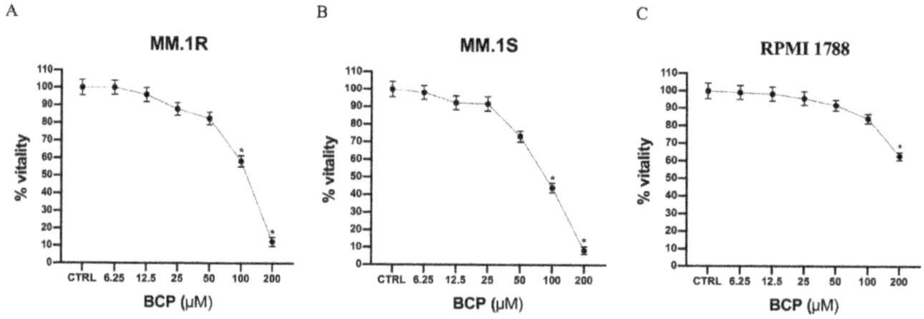

Figure 1. Cell viability evaluated in MM.1R (**A**), MM.1S (**B**), and RPMI 1788 (**C**) cell lines treated with BCP using MTT assays. Values are expressed as percentages of viability reduction compared with control cells. The data are expressed as means ± SEM; n = 3 experiments; * $p < 0.05$ vs. Ctrl.

Images obtained from the FDA/PI staining also showed cell viability: live cells were bright green and nonviable cells were red. Notably, untreated MM.1S cells stained with

FDA showed bright fluorescence, but a low level of fluorescence was observed with PI labeling; MM.1R cells treated with BCP at concentrations of 50 and 100 µM for 24 h showed few cells stained with FDA but many nuclei stained with PI (Figure 2A–F). Overlapping results were obtained in the MM.1S cell line (Figure 2G–N). The graphs presented in Figure 2 O, P represent the cell counts of MM.1R and MM.1S positive cells. BCP at a concentration of 50 µM increased the number of PI-positive cells in both cell lines ($p < 0.05$ vs. CTRL) and reduced the number of positive FDA cells only in MM.1S cells ($p < 0.05$ vs. CTRL). BCP at a concentration of 100 µM significantly increased the number of PI-positive cells ($p < 0.0001$ vs. CTRL) and strongly reduced the number of FDA-positive cells in both cell lines ($p < 0.05$ vs. CTRL).

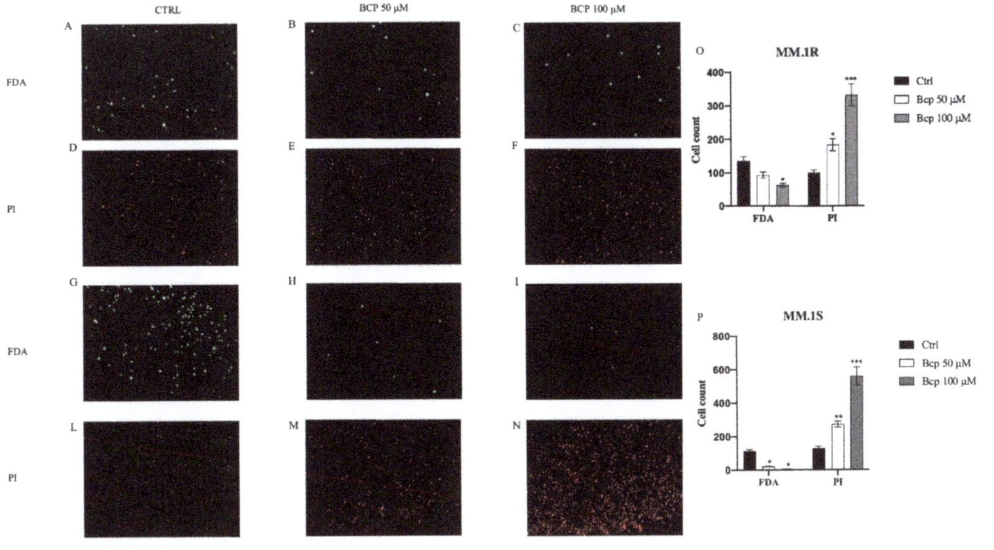

Figure 2. The figure represents the apoptotic process evaluated by FDA/PI staining in MM.1R and MM.1S cell lines treated with BCP. In panels (**A–C**) and (**G–I**), green color reaction indicates viable MM.1R and MM.1S cells, respectively; in panels (**D–F**) and (**L–N**), red reaction indicates MM.1R and MM.1S cells that underwent apoptosis, respectively. Panels (**O**) and (**P**) show the cells counts in MM.1R and MM.1S. The data are expressed as means ± SEM; $n = 3$ experiments; * $p < 0.05$ vs. Ctrl. ** $p < 0.001$ vs. Ctrl. *** $p < 0.0001$ vs. Ctrl.

In addition, a trypan blue assay was performed to confirm the selective antiproliferative effect of BCP on the MM.1S and MM.1R cell lines. The RPMI 1788 cell line, used as normal cells, was treated with BCP at concentrations of 50 and 100 µM for 24 h, thus demonstrating that BCP did not affect the proliferation of normal cells (Figure 3) and confirming the MTT results and BCP-selective effect in the MM cell lines.

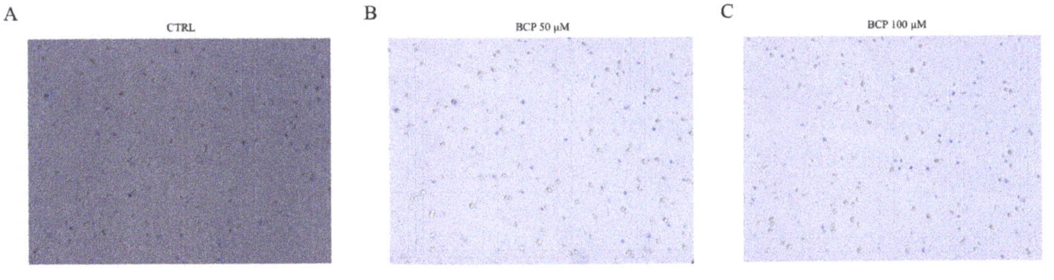

Figure 3. *Cont.*

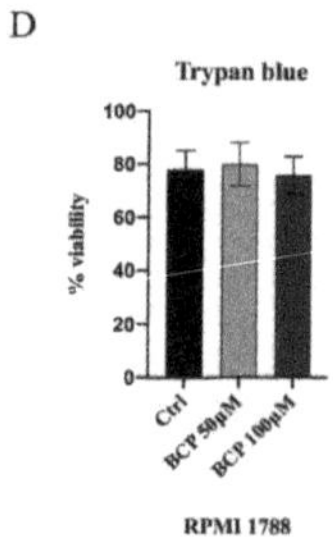

Figure 3. The figure represents the trypan blue staining in RPMI 1788 cells treated with BCP. In panels (**A–C**), blue color reaction indicates RPMI 1788 cells that underwent apoptosis. Panel (**D**) shows the percentage of viable cells. The data are expressed as means ± SEM; *n* = 3 experiments.

3.2. BCP Treatment Induces Apoptotic Pathways in MM.1S and MM.1R Cell Lines

Bcl-2, Bax, and caspase-3 protein expression were studied using Western blot analysis to evaluate whether BCP induces the apoptotic pathway in MM.1S (Figure 4A–C, Figure S1) and MM.1R (Figure 4D–F, Figure S1) cancer cells. BCP significantly increased caspase-3 and Bax, whereas it reduced Bcl-2 expression, compared with untreated cells in both MM.1S and MM.1R following 24 h of treatment especially at a concentration of 100 µM, thus indicating that BCP induced the apoptotic process in MM cancer cells ($p < 0.05$ vs. CTRL; Figure 4).

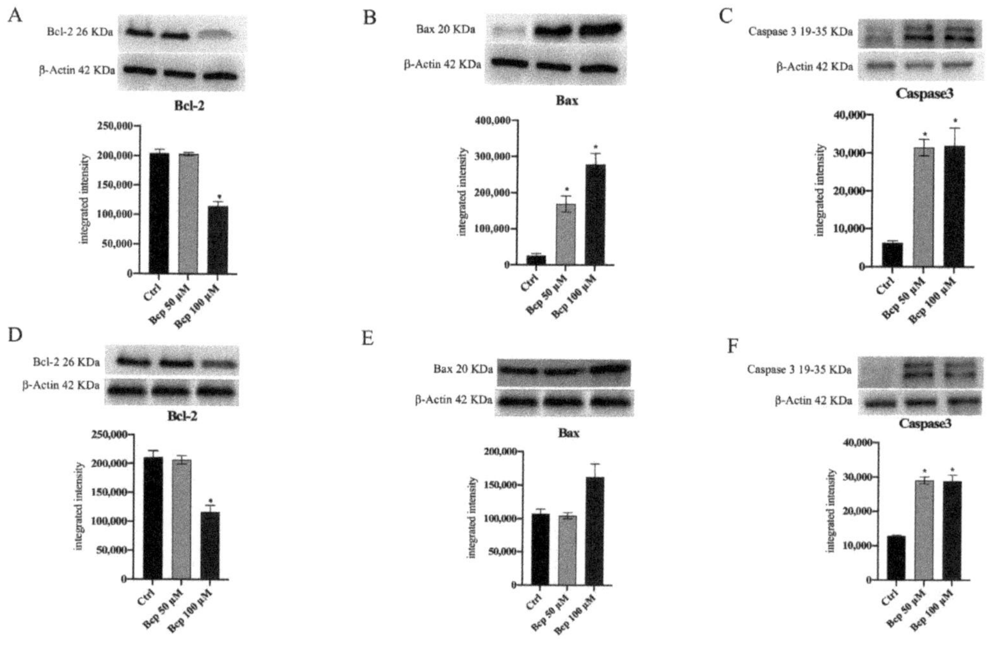

Figure 4. The graphs represent Bcl-2 (**A**), Bax (**B**), and caspase 3 (**C**) protein expression in MM.1S cells and protein expression of Bcl-2 (**D**), Bax (**E**), and caspase3 (**F**) in MM.1R cells treated with BCP. The data are expressed as means ± SEM; $n = 3$ experiments; * $p < 0.05$ vs. Ctrl.

3.3. *BCP Has a Significant Anti-Proliferative Effect through Akt and Wnt/β-Catenin Modulation*

Wnt1 protein levels as well as p-Akt and β−catenin protein expression were evaluated to investigate BCP's anti-proliferative effects in MM.1S and MM.1R cancer cells. BCP treatment caused a marked reduction in Wnt1 in the MM.1S cell line ($p < 0.05$ vs. CTRL; Figure 5), particularly at a concentration of 100 μM. Similar results were obtained in the MM.1R cancer cell line: BCP significantly reduced Wnt1 following 24 h of treatment compared with untreated cells ($p < 0.05$ vs. CTRL; Figure 5). In addition, both cell lines treated with BCP at a concentration of 100 μM showed a significant decrease in p-Akt and β-catenin protein expression, confirming that BCP treatment may have an anti-proliferative effect through Wnt1, p-Akt, and β-catenin reduction ($p < 0.05$ vs. CTRL; Figure 5 and Figures S2–S5). Wnt1, p-Akt, and β-catenin reduction was reversed by the treatment with the CB2R antagonist AM630, which abrogated BCP's effects, thus demonstrating that BCP's mechanism of action was related to CB2 receptor modulation.

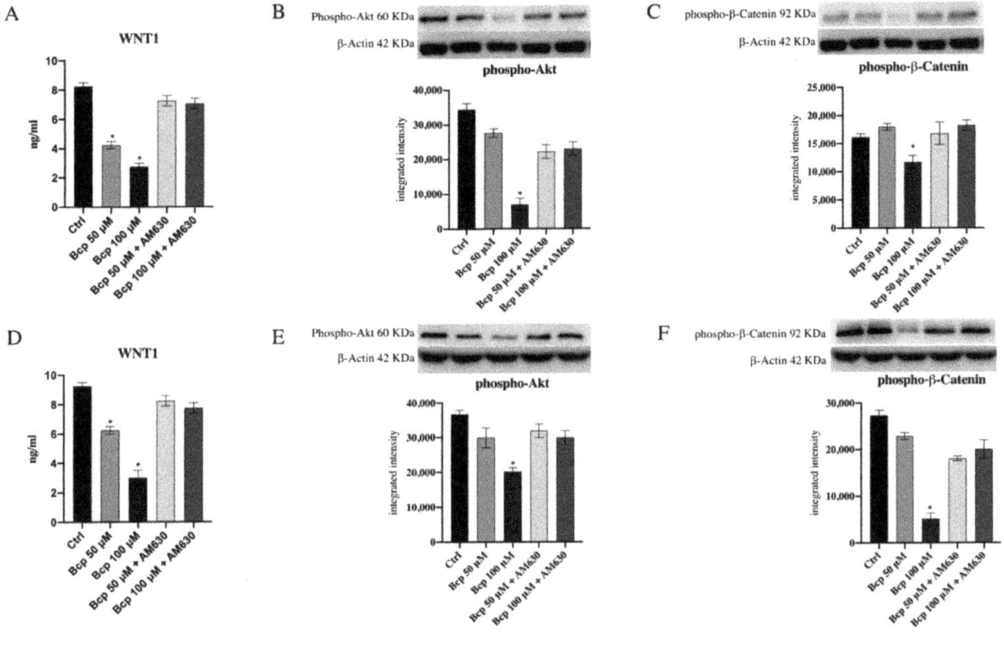

Figure 5. The graphs represent protein levels of Wnt1 (**A**), p-Akt (**B**), and p-β-Catenin (**C**) in MM.1S cells and Wnt1 (**D**), p-Akt (**E**), and p-β-Catenin (**F**) protein levels in MM.1R cells treated with BCP. The data are expressed as means ± SEM; $n = 3$ experiments; * $p < 0.05$ vs. Ctrl.

The reduction in β-catenin activation following BCP treatment was also observed in immunofluorescence. Control cells showed positive staining for β-catenin; this staining pattern was appreciable around the nuclei and at the plasma membrane level (Figure 6A,B). The images in Figure 6C (Figure S6) and D show a very low β-catenin staining pattern, thus confirming BCP's efficacy in reducing β-catenin activation.

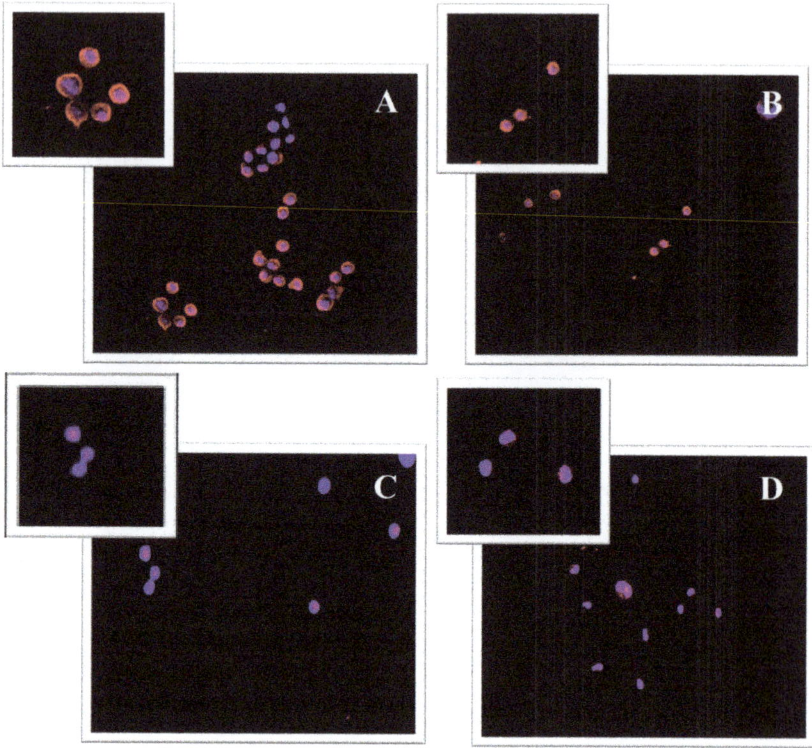

Figure 6. Panel of immunofluorescence staining for β-catenin (red fluorescence). β-catenin fluorescence pattern in control cells, MM.1S (**A**), and MM.1R (**B**) is mainly distributed at the perinuclear and plasma membrane level, as clearly shown in the magnifications in the left corners; MM.1 S cells treated with BCP for 24 h showed a strong reduction in β-catenin staining (**C**); BCP treatment for 24 h caused a significant β-catenin fluorescence reduction in MM.1R treated cells (**D**).

3.4. BCP Anti-Proliferative Effect Is Carried out through Cell Cycle Inhibition

The hypothesis that BCP might exert an anti-proliferative effect in MM cancer cells was further confirmed by the results obtained for cyclin D1 expression and the levels of its kinases, CDK 4 and 6. BCP treatment, particularly at a concentration of 100 μM, significantly reduced CDK4 and CDK6 levels both in MM.1S and MM.1R cells compared with untreated cells ($p < 0.05$ vs. CTRL; Figure 7). As expected, cyclin D1 protein expression was downregulated when MM.1S and MM.1R cells were treated with BCP at a concentration of 100 μM following 24 h of treatment ($p < 0.05$ vs. CTRL; Figure 7 and Figures S6 and S7).

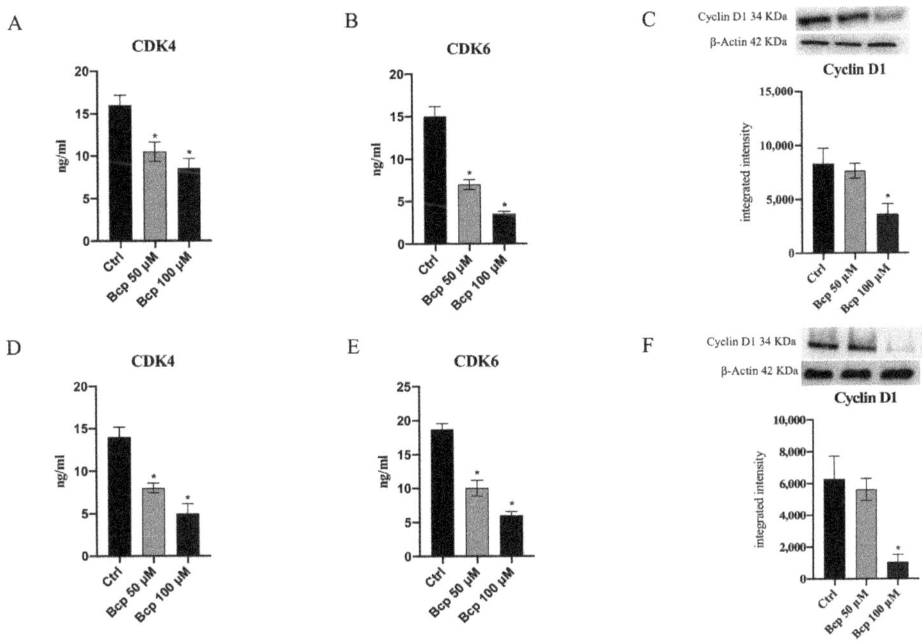

Figure 7. The graphs represent CDK4 (**A**), CDK6 (**B**), and cyclin D1 (**C**) protein levels in MM.1S cells. CDK4 (**D**), CDK6 (**E**), and cyclin D1 (**F**) protein levels in MM.1R cells treated with BCP. The data are expressed as means ± SEM; $n = 3$ experiments; * $p < 0.05$ vs. Ctrl.

4. Discussion

In the past years, several efforts have been made by the scientific community to characterize the role of the ECS in several body areas and to understand if cannabinoid receptors might be considered as effective therapeutic targets. The use of the cannabis plant and its derivatives might represent a new therapeutic window for the management of diseases for which there is no effective therapy, such as cancers, and have a significant impact on medicine and the global economy. Cannabinoids have shown anti-emetic effects in cancer patients as well as significant anti-neoplastic effects in solid tumors, such as glioma and breast cancer [30–32]. The exact mechanism of action is not completely understood, but the therapeutic approach is mainly based on the wide distribution of cannabinoid receptors. MM cells express cannabinoid receptors, as demonstrated by flow cytometry analysis [10,33], and experimental studies have demonstrated that both cannabidiol and different cannabinoid derivatives induce apoptosis in MM cell lines through a caspase-dependent mechanism [7,10].

In the present experimental setting, BCP, a natural CB2R agonist, was evaluated for its anti-proliferative and anti-neoplastic effects in MM.1S and MM.1R cells; in particular, MM.1R cells respond less to chemotherapy and represent a condition observed in cancer patients in advanced stages of the disease [34]. Our team already revealed that BCP reduced cell viability in glioma cell lines and glioma-derived stem-like cells, thus demonstrating that BCP might be used in conditions of resistance [13]. BCP is a safe compound; in fact, it did not affect healthy cells, such as human gingival fibroblasts and human oral mucosa epithelial cells, as already demonstrated in our previous study [25]; in addition, another CB2 agonist, WIN-55,212–2 mesylate, was not only effective in reducing cancer cells proliferation but was also selective toward cancer cells and not control cells (healthy cells) [10], thus supporting the hypothesis that BCP might be used in the clinical practice, affecting cancer cells and remaining safe for normal cells. In accordance with our experimental hypothesis, it has been previously confirmed that cannabinoid use may selectively stimulate apoptosis in MM cells through a caspase-2-dependent mechanism, but what is even more interesting is that cell death was only activated in MM cells and did not affect normal cells; moreover, cannabinoid-induced apoptosis was inhibited by blocking CB2R [10,33].

BCP also proved effective in MM.1S cells and the more resistant MM.1R cell line at concentrations of 50 μM and 100 μM, thus reducing the cell viability of cancer cells and not affecting normal cells, as demonstrated by the MTT assay and trypan blue staining; in particular, the fluorescent marking with FDA confirmed the MTT results and demonstrated that BCP significantly reduced the number of viable cells. This antiproliferative effect is mainly due to the activation of apoptosis as a cell death mechanism. In fact, the triggering of Bax and caspase-3 following BCP treatment in both cell lines pointed out that BCP anti-neoplastic activity might be ascribed to a caspase-dependent mechanism of cell death and p53-mediated apoptosis through Bax stimulation. In addition, Bcl-2, which usually promotes cell survival and is considered an anti-apoptotic protein [35], was significantly reduced in treated cancer cells in favor of apoptotic markers, thus confirming BCP's pro-apoptotic effect. Cannabinoids were able to induce apoptosis in melanoma, glioma, breast cancer, and MM cells through a molecular mechanism that provides for Akt modulation, which is one of the most strongly involved pathways in response to cannabinoid receptor stimulation [15,36].

Phosphatidylinositol-3-kinase (PI3K)/Akt and the mammalian target of rapamycin (mTOR) signaling pathway, which controls cell proliferation, is abnormally activated in several cancers and also in MM patients [37]; therefore, a drug that inhibits this pathway might be effective in the treatment of MM. BCP treatment markedly reduced Akt expression, particularly at a concentration of 100 μM, in both cell lines compared with untreated cells, thus providing an important translational relevance since Akt overexpression often correlates with poor outcomes [38]. PI3K/Akt/mTOR is a sophisticated pathway that is interconnected with other signaling pathways, such as Wnt/β-catenin signaling. Wnt/β-catenin pathway activation is involved in both normal development and aberrant cell proliferation; in fact, a β-catenin increase may exert oncogenic effects in different tumors [39,40]. BCP's anti-proliferative effect was established by the results obtained from Wnt1 and β-catenin expression: a significant decrease was observed in the treated MM.1R and MM.1S cell lines compared with untreated cancer cells. These anti-proliferative effects were abrogated when MM.1 cells were treated with both BCP and the CB2R antagonist AM630, thus demonstrating that BCP's mechanism of action is strictly related to CB2R modulation since AM630 antagonizes this specific receptor. MM.1 cells treated with BCP showed a significant reduction of the positive fluorescence of β-catenin compared with controls (tumor cells). These data indicate that BCP's anti-proliferative effect may be due to the complex modulation of the Akt and Wnt/β-catenin pathways through the essential stimulation of the apoptotic mechanism.

The cyclin D1 gene is a target for β-catenin and is accountable for the progression of cells into the proliferative stage of the cell cycle [41]. In fact, β-catenin-mediated signaling depends on its accumulation and consequent translocation into the nucleus, where it regulates gene transcription. Increased β-catenin levels were associated with malignancies, and this increase is considered one of the features of MM, thus promoting tumor progression through cell cycle activation [42]. The cell cycle is a process that is regulated by different cyclins and their CDKs; the likelihood of developing cancer dramatically increases when the precise balance between cyclins and CDKs is impaired [43]. One of the main alterations observed in cancer concerns cyclin D and CDK4/6 overexpression, and in particular, cyclin D alteration is one of the key hallmarks of MM [44,45]. For this reason, targeting these cell cycle regulators may represent a promising therapeutic approach for the management of myeloma. Surprisingly, in our experimental model, we observed that BCP treatment induced the reduction of cyclin D1 and its kinases, CDK4 and CDK6, in both the MM.1S and MM.1R cell lines compared with untreated cells, further demonstrating BPC's antiproliferative effects through cell cycle modulation, probably as a consequence of β-catenin reduction (Figure 8).

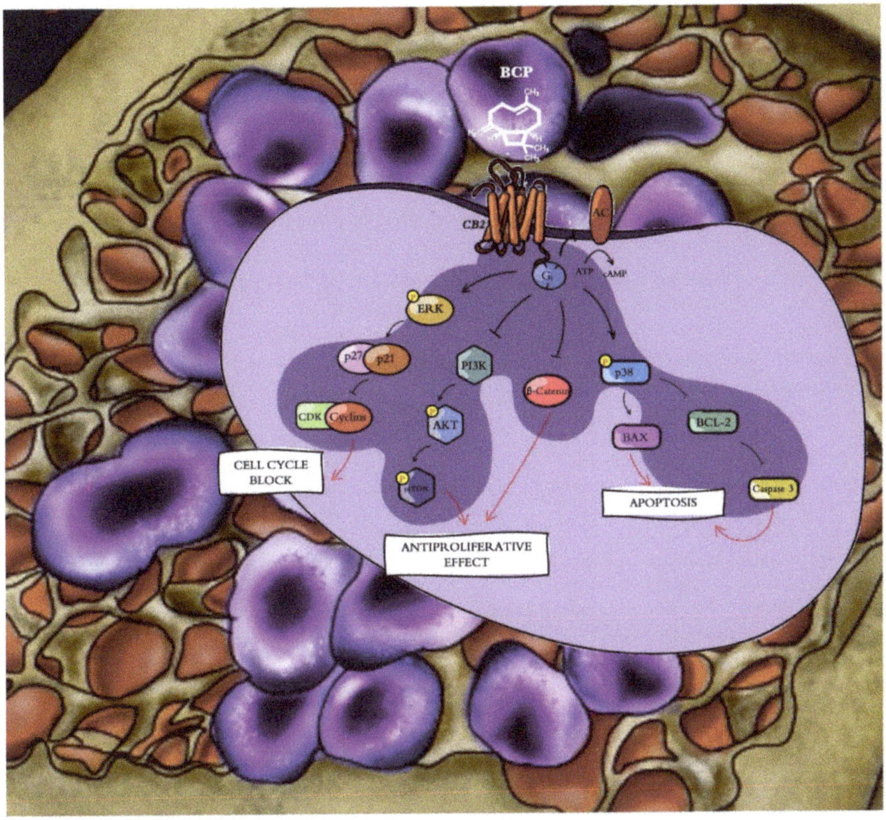

Figure 8. Beta-caryophyllene (β-caryophyllene, BCP) selectively binds cannabinoid type 2 receptor (CB2R), thus inducing an antiproliferative effect through (i) cell cycle modulation by reducing cyclin D1 and Cdk 4/6 expression, (ii) apoptosis activation by increasing Bax and caspase 3 and reducing Bcl-2 expression, and (iii) Akt and β-catenin inhibition.

5. Conclusions

MM is considered an incurable plasma cell cancer; blocking cell proliferation and consequently cell progression in terms of invasion may represent an interesting approach to improve anti-myeloma therapy. On one hand, BCP was able to induce the apoptotic mechanism, activating the molecules involved in apoptosis; moreover, BCP regulated cell proliferation through sophisticated crosstalk between Akt, β-catenin, and cyclin D/CDK 4/6 in a concentration-dependent manner. However, in vivo experimental approaches should be developed to confirm the results described so far and demonstrate that BCP might represent an interesting alternative or additional therapeutic approach to conventional chemotherapy for the treatment of multiple myeloma.

Supplementary Materials: The following are available online at https://www.mdpi.com/article/10.3390/cancers13225741/s1, Figure S1: Original western blots for Figure 4A–F, Figure S2: Original Western blots for Figure 5B, Figure S3: Original Western blots for Figure 5C, Figure S4: Original Western blots for Figure 5E, Figure S5: Original Western blots for Figure 5F, Figure S6: Original Western blots for Figure 7C, Figure S7: Original figure blots for Figure 7F.

Author Contributions: Conceptualization, F.M. and G.P.; formal analysis, R.C.; funding acquisition, F.S.; methodology, L.M. and D.A.; supervision, N.I.; validation, G.V., A.A., and A.H.E.; writing—original draft, F.M.; writing—review and editing, A.B. and F.S. All authors have read and agreed to the published version of the manuscript.

Funding: This work was supported by departmental funding provided to Francesco Squadrito.

Institutional Review Board Statement: Not applicable.

Informed Consent Statement: Not applicable.

Data Availability Statement: The datasets generated for this study are available on request to the corresponding author.

Acknowledgments: The authors would like to thank Rita Lauro for the brilliant graphic contribution to the cartoon-type figure in the present study.

Conflicts of Interest: The authors declare no conflict of interest.

References

1. Siegel, R.L.; Miller, K.D.; Jemal, A. Cancer statistics. *CA Cancer J. Clin.* **2019**, *69*, 7–34. [CrossRef]
2. Kuehl, W.M.; Bergsagel, P.L. Molecular pathogenesis of multiple myeloma and its premalignant precursor. *J. Clin. Investig.* **2012**, *122*, 3456–3463. [CrossRef]
3. Bianchi, G.; Anderson, K.C. Understanding biology to tackle the disease: Multiple myeloma from bench to bedside, and back. *CA Cancer J. Clin.* **2014**, *64*, 422–444. [CrossRef]
4. Khodadadi, L.; Cheng, Q.; Radbruch, A.; Hiepe, F. The Maintenance of Memory Plasma Cells. *Front. Immunol.* **2019**, *10*, 721. [CrossRef]
5. Galiègue, S.; Mary, S.; Marchand, J.; Dussossoy, D.; Carrière, D.; Carayon, P.; Bouaboula, M.; Shire, D.; Le Fur, G.; Casellas, P. Expression of central and peripheral cannabinoid receptors in human immune tissues and leukocyte subpopulations. *Eur. J. Biochem.* **1995**, *232*, 54–61. [CrossRef]
6. Xie, X.-Q.; Feng, R.; Yang, P. Novel Cannabinoid Receptor 2 (CB2) Inverse Agonists and Therapeutic Potential for Multiple Myeloma and Osteoporosis Bone Diseases. US Patent 61/576,041, 15 December 2012.
7. Feng, R.; Tong, Q.; Xie, Z.; Cheng, H.; Wang, L.; Lentzsch, S.; Roodman, G.D.; Xie, X.Q. Targeting cannabinoid receptor-2 pathway by phenylacetylamide suppresses the proliferation of human myeloma cells through mitotic dysregulation and cytoskeleton disruption. *Mol. Carcinog.* **2015**, *54*, 1796–1806. [CrossRef]
8. Jordà, M.A.; Verbakel, S.E.; Valk, P.J.; Vankan-Berkhoudt, Y.V.; Maccarrone, M.; Finazzi-Agrò, A.; Löwenberg, B.; Delwel, R. Hematopoietic cells expressing the peripheral cannabinoid receptor migrate in response to the endocannabinoid 2-arachidonoylglycerol. *Blood* **2002**, *99*, 2786–2793. [CrossRef] [PubMed]
9. Tam, J.; Ofek, O.; Fride, E.; Ledent, C.; Gabet, Y.; Müller, R.; Zimmer, A.; Mackie, K.; Mechoulam, R.; Shohami, E.; et al. Involvement of neuronal cannabinoid receptor CB1 in regulation of bone mass and bone remodeling. *Mol. Pharmacol.* **2006**, *70*, 786–792. [CrossRef] [PubMed]
10. Barbado, M.V.; Medrano, M.; Caballero-Velázquez, T.; Álvarez-Laderas, I.; Sánchez-Abarca, L.I.; García-Guerrero, E.; Martín-Sánchez, J.; Rosado, I.V.; Piruat, J.I.; Gonzalez-Naranjo, P.; et al. Cannabinoid derivatives exert a potent anti-myeloma activity both in vitro and in vivo. *Int. J. Cancer* **2017**, *1403*, 674–685. [CrossRef] [PubMed]
11. Hashiesh, H.M.; Sharma, C.; Goyal, S.N.; Sadek, B.; Jha, N.K.; Kaabi, J.A.; Ojha, S. A focused review on CB2 receptor-selective pharmacological properties and therapeutic potential of β-caryophyllene, a dietary cannabinoid. *Biomed Pharmacother.* **2021**, *140*, 111639. [CrossRef]
12. Di Sotto, A.; Mancinelli, R.; Gullì, M.; Eufemi, M.; Mammolam, C.L.; Mazzanti, G.; Di Giacomo, S. Chemopreventive Potential of Caryophyllane Sesquiterpenes: An Overview of Preliminary Evidence. *Cancers* **2020**, *12*, 3034. [CrossRef] [PubMed]
13. Irrera, N.; D'Ascola, A.; Pallio, G.; Bitto, A.; Mannino, F.; Arcoraci, V.; Rottura, M.; Ieni, A.; Minutoli, L.; Metro, D.; et al. β-Caryophyllene Inhibits Cell Proliferation through a Direct Modulation of CB2 Receptors in Glioblastoma Cells. *Cancers* **2020**, *12*, 1038. [CrossRef]
14. Ellert-Miklaszewska, A.; Kaminska, B.; Konarska, L. Cannabinoids down-regulate PI3K/Akt and Erk signalling pathways and activate proapoptotic function of Bad protein. *Cell Signal.* **2005**, *17*, 25–37. [CrossRef]
15. Velasco, G.; Sanchez, C.; Guzman, M. Anticancer mechanisms of cannabinoids. *Curr. Oncol.* **2016**, *23*, S23–S32. [CrossRef] [PubMed]
16. Sharma, C.; Al Kaabi, J.M.; Nurulain, S.M.; Goyal, S.N.; Kamal, M.A.; Ojha, S. Polypharmacological Properties and Therapeutic Potential of β-Caryophyllene: A Dietary Phytocannabinoid of Pharmaceutical Promise. *Curr. Pharm. Des.* **2016**, *22*, 3237–3264. [CrossRef]
17. Ramachandhiran, D.; Sankaranarayanan, C.; Murali, R.; Babukumar, S.; Vinothkumar, V. β-Caryophyllene promotes oxidative stress and apoptosis in KB cells through activation of mitochondrial-mediated pathway—An in-vitro and in-silico study. *Arch. Physiol. Biochem.* **2019**, *4*, 1–15. [CrossRef]

18. Irrera, N.; D'Ascola, A.; Pallio, G.; Bitto, A.; Mazzon, E.; Mannino, F.; Squadrito, V.; Arcoraci, V.; Minutoli, L.; Campo, G.M.; et al. β-Caryophyllene Mitigates Collagen Antibody Induced Arthritis (CAIA) in Mice Through a Cross-Talk between CB2 and PPAR-γ Receptors. *Biomolecules* **2019**, *9*, 326. [CrossRef]
19. Hashiesh, H.M.; Meeran, M.F.N.; Sharma, C.; Sadek, B.; Kaabi, J.A.; Ojha, S.K. Therapeutic Potential of β-Caryophyllene: A Dietary Cannabinoid in Diabetes and Associated Complications. *Nutrients* **2020**, *12*, 2963. [CrossRef]
20. Sköld, M.; Karlberg, A.T.; Matura, M.; Börje, A. The fragrance chemical beta-caryophyllene-air oxidation and skin sensitization. *Food Chem. Toxicol.* **2006**, *44*, 538–545. [CrossRef]
21. Lou, J.; Teng, Z.; Zhang, L.; Yang, J.; Ma, L.; Wang, F.; Tian, X.; An, R.; Yang, M.; Zhang, Q.; et al. β-Caryophyllene/Hydroxypropyl-β-Cyclodextrin Inclusion Complex Improves Cognitive Deficits in Rats with Vascular Dementia through the Cannabinoid Receptor Type 2 Mediated Pathway. *Front. Pharmacol.* **2017**, *8*, 2. [CrossRef] [PubMed]
22. Santos, P.S.; Souza, L.K.M.; Araújo, T.S.L.; Medeiros, J.V.R.; Nunes, S.C.C.; Carvalho, R.A.; Pais, A.C.C.; Veiga, F.J.B.; Nunes, L.C.C.; Figueiras, A. Methyl-β-cyclodextrin Inclusion Complex with β-Caryophyllene: Preparation, Characterization, and Improvement of Pharmacological Activities. *ACS Omega* **2017**, *2*, 9080–9094. [CrossRef]
23. Santos, P.S.; Oliveira, T.C.; Júnior, L.M.R.; Figueiras, A.; Nunes, L.C.C. β-caryophyllene Delivery Systems: Enhancing the Oral Pharmacokinetic and Stability. *Curr. Pharm. Des.* **2018**, *24*, 3440–3453. [CrossRef] [PubMed]
24. Gertsch, J.; Leonti, M.; Raduner, S.; Racz, I.; Chen, J.Z.; Xie, X.Q.; Altmann, K.H.; Karsak, M.; Zimmer, A. Beta-caryophyllene is a dietary cannabinoid. *Proc. Natl. Acad. Sci. USA* **2008**, *105*, 9099–9104. [CrossRef]
25. Picciolo, G.; Pallio, G.; Altavilla, D.; Vaccaro, M.; Oteri, G.; Irrera, N.; Squadrito, F. β-Caryophyllene Reduces the Inflammatory Phenotype of Periodontal Cells by Targeting CB2 Receptors. *Biomedicines* **2020**, *8*, 164. [CrossRef]
26. Ceravolo, I.; Mannino, F.; Irrera, N.; Squadrito, F.; Altavilla, D.; Ceravolo, G.; Pallio, G.; Minutoli, L. Health Potential of *Aloe vera* against Oxidative Stress Induced Corneal Damage: An "In Vitro" Study. *Antioxidants* **2021**, *10*, 318. [CrossRef] [PubMed]
27. Pizzino, G.; Irrera, N.; Galfo, F.; Pallio, G.; Mannino, F.; D'amore, A.; Pellegrino, E.; Ieni, A.; Russo, G.T.; Calapai, M.; et al. Effects of the antagomiRs 15b and 200b on the altered healing pattern of diabetic mice. *Br. J. Pharmacol.* **2018**, *175*, 644–655. [CrossRef] [PubMed]
28. Pallio, G.; Micali, A.; Benvenga, S.; Antonelli, A.; Marini, H.R.; Puzzolo, D.; Macaione, V.; Trichilo, V.; Santoro, G.; Irrera, N.; et al. Myo-inositol in the protection from cadmium-induced toxicity in mice kidney: An emerging nutraceutical challenge. *Food Chem. Toxicol.* **2019**, *132*, 110675. [CrossRef] [PubMed]
29. Irrera, N.; Arcoraci, V.; Mannino, F.; Vermiglio, G.; Pallio, G.; Minutoli, L.; Bagnato, G.; Anastasi, G.P.; Mazzon, E.; Bramanti, P.; et al. Activation of A2A Receptor by PDRN Reduces Neuronal Damage and Stimulates WNT/β-CATENIN Driven Neurogenesis in Spinal Cord Injury. *Front. Pharmacol.* **2018**, *9*, 506. [CrossRef]
30. Warr, D.; Hesketh, P. Cannabinoids as antiemetics: Everything that's old is new again. *Ann. Oncol.* **2020**, *31*, 1425–1426. [CrossRef] [PubMed]
31. McAllister, S.D.; Soroceanu, L.; Desprez, P.Y. The Antitumor Activity of Plant-Derived Non-Psychoactive Cannabinoids. *J. Neuroimmune Pharmacol.* **2015**, *10*, 255–267. [CrossRef]
32. Hinz, B.; Ramer, R. Anti-tumour actions of cannabinoids. *Br. J. Pharmacol.* **2019**, *176*, 1384–1394. [CrossRef]
33. Garofano, F.; Schmidt-Wolf, I.G.H. High Expression of Cannabinoid Receptor 2 on Cytokine-Induced Killer Cells and Multiple Myeloma Cells. *Int. J. Mol. Sci.* **2020**, *21*, 3800. [CrossRef] [PubMed]
34. Greenstein, S.; Krett, N.L.; Kurosawa, Y.; Ma, C.; Chauhan, D.; Hideshima, T.; Anderson, K.C.; Rosen, S.T. Characterization of the MM.1 human multiple myeloma (MM) cell lines: A model system to elucidate the characteristics, behavior, and signaling of steroid-sensitive and resistant MM cells. *Exp. Hematol.* **2003**, *31*, 271–282. [CrossRef]
35. Li, X.; Dou, J.; You, Q.; Jiang, Z. Inhibitors of BCL2A1/Bfl-1 protein: Potential stock in cancer therapy. *Eur. J. Med. Chem.* **2021**, *220*, 113539. [CrossRef]
36. Gugliandolo, A.; Pollastro, F.; Bramanti, P.; Mazzon, E. Cannabidiol exerts protective effects in an in vitro model of Parkinson's disease activating AKT/mTOR pathway. *Fitoterapia* **2020**, *143*, 104553. [CrossRef]
37. Ramakrishnan, V.; Kumar, S. PI3K/AKT/mTOR pathway in multiple myeloma: From basic biology to clinical promise. *Leuk. Lymphoma* **2018**, *59*, 2524–2534. [CrossRef]
38. Bongiovanni, D.; Saccomani, V.; Piovan, E. Aberrant Signaling Pathways in T-Cell Acute Lymphoblastic Leukemia. *Int. J. Mol. Sci.* **2017**, *18*, 1904. [CrossRef]
39. Gao, J.; Yu, S.R.; Yuan, Y.; Zhang, L.L.; Lu, J.W.; Feng, J.F.; Hu, S.N. MicroRNA-590-5p functions as a tumor suppressor in breast cancer conferring inhibitory effects on cell migration, invasion, and epithelial-mesenchymal transition by downregulating the Wnt-β-catenin signaling pathway. *J. Cell. Physiol.* **2019**, *234*, 1827–1841. [CrossRef]
40. He, L.; Zhou, H.; Zeng, Z.; Yao, H.; Jiang, W.; Qu, H. Wnt/β-catenin signaling cascade: A promising target for glioma therapy. *J. Cell. Physiol.* **2019**, *234*, 2217–2228. [CrossRef] [PubMed]
41. Montalto, F.I.; De Amicis, F. Cyclin D1 in Cancer: A Molecular Connection for Cell Cycle Control, Adhesion and Invasion in Tumor and Stroma. *Cells* **2020**, *9*, 2648. [CrossRef]
42. Van Andel, H.; Kocemba, K.A.; Spaargaren, M.; Pals, S.T. Aberrant Wnt signaling in multiple myeloma: Molecular mechanisms and targeting options. *Leukemia* **2019**, *33*, 1063–1075. [CrossRef] [PubMed]

43. Ding, L.; Cao, J.; Lin, W.; Chen, H.; Xiong, X.; Ao, H.; Yu, M.; Lin, J.; Cui, Q. The Roles of Cyclin-Dependent Kinases in Cell-Cycle Progression and Therapeutic Strategies in Human Breast Cancer. *Int. J. Mol. Sci.* **2020**, *21*, 1960. [CrossRef]
44. Gao, X.; Leone, G.W.; Wang, H. Cyclin D-CDK4/6 functions in cancer. *Adv. Cancer Res.* **2020**, *148*, 147–169. [CrossRef] [PubMed]
45. Misiewicz-Krzeminska, I.; Sarasquete, M.E.; Vicente-Dueñas, C.; Krzeminski, P.; Wiktorska, K.; Corchete, L.A.; Quwaider, D.; Rojas, E.A.; Corral, R.; Martín, A.A.; et al. Post-transcriptional Modifications Contribute to the Upregulation of Cyclin D2 in Multiple Myeloma. *Clin. Cancer Res.* **2016**, *22*, 207–217. [CrossRef] [PubMed]

cancers MDPI

Review

Sulforaphane: A Broccoli Bioactive Phytocompound with Cancer Preventive Potential

Anna E. Kaiser, Mojdeh Baniasadi, Derrek Giansiracusa, Matthew Giansiracusa, Michael Garcia, Zachary Fryda, Tin Lok Wong and Anupam Bishayee *

Lake Erie College of Osteopathic Medicine, Bradenton, FL 34211, USA; alish56890@med.lecom.edu (A.E.K.); mbaniasadi67397@med.lecom.edu (M.B.); dgiansirac01847@med.lecom.edu (D.G.); mgiansirac27767@med.lecom.edu (M.G.); mgarcia64879@med.lecom.edu (M.G.); ZFryda56890@med.lecom.edu (Z.F.); twong76647@med.lecom.edu (T.L.W.)

* Correspondence: abishayee@lecom.edu or abishayee@gmail.com

Simple Summary: As of the past decade, phytochemicals have become a major target of interest in cancer chemopreventive and chemotherapeutic research. Sulforaphane (SFN) is a metabolite of the phytochemical glucoraphanin, which is found in high abundance in cruciferous vegetables, such as broccoli, watercress, Brussels sprouts, and cabbage. In both distant and recent research, SFN has been shown to have a multitude of anticancer effects, increasing the need for a comprehensive review of the literature. In this review, we critically evaluate SFN as an anticancer agent and its mechanisms of action based on an impressive number of in vitro, in vivo, and clinical studies.

Abstract: There is substantial and promising evidence on the health benefits of consuming broccoli and other cruciferous vegetables. The most important compound in broccoli, glucoraphanin, is metabolized to SFN by the thioglucosidase enzyme myrosinase. SFN is the major mediator of the health benefits that have been recognized for broccoli consumption. SFN represents a phytochemical of high interest as it may be useful in preventing the occurrence and/or mitigating the progression of cancer. Although several prior publications provide an excellent overview of the effect of SFN in cancer, these reports represent narrative reviews that focused mainly on SFN's source, biosynthesis, and mechanisms of action in modulating specific pathways involved in cancer without a comprehensive review of SFN's role or value for prevention of various human malignancies. This review evaluates the most recent state of knowledge concerning SFN's efficacy in preventing or reversing a variety of neoplasms. In this work, we have analyzed published reports based on in vitro, in vivo, and clinical studies to determine SFN's potential as a chemopreventive agent. Furthermore, we have discussed the current limitations and challenges associated with SFN research and suggested future research directions before broccoli-derived products, especially SFN, can be used for human cancer prevention and intervention.

Keywords: broccoli; isothiocyanates; sulforaphane; cancer; prevention; intervention; molecular mechanisms

Citation: Kaiser, A.E.; Baniasadi, M.; Giansiracusa, D.; Giansiracusa, M.; Garcia, M.; Fryda, Z.; Wong, T.L.; Bishayee, A. Sulforaphane: A Broccoli Bioactive Phytocompound with Cancer Preventive Potential. *Cancers* **2021**, *13*, 4796. https://doi.org/10.3390/cancers13194796

Academic Editor: David Wong

Received: 13 August 2021
Accepted: 22 September 2021
Published: 25 September 2021

1. Introduction

The development of cancer is a multifactorial process involving cellular mutations, which lead to unrestricted cell growth, thus causing many deleterious effects on the body due to the invasion of malignant cells and metastasis to distant sites, causing widespread organ dysfunction. As a result, cancer is a leading cause of morbidity and mortality across the world [1], which poses a significant burden for our society [2]. Due to the high prevalence of cancer, the utilization of naturally occurring compounds to prevent, inhibit, or reverse tumor development is of high interest in the scientific community. The use of various agents, including natural dietary compounds, is known as cancer chemoprevention, and its major goal is to slow the onset of cancer development and/or to suppress its growth [3]. This brings up an important concept known as "green chemoprevention", which is defined as the consumption of whole plant foods or their extracts for cancer prevention [4].

A diet high in fruits and vegetables alone can reduce total cancer risk by as much as 14% [5]. Therefore, it is suggested that consuming a well-balanced diet containing a wide variety of vegetables, fruits, whole grains, and other plant-based foods prevents the progression or development of cancer [6,7]. The cancer-preventive potential of dietary agents is believed to be due to the synergy or interactions among bioactive food components or plants' secondary metabolites [8]. Over 5000 phytochemicals have been isolated from a variety of plants and are identified in vegetables, fruits, whole grains, legumes, and nuts, but most of them remain unknown [8]. Phytochemicals can be divided into specific categories according to their chemical structures, and the most important of these compounds are phenolics and polyphenols, terpenoids, alkaloids, and sulfur-containing compounds. It has been determined that dietary phytochemicals exert cancer-preventive and therapeutic activities through antioxidant, anti-inflammatory, immunomodulatory, antiproliferative, cell cycle-regulatory, cell death-inducing, autophagy-regulating, anti-invasive, antimigratory, and antiangiogenic effects, as well as modulation of various cell signaling pathways [9–16]. Recently, we have provided a broad overview of the recent development of preclinical and clinical research on the cancer-preventive and therapeutic potential of various dietary agents and bioactive food components [17–23].

A multitude of studies has shown that ingestion of cruciferous vegetables (plants belonging to the Cruciferae family) may lower overall cancer risk, especially for breast, colorectal, bladder, lung, and prostate cancer [24–28]. This is especially true with vegetables in the *Brassica* genus, including broccoli (*Brassica oleracea*), Brussels sprouts, cabbage, cauliflower, and bok choy. Sulfur-containing organic compounds, especially isothiocyanates (ITCs) found within these vegetables, are an important group of phytochemicals that have been shown to have a variety of health benefits. The precursor glucosinolates are metabolized into ITCs by the action of plant myrosinase (EC 3.2.1.147), a β-thioglucoside glucohydrolase, via hydrolysis. ITCs are also released by cutting or chewing, boiling, or by the action of intestinal microflora present in humans [29]. Different glucosinolates produce a variety of distinct ITCs. For example, glucoraphanin (GFN, 4-methylsulfinylbutyl glucosinolate) is the glucosinolate precursor molecule to sulforaphane (SFN, 1-isothiocyanato-4-(methanesulfinyl) butane, Figure 1A). Among the cruciferous vegetables, broccoli and broccoli sprouts have been shown to contain the highest concentration of glucoraphanin, which is also abundant in cabbage, cauliflower, and Brussels sprouts (Figure 1B). Preclinical and clinical studies during the last several decades suggest that ITCs can inhibit carcinogenesis and suppress cancer growth through the regulation of multiple signaling pathways involved in carcinogen biotransformation and detoxification, inflammation, cell cycle, apoptosis, and epigenetic regulation [30–36].

SFN contains an isothiocyanate functional group (-N=C=S) and a methylsulfonyl side chain (R-(S-O)-R), allowing it to be a water-soluble compound, and its pharmacological activity is increased at the neutral pH of the intestine [37]. In the liver, SFN is metabolized via glutathione (GSH) conjugation to the bioactive compound SFN-N-acetylcysteine that reacts with thiol groups of amino acid residues in a variety of proteins [38]. SFN is known to exert various biological and pharmacological activities, including antioxidant [39], anti-inflammatory, immunomodulatory, and antimicrobial effects [40,41], and is reported to confer various health-promoting and disease-mitigating properties. The beneficial effects of SFN include protection against and/or prevention of gastric ulcer [42], cardiovascular diseases [43], chronic kidney disease [44], aging, and neurodegenerative diseases, including Parkinson's disease, Alzheimer's disease, and multiple sclerosis [45–47].

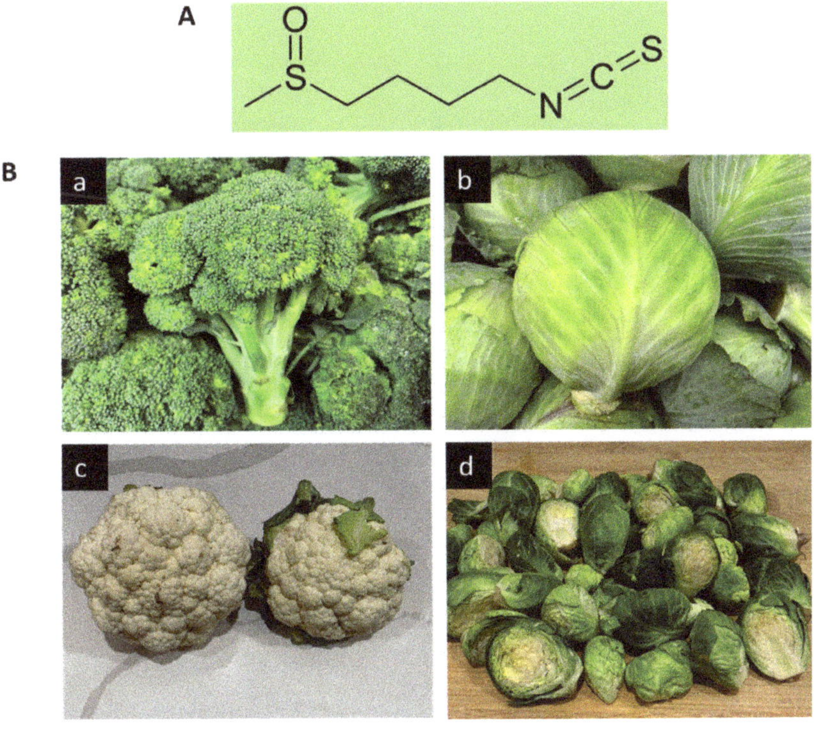

Figure 1. SFN and it various sources. (**A**) Molecular structure of SFN. (**B**) Dietary sources of SFN: (**a**) broccoli, (**b**) cabbage, (**c**) cauliflower, and (**d**) Brussels sprouts.

Zhang et al. [48] isolated SFN from broccoli, and later its cancer-preventive potential was demonstrated by the same group [49]. Based on studies conducted using cell lines, animal models, and human subjects during the last few decades, SFN is considered a chemopreventive agent with encouraging antineoplastic activities. Although several prior publications provide an excellent overview of the effect of SFN in cancer [50–59], these reports represent narrative reviews that focused mainly on SFN's source, biosynthesis, and mechanisms of action in modulating specific pathways involved in cancer without a comprehensive review of SFN's role or value for prevention of various human malignancies. Several other reviews exclusively focus on a particular cancer type, such as breast [60], bladder [61], or prostate cancer [62]. In addition, more recent review articles [63–65] focused on delivery system and synergistic effects of SFN with other anticancer drugs rather than SFN's individual action as a chemopreventive agent. Therefore, the goal of our systematic study is to present an up-to-date and critical review of SFN's efficacy in preventing the development or inhibiting the progression of various cancers types with an in-depth analysis of underlying cellular and molecular mechanisms of action. Furthermore, we discuss the current limitations and challenges of utilizing SFN as a dietary compound in humans for cancer prevention and intervention and make suggestions for the future directions of research.

2. Bioavailability and Pharmacokinetics of SFN

Phytochemicals are molecules obtained from different kinds of plants that are used for the treatment of diseases in both traditional and modern medicine, and those with poor bioavailability may have limited utility as therapeutic agents [66]. Therefore, understanding the metabolism, pharmacokinetics, and bioavailability of phytochemicals, such as SFN, is vital when considering them as therapeutic agents. SFN-rich powders have been made by drying out broccoli sprout or seed extracts. However, the encapsulation and use of these preparations are extremely expensive and challenging to use in clinical trials due to their instability and required freezing to maintain potency. On a positive note, broccoli and broccoli sprouts possess another major phytochemical of interest, GFN. GFN, a water-soluble glucosinolate and relatively inert precursor of SFN, is contained within broccoli, with the highest amounts present in the seeds and developing florets [67].

GFN is hydrolyzed in vivo to SFN via the myrosinase, which is present in gut bacteria as well as the plant itself [68]. This conversion ranges from 1–40%, with a mean of about 10% [69]. This is attributed to a wide variety of factors that include but are not limited to the mode of delivery, both intra- and inter-individual variations in metabolism and in the microbiome composition and performance of the individuals' gut, as well as a number of other factors [69]. Studies have been conducted using jejunum from humans in situ, which found that SFN is well absorbed by enterocytes, where it is conjugated with GSH and then secreted back into the lumen [70].

In vivo, SFN is able to be converted to another ITC, erucin, which is a more favorable form in certain tissues [71]. After consumption, SFN is metabolized to cysteine, cysteinyl-glycine, and finally, N-acetylcysteine (mercapturic acid), all of which are then rapidly excreted in the urine [72]. The excretion process is essentially complete 10–12 h after administration, with maximum concentrations appearing 2–6 h after dosing [72]. Another study reported that SFN is eliminated with small variations between individuals with a typical urinary excretion of 70–90% of the dose [57].

Bricker et al. [73] conducted an experiment where mice were treated with four diets ranging from nonheated broccoli sprout powders (BSP), mildly heated BSP at 60 °C, 5 min steamed BSP, or 3 mmol purified SFN. SFN concentrations in bladder, kidney, skin, lung, liver, and plasma were quantified using high-performance liquid chromatography with tandem mass spectrometry, which showed that mild heating resulted in the greatest ITC metabolite concentrations in vivo followed by the nonheated and steamed BSP diets. They also observed interconversion between SFN and erucin species or their metabolites and reported that erucin is the favored form in the bladder, kidney, and liver, even when only SFN was consumed.

A separate study on rats with oral and intravenous (i.v.) SFN found that the main pathway for metabolic clearance involved conjugation with GSH followed by concurrent processing of the conjugate to mercapturic acid [74]. They measured an absolute bioavailability of 82% between both groups with a dose of 0.5 mg/kg. This study also found that SFN peak plasma concentrations were reached about 1 h after oral administration and within minutes after the i.v. administration. The only time the absorption rate constant decreased was at the highest doses (28 μmol/kg), where the oral bioavailability dropped as low as 20%, indicating that SFN may be absorbed in a carrier-mediated transport mechanism that becomes saturated at high doses. Following i.v. and oral dosing, a rapid drop is observed in the plasma concentrations of SFN, likely reflecting its cellular uptake. This study also shows that the elimination of SFN is illustrated by a long terminal phase, where no major differences in plasma concentrations were apparent between 6 and 24 h following i.v. and oral administrations at lower doses.

Pharmacokinetic studies of SFN have been recorded via cyclocondensation of SFN and its metabolites (dithiocarbamates) with 1,2-benzenedithiol [75]. This highly sensitive method allows for the measurement of SFN and its metabolites in the blood, urine, plasma, and tissues of rodents and humans in the picomolar range [75]. Another study found that after oral administration of 150 μmol SFN to 10-week-old female Sprague Dawley rats, the concentration of dithiocarbamate reached a maximum plasma concentration (C_{max}) of 60 μM 1 h after dosing, with an elimination half-life of 6.7 h [76].

There have also been several clinical studies elaborating the bioavailability of SFN in humans; however, due to it being difficult to deliver SFN in an enriched and stable form for direct human intake, many researchers use GFN as it is much more reproducible and economical. However, the conversion of GFN to SFN is slow and has high inter-individual variations, with the urinary excretion of SFN typically ranging from 2 to 15% when only GFN is used [69]. Fahey et al. [67] found that co-administering GFN with the enzyme myrosinase in a commercially prepared diet supplement produced an equivalent output of SFN metabolites in the human subjects' urine to that which was produced when given an equal dose of GFN in a boiled and lyophilized extract of broccoli sprouts [67]. These investigators also found that when the broccoli sprouts or seeds are administered directly to human subjects without prior extraction and inactivation of endogenous myrosinase, SFN in those preparations are 3–4-fold more bioavailable than SFN from GFN delivered without active plant myrosinase. Fahey et al. [69] found that when adding myrosinase to GFN-rich broccoli extracts, the bioavailability of SFN reached levels of about 35–40%. A similar study showed that participants given broccoli sprouts with already-formed ITCs had a larger bioavailability of SFN as well as increased cumulative excretion of its conjugates when compared to broccoli sprout samples with glucosinolates and inactivated myrosinase [77].

Pharmacokinetic studies found that in oral administration of 200 μmol broccoli sprout ITC (SFN) to four healthy human subjects, the C_{max} of dithiocarbamate was 1.91 ± 0.24 μM 1 h following the dosing, with a half-life of 1.77 ± 0.13 h, and clearance of 369 ± 53 mL/min [78]. A separate study was conducted involving 20 participants administered 200 μmol SFN as SFN-rich powder in capsules reported a C_{max} of 0.7 ± 0.2 μM at 3 h, with a half-life of 1.9 ± 0.4 h for the elimination of SFN equivalents measured by mass spectrometry [79].

In all, SFN is a readily bioavailable and promising agent of interest when considering this phytochemical as a preventative anticancer agent. Although its bioavailability ranges significantly when measured as a metabolite of its precursor, GFN, a co-administration of myrosinase, helps to increase the bioavailability significantly. This elaborates the importance of having myrosinase-producing gut bacteria to aid in uptake and bioavailability when ingested in broccoli. The encouraging results from the pure SFN studies with rats underscore the importance of further human studies regarding the bioavailability of this phytochemical. The results of these studies can then be used to further our knowledge of the best way to utilize SFN as a cancer-preventive agent.

3. Toxicity Studies

Xue et al. [80] demonstrated that concentrations of 20–40 μM SFN induced apoptosis and cytotoxicity in human endothelial cells via inhibition of p38 mitogen-activated protein kinase (MAPK), mitogen-activated protein kinase kinase-1 (MAP3K-1), protein phosphatase M3/6, and activation of extracellular signal-related kinase 1/2 (ERK 1/2) and Jun NH_2-terminal kinase (JNK). Gross-Steinmeyer et al. [81] used SFN on cultured hepatocytes from viable human liver transplants. They determined that exposing human hepatocytes to 10 and 50 μM SFN for 48 h yielded no significant cytotoxicity. Clarke et al. [71] described the effects of 15 μM SFN in normal prostate epithelial cells, which, interestingly, produced no change in expression of p21 and only slight increases of histone deacetylase (HDAC) activity. In this study, normal HDAC activity is an important measurement because it concludes that SFN does not alter the cell cycle in normal, healthy cell lines and therefore is non-cytotoxic. Similarly, p21 increases apoptosis, and hence no change in its expression suggests that SFN does not cause cytotoxicity in normal cells [71]. According to Abbauoui et al. [82], the use of 5, 10, 15, and 20 μM of SFN resulted in no change in survivin expression in normal urothelial cells. Arcidiacono et al. [83] administered 1–5 μg/mL of SFN over 24 h and 48 h periods to normal human epidermal melanocytes and recorded a reduction in cell viability only at the highest concentration (5 μg/mL) used in this study.

An in vivo study conducted by Cornblatt et al. [76] administered a single oral intake of 150 μmol SFN to 10-week-old female Sprague Dawley rats and observed SFN accumulation in mammary tissue with no adverse effects. In mice, dietary SFN at an average daily dose of 7.5 μmol for 21 days had no adverse effects on animal health, food intake, or body weight [84]. This dose was calculated to be the equivalent to the consumption of

1 cup (68 g) of broccoli sprouts in humans [84]. Socała et al. [85] found that at extremely high doses (250–300 mg/kg), SFN caused sedation and muscle impairment in mice. This study concluded that the lethal dose of SFN was 212.67 mg/kg, the therapeutic dose was 191.58 mg/kg, and it also demonstrated that dietary levels of SFN daily showed no changes in animal health, weight, or food intake. Additionally, Castro et al. [86] treated mice with intraperitoneal (i.p.) injection of 50 mg/kg SFN and found no apparent toxicities indicated by lack of change in body weight over 36 days.

Clinical trials on humans have indicated that SFN is relatively safe and free of adverse effects at low doses and minimally harmful at higher doses. However, the Food and Drug Administration limits some clinical trials to 200 μmol of SFN, so more extreme dosages have not been tested [87]. Shapiro et al. [88] showed that consistent dosage in humans of 100 μmol broccoli sprout extract (BSE) or 25 μmol SFN every 8 h for 7 days had no adverse effects measured via thirty-two different parameters in hematological testing. Alumkal et al. [87] determined through a clinical trial that SFN had negligible adverse effects at a dosage of 200 μmol, with the exception of one incident of grade 2 constipation. The study explained that a higher dosage of SFN would likely be of greater benefit but has not been tested yet. Another clinical trial conducted by Tahata et al. [89] found no dose-limiting toxicities of BSE; however, grade 2 nausea occurred in one patient in the 200 μmol SFN dosage group. Zhang et al. [90] conducted a double-blind study with BSE containing 200 μmol SFN and a placebo. Out of the 98 participants, only 3 had adverse effects; two developed headaches and bloating, and the third was in the placebo group. Yagashita et al. [57] found that following oral administration of 100 μmol SFN, patients reported a harsh burning sensation in the back of their throat and posterior aspect of the tongue. At higher doses, patients reported gastrointestinal discomfort, nausea, and heartburn, similar to other clinical trials.

Jeffery and Keck [91] concluded that 3–5 servings of cruciferous vegetables (such as broccoli) per week decreased the risk of developing cancer by over 30%. Even so, many clinical studies have administered SFN in greater concentration than would be found in those 3–5 servings of broccoli and have had success in demonstrating its anticarcinogenic effects with little toxicity. At higher dosages, mild side effects have been reported; therefore, more research on the safety of SFN is warranted. Further research must be performed in order to provide a definitive parameter on safe, maximally effective dosages as well as possible effects of metabolites.

4. Sulforaphane in Cancer Prevention and Intervention

4.1. Literature Search Methodology

This review evaluates primary research articles that exemplify the anticancer properties of SFN in various cancer models. We have employed the Preferred Reporting Item for Systemic Review and Meta-Analysis (PRISMA) criteria [92] for searching and collecting relevant articles. Primary literature was identified by utilizing PubMed, ScienceDirect, and Scopus, and there were no time restraints on the year of publication. The last search was conducted in April 2021. Various combinations of keywords, such as sulforaphane, broccoli, phytochemicals, cancer, prevention, chemopreventive, tumor, apoptosis, in vitro, in vivo, and clinical studies, were utilized for literature search. Only articles published in the English language were considered for inclusion. Reviews, systemic reviews, meta-analyses, letters to editors, book chapters, conference abstracts, and unpublished observations were excluded. The authors focused specifically on preclinical studies that utilized SFN and excluded reports that used broccoli, kale, watercress, and cauliflower extracts, natural and synthetic analogs of SFN, SFN precursors, and combinations of SFN with other phytochemicals or drugs. However, papers that used SFN in combination with another agent were only included if SFN alone showed statistically significant anticancer properties. Clinical trials utilizing SFN, SFN precursors, and cruciferous vegetable extracts/constituents were searched using clinicaltrials.gov. After reading the abstract to determine relevance, the authors accessed articles through a variety of sources. The full articles were then assessed for in-depth evaluation, and the pertinent information has been summarized and reviewed in the following sections. The overview of literature search and study selection is depicted in Figure 2.

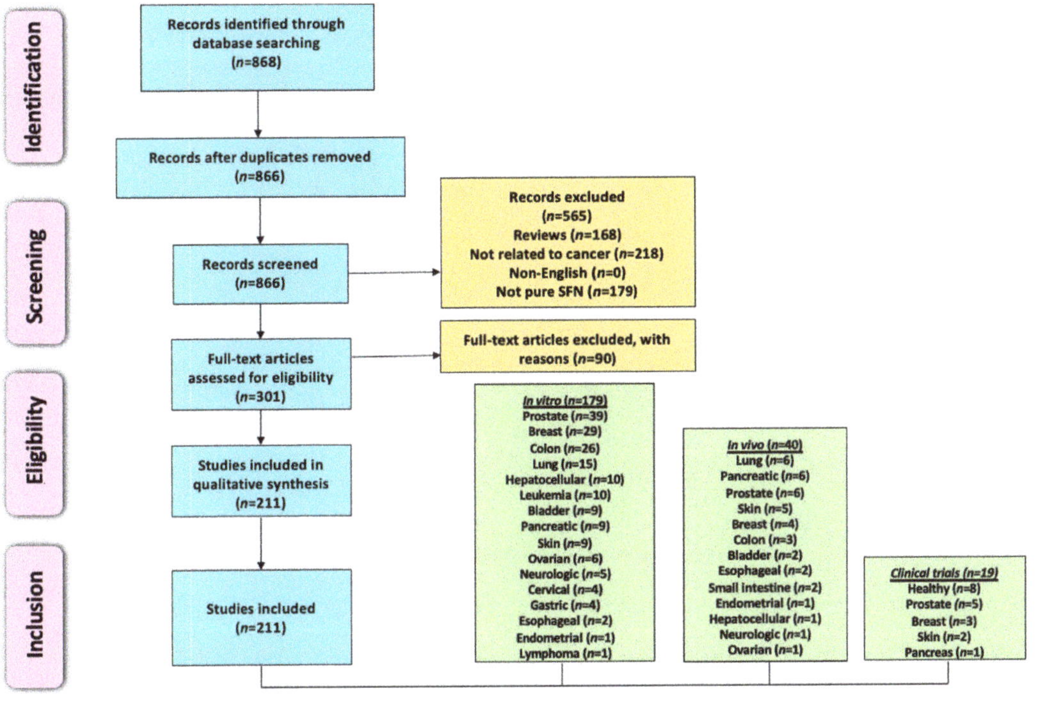

Figure 2. A PRISMA flow diagram depicting the literature search and study selection process relevant to anticancer potential of sulforaphane. The total number of in vitro, in vivo, and clinical studies (238) is greater than the number of studies included in this work (211) because numerous publications contained results from more than one organ-specific cancer or study type (i.e., in vitro, in vivo, or clinical).

4.2. Preclinical Studies (In Vitro and In Vivo)

4.2.1. Breast Cancer

One of the earliest studies to investigate the in vitro cytotoxic effects of SFN on human breast cancer cells was conducted by Tseng et al. [93]. These investigators found inhibition of cell growth when estrogen receptor (ER)-positive and progesterone receptor (PR)-positive MCF-7 cells were exposed to SFN (Table 1). However, involved mechanisms of action were not elucidated. In another study, SFN inhibited proliferation of MCF-7 cells by inducing mitotic arrest in the G2/M phase, increasing cyclin B1 protein and histone H1 phosphorylation, indicating inappropriate cdc2 kinase (CDK1) activation, and inhibiting tubulin polymerization rate [94]. The same researchers [95] uncovered similar mechanisms of inhibited cell growth in F3II sarcomatoid mammary carcinoma cells exposed to SFN. Additionally, Azarenko et al. [96] exposed MCF-7 breast cancer cells to SFN and reported inhibited cell proliferation with a decreased number and size of microtubules at SFN concentrations $\geq$25 μM.

Table 1. Potential antineoplastic effects and underlying mechanisms of action of SFN based on in vitro studies.

Cell Lines Used	Conc. and Duration	Anticancer Effects	Mechanisms	References
Breast cancer				
MCF-7	0.1–100 μM (1–48 h)	Increased cytotoxicity	Not reported	Tseng et al., 2004 [93]
MCF-7	5–30 μM (6–24 h)	Suppressed cell proliferation	↑G2/M phase arrest; ↑cyclin B1; ↑H1 phosphorylation; ↓tubulin polymerization	Jackson and Singletary, 2004 [94]
F3II	5–30 μM (12–48 h)	Inhibited cell growth	↑G2/M phase arrest; ↑cdc2 kinase activity; ↓tubulin polymerization; ↑apoptosis; ↓Bcl-2; ↓PARP; ↑caspase-3-like activity	Jackson and Singletary, 2004 [95]
MCF-7	2.5–50 μM (20–72 h)	Inhibited cell proliferation	↑G2/M phase arrest; ↑microtubule dysfunction; ↑tubulin acetylation; ↓tubulin polymerization	Azarenko et al., 2008 [96]
MDA-MB-231, MDA-MB-468	5–50 μM (3–24 h)	Inhibited cell growth and invasion	↑Apoptosis; ↑USP14; ↑UCHL5; ↑Ub-Prs	Ahmed et al., 2018 [97]
MDA-MB-231, MDA-MB-468, BT-474, MCF-7	1–25 μM (24, 72 h)	Decreased cell growth	↓HDAC5; ↓HDAC5; ↓USF1; ↓USF1; ↓luciferase; ↓LSD1; ↑H3K4me1/2; ↑ AcH3K9; ↓USP28; ↑*CTDSPL*; ↑*GLPR1*; ↑*CYLD*; ↑*TFP12*; ↑*PPP2R1B*; ↑*ISG15*; ↑*EGLN3*	Cao et al., 2018 [98]
MCF-7, MDA-MB-231	5 μM (24–72 h)	Inhibited cell growth	↑G2-M phase arrest; ↓*CCND1*; ↓*CDK4*; ↓HDAC2; ↓HDAC3; ↓HMT; ↑p53; ↑p21; ↑H3K4Me3	Royston et al., 2018 [99]
MDA-MB-231, MCF-7, T47D, MDA-MB-468	5–25 μM (24–72 h)	Inhibited cell growth	↑G2-M phase arrest; ↓cyclin B1 (MDA-MB-231 and MCF-7); ↑apoptosis; ↓global HDAC; ↓EGFR; ↓HER-2	Pledgie-Tracy et al., 2007 [100]
MCF-7, MDA-MB-231, SK-BR-3	5–20 μM (24 h)	Induced cytotoxicity	↑p21; ↑oxidative stress; ↑carbonylation of lamin A/C; ↓lamin B1; ↓nucleolar RRN3; ↑nuclear RRN3; ↓NOP2; ↓WDR12	Lewinska et al., 2017 [101]
MCF-7, MDA-MB-231, SK-BR-3	2.5–20 μM (24 h)	Inhibited cell proliferation	↑Apoptosis; ↑G2/M phase arrest (MCF-7 and MDA-MB-231); ↑G0/G1 phase arrest (SK-BR-3); ↑p53; ↑p21; ↓CCNA2; ↓CCNB1; ↓CCNB2; ↓CCND3; ↓CCNE1, CCND1; ↓CCND2; ↓CCNH; ↓p-ERK1/2 (MDA-MB-231); ↑ROS; ↑DNA DSBs; ↑DNA SSBs; ↓Akt signaling; ↓ATP; ↓AMPK activation; ↓5-mdC; ↑HDAC5; ↓HDAC6-10; ↓DNMT1; ↓DNMT3B	Lewinska et al., 2017 [102]
MCF-7, MDA-MB-231	1–100 μM (24–72 h)	Induced cell death	↑Apoptosis; ↑S phase cells; ↑G2/M phase cells; ↑p21; ↑p27; ↓cyclin A; ↓cyclin B1; ↓CDC2; ↑caspase-3; ↓Bcl-2; ↑autophagy; ↑LC3-I; ↑LC3-II	Kanematsu et al., 2010 [103]

Table 1. *Cont.*

Cell Lines Used	Conc. and Duration	Anticancer Effects	Mechanisms	References
MCF-7, SK-BR-3, MDA-MB-231, MDA-MB-468	5–30 µM (24 h)	Inhibited cell proliferation	↑Autophagosomal vacuoles; ↓mTOR; ↓S6K1; ↓p-Akt	Pawlik et al., 2013 [104]
MDA-MB-231, BT549, MDA-MB-468	10, 25 µM (16–72 h)	Inhibited cell growth	↑Autophagy; ↓P62; ↑Beclin1; ↑LC3-II; ↓HDAC6; ↑PTEN; ↓Akt	Yang et al., 2018 [105]
MDA-MB-231, MDA-MB-436, MDA-MB-468, MDA-MB-453	1–60 µM (24–72 h)	Inhibited cell proliferation	↑Apoptosis; ↑G2/M phase arrest; ↑*Egr1*; ↑*NQO1*; ↑*SL7A11*; ↑*G6PD*; ↑*GCLM*; ↑*SCD*; ↑*ID1*; ↑*IGFBP3*; ↓cyclin B1; ↓Cdc2; ↓p-Cdc2; ↓Cdc25c	Yang et al., 2016 [106]
ZR-75-1	6.25–25 µM (4–72 h)	Inhibited cell growth	↑G1/S phase arrest; ↓CDK2; ↓CDK4; ↓CDK6; ↓CDK2; ↓CDK4; ↓SERTAD1; ↓CCDN2; ↓HDAC3; ↓SERTAD; ↓CCDN2; ↓HDAC3	Cheng et al., 2019 [107]
SH, SHR	5–20 µM (72 h)	Decreased cell proliferation	↑Apoptosis; ↑S-phase arrest (SH cells); ↑S-phase and G2/M-phase arrest (SHR cells); ↓HDAC1; ↑global histone H3 acetylation; ↑DCBLD2; ↓*Septin 9*	Li et al., 2016 [108]
MCF-7, ZR-75-1	2.5–30 µM (24–72 h, 7 days)	Decreased cell proliferation	↓ERα; ↓PR; ↑PSMB5	Ramirez and Singletary, 2009 [109]
T47D, MCF-7, BT-474	2–50 µM (96 h)	Decreased cell viability	↑Apoptosis; ↑PARP cleavage	Pawlik et al., 2016 [110]
MCF-7	25 µM 24–72 h	Inhibited cell proliferation	↑Apoptosis; ↑caspase-7; ↑PARP cleavage; ↓Bcl-2; ↑Bax; ↓ERK1/2 MAPK; ↑p38 MAPK	Jo et al., 2007 [111]
MCF-7	0.01–75 µM (24 and 48 h)	Decreased cell viability	↑Apoptosis; ↓Bcl-2; ↓COX-2	Hussain et al., 2013 [112]
MCF-7, MDA-MB-231	5–20 µM (72 h)	Decreased cell viability	↑Apoptosis; ↓CYP1A1 protein (all cell lines); ↓CYP19 (MCF-7); ↑CYP19; ↑aromatase (MDA-MB-231); ↑CYP1A2 (MDA-MB-231)	Licznerska et al., 2015 [113]
MCF-7, MDA-MB-231	10–70 µM (96 h)	Inhibited cell growth	↑Apoptosis; ↑p53 (MCF-7); ↓PTEN methylation; ↑RARβ2; ↑p21	Lubecka-Pietruszewska et al., 2015 [114]
MCF-7, MDA-MB-231	5–20 µM (3–15 days)	Inhibited cell proliferation	↑Apoptosis; ↓*h*TERT; ↓telomerase activity; demethylation of CpGs of the CTCF binding site; ↑ac-H3; ↑ac-H3K9; ↓tri-me-H3K27; ↓tri-me-H3K9, ↓DNMT1; ↓DNMT3a	Meeran et al., 2010 [115]

Table 1. *Cont.*

Cell Lines Used	Conc. and Duration	Anticancer Effects	Mechanisms	References
MCF-7, MDA-MB-231	1–20 μM (24 h)	Inhibited cell proliferation	↑Apoptosis; ↓HSP70; ↓HSP90; ↓HSF1; ↑p53; ↑p21; ↑AIF; ↑Bax; ↑Bad; ↓Bcl-2; ↑caspase-3; ↑caspase-8; ↑caspase-9	Sarkar et al., 2012 [116]
MCF-7	10 μM (45 min, 6 h)	Inhibited cell growth	↑Nrf2; ↑NQO1; ↑HMOX1; ↑H3K9Ac:H3	Lo and Matthews, 2013 [117]
MCF-7	1–12 μM (4–24 h)		↑TrxR1	Wang et al., 2005 [118]
MDA-MB-231, MDA-MB-468, BT-549, BT-474, SKBR3, HS578T	20–60 μM (16, 24 h)	Decreased cell proliferation	↑Nrf2; ↓RON	Thangasamy et al., 2011 [119]
MCF-7, MDA-MB-231	1–20 μM (24 h)	Decreased cell viability and migration	↑CAV1; ↑CAV1; ↑condensed chromatin	Deb et al., 2014 [120]
MDA-MB-231-Luc-D3H1, JygMC(A)	2.5–20 μM (48 h)	Decreased cell proliferation	↓Primary tumorspheres; ↓secondary tumorspheres; ↓tertiary tumorspheres; ↓CR1; ↓CR3; ↓GRP78; ↓Alk4	Castro et al., 2019 [86]
Gastrointestinal tract and associated cancers				
Esophageal cancer				
OE33, FLO-1	1–12.5 μM (0.5–5 h)	Inhibited cell growth	↑Apoptosis; ↑G1 phase arrest; ↓HSP90; ↑p21	Qazi et al., 2010 [121]
EC9706, ECa109	10–60 μM (3–72 h)	Inhibited cell proliferation and induced autophagy	↑Apoptosis; ↑caspase-9; ↑LC3B-II; ↓p62; ↑Nrf2	Lu et al., 2020 [122]
Gastric cancer				
AGS	2.0–6.75 μM (3–24 h)	Decreased cell growth and migration	↑Apoptosis; ↑ROS; ↑Bax; ↓Bcl-2; ↑cyt c; ↑caspase-8; ↑PARP-1 cleavage; ↑SFE; ↑p-JNK; ↑p-P-38; ↓p-ERK1/2	Mondal et al., 2016 [123]
AGS	2.5–20 μM (24, 48 h)	Inhibited cell viability	↑Apoptosis; ↑G2/M phase arrest; ↑cyclin B1; ↑p53; ↑p21; ↑p-H3; ↑PARP cleavage; ↑p-AMPK; ↓cyt c; ↓MMP	Choi et al., 2018 [124]
MGC803, AGS	2–32 μM (24–48 h)	Inhibited cell proliferation	↑Apoptosis; ↑G2/M phase arrest; ↓SMYD2; ↓SMYD3 mRNA; ↓*CYR61*; ↓*MYL9*	Dong et al., 2018 [125]
AGS, MKN45	31–250 μM (48 h)	Inhibited cell growth	↑Apoptosis; ↑CDX1; ↑CDX2	Kiani et al., 2018 [126]

Table 1. *Cont.*

Cell Lines Used	Conc. and Duration	Anticancer Effects	Mechanisms	References
		Colon cancer		
SW620	5–100 μM (24–72 h)	Decreased cell proliferation	↑Apoptosis; ↑caspase-3; ↑double-strand DNA breaks	Andělová et al., 2007 [127]
SW620	20 μM (12–48 h)	Inhibited cell proliferation	↑Apoptosis; ↑caspase-9; ↑caspase-3; ↑caspase-7; ↑ATM kinase; ↑Chk2 kinase; ↑JNK	Rudolf et al., 2009 [128]
SW480	1–20 μM (3–48 h)	Inhibited cell proliferation	↑Apoptosis; ↑caspase-3; ↑caspase-7; ↑caspase-9; ↑ERK; ↑p53; ↓Bcl-2; ↑Bax/Bcl-2 ratio; ↑ROS; ↑MDA	Lan et al., 2017 [129]
HT-29	5–30 μM (24–96 h)	Inhibited cell growth	↑Apoptosis; ↑G2/M phase arrest; ↑cyclin A; ↑cyclin B1; ↑Bax; ↑PARP cleavage	Gamet-Payrastre et al., 2000 [130]
40-16, 379.2	0.4–50 μM (10–72 h)	Decreased cell growth	↑Apoptosis; ↑PARP cleavage; ↓Pro-C9; ↓Pro-C7; ↓Bax; ↓Bcl-xL	Pappa et al., 2006 [131]
40-16	5, 10 μM (24–72 h)	Inhibited cell growth	↑PARP cleavage; ↑subG1 phase arrest	Pappa et al., 2007 [132]
HCT-116	0.5–100 μM (16–48 h)	Suppressed cell growth	↑Apoptosis; ↑histone H2A.X phosphorylation; ↑caspase-9; ↑caspase-3; ↑JNK; ↑Bid; ↑Bax; ↓Bcl-2	Rudolf and Cervinka, 2011 [133]
HCT-116, HT-29, DLD1, KM12, SNU-1040	2.5, 5 μM (24–72 h)	Inhibited cell proliferation	↑Apoptosis; ↑PARP cleavage; ↑G2/M phase arrest; ↑CDK1; ↑CDC25B; ↑MK2; ↑P38; ↑p-JNK; ↓microtubule polymerization	Byun et al., 2016 [134]
HT-29	6.25–100 μM (4–36 h)	Inhibited cell growth	↑G1 phase arrest; ↓*cyclin D1*; ↓*cyclin A*; ↓*c-myc*; ↑P21; ↑ERK; ↑JNK; ↑p38	Shen et al., 2006 [135]
CT116	5–15 μM (72 h)	Inhibited cell viability	↑Apoptosis; ↑G2 phase arrest; ↑p-SAPK; ↓c-Myc	Zeng et al., 2011 [136]
40-16	0.4–50 μM (3–48 h)	Inhibited cell proliferation	↑G2/M phase arrest (6, 12, and 24 h); ↑subG1 phase arrest (48 h); ↓GSH	Pappa et al., 2007 [137]
HT-29	15 μM (48 h)	Inhibited cell growth	↑Apoptosis; ↓p-cdc2; ↑p21; ↑G2/M phase arrest; ↑Rb phosphorylation; ↑Rb protein	Parnaud et al., 2004 [138]
WiDr	2.5–80 μM (16 h)	Inhibited cell proliferation	↑Apoptosis; ↑autophagy; ↑LC3-1; ↑LC3-II; ↓Bcl-2	Nishikawa et al., 2010 [139]
DLD-1, HCT116, LoVo	5–20 μM (24 h)	Inhibited cell proliferation	↓SKP2 mRNA; ↓SKP2 protein; ↑$p27^{KIP1}$; ↑Akt; ↑ERK	Chung et al., 2015 [140]

Table 1. *Cont.*

Cell Lines Used	Conc. and Duration	Anticancer Effects	Mechanisms	References
Caco-2	1–50 μM (2, 24 h)	Inhibited cell viability	↑KLF4; ↑p21; ↓CDX-2; ↓KLF5; ↓AMACR	Traka et al., 2005 [141]
HCT-116, HT29	15 μM (6 h)	Inhibition of cell growth and migration	↑p53; ↓Wnt/β-catenin; ↑Nrf2; ↑*NMRAL2P*	Johnson et al., 2017 [142]
Caco-2	5–25 μM (6–36 h)	Induced autophagy	↑LC-II; ↑UGT1A1; ↑UGT1A8; ↑UGT1A10 mRNA; ↑Nrf2	Wang et al., 2014 [143]
Caco-2	0.5–20 μM (48 h)	Decreased cell viability	↑MRP2	Harris and Jeffery, 2008 [144]
HTC-116, HT-29, SW48, SW480	15 μM (24 h)	Decreased cell viability	↑G2/M phase arrest; ↓HDAC3; ↓HDAC6; ↑p-H2AX; ↑p-ATR; ↑CtIP acetylation	Rajendran et al., 2013 [145]
RKO, HCT-116	2.5–20 μM (72 h)	Inhibited cell growth	↑Apoptosis; ↓miR-21; ↓HDAC mRNA; ↓hTERT mRNA	Martin et al., 2018 [146]
HCT-116, SW480	0.9–60 μM (24 h)	Decreased cell proliferation	↑pH2AX; ↑pRPA32; ↑p300; ↑histone H4 acetylation	Okonkwo et al., 2018 [147]
HT-29	0.25–10 μM (24 h)	Inhibited cell growth	↓TNF-α; ↓IL-1β; ↓IL-6; ↓IFN-γ; ↓IL-1β	Bessler and Djaldetti, 2018 [148]
HT-29	10–50 μM (24, 48 h)	Suppressed cell growth and migration	↑Apoptosis; ↑subG1 phase arrest; ↑caspase-3; ↓COX-2; ↓HIF-1; ↓VEGF; ↓CXCR4; ↓PGE2	Tafakh et al., 2018 [149]
Caco-2	5–100 μM (24, 72 h)	Inhibited cell proliferation	↑p-ERK1/2; ↑p-Akt; ↑NQO1; ↑UGT1A1; ↓MRP2	Jakubikova et al., 2005 [150]
HCT-116, LoVo, Caco-2, HT-29	1–15 μM (72 h)	Decreased cell growth	↑Apoptosis; ↑ROS; ↓procaspase-8	Kim et al., 2010 [151]
HCT-116	12.5–50 μM (1–24 h)	Inhibited cell migration	↓HIF-1α; ↓VEGF; ↓HO-1; ↓GLUT1	Kim et al., 2015 [152]
		Hepatocellular cancer		
HepG2, Hepa1c1c7	5–100 μM (24 h)	Exhibited cell cytotoxicity	↑ERK2; ↑MAPK pathway	Yu et al., 1999 [153]

Table 1. *Cont.*

Cell Lines Used	Conc. and Duration	Anticancer Effects	Mechanisms	References
HepG2	100 µM (24 h)	Reduced cell viability and promoted cell death	↑Apoptosis; ↑MT-I RNA; ↑MT-II RNA, ↑MT protein expression; ↑Nrf2; ↑p38; ↑JNK/MAPK pathways; ↑caspase-3; ↑PARP cleavage; ↑Bax; ↓Bcl-2; ↓Bcl-xL	Yeh and Yen, 2005 [154]
HepG2	5–30 µM (48 h)	Inhibited cell viability and promotes cell death	↑Apoptosis; ↑caspase-3; ↑Bax; ↓Bcl-2; ↓Bcl-xL; ↓PARP; ↓β-catenin	Park et al., 2007 [155]
HepG2	20 µM (24 h)	Reduced cellular proliferation	↑HO-1; ↑ARE; ↑Nrf2; ↑ERK1/2; ↓Keap1; ↓p38 MAPK; ↓p-MKK3/6	Keum et al., 2006 [156]
Huh-7, SNU-449, NCTC	20–60 µM (24 h)	Reduced cell viability and promoted cell cycle arrest	↑Apoptosis; ↑G2/M phase arrest; ↑caspase-3; ↑caspase-8; ↑caspase-9; ↓PFKFB4; ↓HIF-1α; ↓VEGF	Jeon et al., 2011 [157]
HepG2	1.25–20 µM (24 h)	Reduced cellular proliferation, adhesion, migration, and invasion	↓STAT3; ↓HIF-1α; ↓VEGF	Liu et al., 2017 [158]
Hep3B	5–20 µM (24, 48 h)	Decreased cell viability and promoted cell death	↑Apoptosis; ↓telomerase; ↓hTERT; ↓Akt; ↑ROS	Moon et al., 2010 [159]
HepG2	10–80 µM (48 h)	Inhibited cell proliferation, migration, and invasion	↑Apoptosis; ↓TGF-β–induced EMT; ↓Vimentin; ↑E-Cadherin; ↑GO/G1 arrest; ↑ROS	Wu et al., 2016 [160]
HepG2	80 µM (24–72 h)	Inhibited cell proliferation and promoted cell death	↑Apoptosis; ↑Bip/GRP78; ↑XBP-1; ↑caspase-12; ↑Bid; ↑CHOP/GADD153	Zou et al., 2017 [161]
Hepa 1c1c7, HepG2	1–40 µM (24 h)	Reduced cell viability	↑CYP1A1; ↑AhR transformation; ↑AhR binding to XRE	Anwar-Mohamed and El-Kadi, 2009 [162]
		Pancreatic cancer		
MIA PaCa-2, PANC-1	5–40 µM (24–72 h)	Promoted cell cycle arrest and death	↑Apoptosis; ↑caspase-3, ↑caspase-8, ↑G2-M arrest, ↑ROS	Pham et al., 2004 [163]
AsPC-1, BxPc-3, MIA PaCa-2, PANC-1	0.1–100 µM (12–48 h)	Inhibited cell proliferation and promoted cell death	↑Apoptosis; ↓Akt; ↓Cdk4; ↓p53; ↑proteasomal degradation of HSP90 client proteins; ↑caspase-3; ↓HSP90-p50Cdc37 complex	Li et al., 2012 [164]
AsPC-1, BxPc-3, Capan-1, MIA PaCa2	10 µM (24, 48 h)	Reduced cell viability	↑Apoptosis; ↓NF-κB binding	Kallifatidis et al., 2009 [165]
ASPC, PANC-1, and human pancreatic CSCs	5–20 µM (1–7 days)	Reduced cellular proliferation and promoted cell death	↑Apoptosis; ↓Bcl-2, ↑caspase-3; ↓Nanog; ↓Oct-4; ↓PDGFα; ↓Smo; ↓Gli1; ↓Gli2	Rodova et al., 2012 [166]

Table 1. *Cont.*

Cell Lines Used	Conc. and Duration	Anticancer Effects	Mechanisms	References
AsPC-1, BxPc-3, PANC-1, MIA PaCa-2	10 nM (24 h)	Promoted cell death	↑Apoptosis; ↑miR-365a-3p	Yin et al., 2019 [167]
AsPC-1, BxPc-3, PANC-1	10 μM (24 h)	Promoted cell death	↑miR-135b-5p; ↑RASAL2	Yin et al., 2019 [168]
PANC-1, MIA PaCa-2	1–100 μM (24–72 h)	Inhibited cellular proliferation, invasion, and migration	↑Apoptosis; ↑ROS; ↑AMPK; ↑E-Cadherin; ↓N-Cadherin; ↓Vimentin; ↑Nrf2; ↑HO-1	Chen et al., 2018 [169]
BxPc-3, AsPC-1	10 μM (24 h)	Reduced cell viability	↑E-Cadherin; ↑GJIC; ↑Cx43; ↓c-Met; ↓CD133	Forster et al., 2014 [170]
PANC-1	10 μM (24 h)	Exhibited cytotoxicity	↑Cx43; ↑GJA1 mRNA; ↑GJIC; ↓miR30a-3p	Georgikou et al., 2020 [171]
		Gynecological cancers		
		Cervical cancer		
HeLa	5–30 μM (48 h)	Decreased cell viability	↑Apoptosis; ↑sub-G1 phase arrest; ↑Bax; ↓Bcl-2; ↓Bcl-xL; ↓pro-caspase-3; ↓PARP; ↓β-catenin	Park et al., 2007 [156]
HeLa	0.01–100 μM (24 h)	Inhibited cell growth	↑Apoptosis; ↑caspase-3; ↓Bcl-2; ↓COX-2; ↓IL-1β	Sharma et al., 2011 [172]
HeLa	2.5 μM (24–72 h)	Inhibited cell growth	↓DNMT; ↓DNMT3B; ↓HDAC1; ↑RARβ; ↑CDH1; ↑DAPK1; ↑GSTP1	Khan et al., 2015 [173]
HeLa	6.25–25 μM (24, 72 h)	Decreased cell proliferation	↑G2/M phase arrest; ↑MPM-2; ↓cyclin B1; ↓cyclin B1/CDC2 complex; ↑CDC25C/p-CDC25C ratio; ↑GADD45β	Cheng et al., 2016 [174]
		Endometrial cancer		
MFE280, KLE, Ishikawa, Hec1B, Hec1A, MFE296, AN3CA	1–32 μM (24–72 h)	Inhibited cell viability	↑Apoptosis; ↑G2/M phase arrest; ↓ATP; ↑p21; ↑p27; ↑Cdc2 phosphorylation, ↑caspase-3; ↑Bax; ↓Bcl-2; ↓Cox IV; ↓MEK; ↓ERK	Rai et al., 2020 [175]
		Ovarian cancer		
SKOV3	10–100 μM (12, 24 h)	Inhibited cell growth	↑Apoptosis; ↓Akt; ↓p-Akt; ↓PI3K; ↓cyclin D1; ↓cdk4; ↓cdk6	Chaudhuri et al., 2007 [176]
OVCAR3, SKOV3	2–50 μM (24–72 h)	Reduced cell proliferation	↑Apoptosis; ↑G1 phase arrest	Chuang et al., 2007 [177]

Table 1. *Cont.*

Cell Lines Used	Conc. and Duration	Anticancer Effects	Mechanisms	References
MDAH 2274, SKOV3	5–20 µM (12–72 h)	Induced growth arrest and inhibited cell migration	↑Apoptosis; ↑G1 phase arrest; ↓RB; ↓p130; ↑p107; ↓E2F-1; ↓E2F-2; ↓E2F-3; ↓G1 phase; ↓cyclins; ↓CDKs; ↑non-phosphorylated RB; ↓E2F-1	Bryant et al., 2010 [178]
OVCAR3, OVCAR4, OVCAR5, SKOV3	100 µM (72 h)	Inhibited cell proliferation	↑p38; ↑ERK; ↑JNK (OVCAR3 and SKOV3); ↑thioredoxin reductase (OVCAR3)	Kim et al., 2017 [179]
A2780, SKOV3	2–200 µM (6, 24 h)	Decreased cell growth	↑Apoptosis; ↑HSP27; ↑JNK; ↑MEK1; ↑p38; ↑$p90^{rsk}$ phosphorylation; ↑IP_3R2; ↑NFR2; ↑CHOP; ↑ATF4; ↑GCLC; ↑HMOX1; ↑NQO-1	Hudecova et al., 2016 [180]
PA-1	6.25, 12.5 µM (24, 72 h)	Inhibited cell proliferation	↑G2/M phase arrest; ↓CDC2; ↓cyclin B1/CDC2 complex	Chang et al., 2013 [181]
		Hematological cancers		
		Leukemia		
Jurkat T	3–30 µM (24–72 h)	Decreased cell proliferation	↑Apoptosis; ↑G2/M phase arrest	Fimognari et al., 2002 [182]
Jurkat T	3–30 µM (24, 48 h)	Reduced cell viability	↑Apoptosis; ↑G2/M phase arrest; ↑p53; ↑Bax; ↓cyclin D3; ↓CDK4; ↓CDK6	Fimognari et al., 2003 [183]
HL60	10–110 µM (24–72 h)	Inhibited cell viability	↑Apoptosis	Fimognari et al., 2008 [184]
U937	1–5 µM (48 h)	Reduced cell growth	↑Apoptosis; ↑sub-G1 phase arrest; ↑Bax; ↓Bcl-2; ↑caspase-3; ↑PARP cleavage; ↑ROS; ↑MMP	Choi et al., 2008 [185]
U937, HL60, NB-4, KG-1	15–60 µM (24, 48 h)	Decreased cell proliferation	↑Apoptosis; ↓miR-155	Koolivand et al., 2018 [186]
HL60	6–10 µM (10–48 h)	Decreased cell viability	↑G2/M phase arrest; ↑ROS ↑intracellular Ca^{2+}; ↑caspase-3; ↑caspase-8; ↑caspase-9; ↑Bax; ↑Bid; ↑Fas; ↑Fas-L; ↑Endo G; ↑AIF; ↑cyt c; ↓Bcl-xL; ↑FADD	Shang et al., 2016 [187]
HL60	1–25 µM (24, 48 h)	Inhibited cell viability	↑Apoptosis; ↑NQO1; ↓NQO1; ↓Keap1; ↑Nrf2; ↓PARP; ↓pro-caspase-2; ↓pro-caspase-3; ↓p50; ↑Bax; ↓Bcl-2; ↓NF-κB	Wu et al., 2016 [188]
Nalm-6, REH, RS4	2–40 µM (24, 48 h)	Reduced cell growth	↑Caspase-3; ↑caspase-8; ↑caspase-9; ↑PARP cleavage; ↑G2/M phase; ↑S phase arrest; ↑p21; ↑cyclin B1; ↓Akt; ↓p-mTOR	Suppipat et al., 2012 [189]

Table 1. *Cont.*

Cell Lines Used	Conc. and Duration	Anticancer Effects	Mechanisms	References
B1647	10, 30 µM (24 h)	Inhibited cell proliferation	↓AQP8; ↓ROS; ↑Nox4	Prata et al., 2018 [190]
L-1210	1–5 µM (24, 48 h)	Induced cell growth arrest	↑Apoptosis; ↑DNA strand breaks; ↑PS externalization	Misiewicz et al., 2003 [191]
Lymphoma				
B-lymphoma cells	1–10 µM (24 h)	Inhibited cell growth	↑Caspase-3; ↑caspase-7; ↑caspase- 9; ↑PARP cleavage; ↓p38 MAPK; ↓Akt	Ishiura et al., 2019 [192]
Lung cancer				
A549	1–100 µM (24 h)	Induced mitotic arrest and promoted cell death	↑Apoptosis; ↑G1/S arrest; ↑G2/M arrest; ↓tubulin polymerization; ↑ROS; ↓GSH	Mi and Chung, 2008 [193]
LTEP-A2	6.25–50 µM (3–72 h)	Inhibited cellular proliferation	↑Apoptosis; ↑G2/M arrest	Liang et al., 2008 [194]
A549	30–90 µM (24 h)	Decreased cell proliferation	↑G2/M phase; ↓G0/S phase; ↑p21; ↓cyclin D1	Zuryn et al., 2016 [195]
H1299	5–15 µM (24, 48 h)	Promoted cell cycle arrest and decreased cell viability	↑Apoptosis; ↑necrosis; ↑G2/M phase; ↓G0/S phase; ↓cyclin B1; ↑cyclin D1; ↑cyclin K	Zuryn et al., 2019 [196]
A549, H1299	5–15 µM (48 h)	Promoted cell cycle arrest and cell death	↑Apoptosis; ↑H3 acetylation; ↑H4 acetylation; ↑p53; ↑p21; ↑Bax; ↑G0/G1 arrest; ↑G2/M arrest; ↓HDAC	Jiang et al., 2016 [197]
A549	2.5, 5 µM (5 days)	Decreased cell viability	↑H3K4me1; ↓miR-9-3; ↓DNMT3a; ↓HDAC1; ↓HDAC3; ↓HDAC6; ↓CDH1; ↓CpG methylation	Gao et al., 2018 [198]
A549, H1299	1–15 µM (7 days)	Inhibited cell proliferation and the formation of tumorspheres	↑Apoptosis; ↓miR-19a; ↓miR-19b; ↓Wnt/β-catenin pathway; ↑Bax; ↑caspase-3; ↑caspase-8; ↑caspase-9; ↓CD133; ↓CD44; ↓ALDH1A1; ↓nanog; ↓oct4; ↓PCNA; ↓cyclin D1	Zhu et al., 2017 [199]
H1299, 95C, 95D	0.5–100 µM (24, 48 h)	Inhibited cell proliferation, migration, and invasion	↓miRNA-616-5p; ↓β-catenin; ↓N-cadherin; ↓vimentin	Wang et al., 2017 [200]
A549, CL1-5	10–40 µM (72 h)	Reduced cell viability and aggregation	↑Apoptosis; ↑chromatin condensation; ↑anoikis, ↑annexin V binding; ↑PS externalization; ↑p53; ↑p21; ↑Bad; ↑Bax; ↑cleaved PARP, ↓procaspase-3; ↓procaspase-7; ↓procaspase-9; ↓p-FAK; ↓p-Akt; ↓β-catenin	Tsai et al., 2019 [201]

Table 1. *Cont.*

Cell Lines Used	Conc. and Duration	Anticancer Effects	Mechanisms	References
XWLC-05	0.5–5 μg/L (24, 48, 72 h)	Promoted cell cycle arrest and death	↑Apoptosis; ↑G2/M phase; ↓G0/S phase; ↑p73; ↑PUMA; ↑Bax; ↑caspase-9; ↓Bcl-2; ↓p53	Zhou et al., 2017 [202]
Cadmium-transformed BEAS-2BR	2.5, 5, 10 μM (24 h)	Exhibited cytotoxicity	↑Apoptosis; ↓apoptosis resistance; ↑autophagy; ↑caspase-3; ↑C-PARP; ↓constitutive Nrf2; ↓Bcl-2	Wang et al., 2018 [203]
PC9/gef, H1975, A549, CL1-5, H3255	5–20 μM (48 h)	Reduced cell proliferation	↓pEGFR; ↓p-Akt; ↓p-STAT3; ↑proteasome activity	Chen et al., 2015 [204]
A549, H1299	0.5–5 μM (72 h)	Reduces cellular proliferation, migration, and invasion	↑ERK5; ↑p-ERK5 ↑E-Cadherin; ↑ZO-1; ↓pc-jun; ↓pc-Fos; ↓N-Cadherin; ↓Snail1; ↓MMP-2	Chen et al., 2019 [205]
SK-1, A549	5–30 μM (24 h)	Decreased cell viability and promoted cell death	↑Apoptosis; ↑ERK1/2; ↑Bax; ↑caspase-3; ↑26S proteasome activity; ↓Bim	Geng et al., 2017 [206]
HBE exposed to 2% TS and A549	1–40 μM (1–7 days)	Inhibited TS-induced, CSC-like properties	↓CD133; ↓ALDH1A1; ↓Oct4; ↓Nanog; ↓IL-6; ↓NICD; ↓Hes1; ↓ΔNp63α	Xie et al., 2019 [207]
		Neurological cancer		
T98G and U87MG	20, 40 μM (24, 48 h)	Decreased cell viability and promoted cell death	↑Apoptosis; ↑intracellular Ca^{+2}; ↑Bax:Bcl2; ↑caspase-3; ↑caspase-9; ↑caspase-12; ↑cyt. c; ↑calpain; ↑α-spectrin degradation; ↑ICAD cleavage; ↑AIF; ↑Smac; ↑Diablo; ↓IAPs; ↓NF-κB	Karmakar et al., 2006 [208]
U87, U373, U118, SF767	5–50 μM (24, 48 h)	Inhibited cell survival and promoted cell death	↑Apoptosis; ↑ROS; ↑DNA double-strand breaks; ↑γ-H2AX ↑caspase-3; ↑caspase-7; ↑caspase-9	Bijangi-Visheshsaraei et al., 2017 [209]
U87 and U251	1–50 μM (24, 48 h)	Reduced cell viability and promoted cell death	↑Apoptosis; ↑caspase-3; ↑Bax; ↑ROS; ↓Bcl-2; ↓p-STAT3	Miao et al., 2017 [210]
U251MG	10–40 μM (24 h)	Reduced cell viability and invasion	↑Apoptosis; ↑Bad; ↑Bax; ↑cyt. c; ↑Annexin V-binding capacity; ↓Bcl-2; ↓survivin; ↓invasion; ↓MMP-2; ↓MMP-9; ↓Galectin-3	Zhang et al., 2016 [211]
U87MG, U373MG	10–90 μM (24 h)	Decreased cell proliferation, migration, and invasion	↑ERK1/2; ↑CD44v6; ↓MMP-2	Li et al., 2014 [212]
		Skin cancer		
ME-18	1–5 μM (24, 48 h)	Induced cell growth arrest	↑Apoptosis; ↑DNA strand breaks; ↑PS externalization	Misiewicz et al., 2003 [191]

Table 1. *Cont.*

Cell Lines Used	Conc. and Duration	Anticancer Effects	Mechanisms	References
A375, 501MEL	1–5 μg/mL (2–48 h)	Suppressed cell growth, invasion, and metastasis	↑Apoptosis; ↑MDM2; ↑BAX; ↑PUMA; ↑GADD45A; ↓CDKN1A; ↑FAS; ↑caspase-3; ↑caspase-8; ↑caspase-9; ↓Bcl2; ↑BBC3; ↓ADORA1; ↑HMOX1; ↑TXNRD1; ↑GGLC; ↑GCLM;↑AKR1B10; ↑G6PD; ↑HTRA3; ↓FST; ↓ITGB4; ↓PLAT; ↓ITGB2; ↓G2/M phase; ↑CDKN1A; ↑EGR1; ↑GADD45B; ↑ATF3	Arcidiacono et al., 2018 [83]
A375	2 μg/mL (24–72 h)	Shifted growth factor receptor ratio from prosurvival to proapoptotic	↑Apoptosis	Arcidiacono et al., 2018 [213]
A375	0.1–100 μM (24, 48 h)	Decreased cell survival	↑Apoptosis; ↑caspase-3; ↑caspase-4; ↑caspase-6; ↑caspase-7; ↑caspase-8; ↑caspase-9	Mantso et al., 2016 [214]
A375 and WM793	1–20 μM (24, 48 h)	Reduced spheroid formation, migration, and invasion	↑Apoptosis; ↓Ezh2; ↓H3K27me3; ↓Bmi-1; ↓Suz12	Fisher et al., 2016 [215]
B16F-10	1–5 μg/mL	Reduced cell viability and proliferation	↑Apoptosis; ↑caspase-3; ↑caspase-9; ↑Bax; ↑p53; ↓caspase-8; ↓Bcl-2; ↓Bid; ↓NF-κB; ↓IL-1β; ↓IL-6; ↓TNF-α; ↓IL-12p40; ↓GM-CSF; ↓p65; ↓p50; ↓c-Fos; ↓ATF-2; ↓CREB; ↓c-Rel	Hamsa et al., 2011 [216]
B16	20–50 μM (24–72 h)	Reduced cell viability	↓HDAC	Enriquez et al., 2013 [217]
B16 and S91	20–50 μM (24–72 h)	Inhibited cell growth and proliferation	↓HDAC	Do et al., 2010 [218]
Bowes and SK-MEL-28	5–100 μM (2–48 h)	Decreased cellular proliferation	↑Apoptosis; ↑p-p38 kinase; ↑p53; ↑PUMA; ↑Bax; ↑ROS	Rudolf et al., 2014 [219]
		Urogenital cancers		
		Bladder cancer		
T24	5–20 μM (24, 48 h)	Inhibited cell proliferation	↑Apoptosis; ↓S and G2/M phase cells; ↑p27	Shan et al., 2006 [220]
T24	50–20 μM (4–24 h)	Decreased cell growth	↓COX-2; ↑nuclear NF-κB translocation; ↑p38	Shan et al., 2009 [221]
T24	5–20 μM (10, 24 h)	Inhibited cell growth	↑TR-1 mRNA; ↑GSTA1 mRNA; ↓COX-2	Shan et al., 2010 [222]

Table 1. *Cont.*

Cell Lines Used	Conc. and Duration	Anticancer Effects	Mechanisms	References
T24	5–20 μM (24 h)	Decreased cell invasion and migration	↑E-cadherin; ↓Snail; ↓ZEB1; ↑miR200c	Shan et al., 2013 [223]
T24	10, 20 μM (24 h)	Inhibited cell growth	↑Apoptosis; ↑caspase-3; ↑caspase-9; ↑PARP cleavage; ↓XIAP; ↓cIAP-1; ↓cIAP-2; ↑Bax; ↑cyt. c; ↑ER stress; ↑*GRP78*; ↑*CHOP*; ↑ROS; ↑Nrf2; ↓Keap1; ↑HO-1	Jo et al., 2014 [224]
RT4, J82, UMUC3	5–100 μM (48 h)	Inhibited cell proliferation	↑Apoptosis; ↓NHU; ↑G2/M phase arrest; ↑caspase-3; ↑caspase-7 activity; ↑PARP cleavage; ↓survivin; ↓EGFR; ↓HER2/neu	Abbaoui et al., 2012 [82]
RT4, J82, UMUC3	4–20 μM (3–48 h)	Decreased cell growth	↓HDAC; ↑p21 (RT4 cells); ↓thymidylate synthase; ↓histone H1 phosphorylation; ↑PP1β; ↑PP2A	Abbaoui et al., 2017 [225]
BIU87	10–80 μM (24 h)	Decreased cell proliferation	↑Apoptosis; ↑G2/M phase arrest; ↑IGFBP-3 mRNA; ↓NF-κB	Dang et al., 2014 [226]
5637	20 μM (4–48 h)	Suppressed cell growth	↑Apoptosis; ↑G2/M phase arrest; ↑histone H3 phosphorylation; ↑cyclin B1; ↑Cdk1; ↑caspase-3; ↑PARP cleavage; ↑MMP loss; ↑ROS	Park et al., 2014 [227]
		Prostate cancer		
LNCaP, MDA PCa 2a, MDA PCa 2b, PC-3, TSU-Pr1	0.1–0.15 μM (1–72 h)	Reduced cellular proliferation	↑NQO1; ↑QR; ↑γ-GCS-L; ↑GSH; ↑microsomal GST; ↑α-class GSTs	Brooks et al., 2001 [228]
DU145, LNCaP, PC-3, and CWR22Rv1	20, 40 μM (12, 24 h)	Reduced cell viability	↑Apoptosis; ↓p-STAT3; ↓IL-6-induced STAT3 phosphorylation; ↓JAK2; ↓pSTAT3 nuclear translocation; ↓STAT3 dimerization; ↓Bcl-2; ↓cyclin D1; ↓survivin; ↓Mcl-1	Hahm et al., 2010 [229]
LNCaP, PC-3	10–40 μM (2–24 h)	Reduced cell growth and proliferation	↑Apoptosis; ↑p53; ↑Bax; ↑E2F1; ↑Apaf-1; ↓Bak; ↓Bcl-xL; ↓NF-κB; ↓cIAP1; ↓cIAP2; ↓XIAP	Choi et al., 2007 [230]
LNCaP	1, 10 μM (24–72 h)	Reduced cell viability and growth	↑Apoptosis; ↓Bcl-xL; ↓glycolysis; ↓HIF-1α; ↓nuclear AR; ↓PSA	Carrasco-Pozo et al., 2019 [231]
LNCap, C4-2	1–40 μM (24, 48 h)	Inhibited androgen-stimulated cell growth and proliferation	↑Transcriptional repression of AR; ↓total AR; ↓Ser210/213 phosphorylated AR; ↓intracellular PSA; ↓secreted PSA	Kim and Singh, 2009 [232]
PC-3, LNCaP	40 μM (16 h)	Reduced cell viability and promoted cell death	↑Apoptosis; ↑autophagy; ↑LC3; ↑cyt. c	Herman-Antosiewicz et al., 2006 [233]

Table 1. *Cont.*

Cell Lines Used	Conc. and Duration	Anticancer Effects	Mechanisms	References
LNCaP, PC-3	20 µM (24 h)	Inhibited cell growth and proliferation	↑Apoptosis; ↑autophagy; ↑LC3 cleavage; ↑ROS; ↑G2/M phase arrest; ↑cyt. c; ↑Bax; ↓Bcl-2; ↓respiratory chain activity	Xiao et al., 2009 [234]
LNCaP, PC-3	150, 300 µM (4 h)	Decreased cell proliferation	↑Apoptosis; ↑autophagy; ↑LC3-II; ↓p62	Watson et al., 2015 [235]
DU145	5–20 µM (24, 48 h)	Inhibited cell viability	↑Apoptosis; ↑G2/M phase arrest; ↑PARP cleavage; ↑ROS; ↑JNK	Cho et al., 2005 [236]
PC-3	10–40 µM (24 h)	Reduced cell viability and proliferation	↑Apoptosis; ↑DNA double-strand breaks; ↑S-phase arrest	Hac et al., 2020 [237]
LNCaP	20–100 µM (24 h)	Decreased cell viability and growth	↑Apoptosis; ↑PARP cleavage; ↑caspase-3; ↓PGM3	Lee et al., 2010 [238]
PC-3	20–100 µM (24–72 h)	Reduced cell survival and proliferation	↑Apoptosis; ↑G0/G1 arrest; ↑caspase-3; ↑caspase-8; ↑caspase-9; ↑Bax; ↑PARP cleavage; ↓Bcl-2	Singh et al., 2004 [239]
PC-3, DU145	10–40 µM (1–24 h)	Reduced cell viability	↑Apoptosis; ↑caspase-3; ↑caspase-9; ↑Bid cleavage; ↑PARP cleavage; ↑Fas; ↑cyt. c; ↑disruption of mitochondrial membrane potential; ↑ROS; ↓GSH	Singh et al., 2005 [240]
PC-3	5–20 µM (24–96 h)	Reduced cell viability	↑Apoptosis; ↑NRF1; ↑mitochondrial fission; ↑Bax; ↑PGC1α; ↓HIF-1α	Negrette-Guzmán et al., 2017 [241]
22Rv1	5–50 µM (3–24 h)	Inhibited cell growth	↑Apoptosis; ↓USP14 and UCHL5 active sites; ↑USP14; ↑UCHL5 protein; ↑Ub-Prs	Ahmed et al., 2018 [97]
LNCaP, PC-3	15 µM (6, 24 h)	Inhibited cell proliferation	↑HO-1; ↑NQO1; ↓BMX; ↓CDK2; ↓PLK1; ↓Sp1	Beaver et al., 2014 [242]
LNCaP	10, 25 µM (2–72h)	Reduced cell growth	↑Apoptosis; ↑NQO1; ↑LTB4DH; ↑ME1; ↑TXNRD1; ↑GSTM1; ↑MGST1; ↑SOD1; ↑PRDX1; ↑GCLM; ↓Jun; ↑G2/M arrest	Bhamre et al., 2009 [243]
LNCaP, PC-3	15 µM (24, 48 h)	Inhibited cellular growth	↑Ac-H3 at P21 promoter; ↑p21; ↑G2/M phase arrest; ↑HO-1; ↑NQO1; ↓HDAC3; ↓HDAC4; ↓HDAC6	Clarke et al., 2011 [71]
LNCaP, VCaP	10–20 µM (12, 24 h)	Decreased cell viability	↑HSP90 acetylation; ↓AR; ↓HDAC6; ↓ERG	Gibbs et al., 2009 [244]
LNCaP, PC-3	15 µM (48 h)	Promoted cell cycle arrest and death	↓HDAC activity; ↑Ac-H3; ↑Ac-H4; ↑caspase-3; ↑G2/M arrest	Myzak et al., 2006 [245]

Table 1. *Cont.*

Cell Lines Used	Conc. and Duration	Anticancer Effects	Mechanisms	References
TRAMP C1		Exhibited cytotoxicity	↑Nrf2; ↑NQO-1; ↑Ac-H3; ↓DNMT1; ↓DNMT3a; ↓HDAC1; ↓HDAC4; ↓HDAC5; ↓HDAC7	Zhang et al., 2013 [246]
LNCaP, PC-3	15 µM (3–24 h)	Decreased cellular proliferation	Altered ~100 lncRNA's expression	Beaver et al., 2017 [247]
PC-3, LNCaP	10, 20 µM (8–24 h)	Reduced cell proliferation and migration	↓Notch1; ↓Notch2; ↓Notch4; ↑DNA fragmentation	Hahm et al., 2012 [248]
PC-3, LNCaP	15, 30 µM (24, 48 h)	Decreased cellular proliferation	↓DNMT1; ↓DNMT3b; ↓cyclin-D2-promoter methylation; ↑cyclin D2	Hsu et al., 2011 [249]
LNCaP, PC-3	15 µM (48 h)	Exhibited cytotoxicity	↓DNMT1; ↓DNMT3b; ↑CCR4; ↑TGFBR1	Wong et al., 2014 [250]
LNCaP, PC-3	2.5–20 µM (24 h)	Decreased cell viability and proliferation	↑Apoptosis; ↓pCSC; ↓CD24; ↓ITGA6; ↓ZEB2; ↓c-Myc	Vyas et al., 2016 [251]
LNCaP, PC-3	15 µM (6–24 h)	Decreased cell viability	↑SUV39H1 post-translational modification; ↓H3K9me3; ↓chromatin-associated SUV39H1	Watson et al., 2014 [252]
LNCaP, 22Rv1, PC-3	5, 10 µM (24 h)	Decreased cell viability	↓Glycolysis; ↓HKII; ↓LDHA; ↓PMK2	Singh et al., 2019 [253]
DU145	5–40 µM (24 h)	Decreased cell viability, migration, and invasion	↓Pseudopodia; ↓MMP-2; ↑p-ERK1/2; ↑E-Cadherin; ↓CD44v6	Peng et al., 2015 [254]
PC-3, DU145	10, 20 µM (24 h)	Decreased cell proliferation and migration	↑Apoptosis; ↑Vimentin; ↑PAI-1; ↓E-cadherin	Vyas and Singh, 2014 [255]
PC-3	40 µM (3–24 h)	Inhibited cell viability	↑Autophagy; ↓S6K1 phosphorylation; ↑LC3	Hac et al., 2015 [256]
PC-3	5–50 µM (24 h)	Decreased cell viability	↑H2S; ↑p38; ↑JNK	Pei et al., 2011 [257]
PC-3	10–40 µM (2–24 h)	Decreased cell survival	↓Protein synthesis; ↓[3H]-leucine incorporation; ↓mTOR signaling; ↑S6K1 dephosphorylation; ↓survivin	Wiczk et al., 2012 [258]
PC-3	1–40 µM (24 h)	Decreased cell viability	↓NF-κB; ↓p65 nuclear translocation; ↓VEGF; ↓cyclin-D1; ↓Bcl-xL; ↓IKKα phosphorylation; ↓IKKβ phosphorylation	Xu et al., 2005 [259]

Table 1. *Cont.*

Cell Lines Used	Conc. and Duration	Anticancer Effects	Mechanisms	References
PC-3	5–40 µM (6–24 h)	Reduced cell viability	↑AP-1; ↑p-ERK1/2; ↑p-JNK1/2; ↑p-Elk-1; ↑p-c-Jun	Xu et al., 2006 [260]
DU145	5–40 µM (24 h)	Inhibited angiogenesis	↓HIF-1α; ↑JNK signaling; ↑ERK signaling; ↓VEGF	Yao et al., 2008 [261]
LNCaP, 22Rv1	5, 10 µM (8–24 h)	Inhibited cell proliferation	↓ACC1; ↓FASN; ↓CPT1A; ↓ACADVL; ↓ACADM; ↓HADHA; ↓SREBP1	Singh et al., 2018 [262]
LNCaP	10–60 µM (24 h)	Promoted cell cycle arrest and death	↑G2/M arrest; ↑S phase arrest; ↑mitotic arrest; ↓cyclin D1; ↓cyclin E1; ↓Cdk4; ↓Cdk6; ↓Cdk1; ↓Cdc25C; ↑cyclin B1; ↑p53; ↑p21	Herman-Antosiewicz et al., 2007 [263]
LNCaP, DU-145	15 µM (24 h)	Reduced cellular proliferation	↓hTERT; ↓G0/G1 transition; ↓S phase; ↓NF-κB; ↓HDAC inhibitor activity; ↓H3K4me2 signal; ↓MeCP2; ↑H3K18Ac signal ↑DNMT1; ↑DNMT3a; ↑Pan-acetylated H3; ↑Pan-acetylated H4	Abbas et al., 2016 [264]

Symbols: ↑, increased or upregulated; ↓decreased or downregulated.

Ahmed et al. [97] conducted a study to determine the cytotoxic effect of SFN on MDA-MB-231 and MDA-MB-468 breast cancer cells (both are ER- and PR-negative). SFN showed antiproliferative and anti-invasive effects through increased apoptosis; elevated total ubiquitinated proteins (Ub-Prs); inhibition of the activity of the deubiquitinating enzyme (DUBs), ubiquitin-specific protease 14 (USP14), and ubiquitin C-terminal hydrolase L5 (UCHL5); and increased USP14 and UCHL5 proteins. Overall, this study indicated that inhibition of the proteasomal cysteine DUBs activates a feedback reaction that increases the levels of USP14 and UCHL5 proteins and that specific 19S-DUB inhibitors are novel anticancer targets of SFN.

Cao et al. [98] exposed MDA-MB-231, MDA-MB-468, BT-474, and MCF-7 breast cancer cells to SFN and found decreased cell growth via inhibition of the transcription of epigenetic regulator HDAC5 by blockage of the promotor region. This resulted in destabilization of the flavin adenine dinucleotide-dependent histone demethylase 1 (LSD1) protein, indicating that the HDAC5-LSD1 axis is an effective target of SFN in breast cancer cells. Similarly, Royston et al. [99] observed decreased HDACs (HDAC2 and HDAC3) as well as cell cycle arrest in MCF-7 and MDA-MB-231 cells following SFN exposure. This study also showed that SFN decreased histone methyltransferase (HMT) activity in MCF-7 cells, and there was an increase in two tumor suppressors, p53 and p21. Similar cell cycle dysfunctions were noted in MDA-MB-231 and MCF-7 cell lines in a study conducted by Pledgie-Tracy et al. [100], who observed that SFN at concentrations 5 μM and higher inhibited the growth of MDA-MB-231, MCF-7, T47D (ER-positive), and MDA-MB-468 cells. Specifically, MDA-MB-231 and MCF-7 cells were arrested in the G2/M phase in parallel with an increase in cyclin B1 protein expression, and SFN was shown to inhibit global HDAC activity in all cell lines.

Lewinska et al. [101] examined anticancer properties of SFN against MCF-7, MDA-MB-231, and SK-BR-3 (ER-negative, PR-negative, and human growth factor receptor (HER)-positive) cell lines, and found that SFN decreased cell proliferation, which was accompanied by an increase in p21, determined to be p53-independent. Overall, SFN was shown to induce oxidant-based nucleolar stress, which was demonstrated by an increase in superoxide levels, increased protein carbonylation, and changes in nuclear morphology. Lewinska et al. [102] later supported these results by finding elevated levels of p21 in the same three cell lines, as well as increased p53 in MCF-7 cells only. This is the first study to report that SFN-induced cell cycle arrest is permanent, supported by an increase in senescence-associated β-galactosidase staining. Finally, an increase in reactive oxygen species (ROS), genotoxicity, and a decrease in Akt signaling led to apoptosis in all three cell lines.

SFN induced growth inhibition in a time- and concentration-dependent manner in MCF-7 and MDA-MB-231 cells via increased cells in the S and G2/M phases; changes in cell cycle regulatory molecules, such as an increase in p21 and p27; as well as a decrease in cyclin A, cyclin B1, and CDC2 proteins [103]. This study is one of the first to uncover the autophagy-inducing effect of SFN in MDA-MB-231 cells, supported by the formation of autophagosomes, autolysosomes, accumulation of acidic vesicular organelles (AVOs), and an increased level of LC3-II. Later, Pawlik et al. [104] supported these results, showing that SFN induced autophagosomal lysosomes in MCF-7, MDA-MB-231, MDA-MB-468, and SK-BR-3 cells. This effect of SFN has been linked to targets in the pro-survival pathway, indicated by decreases in Akt and S6KI phosphorylation.

Yang et al. [105] demonstrated that 25 μM SFN induced autophagy in three triple-negative (ER-negative, PR-negative, and HER2-negative) breast cancer cell lines, namely, MDA-MB-231, BT549, and MDA-MB-468, as well as suppressed HDAC6 expression, resulting in phosphatase and tensin homolog (PTEN) activation. Another study found decreased expression of cyclin B1, CDC2, p-CDC2, and CDC25C, which may be due to SFN-induced upregulation of the tumor-suppressor gene *Egr1* in various breast cancer cells [106].

Additional cell lines have been exposed to SFN to determine how this phytochemical impacts the cell cycle. Cheng et al. [107] investigated the effects of SFN on ZR-75-1 (ER-positive, PR-positive, and HER2-positive) cell survival and found that SFN decreased cell viability in a concentration-dependent manner. G1/S arrest was observed with concomitant downregulation of CDK2 and CDK4 protein levels at 12.5 and 25 μM SFN. Li et al. [108] transfected normal human mammary epithelial cells to create ER-SH (precancerous) cells and SHR (completely transformed breast cancer) cells. SFN inhibited cell growth in both cell lines, and cell cycle arrest was noted. Additionally, a decrease in HDAC1 was observed, which resulted in an increase in global and local histone acetylation. The ZR-75-1 cell line was used in another study along with MCF-7 cells [109]. Suppression of cell growth was identified in both cell lines after exposure to 30 μM SFN. Additionally, ERα protein expression was significantly inhibited in both cell lines, and Erα mRNA expression and gene transcription were significantly decreased in MCF-7 cells. This was the first study to indicate that regulation of ERα mRNA may be due to SFN inhibition of ERα transcription.

Many other studies have explored the mechanisms behind SFN-induced apoptosis. Pawlik et al. [110] introduced SFN to three ER-positive breast cancer cell lines, namely, T47D, MCF-7, and BT-474, and found decreased cell growth in a concentration-dependent manner, as well as increased PARP cleavage, indicating induced apoptosis. Additional mechanisms that have been attributed to apoptosis include an increase in PARP and caspase-7 cleavage, decreased Bcl-2 protein with increased Bax protein, and an increase in p38 activity with concomitant inhibition of ERK1/2 activity [111]. SFN-induced inhibition of *Bcl-2* was also observed in a study conducted by Hussain et al. [112]. After SFN exposure, they observed decreased viability of MCF-7 cells, and apoptosis was confirmed via observation of morphological changes. Additionally, SFN downregulated the anti-apoptotic gene *Bcl-2* and the proinflammatory gene cyclooxygenase-2 (*COX-2*). Licznerska et al. [113] exposed MCF-7 and MDA-MB-231 lines to SFN and observed decreased cell viability, induction of apoptosis, and reduced cytochrome P-450 (CYP) 1A1 protein levels. In the MCF-7 cell line, SFN reduced *CYP19* expression and protein levels. However, in MDA-MB-231 cells, SFN increased *CYP19* expression and protein levels, increased CYP1A2 protein levels, and increased aromatase protein. Lubecka-Pietruszewski et al. [114] explored additional proapoptotic mechanisms of SFN in MCF-7 and MDA-MB-231 cell lines. They found elevated *PTEN* and *RARbeta2* expression in both cell lines induced through promotor DNA methylation mechanisms. Additionally, Meeran et al. [115] demonstrated that SFN inhibited proliferation of the same cell lines, which was attributed to decreased human telomerase reverse transcriptase (*hTERT*) via epigenetic modification of the *hTERT* promotor. Finally, Sarkar et al. [116] observed SFN-induced cell growth inhibition and apoptosis in the same cell lines due to decreased expression of heat shock protein 70 (HSP70), HSP90, and heat shock factor 1 (HSF1), increased *p53* and *p21* expression, and increased expression of Bax and Bad with concomitantly decreased expression of Bcl-2.

SFN has also been shown to inhibit cell proliferation by additional cellular mechanisms. Lo and Matthews [117] exposed MCF-7 breast cancer cells to SFN and observed an increase in nuclear factor erythroid-2-related factor 2 (Nrf2), NADPH-dependent oxidoreductase 1 (NQO1), and heme oxygenase 1 (HMOX1) mRNA, indicating that SFN plays an important role in protecting cells from oxidative stress by upregulating phase II detoxifying enzymes. Similarly, Wang et al. [118] exposed the same cell line to SFN and found an increase in thioredoxin reductase 1 (TrxR1) mRNA expression, which plays an important role in protection against oxidative stress. Thangasamy et al. [119] explored the effects of SFN-induced Nrf2 expression on the tyrosine kinase receptor, recepteur d′ origine nantais (RON), also known as macrophage-stimulating 1 receptor, in MDA-MB-231, MDA-MB-468, BT-549, BT-474, SKBR3, and HS578T breast cancer cells. With increased Nrf2 stabilization, RON expression decreased via decreased promoter activity. This was the first evidence depicting SFN-induced decreases in the oncogene RON via Nrf2. In another study, SFN decreased the viability of MCF-7 and MDA-MB-231 cells in parallel with an increase in mRNA and protein expression of the tumor suppressor and oncogene CAV1 [120]. Finally, Castro et al. [86] exposed two triple-negative breast cancer cell lines, MDA-MB-231-Luc-D3H1, and the mouse mammary carcinoma cell line, JygMC(A), to SFN, and found inhibited cell proliferation as well as a decrease in the number of primary, secondary, and tertiary tumorspheres in both cell lines, indicating a reduced capacity for self-renewal.

The anticancer effects of SFN on breast cancer have also been explored in many in vivo studies. Jackson and Singletary [95] subcutaneously injected F3II sarcomatoid mammary carcinoma cells into BALB/c mice. Five days later, lateral tail vein injections of 15 nmol SFN were administered daily for 13 days, after which tumors were excised and examined. The experimenters found significantly smaller tumors in SFN-injected mice versus control mice, as well as reduced proliferating cell nuclear antigen (PCNA) and elevated PARP fragment (Table 2). The BALB/c mice were used in another study, where they were xenografted with MDA-MB-231-luc-D3H1 cells [86]. Daily 50 mg/kg SFN (i.p.) injections were administered for 2 weeks prior to xenograft in one group of mice and for 3 weeks after xenograft in another experimental group. Results showed a 29% decrease in tumor volume in the pretreatment group and a 50% reduction in tumor volume in the posttreatment group when compared to the control. Mechanistic results include decreased expression of *ALDH1A1, NANOG, CR1, GDF3, FOXd3, NOTCH4,* and *WNT3* genes. Kanematsu et al. [265] transplanted BALB/c mice with KPL-1 cells (ER-positive, PR-negative, and HER2-negative) and injected (i.p.) either 25 or 50 mg/kg SFN 5 days per week for 4 weeks. SFN suppressed the growth of the tumor cells, possibly via induction of apoptosis in a dose-dependent manner. Yang et al. [106] implanted MDA-MB-453 cells into nude mice, and the animals were then treated with 100 mg/kg SFN via i.v. injection daily for 15 days. A significant decrease in tumor weights was observed in the experimental group compared to the control, and an increase in *Egr1* expression was noticed along with a decrease in *cyclinB1* and *CDC25c* expression.

Table 2. Potential antineoplastic effects and underlying mechanisms of action of SFN based on in vivo studies.

Animal Tumor Models	Anticancer Effects	Mechanisms	Dose (Route)	Duration	References
		Breast cancer			
BALB/c mice injected with F3II cells	Suppressed tumor development	↓PCNA; ↑PARP fragment	15 nmol, daily (i.v.)	13 days	Jackson and Singletary, 2004 [95]
Nude female BALB/c mice xenografted with MDA-MB-231-Luc-D3H1 cells	Inhibited tumor growth	↓*ALDH1A1*; ↓*NANOG*; ↓*CR1*; ↓*GDF3*; ↓*FOXD3*; ↓*NOTCH4*; ↓*WNT3*	50 mg/kg (i.p.)	3, 5 weeks	Castro et al., 2019 [86]
Female athymic BALB/c mice transplanted with KPL-1 cells	Suppressed tumor growth	↑Apoptotic ratio	25, 50 mg/kg (i.p.)	26 days	Kanematsu et al., 2011 [265]
Nude mice xenografted with MDA-MB-453 cells	Reduced tumor size	↑*Egr1*; ↓*cyclin B1*; ↓*CDC25c*	100 mg/kg (i.v.)	15 days	Yang et al., 2016 [106]
		Gastrointestinal tract and associated cancers			
		Esophageal cancer			
SCID mice inoculated with BEAC and FLO-1 cells	Reduced tumor size	Not reported	0.75 mg/day (s.c.)	2 weeks	Qazi et al., 2010 [121]
Male BALB/c mice inoculated with ECa109 cells	Decreased tumor size	↑LC3B-II; ↓P62	5 mg/kg, every other day (i.p.)	2 weeks	Lu et al., 2020 [122]
		Small intestine			
Male Apc$^{Min/+}$ mice	Decreased tumor number and size	↑Apoptosis; ↓p-JNK; ↓p-ERK; ↓p-Akt	300 and 600 ppm/day (via diet)	3 weeks	Hu et al., 2006 [266]
Male Apc$^{Min/+}$ mice	Reduced tumor size	↑Apoptosis; ↑p21; ↑caspase-3; ↑caspase-9; ↑COX-2; ↓p-Akt	300 and 600 ppm/day (via diet)	3, 10 weeks	Shen et al., 2007 [267]
		Colon cancer			
Nude male mice xenografted with HCT116 cells	Suppressed tumor growth; decreased tumor size	↑CDK1; ↑MK2; ↑p38 phosphorylation	1 and 5 mg/kg/day (i.p.)	13 days	Byun et al., 2016 [134]
Male C57BL/6J$^{+/Min}$ mice	Inhibited tumor growth	↓HDAC; ↑acetylated histone H4; ↑p21; ↑Bax	~6 µmol/day (via diet)	10 weeks	Myzak et al., 2006 [245]
Male WT and Nrf2 mice induced tumors with DMT	Reduced tumor size	↓HDAC; ↓HDAC3 protein; ↑global histone H4 acetylation	400 ppm/day or alternate days (via diet)	25, 35 weeks	Rajendran et al., 2015 [268]

Table 2. *Cont.*

Animal Tumor Models	Anticancer Effects	Mechanisms	Dose (Route)	Duration	References
		Hepatocellular cancer			
Female BALB/c athymic mice inoculated with HepG2 cells	Reduced tumor growth and volume	Not reported	50 mg/kg, every 2 days (i.p.)	13 days	Wu et al., 2016 [160]
		Pancreatic cancer			
Male Syrian Hamster injected with BOP to initiate carcinogenesis	Prevented pancreatic carcinogenesis	Not reported	80 ppm/day (p.o.)	3 weeks	Kuroiwa et al., 2006 [269]
Male SCID mice inoculated with PANC-1	Decreased tumor growth	Not reported	250–500 μmol/kg/d (i.p.)	3 weeks	Pham et al., 2004 [163]
Female athymic (nu/nu) mice inoculated with Mia Paca-2	Inhibited tumor growth	Not reported	25 or 50 mg/kg (5× per week i.p.)	4 weeks	Li et al., 2012 [164]
Male NOD/SCID/IL2Rγ mice inoculated with human pancreatic CSCs	Reduced tumor growth	↓Smo; ↓Gli 1; ↓Gli 2; ↓Oct-4; ↓VEGF; ↓PDGFα; ↓Bcl-2; ↓XIAP; ↑E-Cadherin	20 mg/kg/day (5× per week p.o.)	6 weeks	Li et al., 2013 [270]
Nude mice inoculated with MIA-PaCa2	Blocked tumor growth and angiogenesis	↑Apoptosis; ↓NK-κB binding	4.4 mg/kg (i.p.) on days 4, 5, and 6 after tumor transplant	1 week	Kallifatidis et al., 2009 [165]
BALB/c nude mice (transgenic pancreatic cancer mice)	Reduced tumor volume and weight	↑Nrf2; ↓Ki-67; ↑p-AMPK	50 mg/kg, every other day (i.p.)	120 days	Chen et al., 2018 [169]
		Gynecological cancers			
		Endometrial cancer			
Female SCID mice inoculated with Ishikawa cells	Reduced tumor volume	↑Apoptosis	50 mg/kg once a day (i.p.)	30 days	Rai et al., 2020 [175]
		Ovarian cancer			
Athymic mice inoculated with A2780 cells	Inhibited tumor growth	↑IP_3R	40 mg/kg, once a day (i.p.)	7 days	Hudecova et al., 2016 [180]
		Lung cancer			
A/J mice treated with benzopyrene and NNK	Inhibited cellular proliferation. Reduced tumor size and weight	↑Apoptosis; ↑casspase-3; ↓PCNA	1.5 and 5 μmol/g (p.o.)	42 weeks	Conaway et al., 2005 [271]

Table 2. *Cont.*

Animal Tumor Models	Anticancer Effects	Mechanisms	Dose (Route)	Duration	References
Nude mice inoculated with LTEP-A2 cells	Reduced tumor weight	↑Apoptosis; ↑G2/M arrest	25–100 mg/kg, 3 doses/week (i.p.)	9 days	Liang et al., 2008 [194]
NOD/SCID mice inoculated with A549 cells	Reduced tumor volume and weight	↑Apoptosis; ↑H3 acetylation, ↑H4 acetylation; ↑p53; ↑p21; ↑Bax; ↑G0/G1 arrest; ↑G2/M arrest; ↓HDAC	9 µM/mice/day on alternate days (p.o.)	28 days	Jiang et al., 2016 [197]
BALB/c nu/nu male mice inoculated with NSCLC	Reduced tumor volume	↓EGFR	10 µmol/kg, 5 doses/week (i.t.)	21 days	Chen et al., 2015 [204]
BALB/c nude female inoculated with H1299	Reduced tumor weight and volume and inhibited cell migration and invasion	↑ERK5; ↑pERK5; ↑E-Cadherin; ↑ZO-1; ↓pc-jun; ↓pc-Fos; ↓N-Cadherin; ↓Snail1	25 and 50 mg/kg every 3 days (i.p.)	21 days	Chen et al., 2019 [205]
Nude male BALB/c mice inoculated with H1299 and 95D cells	Decreased the incidence of lung metastasis	↓miRNA-616-5p; ↓β-catenin; ↓N-cadherin; ↓Vimentin	25 or 50 mg/kg, every 3 days (i.v.)	4 weeks	Wang et al., 2017 [200]
		Neurological cancer			
Female NSG mice inoculated with GBM10 cells	Inhibited tumor growth	Not reported	100 mg/kg for 5-day cycles (p.o.)	3 weeks	Bijangi-Vishehsaraei et al., 2017 [209]
		Skin cancer			
C57BL/6 mice injected with B16F-10 melanoma cells	Inhibited tumor growth and lung metastasis	↓Lung hydroxyproline; ↓lung uronic acid; ↓lung hexosamine; ↓serum sialic acid; ↓serum GGT; ↑IL-2; ↑IFN-γ; ↓IL-1β; ↓IL-6; ↓TNF-α	500 µg/kg (i.p.)	10 days	Thejass and Kuttan, 2006 [272]; Thejass and Kuttan, 2007 [273]
C57BL/6 mice inoculated with B16 cells	Reduced tumor volume	↓HDAC	500 µmol/kg, 3 doses/week (i.p.)	4 weeks	Do et al., 2010 [218]
C57Bl/6 mice inoculated with B16 cells	Inhibited tumor growth and reduced volume	↓HDAC	500 µmol/kg, 3 doses/week (i.p.)	4 weeks	Enriquez et al., 2013 [217]

Table 2. *Cont.*

Animal Tumor Models	Anticancer Effects	Mechanisms	Dose (Route)	Duration	References
NSG mice inoculated with A375	Reduced tumor formation and volume	↑Apoptosis; ↓Ezh2; ↓H3K27me3; ↓MMP-9; ↓MMP-2; ↑TIMP3; ↑PARP cleavage; ↑procaspase-8; ↑procaspase-9	10 µmol/kg, 3 doses/week (p.o.)	6 weeks	Fisher et al., 2016 [215]
		Urogenital cancers			
		Bladder cancer			
Nude female athymic mice xenografted with UMUC3 cells	Inhibited tumor growth	Not reported	295 µmol/kg (p.o.)	2 weeks	Abbaoui et al., 2012 [82]
Male athymic mice xenografted with UMUC3 cells	Suppressed tumor growth	↑Apoptosis; ↑caspase-3; ↑cyt. c; ↓survivin	12 mg/kg (p.o.)	5 weeks	Wang and Shan, 2012 [274]
		Prostate cancer			
Nude male athymic BALB/c (nu/nu) mice xenografted with PC-3 cells	Reduced tumor growth	↑Apoptosis; ↑Bax; ↑Ac-H3; ↑Ac-H4; ↓HDAC	443 mg/kg/day (p.o.)	3 weeks	Myzak et al., 2007 [84]
Male and female athymic mice PC-3 xenograft	Inhibited tumor growth	↑Apoptosis; ↑Bax	5.6 µmol, 3 times/week (p.o.)	3 weeks	Singh et al., 2004 [240]
Male TRAMP [C57BL/6xFVB]F1 hybrid	Decreased cell proliferation and pulmonary metastasis	↑Apoptosis; ↑E-Cadherin; ↑Bad; ↑Bak; ↑Bid; ↑Bax; ↑NK cell cytotoxicity; ↑PARP cleavage; ↓Mcl-1; ↑T-cell infiltration	6 µmol, 3 times/week (p.o.)	17–19 weeks	Singh et al., 2009 [275]
PTEN^ L/L;PB-Cre4 mice	Inhibited cell viability and proliferation	↑Apoptosis; ↑cell cycle arrest; ↑caspase-3; ↑caspase-7; ↑cyclin B1; ↓cyclin D2	0.1, 1 µmol/g/day (p.o.)	8 weeks	Traka et al., 2010 [276]
TRAMP mice	Inhibited tumor growth	↓ACC1; ↓FASN; ↓acetyl-coA; ↓total FFA; ↓phospholipids	Not specified	Not specified	Singh et al., 2018 [262]
TRAMP and Hi-Myc mice with prostate adenocarcinoma	Decreased tumor size	↓Glycolysis; ↓HKII; ↓PKM2; ↓LDHA; ↓lactate	1 mg, 3 times/week (p.o.)	5 weeks	Singh et al., 2019 [253]

Symbols: ↑, increased or upregulated; ↓decreased or downregulated.

4.2.2. Gastrointestinal Tract and Associate Cancers

Esophageal Cancer

SFN has shown anticancer properties in a variety of gastrointestinal tract cancers. Qazi et al. [121] exposed esophageal cancer cell lines OE33 and FLO-1 to SFN and witnessed inhibited cell growth through apoptosis induction, G1 phase arrest, upregulation of p21, and downregulation of HSP90. Additionally, Lu et al. [122] treated EC9706 and ECa109 esophageal squamous cancer cells with SFN and observed inhibited cell proliferation. Increased apoptosis was attributed to activation of the Nrf2 pathway and was accompanied by increases in caspase-9 and LC3B-II, an autophagosome marker, along with decreased p62.

Qazi et al. [121] also extended their in vitro work to evaluate in vivo efficacy of SFN in mice xenografted with BEAC and FLO-1 tumors. After 2 weeks of daily subcutaneous (s.c.) injections of SFN, tumor growth was significantly reduced compared to the control group; however, anticancer mechanisms were not identified. Lu et al. [122] also extended their in vitro findings into a mouse tumor model. BALB/c male mice inoculated with ECa109 cells were given i.p. injections of 5 mg/kg SFN every other day for 2 weeks. Tumor size was decreased in the SFN experimental group, and tissue evaluation revealed an increase in LC3B-II and a decrease in p62. These results, along with the in vitro findings, support the notion that SFN induces apoptosis and promotes autophagy through modulation of the Nrf2 pathway in esophageal cancer cells.

Gastric Cancer

The antitumor properties of SFN have also been established in gastric carcinoma. Mondal et al. [123] determined that SFN reduced the viability of AGS gastric carcinoma cells by inducing apoptosis, modifying cell morphology, and generating intracellular ROS. Additional apoptotic mechanisms, including increased Bax, cytochrome c (cyt. c), caspase-3, caspase-8 and PARP cleavage, and decreased Bcl-2, were elucidated. Choi et al. [124] observed proapoptotic mechanisms in the same cell line with an increase in G2/M phase arrest and elevated levels of cyclin B1, p53, p21, phosphorylated AMPK (p-AMPK), intracellular ROS, and cytosolic cyt. c. Dong et al. [125] also witnessed concentration-dependent apoptosis and G2/M phase arrest in both AGS and MGC803 cells after SFN exposure. SFN also inhibited the histone methyltransferase suppressor of variegation, enhancer of zeste, trithorax, and myeloid-nervy-DEAF1 domain containing 2 (SMYD2) and SMYD3 mRNA expression, as well as transcriptional and post-transcriptional regulation of SMYD2 and SMYD3. Finally, Kiani et al. [126] elucidated additional apoptotic mechanisms of SFN in both AGS and MKN45 gastric cancer cell lines. The tumor suppressor genes, caudal type homeobox 1 (*CDX1*) and *CDX2*, showed increased expression at 31 μg/mL SFN; however, *CDX2* expression was significantly reduced at concentrations above 125 μg/mL.

Small Intestine Cancer

At least two studies investigated the in vivo anticancer properties of SFN in intestinal neoplasia models using $Apc^{Min/+}$ mice. In one study, the experimental animals consumed 300 and 600 ppm/day SFN via diet over the course of three weeks. Upon tumor assessment, the average number and size of small intestinal polyps in SFN-exposed mice were significantly reduced than the control group in a dose-dependent fashion. Mechanistically, SFN induced apoptosis with a decrease in the expression of p-Akt, p-ERK, and p-JNK [266]. Additionally, Shen et al. [267] fed mice 300 and 500 ppm/day SFN over the course of 10 weeks, and reduced tumor size was mainly contributed to apoptotic mechanisms, including increases in p21, caspase-3, and caspase-9.

Colon Cancer

To understand the effect of SFN in colon cancer, many in vitro studies have been conducted using a variety of human colon cancer cell lines. Andělová et al. [127] demonstrated that SFN inhibited the viability and proliferation of SW620 colon cancer cells in a time- and concentration-dependent manner. They found that SFN also caused DNA damage and chromatin condensation after 24 and 48 h and elevated caspase-3 activity with concentrations of SFN above 20 μM. Using SW620 colon cancer cells, Rudolf et al. [128] explored the mechanisms underlying SFN-mediated apoptosis. Results suggested that SFN-induced apoptosis involves DNA-damage signaling with efficiency dependent on p53 status and caspase-2 activation. Enhanced activity of these pathways may serve to amplify the critical proapoptotic signals interacting with mitochondria, which in turn activates effector caspases. Lan et al. [129] examined the effects of SFN in p53-deficient human colon cancer cells SW480 and found that SFN induced mitochondria-associated apoptosis, increased the Bax/Bcl-2 ratio, and activated caspase-3, caspase-7, and caspase-9. Moreover, SFN-induced apoptosis was associated with increased generation of ROS and activation of ERK and p38 MAPK. All in all, SFN-induced apoptosis was confirmed to be ROS-dependent in association with ERK/p38 rather than p53/p73 signaling pathways.

The aforementioned premise has been supported by the work of Gamet-Payrastre et al. [130], who reported that SFN induced cell cycle arrest, followed by apoptosis, which corresponded to an increased expression of cyclins A and B1 in HT-29 colon carcinoma cells. Additionally, the researchers observed no change in the expression of p53 in SFN-treated cells but did observe increased expression of Bax, cytosolic cyt. c, and cleavage of PARP. Comparably, Pappa et al. [131] reported results of increased PARP cleavage in human colon cancer cell lines 40-16 and 379.2 when treated with SFN, and they also observed previously mentioned p53-independent mechanisms of apoptosis induction. Pappa et al. [132] investigated the impact of SFN in 40-16 colon carcinoma cells, and results supported a relationship between SFN and increased PARP cleavage as well as subG1-phase cell-cycle arrest. Additionally, Rudolf and Cervinka [1] extended the role of SFN independent of p53 in human colon cancer HCT-116 cells. By knocking out p53, they observed SFN-dependent cytotoxicity and proapoptotic activity based on selective activation of JNK, which may have directly influenced the expression of Bax and Bcl-2 while promoting the loss of mitochondrial cyt. c and activation of caspases. These results are important in recognizing the chemopreventive potential of SFN in colon cancer with inactivated or lost p53.

In the available literature, SFN has also been shown to have inhibitory effects on the cell cycle in colon cancer cell lines. For example, Byun et al. [134] investigated the effects of SFN on various human colon cancer cell lines, namely, HT-29, HCT-116, KM12, SNU-1040, and DLD-1. Results showed inhibitory growth effects on all cell lines, and SFN was found to induce G2/M phase cell cycle arrest and apoptosis, concomitant with phosphorylation of CDK1 and CDC25B at inhibitory sites, and upregulation of the p38 and JNK pathways. It was also determined that SFN is a potent inhibitor of microtubule polymerization while generating ROS via GSH depletion. On the contrary, Shen et al. [135] demonstrated that SFN inhibited serum-stimulated growth of HT-29 cells by hindering the cell cycle at the G1 phase, in parallel with upregulation of $p21^{CIP1}$ expression and downregulation of cyclin A, cyclin D1, cyclin E, and c-Myc expression.

Zeng et al. [136] concluded that SFN significantly inhibited the proliferation of HCT-116 human colon cancer cells via reduced G1 phase cell distribution and induced apoptosis via enhanced phosphorylation of stress-activated protein kinase (SAPK) and decreased c-Myc. Further expanding upon G2/M phase cell cycle arrest, Pappa et al. [137] demonstrated a novel biphasic inhibitory cell growth pattern in 40-16 human colon cancer cells treated with SFN. A transient SFN exposure for up to 6 h resulted in reversible G2/M cell cycle arrest, while a minimum continuous exposure time of 12 h was necessary for SFN to irreversibly arrest cells in the G2/M phase and subsequently induce apoptosis. These researchers proposed that the reversible G2/M arrest and cytostatic effects of SFN at low concentrations may be related to an observed decrease in GSH induction. In HT-29 human colon cancer cells, Parnaud et al. [138] observed that SFN-treated cells expressed higher levels of p21 and hyperphosphorylation of Rb, leading to increased apoptosis. Moreover, preincubation of HT-29 cells with roscovitine, a cdc2 kinase inhibitor, blocked SFN-induced apoptosis and G2/M arrest, which emphasized the importance of this kinase in the apoptotic pathway induced by SFN.

Many other studies depict the ability of SFN to induce apoptosis in human colon cancer cells. Nishikawa et al. [139] determined that WiDr human colon cancer cells underwent concentration-dependent autophagy as a defense mechanism against SFN-induced apoptosis, as evidenced by the accumulation of acidic vesicular organelles and recruitment of light chain 3 to autophagosomes. Another interesting facet to the proapoptotic effects of SFN was contributed by Chung et al. [140], who investigated the antiproliferation effects of SFN in relation to the oncoprotein SKP2 in various human colon adenocarcinoma cell lines, such as DLD-1, HCT-116, and LoVo. The antiproliferative effect of SFN was accompanied by downregulation of SKP2, leading to the stabilization and thus upregulation of p27KIP1. SFN treatment also led to the activation of both Akt and ERK, indicating downregulation of SKP2 without Akt or ERK inhibition.

In addition to the proapoptotic effects of SFN summarized in previous sections, other investigators have proposed additional possible anticancer mechanisms of SFN in colon cancer cells. Traka et al. [141] published a transcriptome analysis of human colon Caco-2 cancer cells exposed to physiological concentrations of SFN, recording a >2-fold increase in expression of 106 genes and a >2-fold decrease in expression of 63 genes, supporting the role of SFN in inhibiting cell growth. Most notably, upregulation in several genes associated with antioxidant response element (ARE)-mediated transcription and Nrf2 activation, including NQO1, theoredoxin reductase (TR1), aldo-ketoreductase (AKR), and heme oxygenase 1, was observed. Remarkable genes that experienced significant decreases in expression post-SFN exposure included formyltetrahydrofolate synthase and DNA (cytosine-5-)-methyltransferase 1. Another transcriptomic study conducted by Johnson et al. [142], using SFN-treated human colon cancer cell lines, HT-29 and HCT-116, demonstrated that SFN strongly induced the expression of NQO1, several other Nrf2-dependent targets, and Loc344887 (NMRAL2P), a noncoding RNA that acts as a novel, functional pseudogene for the NmrA-like redox sensor and coregulator of NQO1.

Many other studies have identified additional anticancer mechanisms of SFN that further the understanding of this biochemical. In the investigation of the role of SFN on autophagy, Wang et al. [143] specified that SFN induced autophagy in a concentration- and time-dependent manner in Caco-2 cells. Specifically, the anticancer effects of SFN on Caco-2 cells may be attributed, at least in part, to induction of various phase II enzymes, namely, uridine 5′-diphospho-glucuronosyltrasferase 1A1 (UGT1A1), UGT1A8, and UGT1A10, via nuclear translocation of Nrf2 and human pregnane X receptor (hPXR). Additionally, Harris and Jeffery [144] investigated the effects of SFN on the expression of multidrug resistance protein 1 (MRP1) and MRP2 in the same cell line. SFN at 5 μM significantly increased the expression of MRP2 but showed no effect on the expression of MRP1. The relatively small concentration of SFN required to produce these effects is a significant distinction to understand when considering the possible physiological consequences of consuming SFN in relation to preventing the occurrence of colon cancer.

Continuous efforts to explain the chemoprotective effects of SFN have led researchers to examine its effects in association with other biochemical pathways that may contribute to its anticancer potential. Using human colon cancer cell line HCT-116, Rajendran et al. [145] demonstrated that SFN inhibited HDAC activity and increased HDAC protein turnover, causing susceptibility to SFN-induced DNA damage. As a result, the researchers again offered a model for the differential effects in cancer cells versus non-cancer cells of HDAC inhibition and DNA damage/repair signaling following SFN treatment. Martin et al. [146] supported these results by observing decreased HDAC and hTERT mRNA levels in RKO and HCT-116 cells after SFN exposure. Okonkwo et al. [147] investigated SFN and its structural analogs as modifiers of HDAC and histone acetyltransferase activity (HAT), as well as anticancer effects on human colon cancer cell lines HCT-116 and SW480. In SFN-treated HCT-116 cells, an increase of nuclear pH2AX and pRPA32 levels were observed, suggesting both enhanced DNA damage and repair, respectively. In the SW480 colon cancer cell line, SFN demonstrated increased cytotoxicity when compared to normal CCD112 colon epithelial cells. Additionally, increases in p300, a HAT-associated protein, expression and histone H4 acetylation were observed in both cell lines treated with SFN.

A study conducted by Bessler and Djaldetti [148] addressed the effects of SFN on the inflammatory relationship between human peripheral blood mononuclear cells (PBMCs) and the colon cancer cell lines, HT-29 and RKO. Results showed that while HT-29 and RKO cancer cells stimulated both pro- and anti-inflammatory cytokine production by PBMCs, the addition of SFN exerted a concentration-dependent inhibitory effect on inflammatory cytokine production by these cells, specifically with tumor necrosis factor-α (TNF-α), interleukin-1β (IL-1β), IL-6, IL-2, IL-10, and interferon γc (IFNγc). Tafakh et al. [149] investigated the expression of many genes at the mRNA level in HT-29 cells treated with SFN. Results indicated that SFN preconditioning decreased the expression of COX-2, microsomal prostaglandin E synthase-1 (mPGES-1), hypoxia-inducible factor (HIF-1), vascular endothelial growth factor (VEGF), C-X-C chemokine receptor type 4 (CXCR4), matrix metalloproteinase-2 (MMP-2), and MMP-9. Additional novel findings include decreased PGE_2 generation and inhibited in vitro motility/wound healing activity of HT-29 cells. The researchers concluded that the anticancer effects of SFN were associated with antiproliferative and antimigratory activities arising from the downregulation of the COX-2/mPGES-1 axis.

Although the exact anticancer mechanisms of SFN remain to be fully clarified, additional studies have served to progress the current agenda of understanding the effects of SFN on colon cancer cells. Jakubíková et al. [150] found that at high concentrations, SFN induced accumulation of sub-G1 cells, cell death, and dissipation of mitochondrial membrane potential in Caco-2 cells. Mechanistically, phosphorylation of ERK1/2 and Akt kinases was increased, but SFN had no effect on JNK and p28 activation. These results highlight the importance of phosphatidylinositol 3-kinase/protein kinase B (PI3K/Akt) and mitogen-activated protein kinase/ERK kinase (MEK)/ERK signaling as intracellular mediators in SFN-mediated phase II enzyme transcription and cell cycle arrest in Caco-2 cells. Expanding upon the apoptotic effects of SFN, Kim et al. [151] explored how the oxidation of sulfur in the side chain of SFN affected apoptosis induction in human colon cancer cell lines, HCT-116, LoVo, Caco-2, and HT-29. Researchers found that SFN, which contains oxidized sulfur, elicited a greater growth inhibitory effect in comparison with SFN analogs containing non-oxidized sulfur. The data demonstrated that increased apoptosis induction in HCT-116 cells by SFN was associated with an increase in caspase-8 activation but not with a rise in caspase-9 activity.

Additionally, Kim et al. [152] investigated the relationship between SFN and HIF-1α expression in HCT-116 human colon cancer cells, and results showed a concentration-dependent inhibition of HIF-1α expression and suppression of HIF-1α target gene activation. SFN also inhibited VEGF expression, suggesting that SFN may hinder colon cancer progression and angiogenesis by downregulating the expression of HIF-1α and VEGF.

The vast majority of publications regarding the effects of SFN colon cancer are based on in vitro studies; however, a handful of in vivo studies exist. Expanding on their in vitro findings, Byun et al. [134] reported that SFN markedly suppressed the growth of HCT-116 xenografted tumors in nude male mice. Mechanistically, SFN increased cyclin-dependent kinase 1 (CDK1), MAPK-activated protein kinase 2 (MK2), and p38 phosphorylation. Myzak et al. [245] also expanded their in vitro work by treating $APC^{min/+}$ mice with a single dose of SFN (10 μmol) and reported suppressed tumor growth as well as significant inhibition of HDAC activity with an associated increase in acetylated histones H3 and H4. Additionally, long-term treatment with SFN for 10 weeks in the diet resulted in elevated levels of acetylated histones and $p21^{WAF1}$ in the colon, including acetylated histones specific to the promoter region of *P21* and *Bax* genes. These results suggest that HDAC inhibition by SFN contributes to the chemopreventive and chemotherapeutic mechanisms of SFN in vivo. Similarly, Rajendran et al. [268] investigated the antitumor capability of SFN to induce Nrf2-dependent pathways and inhibit HDAC activity in vivo. By treating wild type

(WT) and Nrf2-deficient (Nrft2$^{-/+}$) mice with the colon carcinogen dimethylhydrazine (DMH) and subsequent dietary SFN (400 ppm) treatment, researchers demonstrated that WT mice were more susceptible to colon tumor induction than Nrf2$^{-/+}$ mice. WT mice also had higher levels of HDAC on several genes, including cyclin-dependent kinase inhibitor 2a (Cdkn2a/p16). These results ultimately support the role of SFN in inducing Nrf2 pathways in colon cancer models and should lead future studies to focus on Nrf2 as a tumor growth determinant and HDAC inhibitor.

Hepatocellular Cancer

A study conducted by Yu et al. [153] using HepG2 human hepatic cancer and Hepa1c1c7 hepatoma cells found that SFN treatment exhibited cytotoxicity via an increase in the expression of the MAPK/ERK2 signaling pathway. A similar study using HepG2 cell lines showed that SFN treatment demonstrated antiproliferative effects by upregulating metallothionein (MT) genes MT-1 and MT-II and promoting apoptosis, indicated by induction of caspase-3, Bax, and PARP cleavage, as well as decreased levels of Bcl-2 and Bcl-xL expression [154]. Park et al. [155] observed very similar mechanisms within the same cell line. Keum et al. [156] elaborated different antiproliferative mechanisms of SFN in the same cell line and determined that increased ARE caused an increase in heme oxygenase-1 (HO-1) through activation of Nrf2 and suppression of Kelch-like ECH-associated protein 1 (Keap1).

Jeon et al. [157] treated Huh-7, SNU-449, and NCTC hepatic cancer cell lines with SFN and found an increase in apoptosis via induction of caspase-3, caspase-8, and caspase-9. They were also able to show several novel findings, including increased G2/M phase arrest, as well as decreased expression of phosphofructo-2-kinase/fructose-2,6-biphosphatases (PFKFB) and HIF-1α, leading to decreased VEGF and angiogenesis. Liu et al. [158] also showed that SFN treatment in HepG2 resulted in decreased expression of HIF-1α and VEGF, along with decreased expression of signal transducer and activator of transcription 3 (STAT3).

Moon et al. [159] reported treatment of Hep3B hepatic cancer cells with SFN elicited an increase in apoptosis via the production of ROS. They also observed several unique findings, including a decrease in telomerase and hTERT, which may be related to an inhibition of Akt signaling. Wu et al. [160] demonstrated similar results in HepG2 cells as well as the unique findings that SFN treatment decreased expression of Vimentin and increased expression of E-cadherin, suggesting that SFN suppresses epithelial–mesenchymal transition (EMT). Moreover, SFN treatment in HepG2 cells resulted in apoptosis via regulation of several novel pathways, including increased expression of Bip/glucose-regulated protein 78 (GRP78), XBP-1, caspase-12, C/EBP-homologous protein (CHOP)/GADD153, and Bid [161]. These findings, along with the other studies, imply SFN's role in inducing apoptosis in hepatocellular cell lines.

A separate group of researchers investigated SFN's role in activating phase I biotransformation enzymes in Hepa 1c1c7 (murine) and HepG2 cells and found that it reduced cell viability by increasing the expression of CYP1A1 mRNA [162]. They also determined that SFN successfully activated AhR transformation and its subsequent binding to the xenobiotic response element (XRE).

Very limited information is available on in vivo anti-hepatocellular cancer effects of SFN. However, a study was conducted on female BALB/c athymic mice xenografted with HepG2 cells and treated with SFN for 13 days, and the investigators noted a subsequent reduction in tumor growth and volume via an unknown mechanism [160].

Pancreatic Cancer

An early study found that pancreatic cancer cell lines MIA PaCa-2 and PANC-1 treated with SFN resulted in a promotion of cell cycle arrest and death. These effects were mediated via increased apoptosis with subsequent induction of pro-apoptotic proteins (caspase-3 and caspase-8), G2-M arrest, and ROS [163]. A similar study conducted with the aforementioned cell lines along with AsPC-1 and BxPc-3 cells found cell cycle arrest via suppressed Akt signaling and CDK4 expression as well as a rise in the proteasomal degradation of HSP90 client proteins [164]. Another group of researchers found that SFN treatment of AsPC-1, BxPc-3, Capan-1, and MIA PaCa-2 cells reduced overall cell viability by increasing apoptosis, but also by decreasing nuclear factor-κB (NF-κB) binding [165]. Rodova et al. [166] found similar results of increased apoptosis in ASPC, PANC-1, and human pancreatic cancer stem cells (CSCs) through various mechanisms, including increased caspase-3, decreased Bcl-2, and decreased Nanog, Oct4, Smo, and Hedgehog (Hh) signaling.

Yin et al. [167] treated AsPC-1, BxPc-3, PANC-1, and MIA PaCa-2 cell lines with SFN and demonstrated increased apoptosis through a novel mechanism of increased miR-365a-3p. Moreover, elevated expression of miR135b-5p was identified in a separate study, which ultimately led to the upregulation of the RASAL2 tumor suppressor gene involved in the inhibition of tumor growth [168]. Chen and colleagues [169] noted inhibition of cellular proliferation, invasion, and migration of PANC-1 and MIA PaCa-2 cells treated with SFN. This was demonstrated via an increase in apoptosis, AMPK signaling, ROS production, E-Cadherin, HO-1 and Nrf-2, and a decrease in Vimentin and N-cadherin.

Forster et al. [170] reported a reduction in cell viability in BxPc-3 and AsPC-1 pancreatic cell lines, which was contributed to increased E-Cadherin, Cx43, gap junctional intercellular communication (GJIC), as well as decreased expression of cancer stem cell markers c-Met and CD133. These mechanisms aligned with those reported by Georgikou et al. [171], who noted increased Cx43 and GJIC, increased expression of the GJA1 mRNA gene whicthath encodes Cx43, and decreased miR30a-3p in PANC-1 cells.

Several in vivo studies have been conducted to elaborate on SFN's antiproliferative effect against various pancreatic cancer cell lines. Kuroiwa et al. [269] reported that SFN prevented N-nitrosobis(2-oxopropyl) amine (BOP)-induced pancreatic carcinogenesis in male Syrian hamsters via an unknown mechanism. Pham et al. [163] exposed male severe combined immunodeficiency (SCID) mice inoculated with PANC-1 cells to SFN over the course of 3 weeks and reported decreased tumor growth. Another study treated female athymic (nu/nu) mice inoculated with MIA PaCa-2 with SFN and reported inhibition of tumor growth [164]. Reduced tumor growth was also reported in a study utilizing male NOD/SCID/IL2Rγ mice inoculated with human pancreatic CSCs when treated with SFN for 6 weeks [270]. Mechanistically, they noted an upregulation in E-Cadherin, as well as a decrease in VEGF, Bcl-2, Smo, Gli1/2, and PDGFα [270]. Kallifatidis et al. [165] conducted a study exposing nude mice inoculated with MIA PaCa-2 cells to SFN and reported inhibition in tumor growth and angiogenesis and increased apoptosis concomitant with decreased NK-κB expression. Chen et al. [169] treated BALB/c nude mice with SFN and reported a reduction in tumor volume and weight via activation of AMPK signaling. They also reported a strengthening of Nrf-2 nuclear localization, implying SFN's potential for cancer prevention and treatment.

4.2.3. Gynecological Cancers

Cervical Cancer

All in vitro studies examining the effect of SFN on cervical cancer were performed using HeLa cells. Park et al. [156] exposed HeLa cells to SFN and observed inhibited cell viability, increased formation of apoptotic bodies, increased accumulation of cells in the sub-G1 phase, and downregulated Bcl-1/Bcl-xL and c-inhibitor of the apoptosis (cIAP-1). Another study reported that SFN resulted in 50% inhibition of HeLa cell growth following SFN treatment at 12 μM. Mechanistically, SFN induced a concentration-dependent increase in caspase-3 and a downregulation of Bcl-2, COX-2, and IL-1β [172]. A subsequent study by Khan et al. [173] found that SFN inhibited DNA methyltransferase (DMNT), downregulated DNMT3B, and decreased HDAC activity by directly interacting with HDAC1 in HeLa cells. This study concluded that SFN has potential antitumorigenic effects and may reactivate silencing of tumor suppressor genes epigenetically by altering methylation. Moreover, Cheng et al. [174] determined that SFN treatment of HeLa cells decreased their survival and proliferation by inducing cell arrest in the G2/M and G1 phases as well as decreasing cyclin B1 and cyclin B1/CDC2 complexes.

Endometrial Cancer

Recently, Rai et al. [175] investigated the effects of SFN on MFE280, KLE, Ishikawa, Hec1B, Hec1A, MFE296, and AN3CA endometrial cells. Inhibition of proliferation and induction of apoptosis was observed along with G2/M phase arrest, which was attributed to both the suppression of the PI3K/Akt/mTOR pathway and increased phosphorylation of MEK and ERK, leading to decreased MEK and ERK expression. This was the first study to imply that SFN has anticancer properties against endometrial cancer.

Rai et al. [175] also expanded their investigation to an in vivo Ishikawa xenograft mouse model and observed decreased tumor volume via apoptotic mechanisms after i.p. administration of 50 mg/kg SFN daily for 16 days. The antitumor effect was superior to that of paclitaxel (10 mg/kg, once every seven days).

Ovarian Cancer

One of the earliest studies to investigate the in vitro cytotoxic effect of SFN on ovarian cancer was conducted by Chaudhuri et al. [176]. The findings revealed the antiproliferative effect of SFN on SKOV3, C3, and T3 cells with decreased cell survival and loss of cell viability with increased concentration. Mechanistically, SFN had an impact on the PI3K/Akt pathway by downregulating the steady-state level of the total and active Akt protein, cyclin D1, cdk4, and cdk6 levels in all three cell lines. In another study, exposure of OVCAR-3 and SKOV-3 cells to SFN for a two-day period significantly reduced cell viability and the accumulation of cells in the G1 phase, and cell apoptosis was identified after 4 h of SFN treatment [177]. Bryant et al. [178] exposed SKOV3 and MDAH-2774 cells to SFN, which resulted in a concentration-dependent inhibition of cancer cell proliferation. Additionally, SFN induced apoptosis and increased S phase cells and G1 arrest in MDAH-2774 cells. Kim et al. [179] reported the effect of SFN on cell growth at 72 h in OVCAR3, OVCAR4, OVCAR5, and SKOV3 cell lines and found that SFN was effective at inhibiting cancer cell growth via activation of p38 and ERK. In a separate study, SFN treatment over a 24 h period induced apoptosis in SKOV3 and A2780 ovarian cancer cell lines. Further investigation uncovered an increase in type 1 inositol 1,4,5- triphosphate receptor (IP_3R1) and Nrf2 protein expression with a resultant increase in Nrf2-regulated genes, such as the catalytic subunit of glutamate-cysteine ligase (GCLC), HMOX1, and NQO-1. Additional findings in the A2780 cell line include increased ROS and increased phosphorylation of HSP27, JNK, mitogen-activated protein kinase 1 (MEK1), p38, p90RSK, and c-JUN [180]. Finally, Chang et al. [181] reported that SFN treatment decreased cell survival and proliferation, increased cell accumulation in the G2/M phase, and downregulated cell division cycle protein 2 (CDC2), causing dissociation of the cyclin B1/CDC2 complex in PA-1 ovarian cancer cells.

The only study investigating the in vivo anticancer effect of SFN on ovarian cancer was conducted by Hudecova et al. [180]. Athymic nude mice with A2780 ovarian cancer xenografts received 40 mg/kg SFN (i.p.) for 7 days, after which tumor size was significantly reduced compared to the control. These results were attributed to increased IP_3R1, supporting the in vitro results as mentioned earlier.

4.2.4. Hematological Cancers

Leukemia

Fimognari et al. [182] performed one of the earliest studies to investigate the in vitro effect of SFN on leukemia in which SFN arrested Jurkat cells in the G2/M phase. SFN induced apoptosis in a time- and concentration-dependent manner with the appearance of decreased DNA content as well as increased expression of p53 and Bax proteins. In a subsequent study, Fimognari et al. [183] supported these findings with very similar results in the same cell line. In addition, cyclin D3 was significantly decreased, while the expression of cyclin D2, CDK4, and CDK6 was slightly decreased. A further study by Fimognari et al. [184] reported that SFN induced differentiation in HL-60 promyelocytic leukemia cells, including granulocytes and macrophages, via apoptosis. Choi et al. [185] reported that SFN inhibited the viability of U937 cells, induced apoptosis, caused accumulation of cells in the sub-G1 phase, downregulated Bcl-2, increased expression of caspase-3, stimulated the release of ROS, and hyperpolarized the mitochondrial membrane in a concentration-dependent manner. Koolivand et al. [186] reported that treatment of U937, KG-1, HL-60, and NB-4 acute myeloid leukemia cells with SFN decreased live cells and increased mortality rates in a concentration- and time-dependent manner. In addition, increased concentrations of SFN induced primary apoptosis of HL-60 cells, and SFN significantly decreased the expression of miR-155 in all four cell lines. Moreover, a study by Shang et al. [187] revealed the effect of SFN on HL-60 cells and reported antiproliferative effects previously reported, but also noted increased Fas-associated death domain (FADD), which is indicative of apoptosis. A similar study that focused on the effect of SFN on HL-60 cells reported that SFN induced NQO1 expression in cells containing NQO1*2 genotype and SFN downregulated cytosolic Keap1, accompanied by increased nuclear Nrf2. Prolonged exposure of HL-60 to SFN resulted in inhibition of cell proliferation due to cell cycle arrest and apoptosis caused by induction of p-H2AX expression, PARP cleavage, and caspase-mediated cell death [188]. Suppipat et al. [189] utilized different leukemia cell lines, namely, Nalm-6, Nalm-6 human pre-B cells, and REGM and RS-4 pre-B ALL cells, and observed decreased cell viability and accumulation of cells in the G2/M cell cycle phase after exposure to SFN. A study by Prata et al. [190] revealed that SFN has cytotoxic effects at 30 μM in leukemia B1647 cells and significantly decreased cell viability. Moreover, 10 μM of SFN significantly decreased aquaporin-8 (AQP8) both at transcriptional and protein levels, decreased intracellular ROS levels, and lowered the level of Nox-2. Misiewicz et al. [191] investigated the effect of SFN on the L-1210 leukemia cell line, and the results revealed cell growth arrest, decreased cell viability, and decreased cell density.

Lymphoma

Only one study investigating the in vitro effect of SFN on lymphoma was conducted by Ishiura et al. [192]. In this study, SFN significantly inhibited the proliferation of Kaposi's sarcoma-associated herpesvirus-positive primary effusion lymphoma cell lines (BC2, BC3, and HBL6) and decreased their viability by suppressing p38 MAPK and Akt signaling. In addition, SFN caused the cleavage of caspase-3, caspase-7, caspase-9, and PARP in BC2 and BC3 cells, which indicates that SFN triggers apoptosis via the caspase 9-dependent pathway.

4.2.5. Lung Cancer

A preliminary study conducted by Mi and Chung [193] examined the effect of SFN on the A549 human lung cancer cell line, and they found increased apoptosis and cell cycle arrest at the G1/S and G2/M checkpoints. Furthermore, SFN inhibited cell division by causing a decrease in tubulin polymerization; therefore, preventing mitotic spindle formation during mitosis. Utilizing the LTEP-A2 human lung adenocarcinoma cell line, similar results were obtained, as SFN significantly inhibited cellular proliferation by upregulating apoptosis and halting the cell cycle at the G2/M phase [194]. Zuryn et al. [195] corroborated these results in the A549 cell line and determined that part of the cell cycle arrest was mediated by a decrease in cyclin D1 and upregulation of the CDK inhibitor p21. In a later study, this same group revealed that SFN caused cell cycle arrest by decreasing cyclin B1 and increasing cyclin K in H1299 cells [196]. Similar results were uncovered when A549 and H1299, non-small cell lung cancer cells (NSCLCs), were exposed to SFN, and it was determined that an increase in apoptosis was partially mediated by increased p53 and Bax [197]. Additionally, SFN exposure caused significantly increased H3 and H4 acetylation and decreased HDAC activity. Gao et al. [198] further elucidated SFN's ability to alter the epigenetics of A549 cells, in which SFN showed downregulated HDAC1, HDAC3, HDAC6, decreased CpG methylation, and upregulated histone modifier H3K4me1.

Zhu et al. [199] further elucidated SFN's mechanisms of regulating gene expression, apoptosis, and cellular growth. In A549 and H1299 cell lines, SFN decreased miR-19a and miR-19b and inhibited the transcription regulators Nanog and Oct4. This group determined that apoptosis was upregulated by increased Bax, caspase-3, caspase-8, and caspase-9. Additionally, cellular growth was restricted by the downregulation of the Wnt/β-catenin pathway. Wang et al. [200] observed similar results utilizing the NSCLC cell lines H1299, 95C, and 95D. Tsai et al. [201] determined that A549 and CL1-5 cells treated with SFN showed significantly inhibited growth by downregulation of multiple growth pathways, including β-catenin, Akt, and FAK. In addition to the mechanisms listed previously regarding apoptosis, this team determined that there was increased externalization of phosphatidylserine to the outer lipid bilayer. In another study, SFN increased the proapoptotic factor p53, upregulated modulator of apoptosis (PUMA), Bax, caspase-9, and p73, and simultaneously decreased the antiapoptotic factor Bcl-2 in XWLC-05 cells [202]. Similar antiapoptotic mechanisms were observed in cadmium-transformed BEAS-2BR, bronchial epithelial cells, treated with SFN [203]. Moreover, this group of researchers was the first to determine SFN's ability to induce autophagy and decrease the transcription factor Nrf2 in bronchogenic carcinoma cell lines.

Chen et al. [204] was the first group of researchers to determine SFN's ability to induce proteasomal activity in various NSCLCs, such as PC9/gef, H1975, A549, CL1-5, and H3255. Furthermore, novel mechanisms involving the inhibition of cellular growth were confirmed by observing SFN's ability to significantly decrease the phosphorylation of the epidermal growth factor receptor (EGFR) and STAT3 signal transducer in addition to decreasing p-Akt as previously established. These investigators illustrated for the first time that ERK5 activation via phosphorylation mediates SFN's suppressive effect on human bronchogenic carcinoma cells. Additionally, SFN exhibited significant potential to inhibit cellular adhesion and migration via downregulation of pc-jun, pc-Fos, Snail1, MMP-2, and N-cadherin in spite of SFN inducing expression of tight junction, ZO-1, and cellular adhesion molecule E-cadherin [205]. Geng et al. [206] further confirmed these results by treating SK-1 and A549 cells to SFN and reported an increase in 26S proteasomal activity in addition to upregulation of the ERK1/2 signaling cascade. As previously described, these investigators demonstrated that SFN stimulated apoptosis via an increase in Bax and caspase-3 while decreasing the antiapoptotic factor Bim.

Recently, it has been reported that SFN hinders the acquisition of tobacco-smoke-induced lung cancer stem-cell-like properties via modulation of the IL-6/ΔNp63α/Notch signaling axis [207]. This axis is upregulated in tobacco-smoke-induced lung cancer cell lines HBE and A549, and an increase in ΔNp63α is positively correlated with CD133 and Oct4 expression. SFN administered over a period of 7 days was shown to significantly downregulate ΔNp63α, resulting in a concomitant decrease in CD133 and Oct4. Furthermore, SFN's ability to attenuate the Notch signaling pathway was exemplified by its capability to decrease IL-6, NICD, Hes1, and Nanog expression.

One of the earliest studies to determine SFN's antitumorigenic effects in vivo was performed on A/J mice treated with lung carcinogen benzopyrene and 4-(methylnitrosamino)-1-(3-pyridyl)-1-butanone (NNK). Benzopyrene- and NNK-induced mice were treated with 1.5 and 5 μmol/g SFN (per os, p.o.) for 42 weeks, resulting in a significantly reduced tumor size and weight. Mechanistically, apoptosis was upregulated via increased caspase-3 and downregulated PCNA [271].

Liang et al. [194] utilized nude mice inoculated with LTEP-A2 human lung adenocarcinoma cells to investigate the antitumor effects of SFN. Parenteral administration (i.p.) of 25, 50, and 100 mg/kg SFN for 9 days resulted in a reduced tumor weight via upregulation of apoptosis and increased cell cycle arrest at the G2/M restriction point. Jiang et al. [196] further elucidated SFN's ability to decrease tumor weight in NOD/SCID mice inoculated with A549 human lung cancer cells. SFN (9 μmol/day, p.o.) for 28 days caused an increase in proapoptotic factors p53, p21, and Bax. Furthermore, this team of researchers determined that SFN's capacity to alter chromosomal packaging in vivo was mediated by increased H3 and H4 acetylation and downregulation of HDAC activity. BALB/c nu/nu male mice inoculated with NSCLCs and treated with SFN at a dose of 10 μmol/kg, five times per week, over 21 days, showed significantly reduced tumor volume [204]. This decrease in tumor volume was mediated by decreasing the tumor's response to growth factors via downregulation of the EGFR. In a later study, this same group determined novel mechanisms of SFN's action in vivo using BALB/c nude female mice inoculated with H1299 cells [205]. ERK5 growth signaling pathway was significantly inhibited, thus resulting in a decreased tumor weight and volume. Additionally, cell migration and invasion were hindered by the downregulation of N-cadherin adhesion protein despite the upregulation of E-cadherin and tight junction ZO-1, as previously reported in vitro. Wang et al. [200] corroborated these results utilizing nude male BALB/c mice inoculated with H1299 and 95D cells. Mice treated with SFN every 3 days for 4 weeks at a dose of 25 or 50 mg/kg (i.v.) showed a reduced number of metastatic lung nodules via downregulation of N-cadherin, Vimentin, and β-catenin.

4.2.6. Neural Cancer

There have been only a handful of studies investigating the effect of SFN treatment on neural cell cancers, and the results show promise for anticancer properties. Karmakar et al. [208] performed a study treating glioblastoma cell lines T98G and U87MG with SFN and reported a decrease in cell viability and increase in apoptosis via upregulation of caplain, proapoptogenic mitochondrial protein Smac/Diablo, apoptosis inducible factor (AIF), as well as increased expression of caspase-3, caspase-9, caspase-12, Bax:Bcl-2, cyt. c, and increased intracellular calcium level. This group of researchers also found a reduction in the expression of apoptosis inhibitor proteins and NF-κB. Another study conducted by Bijangi-Visheshsaraei et al. [209] exposed U87, U373, U118, and SF767 cells to SFN and found a decrease in cell survival and promotion of cell death via induction of caspase-3, caspase-9, and caspase-7, and increased production of ROS with a resultant increase in double-stranded DNA breaks. A novel finding in their study showed increased expression of γ-H2AX, a protein that localizes near DNA strand breaks and recruits other proteins to the site of damage. Miao et al. [210] were able to show that treatment with SFN in U87 and U251 glioblastoma cells resulted in inhibition of cell survival and promotion of cell death via many of the above mechanisms. Zhang et al. [211] exposed U251MG glioblastoma cells to SFN and observed a reduction in cell viability and promotion in cell death via increased apoptosis and decreased invasion linked to decreased expression of MMP-2, MMP-9, and Galectin-3. In a separate study, Li et al. [212] treated U87MG and U373MG cells with SFN and documented reduced proliferation, migration, and invasion via decreased expression of MMP-2, as well as an increase in ERK1/2.

Only one study has reported the anticancer potential of SFN using an in vivo glioblastoma model. Bijangi-Visheshsaraei et al. [209] treated female NSG mice inoculated with GBM10 cells with 100 mg/kg SFN for 5-day cycles (p.o.) over 3 weeks and found increased inhibition of tumor growth; however, mechanisms were not revealed.

4.2.7. Skin Cancer

In one of the earliest studies investigating the effects of SFN on skin cancer, Misiewicz et al. [191] treated ME-18 human melanoma cells with SFN and reported arrested cell growth. This was accompanied by increased apoptosis with resultant DNA strand breaks and phosphatidylserine externalization. Arcidiacono et al. [83] also showed suppressed cell growth as well as decreased invasion and metastasis in 501MEL human malignant melanoma cells via increased expression of caspase-3, caspase-8, and caspase-9. They also reported that SFN upregulated the expression of pro-apoptotic genes, including p53, Bax, PUMA, Fas, MDM2, EGR1, GADD45b, ATF3, and CDKN1A. Subsequently, the same research team observed that SFN treatment shifted the growth factor receptor ratio from prosurvival to proapoptotic one, with a measurable increase in apoptosis in A375 human malignant melanoma cells [213].

In a separate study, Mantso et al. [214] demonstrated that when treated with SFN, A375 cells exhibited decreased survival due to an increase in apoptosis with concomitant expression of multiple caspases. Another experiment conducted by Fisher et al. [215] on A375 and WM793 cell lines showed that SFN reduced spheroid migration, formation, and invasion in addition to increased apoptosis via suppression of Ezh2, H3K27me3, Bmi-1, and Suz12.

Hamsa et al. [216] treated B16F-10 melanoma cell lines with SFN and witnessed a reduction in cell viability and increased apoptosis via induction of caspase-3, caspase-8, caspase-9, and Bax, as well as decreased expression in Bcl-2, IL-1β, IL-6, TNF-α, IL-12p40 C-Fos, ATF-2, CREB, and NF-κB. Enriquez et al. [217] also reported a reduction in cell viability when treating B16 murine melanoma cells with SFN with a measurable decrease in HDAC. Decreased HDAC activity was reported in another study conducted on B16 and S91 murine melanoma cells [218]. Additionally, SFN decreased cellular proliferation, promoted oxidative stress, and modulated gene expression in Bowes and SK-MEL-28 human melanoma cell lines [219]. Mechanistically, an increase in apoptosis was observed through upregulation in phosphorylated p38 kinase, p53, PUMA, Bax, and ROS production.

Several in vivo studies elaborate on SFN's in vitro anticancer effects. Thejass and Kuttan [272] treated C57Bl/6 mice with xenografted B16F-10 melanoma tumors with 500 μg/kg (i.p.) SFN over 10 days and reported inhibition of tumor growth and lung metastasis via decreased expression of hydroxyproline, uronic acid, and hexosamine in the lungs as well as decreased sialic acid and γ-glutamyl transpeptidase (GGT) in the serum. Ancillary studies indicate that SFN treatment inhibited the spread of metastatic tumor cells via stimulation of cell-mediated immune response, upregulation of IL-2 and interferon-γ (IFN-γ), and downregulation of several proinflammatory cytokines [273]. Another study was conducted on C57BL/6 mice inoculated with B16 murine melanoma cells and treated with 500 μmol/kg SFN 3 doses/week (i.p.) for 4 weeks and reported a reduction in tumor volume via decreased expression of HDACs [218]. An additional study using the same tumor model and SFN regimen also reported inhibition of tumor growth and reduced cell volume via a decrease in HDAC expression [217]. Fisher et al. [215] conducted an experiment using NSG mice inoculated with A375 melanoma cells and treated with SFN for 6 weeks and noted a decrease in tumor formation and volume. A mechanistic evaluation showed increased apoptosis via decreased MMP-9, MMP-2, H3K27me3, and Ezh2, as well as elevation in the cleavage of procaspase-8, procaspase-9, and PARP.

4.2.8. Urogenital Cancers

Bladder Cancer

Shan et al. [220] was the first group to portray the anticancer properties of SFN in a bladder cancer cell line. SFN inhibited T24 cell growth by inducing early apoptosis, decreasing cells in both the S and G2/M phases, and reducing p27 expression. In a separate study, this group demonstrated SFN's ability to downregulate COX-2 mRNA and protein levels in the T24 cell line, which was shown to be a consequence of increased nuclear NF-κB translocation with a concurrent decrease in COX-2 promotor binding as well as upregulated phosphorylation of p38 [221]. Shan et al. [222] continued this research by establishing SFN's capability of inducing thioredoxin reductase-1 (TR-1) and glutathione S-transferase (GSTA1-1) via activation of p38 MAPK. Furthermore, SFN has been shown to significantly inhibit T24 cell adhesion to matrigel, fibronectin, and laminin and attenuate cell migration [223]. Mechanistically, SFN decreased COX-2, MMP-2, and MMP-9 while upregulating E-cadherin. Suppression of Snail and ZEB1 transcription factors, mediated by increased miR-200c expression, has been linked to the increase in E-cadherin [222].

The T24 bladder carcinoma cell line has been exposed to SFN in another study conducted by Jo et al. [224]. SFN inhibited cell viability and induced apoptosis by activating caspase-3 and caspase-9, increasing PARP cleavage, upregulating Bax, and increasing cytosolic cyt. c levels. Additionally, SFN increased endoplasmic reticulum stress, evident by increased GRP78 and CHOP. SFN-induced apoptosis was also initiated in RT4, J82, and UMUC3 bladder cancer cell lines in a study conducted by Abbaoui et al. [82]. Moreover, the same research group displayed SFN's capability to inhibit HDAC1, HDAC2, HDAC4, and HDAC6 activity; however, histone acetylation status was not significantly altered [225]. These results suggest that SFN-induced HDAC inhibition may not directly impact histone acetylation but instead may act on additional cytoplasmic targets.

SFN-induced apoptosis has been explored in two additional bladder cancer cell lines. BIU87 cells exposed to concentrations greater than 20 μM SFN demonstrated significant inhibition of cell proliferation, which was attributed to apoptosis indicated by an accumulation of cells in the G2/M phase of the cell cycle [226]. Additionally, this study illustrates that SFN-enhanced insulin-like growth factor-binding protein-3 (IGFBP-3) also plays a role in inducing apoptosis in bladder carcinoma. Park et al. [227] documented SFN's capability of inducing apoptosis by disrupting the mitochondrial membrane and mediating intracellular ROS. After the 5637 bladder cancer cell line was exposed to SFN, an increase in G2/M phase arrest was observed along with increased H3 phosphorylation, PARP cleavage, cyclin B1, Cdk1, caspase-3, and a decrease in mitochondrial membrane potential.

SFN has been shown to inhibit bladder tumor growth by inducing apoptosis in two in vivo studies. Abbaoui et al. [82] inoculated nude mice with UMUC3 bladder carcinoma cells, and after 2 weeks of dietary SFN (295 μmol/kg) exposure, there was a significant decrease in tumor weight compared to the control. This study also confirmed detectable SFN levels in the mouse plasma and tumor tissue; however, mechanisms of tumor suppression were not explored. Wang and Shan [274] observed similar antitumorigenic effects in UMUC3 xenografted mice fed 12 mg/kg SFN per day. SFN induced apoptosis, promoted the expression of caspase-3 and cyt. c, and suppressed expression of survivin compared to the control group. This is one of the earliest reports to suggest that survivin is a target of SFN in bladder carcinoma in vivo.

Prostate Cancer

An early study executed by Brooks et al. [228] determined that SFN inhibited cellular proliferation in various human prostate cancer cells by increasing the antioxidant enzymes NQO1, quinone reductase, and GST. Hahm et al. [229] found that SFN reduced viability of DU145, LNCaP, PC-3, and CWR22v1 cells by suppressing the IL-6/JAK/STAT3 pathway and decreasing Bcl-2, which, in turn, enabled apoptosis and decreased cell growth. Choi et al. [230] demonstrated that SFN reduced cellular growth in LNCaP and PC-3 cells by increasing proapoptotic factors Bax and apoptotic protease activating factor-1 (APAF-1) and decreasing antiapoptotic factors BAK, Bcl-xL, cIAP1/2, and XIAP. Additionally, cell cycle regulators p53 and E2F1 were increased. Similarly, Carrasco-Pozo et al. [231] discovered increased apoptosis in LNCaP cells after SFN exposure via decreased BcL-xL, prostate-specific antigen (PSA), nuclear androgen receptor, and HIF-1α. Kim and Singh [232] similarly reported a decrease in LNCap and C4-2 cellular proliferation after SFN exposure due to an increase in transcriptional repression of androgen receptor mRNA, leading to a decrease in Ser210/213 phosphorylated and total androgen receptor.

A study performed by Herman-Antosiewicz et al. [233] found that SFN induced autophagy and apoptosis in PC-3 and LNCaP cells by upregulation of LC-3 cleavage, which stabilizes the autophagosome. Additionally, apoptosis was increased due to an increment in cyt. c release. Xiao et al. [234] also observed LNCaP and PC-3 cell growth inhibition via increased apoptosis with a concomitant increase in Bax, cyt. c, ROS, and LC-3 cleavage. Watson et al. [235] observed similar mechanisms of SFN-induced autophagy.

SFN increased apoptosis and G2/M phase arrest in DU145 human prostate cancer cells by increasing JNK pathway activity, leading to activation of p53 and increased JNK, ROS, and PARP cleavage [236]. Hac et al. [237] also conducted a study exposing PC-3 cells to SFN and observed apoptosis and S-phase arrest most likely caused by an increase in DNA double-stranded breaks. Another study conducted by Lee et al. [238] also documented decreased LNCaP cell viability and growth through an increase in PARP cleavage and caspase-3 after SFN exposure, indicating increased apoptosis. Singh et al. [239,240] showed that SFN reduced PC-3 and DU145 cell survival and proliferation, which was marked by increased caspase-3, caspase-8, caspase-9, and Bax, as well as decreased Bcl-2 with the promotion in PARP cleavage. Negrette-Guzmán et al. [241] determined that SFN resulted in reduced PC-3 cell viability, measured by decreases in PGC1α and HIF-1α along with increases in Bax and NRF1.

Ahmed et al. [97] reported a novel finding that SFN inhibited the growth of 22Rv1 cells by inducing apoptosis through increased USP14 and UCHL5 proteins. Beaver et al. [242] determined that SFN-induced cell growth restriction in LNCaP and PC-3 cells was related to a decrease in CDK2, PLK1, and BMX, which are all required for cell cycle progression. Additionally, SP1 was downregulated, and NQO1 was upregulated. Similarly, a study conducted by Bhamre et al. [243] showed reduced growth of LNCaP cells coinciding with increased G2/M cell cycle arrest and subsequent apoptosis through decreased levels of Jun protein. Additional findings indicated increased levels of NQO1, TXNRD1, GSTM1, MGST1, SOD1, and PRDX1.

A study conducted by Clarke et al. [71] found that SFN inhibited the growth of LNCap and PC-3 cells through downregulation of HDAC3, HDAC4, and HDAC6. All these mechanisms contributed to the inhibition of the cell cycle at the G2/M phase, leading to decreased cell growth and division. Similarly, Gibbs et al. [244] found that SFN decreased the viability of LNCaP and VCaP cells via a decrease in HDAC6, androgen receptor expression, HSP90, and ERG. Another study similarly found decreased levels of HDAC and increased levels of acetylated H3 and H4 leading to G2/M phase arrest [245]. Zhang et al. [246] reported similar results regarding the decreased expression of HDAC and elevated levels of acetylated H3 but also found upregulation of Nrf2 and NQO-1, as well as decreased DNMT3a and DNMT1.

Beaver et al. [247] observed decreased cellular proliferation of LNCaP and PC-3 cells upon SFN treatment, and mechanistically, they found altered expressions of approximately 100 long non-coding RNAs. Hahm et al. [248] exposed LNCaP and PC-3 cells to SFN and also found reduced cell proliferation and migration concomitant with decreased Notch1, Notch2, and Notch4 as well as an increase in DNA fragmentation. After SFN exposure, Hsu et al. [249] observed decreased cellular proliferation of the LNCaP and PC-3 cell lines, and they also saw a decrease in DNMT1 and DNMT3. The investigators also found a decrease in cyclin D2 promoter methylation and consequently an increase in cyclin D2, associated with the prevention of tumor progression. According to Wong et al. [250], similar mechanisms were found to be responsible for SFN's cytotoxicity in the LNCaP and PC-3 cell lines in spite of an increase in CCR4 and transforming growth factor-β (TGF-β) receptor type 1 (TGFBR1), which allow for tumor progression. Vyas et al. [251] also observed decreased cellular proliferation and viability in the same cell lines after SFN exposure due to decreased CD24, ITGA6, ZEB2, and c-Myc. A study conducted by Watson et al. [252] found decreased cell viability in LNCaP and PC-3 cells introduced to SFN as well as an increase in post-translational modification of SUV39H1. This subsequently led to a decrease in H3K9me3-specific histone methyltransferase, resulting in an increase in CD8 + T-cells. Singh et al. [253] reported that SFN resulted in decreased cell viability through decreased glycolysis in LNCaP and 22Rv1 cells. Moreover, there was a decrease in LDHA, which facilitates the glycolytic process by converting pyruvate to lactate and is an important biomarker for cancer progression. Finally, PMK2, a pyruvate kinase important in the glycolysis pathway, was also decreased.

Several studies showed a reduction in prostate cancer cell migration through different and novel mechanisms. Peng et al. [254] revealed that treatment of DU145 cells with SFN resulted in decreased pseudopodia, as well as decreased MMP-2 and CD44v6. This study also showed increased p-ERK1/2 and E-Cadherin. Vyas and Singh [255] determined that SFN decreased cell proliferation and migration of PC-3 and DU145 cell lines with a concomitant reduction in E-Cadherin, as well as an increase in PAI-1 and vimentin.

Hac et al. [256] exposed the PC-3 cell line to SFN and revealed a decrease in S6K1 phosphorylation, which is important for the regulation of mTOR and protein synthesis. LC3, a key protein in autophagy, was shown to be elevated as well. Pei et al. [257] showed an increase in H2S (associated with DNA damage), p38 (involved in cell differentiation, apoptosis, and autophagy), and JNK (implicated in tumor suppression) upon SFN treatment of PC-3 cells. Wiczk et al. [258] conducted a study using SFN and PC-3 cells, which revealed increased S6K1 dephosphorylation leading to decreased levels of mTOR and survivin protein. Two studies conducted by Xu et al. [259,260] revealed that SFN reduced PC-3 cell viability through different mechanisms. The first study reported decreased NF-κB levels, p65 nuclear translocation, VEGF, and IKKα and IKKβ phosphorylation [259]. The second study [260] showed an increase in p-ERK1/2, JNK1/2, and p-c-Jun, which led to reduced cell viability. However, increased AP-1 was also recorded, which is critical in allowing cancer migration and proliferation. ELK1, a factor that is coupled to androgen receptors allowing growth of prostate cancers, was also increased. Yao et al. [261] found that SFN increased JNK and ERK signaling and decreased VEGF and HIF-1α, all contributing to a decrease in proliferation of DU145 cells.

A study conducted by Singh et al. [262] showed inhibited LNCaP and 22Rv1 cellular proliferation through a variety of mechanisms. The effects of SFN on these cells showed a reduction in carnitine palmitoyltransferase 1A, medium-chain acyl-CoA dehydrogenase, hydroxyacyl-CoA dehydrogenase trifunctional multienzyme complex subunit α, and sterol regulatory element-binding protein 1. Herman-Antosiewicz et al. [263] conducted a study that showed that SFN exposure to LNCaP cells promoted cell cycle arrest and decreased proliferation. Mechanistic results revealed decreased levels of cyclin D1, cyclin E1, CDK4, CDK6, CDK1, and CDC25C, as well as increased levels of p53, p21, and cyclin B1. Abbas et al. [264] found that SFN induced cell cycle arrest, mediated via several mechanisms. Decreased hTERT was reported, and there was also a decrease in HDAC-inhibitory activity, allowing histones to be deacetylated to reduce DNA transcription. This study also measured decreased H3K4me2 and MeCP2. This reduction in cellular proliferation was observed even with an increase in H3K18A, a biomarker in cancer progression, as well as increases in DNMT3a, DNMT1, pan-acetylated H3, and H4.

The promising in vitro anticancer effects of SFN have been extended to several in vivo investigations. Myzak and colleagues [84] conducted a study that revealed a reduction in tumor growth in nude, male, athymic BALB/c mice that were xenografted with PC-3 cells and treated with 443 mg/kg/day SFN for 3 weeks. Increases in Bax and acetylated-H3 and -H4 were identified alongside decreased HDAC. Similarly, Singh et al. [240] found inhibited tumor growth in male and female athymic mice with xenografted PC-3 tumors using 5.6 μmol SFN 3 times/week (p.o.) for 3 weeks. Mechanistically, increased apoptosis via increased Bax was identified. Subsequently, Singh et al. [275] found a decrease in tumor cell proliferation and pulmonary metastasis in male TRAMP F1 hybrid mice using 6 μmol SFN in 0.1 PBS 3 times a week (p.o.) for 17–19 weeks. The study also reported increased apoptosis and increases in Bax, Bid, Bak, Bad, and PARP cleavage. Antiapoptotic factor Mcl-1 was decreased, and E-cadherin was also upregulated [275]. Traka et al. [276] revealed inhibition of cell viability and proliferation using 0.1 or 1 μmol/g SFN per day (p.o.) for 8 weeks in PTEN^ L/L and PB-Cre4 mice. Elevated levels of caspase-3, caspase-7, and cyclin B1 were reported, as well as decreased cyclin D2.

Singh et al. [262] treated adenocarcinoma of TRAMP mice SFN, which resulted in tumor growth inhibition. Decreased acetyl CoA carboxylase (ACC1) and FASN, enzymes involved in fatty acid metabolism, were reported. Additionally, fatty acid, acetyl-CoA, and phospholipid levels were decreased. Similarly, Singh et al. [253] introduced 1 mg SFN 3 times per week (p.o.) for 5 weeks to TRAMP and Hi-Myc mice with prostate adenocarcinoma and noted inhibition of tumor growth. The TRAMP mice model overall showed a lower incidence of prostatic intraepithelial neoplasia by 23–28%. A mechanistic evaluation revealed a decrease in hexokinase 2, the rate-limiting enzyme in glycolysis, a decrease in tumor M2-pyruvate kinase, a pyruvate kinase specific for malignant growths, and a decrease in lactate dehydrogenase, an enzyme responsible for anaerobic glycolysis in both mouse models. Additionally, there was significantly suppressed glycolysis in the Hi-Myc mouse model.

4.3. Clinical Studies

Many retrospective (observational), prospective, and interventional clinical studies have been conducted to evaluate cancer-preventive and therapeutic efficacy of broccoli and broccoli-derived products containing GFN and/or SFN. In the following section, we present many of these studies.

Epidemiological studies have suggested that consumption of cooked meat and meat products increases the risk of colorectal cancer [277]. Walters et al. [278] investigated the cancer-preventative capability of cruciferous vegetables by examining excretion of the food-derived carcinogen, 2-amino-1-methyl-6-phenylimidazo[4,5-*b*]pyridine (PhIP), in a group consisting of twenty non-smoking Caucasian males. During phases 1 and 3, participants avoided cruciferous vegetable intake, and during phase 2, participants ingested 250 g each of Brussels sprouts and broccoli per day. At the end of each phase, each participant consumed a meat meal containing 4.9 μg PhIP, and the urinary metabolite of PhIP (N^2-hydroxy-PhIP-N^2-glucuronide) was measured. There was a significant increase in urinary excretion N^2-hydroxy-PhIP-N^2-glucuronide in phase 2 compared to phases 1 and 3 (Table 3). This study demonstrates that consumption of cruciferous vegetables can induce the metabolism of PhIP in humans, underscoring chemopreventive potential.

Due to consumption of foods contaminated with aflatoxin, a dietary hepatocarcinogen, and exposure to high levels of phenanthrene, a polycyclic aromatic hydrocarbon, the residents of Qidong, People's Republic of China, are at an elevated risk for the development of hepatocellular carcinoma. In a randomized, placebo-controlled chemopreventive trial, 200 healthy adults from Qidong drank hot water infusions of 3-day old broccoli sprouts containing 400 μmol of GFN for two weeks. The results indicated an inverse association between the urinary excretion of dithiocarbamates (SFN metabolites) and aflatoxin-DNA adducts or *trans, anti*-phenanthrene tetraol (a metabolite of phenanthrene) in individuals receiving the broccoli drink [279]. In a crossover clinical study conducted by the same research group [280], 50 healthy volunteers from the same region as mentioned above received two broccoli-sprout-derived beverages (enriched with SFN or GFN). It was determined that individuals receiving either one or both beverages had a 20–25% increase in excretion of GSH-derived conjugates of benzene, acrolein, crotonaldehyde (all airborne pollutants) compared with their preinterventional base values, indicating enhanced detoxification of environmental carcinogens. In an extended study by the same group [281] with a larger study population and extended period of intervention, the broccoli sprout beverage elicited rapid and sustained increases in the levels of excretion of GSH conjugates of benzene and acrolein, but not crotonaldehyde, compared to the placebo group [281]. These findings may be valuable in designing a future chemopreventive trial to evaluate the ability of broccoli bioactive food components to prevent environmental carcinogenesis.

Table 3. Clinical studies on broccoli constituents in cancer prevention and intervention.

Study Subjects	Study Type	Study Population	No. of Patients/Control Subjects	Intervention	Status	Main Findings/Objectives	References
Healthy males	Dietary intervention study	United Kingdom	20	Brussels sprouts and broccoli (250 g each)	Completed	Increased urinary excretion of PhIP metabolites in group that did not consume broccoli	Walters et al., 2004 [278]
Healthy adults	Randomized placebo-controlled clinical trial	China	200	Broccoli sprout infusion (400 μmol GFN)	Completed	Showed an inverse association of dithiocarbamate and aflatoxin-DNA adducts	Kensler et al., 2005 [279]
Healthy adults	Crossover clinical trail	China	50	Broccoli sprout beverages (800 μmol GFN or 150 μmol SFN)	Completed	Enhanced urinary excretion of mercapturic acids of acrolein, benzene, and crotonaldehyde	Kensler et al., 2012 [280]
Healthy adults	Randomized, placebo-controlled clinical trial	China	148/143	Broccoli sprout beverages (600 μmol GFN and 40 μmol SFN)	Completed	Increased the excretion of benzene-derived mercapturic acid in individuals with positive *GSTT1* genotype compared to null genotype	Egner et al., 2014 [281]
Healthy adults (smokers and non-smokers)	Randomized crossover study	Italy	20	Broccoli (200 g/day)	Completed	Decreased DNA strand break in both smoker and non-smoker and reduced oxidative purine in the smoker group	Riso et al., 2009 [282]
Health adults (smokers)	Placebo-controlled intervention study	Italy	27	Broccoli (250 g/day, 110 μmol ITC/day)	Completed	Decreased oxidized DNA lesions and suppressed DNA strand breaks in the PBMCs of smokers with higher protections with *GSTM1*-null genotype	Riso et al., 2010 [283]
Healthy volunteers	Pilot clinical trial	United State	10	GFN-rich (600 μmol/L GFN) or SFN-rich (150 μmol/L SFN) BSE	Completed	Upregulated *NQO1* mRNA in oral mucosa	Buamen et al., 2016 [284]
Healthy adults	Randomized clinical trial	United States	20	Fresh broccoli sprouts or BSE (200 μmol SFN)	Completed	Decreased PBMC HDAC activity, especially in higher dose group or following repeated intake	Atwell et al., 2015 [79]

Table 3. *Cont.*

Study Subjects	Study Type	Study Population	No. of Patients/Control Subjects	Intervention	Status	Main Findings/Objectives	References
Breast cancer patients	Double-blinded clinical trial	United States	27/27	Broccoli seed extract with GFN (224 mg or 512 μmol GFN)	Completed	Decreased PBMC HDAC activity and Ki-67 and HDAC3 serum levels	Atwell et al., 2015 [285]
Breast cancer patients	Double-blinded clinical trial	United States	27/27	Cruciferous vegetables	Completed	Increased consumption led to significantly lower Ki-67 levels in breast cancer samples	Zhang et al., 2015 [286]
Breast cancer patients	Non-randomized interventional clinical trial	Belgium, France, Spain, United Kingdom	60	α-cyclodextrin complex of SFN (SFX-01)	Not completed	Showed potential to reverse resistance to endocrine therapy in metastatic breast cancer	Howell et al., 2019 [287]
Pancreatic cancer patients	Double-blinded, randomized pilot trial	Germany	40	Freeze-dried broccoli sprout (90 mg SFN/day, 507.64 μmol/day)	Not completed	Primary goal is to increase the survival of patients with pancreatic ductal adenocarcinoma	Lozanovski et al., 2014 [288]
Prostate cancer patients	Non-randomized trial	United Kingdom	20	Broccoli (400 g/week)	Completed	Broccoli consumption interacted with *GSTM1* genotype and resulted in alterations of TGFβ1 and EGF signaling pathways	Traka et. al., 2008 [289]
Prostate cancer patients	Single-arm trial	United States	20	SFN-rich extract (200 μmol/day)	Completed	Reduced PSA by more than 50% in one patient and registered a smaller decline (<50%) in PSA in seven patients; prolonged PSA doubling time	Alumkal et al., 2015 [87]
Prostate cancer patients	Double-blinded, randomized, placebo-controlled trial	France	38/40	SFN extracted from broccoli seeds (60 mg SFN/day, 338.42 μmol SFN/day)	Completed	Lowered PSA level at months 0, 1, 3, and 6 as well as prolonged PSA doubling time	Cipolla et al., 2015 [290]

Table 3. *Cont.*

Study Subjects	Study Type	Study Population	No. of Patients/Control Subjects	Intervention	Status	Main Findings/Objectives	References
Prostate cancer patients	Randomized double-blinded, controlled trial	United Kingdom	41/20	Broccoli soup (300 mL/week)	Completed	Attenuated the transcriptional changes in the prostate in line with a reduction in the risk of cancer progression	Traka et al., 2019 [291]
At-risk prostate cancer patients	Double-blinded, randomized, controlled trial	United States	48/48	BSE (200 µmol SFN/day)	Completed	Increased HDAC activity in prostate cancer patients; did not alter tissue biomarkers; downregulated *AMACR* and *ARLNC1* genes	Zhang et al., 2020 [90]
Skin cancer patients	Double-blinded, randomized clinical trial	United State	17	BSE (50–200 µmol SFN/day)	Not completed	To evaluate the effect on biomarkers Ki-67, Bcl-2, and STAT3	Kirkwoood et. al., 2016 [292]
Skin cancer patients	Double-blinded, randomized clinical trial	United States	17	BSE (50–200 µmol SFN/day)	Completed	Decreased the levels of pro-inflammatory cytokines (IP-10, MCP-1, MIG, and MIP-1β) and increased tumor suppressor decorin on day 28	Tahata et al., 2018 [89]

A crossover clinical study by Riso et al. [282] evaluated the protective effect of 200 g broccoli intake for 10 days in healthy males, including 10 smokers and 10 non-smokers. Blood samples were collected at 0, 10, 30, and 40 days for assessment of DNA damage, IGF-I, and HDAC. The results showed that the broccoli diet decreased DNA strand breaks in both groups and reduced the oxidized purines only in the smoker group. However, broccoli intake did not alter HDAC activity or IGF-I levels. In the following year, the same group [283] published the results of another study in which 27 healthy smokers consumed steamed broccoli (250 g/day) or a control diet for 10 days. Broccoli intake decreased the level of oxidized DNA lesions and prevented hydrogen peroxide-induced DNA strand breaks in PBMCs from smokers. A higher level of protection was observed in participants with the *GSTM1*-null genotype.

Several epidemiological studies indicate that diets rich in cruciferous vegetables are linked to a reduced risk of oral cancer [293,294]. In a pilot clinical trial in 10 healthy volunteers, consumption of either GFN- or SFN-rich BSE or topical exposure to SFN-rich extract showed upregulation of *NQO1* mRNA in buccal scrapings (oral mucosa), suggesting the chemopreventive potential of SFN against carcinogen-induced oral cancer [284].

In a study conducted by Atwell et al. [79], 20 healthy adults consumed fresh broccoli sprouts or myrosinase-treated BSE, each providing 200 μmol SFN single dose daily, or two 100-μmol doses taken 12 h apart in a divided dose phase. Three chemopreventive mechanistic targets of SFN, namely, HO-1, HDAC, and p21, were measured in the PBMCs. The results indicated that the consumers of both sprouts and BSE had fluctuations in the HDAC activity, with greater decreases in HDAC activity noted in higher-dose or repeated-intake subjects.

In a double-blind, randomized controlled trial, 54 women with abnormal mammograms who were scheduled for breast biopsy consumed 250 mg of broccoli seed extract daily containing 30 mg of GFN (68.57 μmol GFN) or a placebo for 2–8 weeks before their biopsy. Plasma and urine SFN metabolites, PBMC HDAC activity, and tissue biomarkers, such as HDAC3, HDAC6, H3K18ac, H3K9ac, Ki-67, and p21, were measured pre- and post-treatment in benign, ductal carcinoma in situ (DCIS) or invasive ductal carcinoma (IDC) breast tissues. Statistically significant reductions in PBMC HDAC activity, as well as a decrease in Ki-67 and HDAC3 serum levels in benign tissues of the GFN-supplemented group, were observed, indicating that GFN may modulate HDAC activity, resulting in decreased cell proliferation [285]. The same group [286] conducted another study on 54 women with abnormal mammograms who were scheduled for breast biopsy and investigated the relationship between the intake of cruciferous vegetables and selected tumor biomarkers of the previous study. Total cruciferous vegetable intake was assessed using the National Cancer Institute Diet History Questionnaire and Arizona Cruciferous Vegetable Food Frequency Questionnaire, urine and serum ITC levels were estimated, and the biomarkers were measured in breast tissues using immunohistochemistry. Participant cruciferous vegetable intake was 81.7 g/day, and increased total cruciferous vegetable intake was associated with significantly lower Ki-67 levels in breast DCIS tissues but not in benign or IDC tissues. These results suggest that consumption of cruciferous vegetables plays a role in inhibiting breast cancer cell proliferation. A phase II clinical trial is investigating the effect of α-cyclodextrin complex of SFN known as SFX-01 (Evgen Pharma, Alderley Park, United Kingdom) on 60 participants, given over the 18 months. The preliminary results indicate that SFX-01 has the potential to reverse resistance to endocrine therapies in patients with ER+ HER2- metastatic breast cancer [287].

A prospective randomized, double-blind clinical trial is investigating the effect of freeze-dried broccoli sprouts containing 90 mg SFN (507.64 μmol SFN) daily on 40 patients with non-resectable pancreatic ductal adenocarcinoma undergoing palliative chemotherapy for a year. The primary goal of the study is to increase the overall survival of the patients [288]. The final results are not published yet.

Epidemiological studies have suggested that individuals who consume diets rich in cruciferous vegetables are at lower risk of both the incidence and aggressive forms of prostate cancer [295,296]. A clinical trial conducted by Traka et al. [289] investigated the effect of the consumption of 400 g broccoli per week for 12 months on prostate gene expression in 20 males with high-grade prostatic intraepithelial neoplasia. The results indicated that there was a significant difference in gene expression between *GSTM1*-positive and null individuals in the broccoli diet group. The altered genes are associated with the TGF-β1 and epidermal growth factor (EGF) signaling pathway. The findings suggested that consuming broccoli interacts with the GSTM1 genotype through signaling pathways associated with inflammation and carcinogenesis in the prostate. Later, Alumkal et al. [87] performed a study in which a BSE containing 200 μmole SFN was given to 20 men with recurrent prostate cancer for 20 weeks. The findings demonstrated that treatment with SFN-rich extract reduced PSA by more than 50% only in one patient, and a smaller decline in PSA was noted in seven patients. Additionally, there was a significant increase in PSA doubling time (PSADT) due to the intervention. Cipolla et al. [290] performed a double-blinded, randomized, placebo-controlled multicenter trial in which 75 men with increasing PSA levels after radical prostatectomy received 60 mg (338.42 μmol) of oral SFN daily for 6 months followed by 2 months with no treatment. The results showed that the SFN group had lower PSA levels at months 0, 1, 3, and 6, as well as longer PSADT compared to the placebo group. In addition, a PSA increase of more than 20% was noted in the placebo group at 6 months compared to the SFN group. Traka et al. [291] demonstrated the effect of weekly intake of 300 mL portion of soup made from GFN-enriched broccoli or standard broccoli (control) for 12 months on prostate cancer patients who underwent transperineal template biopsy. Gene expression in tissues from the patients was quantified before and after the dietary intervention. The results indicated that the consumption of GFN-rich broccoli soup affected gene expression in the prostate of patients, indicating a reduction in the risk of cancer progression. In another study conducted by Zhang et al. [90], 96 men scheduled for prostate biopsy consumed capsules containing BSE (providing 200 μmol SFN) daily or a placebo with the objective of understanding the impact of SFN on blood HDAC activity, prostate genes expression, and tissue biomarkers, such as histone H3 lysine 18 acetylation (H3K18ac), HDAC3, HDAC6, Ki67, and p21. The results showed a significant increase in urinary and plasma SFN metabolite levels in the extract-treated group but failed to show any significant difference in HDAC activity. However, within the subgroup of subjects with confirmed prostate cancer, the extract treatment significantly increased HDAC activity. In addition, there was no significant difference between the two groups on tissue biomarkers, which was thought to be due to undetectable levels of SFN in prostate tissue. Finally, using biopsy samples, this study detected treatment-related alterations in the expression of six genes, including α-methylacyl-coA racemase (AMACR), androgen receptor-regulated long non-coding RNA (ARLNC1), C1orf64, SLIT1, RP11-672G23-1, and RP1-274L7.1, which may play a role in the development of prostate cancer and are important targets for future studies.

A double-blinded clinical study by Kirkwood et al. [292] is investigating the effect of BSE on 17 individuals for 28 days on patients with a history of melanoma and multiple atypical/dysplastic nevi. Patients randomly received oral BSE (standardized for 50, 100, or 200 μmol SFN) daily for evaluation of its effect on melanoma risk marker STAT3 as well as proliferative marker Ki-67 and apoptotic marker Bcl-2. The final results are not published yet. However, according to a report published by the same group [89], the aforementioned oral regimen of BSE has been implicated in decreasing pro-inflammatory cytokines human interferon-inducible protein 10 (IP-10), monocyte chemoattractant protein 1 (MCP-1), monokine induced by gamma (MIG), and macrophage inflammatory protein 1β (MIP-1β), along with decreased IFN-γ and increased tumor suppressor decorin in skin nevi of patients with a history of melanoma. Additionally, a trend towards decreased nevi size was observed with increased SFN level after the 28-day period; however, measurements were not statistically significant [89].

Although not many clinical studies have investigated the effect of cruciferous vegetables and cruciferous vegetable products on cancer, the research that has been conducted shows promising results, such as decreased cell proliferation, impacts on inflammatory cytokines, and decreases in tumor markers. These studies have opened up varied directions for future research that can more accurately identify the benefit of intake of cruciferous vegetable components, especially SFN.

5. Conclusions and Future Directions

The *Brassica* genus includes broccoli, Brussels sprouts, and cabbage, among other nutritious vegetables that contain organosulfur compounds, including ITCs. SFN has been shown to be the most potent ITC and has been found in the highest concentrations in broccoli and broccoli sprouts. SFN possesses anticancer properties that have lately been a focus of natural product cancer preventative research. The purpose of this review was to provide a systemic analysis of preclinical and clinical studies that examined the anticancer and chemopreventive actions of SFN. This analysis also detailed the bioavailability and toxicity of SFN.

While bioavailability studies are lacking due to SFN instability and the expense of creating SFN products, a substantial amount of in vitro, in vivo, and clinical trials utilizing SFN precursors and metabolites have supported the use of this phytochemical as an anticancer agent. After oral consumption, SFN has been detected in serum and many tissue types indicating its ability to reach a variety of tumors. In vitro and in vivo studies have aided in determining a therapeutic dose of SFN; however, there has been a disconnect in the literature between dosages utilized in animal models and the tolerable doses in humans. Many of the published in vivo studies report chemopreventive effects with doses of SFN that would be unachievable in human subjects. Doses ranging from 5 to 100 mg/kg SFN have been shown to suppress tumor growth in animal models, translating to 350–7000 mg for a 70 kg individual. Additionally, one of the most common delivery methods employed in animal studies was i.p. injection, but most clinical trials aim to investigate oral intake. Future research in animal studies should aim to translate better into clinical trial scenarios to provide more insight into the true anticancer effects of SFN.

One of the most pressing questions in this research is the translation of cruciferous vegetable intake to GFN/SFN dose consumption for cancer prevention. Yagishita et al. [57] have reported an average concentration of 0.38 μmol/gram GFN in raw broccoli from Baltimore supermarkets with a range of 0.005–1.13 μmol/g. Additionally, an average of 0.36 μmol/g GFN has been reported in field/greenhouse-grown broccoli [57]. Most clinical trials utilize doses of GFN ranging from 25 to 800 μmol [57], translating to about 65–2105 g raw broccoli or 3/4 to 23 cups of raw broccoli. The lower end of this range is reasonable to consume daily, but the mid-upper end of this range breaches a realistic boundary, opening the opportunity for GFN/SFN supplements that meet the required chemopreventive doses.

There have been few adverse effects of SFN reported in the literature. One study has reported a lethal dose of SFN determined via oral SFN administration to rats, but such toxic doses have not been established in clinical trials due to maximal dose regulations. Mild adverse effects, such as gastrointestinal distress, nausea, and heartburn, have been reported in clinical trials. However, the reported anticancer properties of SFN greatly outweigh these minute side effects.

It was determined that the vast majority (i.e., 192) of the current literature focusing on anticancer properties of SFN has been preclinical studies, whereas only 19 studies have investigated the effects of products containing SFN and its biogenic precursor in clinical trials. In vitro studies have focused on numerous specific cancer subtypes, while in vivo studies have used only a few organ-specific tumor models. Prostate cancer has been the most investigated cancer type, closely followed by breast cancer, based on published clinical trials. Analysis of the published data has revealed SFN's diverse mechanistic regulation, which includes, but is not limited to, modulation of proliferation, cell death, cell cycle arrest, oxidative stress, inflammation, migration, invasion, and metastasis (Figure 3).

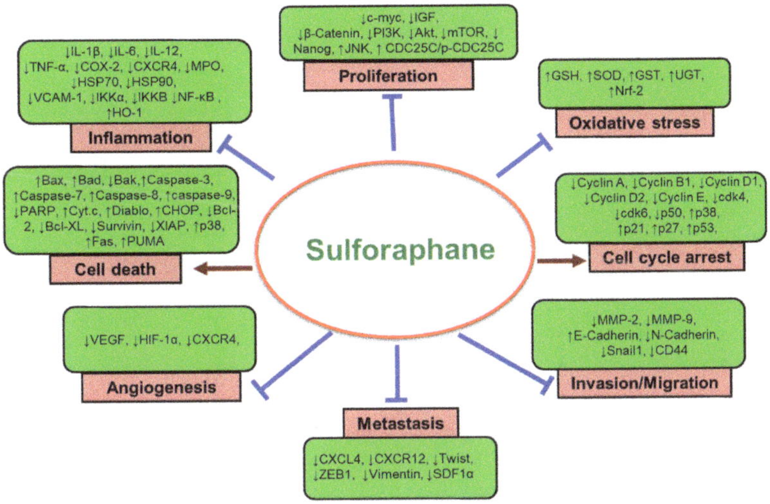

Figure 3. Chemopreventive and anticancer and effects of SFN extrapolated from in vitro and in vivo literature analysis. Symbols: ↑, increased or upregulated; ↓ decreased or downregulated; ⊥, blocked.

In regard to in vitro studies, a few mechanistic pathways of note were consistent between cancer subtypes. It is clear that the Nrf2/Keap pathway plays a significant role in SFN induced cytotoxicity. Mechanistically, SFN has been shown to increase nuclear Nrf2 through two specific pathways. The first is through modification of Keap1 cysteine residues, causing a release of Nrf2 that is able to translocate to the nucleus. The second is through epigenetic modulation of HDACs and DNMTs. SFN has been shown to influence epigenetic modulation through DNA methylation, histone modification, and non-coding RNAs, allowing for increased Nrf2 transcription and translation, again resulting in increased nuclear Nrf2. Within the nucleus, Nrf2 is able to bind to ARE and maf to increase transcription of cytoprotective phase II enzymes (Figure 4). Additionally, apoptosis was induced by SFN in the majority of in vitro studies. Many mechanisms were uncovered, including, but not limited to, increased Bax and Bad, increased caspase-3, caspase-7, caspase-8, caspase-9, and decreased Bcl-2 and Bcl-xL (Figure 5). Modulation of these endpoints indicates that SFN acts on both the intrinsic and extrinsic apoptotic pathways. SFN was also recognized to induce cell cycle arrest in many cancer cell models. Arrest primarily occurred in the G2/M phase but was also noted in the G1/S phase. Likewise, SFN has been shown to modulate angiogenesis and autophagy, contributing to its broad spectrum of antiproliferative actions.

Several directions of future investigation have been identified throughout this systemic review. A substantial number of in vitro studies across cancer subtypes have identified specific anticancer properties of SFN, and it is clear that additional in vivo studies should be performed to support these mechanisms. Similarly, many in vivo studies have utilized various broccoli extracts, but because of its potent nature, it would be beneficial to understand the effects of pure SFN in animal tumor models. While BSE contains GFN that is metabolized to SFN, it is difficult to accurately control and determine the dose of SFN due to differences in gut microbes and liver conjugation enzymes. Therefore, future in vivo studies should focus on utilizing pure SFN to allow for the most accurate translation to human clinical trials.

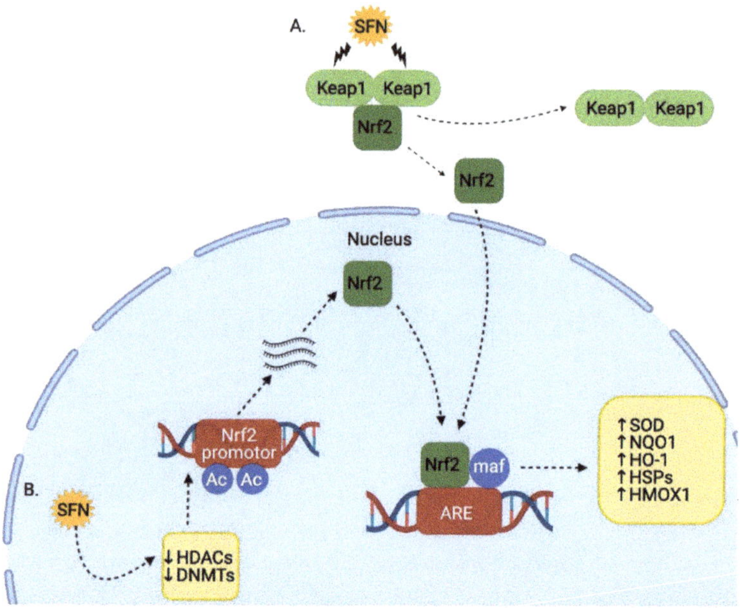

Figure 4. Effect of SFN on Nrf2/Keap1 pathway. (**A**) SFN modifies Keap1 cysteine residues, causing release of Nrf2, which allows it to translocate to the nucleus. (**B**) SFN also induces epigenetic modulation of HDACs and DNMTs, causing increased Nrf2 transcription and translation. Consequently, the increased nuclear Nrf2 binds to ARE and maf to increase transcription of various cytoprotective phase II enzymes. This figure was created using resources available at BioRender.com (accessed on 4 July 2021). Symbols: ↑, increased or upregulated; ↓ decreased or downregulated.

Several anticancer mechanisms have been proposed by a variety of researchers, and some of these mechanisms contradict one another. Therefore, additional studies must be conducted to fully elucidate the molecular targets of SFN as well as identify reliable biomarkers that accurately depict the efficacy of SFN in pre-clinical and clinical studies. Additional cancer types must be explored in clinical trials as only breast, skin, pancreatic, and prostate cancer trials have been published. Furthermore, many of the reported clinical trials utilized a variety of cruciferous vegetable products; however, it would be beneficial to study the effects of pure SFN as it appears to be the phytochemical with the greatest anticancer properties. Greater sample sizes and the use of randomized controlled trials would provide more substantial support for SFN's chemopreventive properties.

This extensive review only included in vitro and in vivo studies that reported the effects of SFN alone on different cancer cell lines. During this work, we came across many published studies (not presented here) that reported significant effects of SFN in combination with other phytochemicals and chemotherapeutic agents. Additionally, many studies have addressed the instability of SFN and have formulated a multitude of delivery systems to increase the bioavailability of SFN. Such delivery systems include microencapsulation, microspheres, nanoparticles, micelles, and liposomes. Analysis of this literature could provide additional knowledge of the anticancer and chemotherapeutic properties of SFN-containing regimens. Based on the overwhelming evidence presented in this in-depth analysis of current research, SFN is a promising antineoplastic and chemopreventive phytochemical that can be utilized as a valuable cancer-fighting agent.

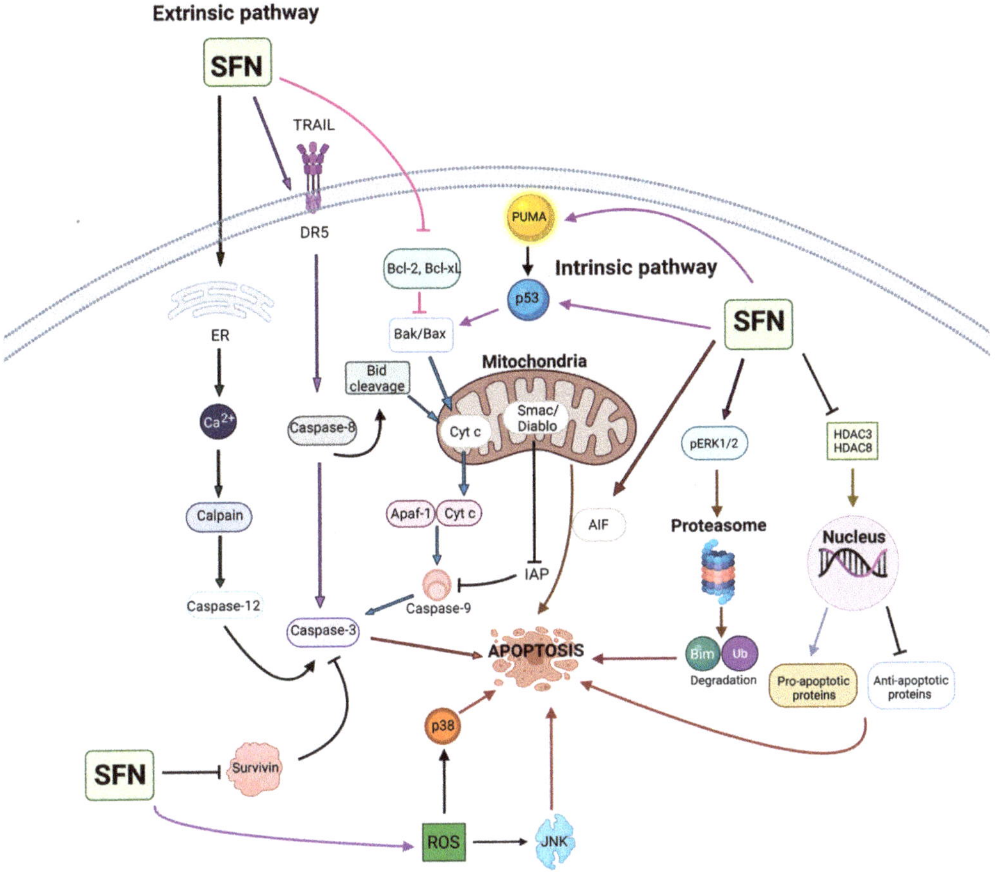

Figure 5. SFN modulates multiple targets in the intrinsic and extrinsic apoptotic pathways. SFN has been found to alter the expression or activate/inactivate various apoptotic mediators and regulators. Symbols: →, increased, upregulated or activated; ⊥, blocked or suppressed. This figure was created using resources available at BioRender.com (accessed on 17 September 2021).

Author Contributions: Conceptualization, A.B.; methodology, A.B.; investigation, A.E.K., M.B., D.G., M.G. (Matthew Giansiracusa), M.G. (Michael Garcia), Z.F. and T.L.W.; writing—original draft preparation, A.E.K., M.B., D.G., M.G. (Matthew Giansiracusa), M.G. (Michael Garcia), Z.F. and T.L.W.; writing—A.B.; supervision, A.B.; project administration, A.B. All authors have read and agreed to the published version of the manuscript.

Funding: This research received no external source of funding.

Acknowledgments: The authors wish to extend our thanks to researchers all over the world who have made significant contributions to our understanding of SFN's potential in cancer prevention and intervention. The authors sincerely regret that we are unable to cite each and every pertinent publication due to space limitations.

Conflicts of Interest: The authors declare no conflict of interest.

Abbreviations

APAF-1	apoptotic protease activating factor-1
ARE	antioxidant response element
BSE	broccoli sprout extract
BSP	broccoli sprout powders
COX-2	cyclooxygenase-2
CYP	cytochrome P-450
CXCR4	C-X-C chemokine receptor type 4
DCIS	ductal carcinoma in situ
DMH	dimethylhydrazine
DMNT	DNA methyltransferase
EMT	epithelial–mesenchymal transition
ER	estrogen receptor
ERK	extracellular signal-related kinase
FADD	Fas-associated death domain
GFN	glucoraphanin
GGT	γ-glutamyl transpeptidase
GSH	glutathione
GST	glutathione S-transferase
HDAC	histone deacytylase
HER	human growth factor receptor
HIF	hypoxia-inducible factor
HMOX1	heme oxygenase 1
HSP70	heat shock protein 70
IDC	invasive ductal carcinoma
IFN-γ	interferon-γ
IL	interleukin
i.p.	intraperitoneal
ITC	isothiocyanate
i.v.	intravenous
JNK	Jun NH_2-terminal kinase
Keap1	Kelch-like ECH-associated protein 1
MAPK	mitogen-activated protein kinase
MEK1	mitogen-activated protein kinase 1
MMP	matrix metalloproteinase
NF-κB	nuclear factor-κB
NQO1	NADPH-dependent oxidoreductase 1
Nrf2	nuclear factor erythroid-2-related factor 2
NSCLCs	non-small cell lung cancer cells
PARP	poly (ADP-ribose) polymerase
PBMCs	peripheral blood mononuclear cells
PCNA	proliferating cell nuclear antigen
PR	progesterone receptor
PRIMSA	Preferred Reporting Item for Systemic Review and Meta-Analysis
PSA	prostate-specific antigen
PTEN	phosphatase and tensin homolog
PUMA	p53 upregulated modulator of apoptosis
ROS	reactive oxygen species
SF	sulforaphane
STAT3	signal transducer and activator of transcription 3
TGF-β	transforming growth factor-β
TNF-α	tumor necrosis factor-α
VEGF	vascular endothelial growth factor
XRE	xenobiotic response element

References

1. Sung, H.; Ferlay, J.; Siegel, R.L.; Laversanne, M.; Soerjomataram, I.; Jemal, A.; Bray, F. Global cancer statistics 2020: GLOBOCAN estimates of incidence and mortality worldwide for 36 cancers in 185 countries. *CA Cancer J. Clin.* **2021**, *68*, 394–424. [CrossRef]
2. Torre, L.A.; Siegel, R.L.; Ward, E.M.; Jemal, A. Global Cancer Incidence and Mortality Rates and Trends—An Update. *Cancer Epidemiol. Biomark. Prev.* **2016**, *25*, 16–27. [CrossRef]
3. Sporn, M.B.; Dunlop, N.M.; Newton, D.L.; Smith, J.M. Prevention of chemical carcinogenesis by vitamin A and its synthetic analogs (retinoids). *Fed. Proc.* **1976**, *35*, 1332–1338.
4. Fahey, J.W.; Talalay, P.; Kensler, T.W. Notes from the field: "green" chemoprevention as frugal medicine. *Cancer Prev. Res.* **2012**, *5*, 179–188. [CrossRef]
5. Aune, D.; Giovannucci, E.; Boffetta, P.; Fadnes, L.T.; Keum, N.; Norat, T.; Greenwood, D.C.; Riboli, E.; Vatten, L.J.; Tonstad, S. Fruit and vegetable intake and the risk of cardiovascular disease, total cancer and all-cause mortality-a systematic review and dose-response meta-analysis of prospective studies. *Int. J. Epidemiol.* **2017**, *46*, 1029–1056. [CrossRef]
6. Amin, A.R.; Kucuk, O.; Khuri, F.R.; Shin, D.M. Perspectives for cancer prevention with natural compounds. *J. Clin. Oncol.* **2009**, *27*, 2712–2725. [CrossRef]
7. Gullett, N.P.; Ruhul Amin, A.R.; Bayraktar, S.; Pezzuto, J.M.; Shin, D.M.; Khuri, F.R.; Aggarwal, B.B.; Surh, Y.J.; Kucuk, O. Cancer prevention with natural compounds. *Semin. Oncol.* **2010**, *37*, 258–281. [CrossRef]
8. Liu, R.H. Health-promoting components of fruits and vegetables in the diet. *Adv. Nutr.* **2013**, *4*, 384S–392S. [CrossRef]
9. Lee, K.W.; Bode, A.M.; Dong, Z. Molecular targets of phytochemicals for cancer prevention. *Nat. Rev. Cancer.* **2011**, *11*, 211–218. [CrossRef]
10. Block, K.I.; Gyllenhaal, C.; Lowe, L.; Amedei, A.; Amin, A.R.M.R.; Amin, A.; Aquilano, K.; Arbiser, J.; Arreola, A.; Arzumanyan, A.; et al. Designing a broad-spectrum integrative approach for cancer prevention and treatment. *Semin. Cancer Biol.* **2015**, *35*, S276–S304. [CrossRef]
11. Tewari, D.; Nabavi, S.F.; Nabavi, S.M.; Sureda, A.; Farooqi, A.A.; Atanasov, A.G.; Vacca, R.A.; Sethi, G.; Bishayee, A. Targeting activator protein 1 signaling pathway by bioactive natural agents: Possible therapeutic strategy for cancer prevention and intervention. *Pharmacol. Res.* **2018**, *128*, 366–375. [CrossRef]
12. Das, B.; Sarkar, N.; Bishayee, A.; Sinha, D. Dietary phytochemicals in the regulation of epithelial to mesenchymal transition and associated enzymes: A promising anticancer therapeutic approach. *Semin. Cancer Biol.* **2019**, *56*, 196–218. [CrossRef]
13. Deng, S.; Shanmugam, M.K.; Kumar, A.P.; Yap, C.T.; Sethi, G.; Bishayee, A. Targeting autophagy using natural compounds for cancer prevention and therapy. *Cancer* **2019**, *125*, 1228–1246. [CrossRef]
14. Tewari, D.; Patni, P.; Bishayee, A.; Sah, A.N.; Bishayee, A. Natural products targeting the PI3K-Akt-mTOR signaling pathway in cancer: A novel therapeutic strategy. *Semin. Cancer Biol.* **2019**, *S1044-579X*, 30405–30455. [CrossRef]
15. Fakhri, S.; Moradi, S.Z.; Farzaei, M.H.; Bishayee, A. Modulation of dysregulated cancer metabolism by plant secondary metabolites: A mechanistic review. *Semin. Cancer Biol.* **2020**, *S1044-579X*, 30040–30047. [CrossRef]
16. Bose, S.; Banerjee, S.; Mondal, A.; Chakraborty, U.; Pumarol, J.; Croley, C.R.; Bishayee, A. Targeting the JAK/STAT Signaling Pathway Using Phytocompounds for Cancer Prevention and Therapy. *Cells* **2020**, *9*, 1451. [CrossRef]
17. Tuli, H.S.; Tuorkey, M.J.; Thakral, F.; Sak, K.; Kumar, M.; Sharma, A.K.; Sharma, U.; Jain, A.; Aggarwal, V.; Bishayee, A. Molecular Mechanisms of Action of Genistein in Cancer: Recent Advances. *Front. Pharmacol.* **2019**, *10*, 1336. [CrossRef]
18. Aggarwal, V.; Tuli, H.S.; Tania, M.; Srivastava, S.; Ritzer, E.E.; Pandey, A.; Aggarwal, D.; Barwal, T.S.; Jain, A.; Kaur, G.; et al. Molecular mechanisms of action of epigallocatechin gallate in cancer: Recent trends and advancement. *Semin. Cancer Biol.* **2020**, *24*, 30107. [CrossRef]
19. Mirza, B.; Croley, C.R.; Ahmad, M.; Pumarol, J.; Das, N.; Sethi, G.; Bishayee, A. Mango (*Mangifera indica* L.): A magnificent plant with cancer preventive and anticancer therapeutic potential. *Crit. Rev. Food* **2020**, *8*, 2125–2151. [CrossRef]
20. De Greef, D.; Barton, E.M.; Sandberg, E.N.; Croley, C.R.; Pumarol, J.; Wong, T.L.; Das, N.; Bishayee, A. Anticancer potential of garlic and its bioactive constituents: A systematic and comprehensive review. *Semin. Cancer Biol.* **2020**, *73*, 219–264. [CrossRef]
21. Nouri, Z.; Fakhri, S.; Nouri, K.; Wallace, C.E.; Farzaei, M.H.; Bishayee, A. Targeting Multiple Signaling Pathways in Cancer: The Rutin Therapeutic Approach. *Cancers* **2020**, *12*, 2276. [CrossRef]
22. Ghanbari-Movahed, M.; Jackson, G.; Farzaei, M.H.; Bishayee, A. A Sstematic Review of the Preventive and Therapeutic Effects of Naringin Against Human Malignancies. *Front. Pharmacol.* **2021**, *12*, 639840. [CrossRef]
23. Wong, T.L.; Strandberg, K.R.; Croley, C.R.; Fraser, S.E.; Nagulapalli Venkata, K.C.; Fimognari, C.; Sethi, G.; Bishayee, A. Pomegranate bioactive constituents target multiple oncogenic and oncosuppressive signaling for cancer prevention and intervention. *Semin. Cancer Biol.* **2021**, *73*, 265–293. [CrossRef]
24. Lin, H.J.; Probst-Hensch, N.M.; Louie, A.D.; Kau, I.H.; Witte, J.S.; Ingles, S.A.; Frankl, H.D.; Lee, E.R.; Haile, R.W. Glutathione transferase null genotype, broccoli, and lower prevalence of colorectal adenomas. *Cancer Epidemiol. Biomark. Prev.* **1998**, *7*, 647–652.
25. Michaud, D.S.; Spiegelman, D.; Clinton, S.K.; Rimm, E.B.; Willett, W.C.; Giovannucci, E.L. Fruit and vegetable intake and incidence of bladder cancer in a male prospective cohort. *J. Natl. Cancer Inst.* **1999**, *91*, 605–613. [CrossRef]
26. Cohen, J.H.; Kristal, A.R.; Stanford, J.L. Fruit and vegetable intakes and prostate cancer risk. *J. Natl. Cancer Inst.* **2000**, *92*, 61–68. [CrossRef]

27. Ambrosone, C.B.; McCann, S.E.; Freudenheim, J.L.; Marshall, J.R.; Zhang, Y.; Shields, P.G. Breast cancer risk in premenopausal women is inversely associated with consumption of broccoli, a source of isothiocyanates, but is not modified by GST genotype. *Nutrition* **2004**, *134*, 1134–1138. [CrossRef]
28. Mori, N.; Shimazu, T.; Sasazuki, S.; Nozue, M.; Mutoh, M.; Sawada, N.; Iwasaki, M.; Yamaji, T.; Inoue, M.; Takachi, R.; et al. Cruciferous Vegetable Intake Is Inversely Associated with Lung Cancer Risk among Current Nonsmoking Men in the Japan Public Health Center (JPHC) Study. *Nutrients* **2017**, *147*, 841–849. [CrossRef]
29. Shapiro, T.A.; Fahey, J.W.; Wade, K.L.; Stephenson, K.K.; Talalay, P. Chemoprotective glucosinolates and isothiocyanates of broccoli sprouts: Metabolism and excretion in humans. *Cancer Epidemiol. Biomark. Prev.* **2001**, *10*, 501–508.
30. Navarro, S.L.; Li, F.; Lampe, J.W. Mechanisms of action of isothiocyanates in cancer chemoprevention: An update. *Food and Funct.* **2011**, *2*, 579–587. [CrossRef]
31. Zhang, Y. The molecular basis that unifies the metabolism, cellular uptake and chemopreventive activities of dietary isothiocyanates. *Carcinogenesis* **2012**, *33*, 2–9. [CrossRef]
32. Gupta, P.; Kim, B.; Kim, S.H.; Srivastava, S.K. Molecular targets of isothiocyanates in cancer: Recent advances. *Mol. Nutr. Food Res.* **2014**, *58*, 1685–1707. [CrossRef]
33. Kumar, G.; Tuli, H.S.; Mittal, S.; Shandilya, J.K.; Tiwari, A.; Sandhu, S.S. Isothiocyanates: A class of bioactive metabolites with chemopreventive potential. *Tumor Biol.* **2015**, *36*, 4005–4016. [CrossRef]
34. Palliyaguru, D.L.; Yuan, J.M.; Kensler, T.W.; Fahey, J.W. Isothiocyanates: Translating the Power of Plants to People. *Mol. Nutr. Food Res.* **2018**, *62*, e1700965. [CrossRef]
35. Singh, D.; Arora, R.; Bhatia, A.; Singh, H.; Singh, B.; Arora, S. Molecular targets in cancer prevention by 4-(methylthio)butyl isothiocyanate—A comprehensive review. *Life Sci.* **2020**, *241*, 117061. [CrossRef]
36. Hudlikar, R.; Wang, L.; Wu, R.; Li, S.; Peter, R.; Shannar, A.; Chou, P.J.; Liu, X.; Liu, Z.; Kuo, H.D.; et al. Epigenetics/epigenomics and prevention of early stages of cancer by isothiocyanates. *Cancer Prev. Res.* **2021**, *14*, 151–164. [CrossRef]
37. Xu, T.; Ren, D.; Sun, X.; Yang, G. Dual roles of sulforaphane in cancer treatment. *Anticancer Agents Med. Chem.* **2012**, *12*, 1132–1142. [CrossRef]
38. Kumar, A.; Sabbioni, G. New biomarkers for monitoring the levels of isothiocyanates in humans. *Chem. Res. Toxicol.* **2010**, *23*, 756–765. [CrossRef]
39. De Figueiredo, S.M.; Binda, N.S.; Nogueira-Machado, J.A.; Vieira-Filho, S.A.; Caligiorne, R.B. The antioxidant properties of organosulfur compounds (sulforaphane). *Recent Pat. Endocr. Metab. Immune Drug Discov.* **2015**, *9*, 24–39. [CrossRef]
40. Houghton, C.A. Sulforaphane: Its "Coming of Age" as a Clinically Relevant Nutraceutical in the Prevention and Treatment of Chronic Disease. *Oxid. Med. Cell. Longev.* **2019**, *2019*, 2716870. [CrossRef]
41. Mahn, A.; Castillo, A. Potential of Sulforaphane as a Natural Immune System Enhancer: A Review. *Molecules* **2021**, *26*, 752. [CrossRef]
42. Zeren, S.; Bayhan, Z.; Kocak, F.E.; Kocak, C.; Akcılar, R.; Bayat, Z.; Simsek, H.; Duzgun, S.A. Gastroprotective effects of sulforaphane and thymoquinone against acetylsalicylic acid-induced gastric ulcer in rats. *J. Surg. Res.* **2016**, *203*, 348–359. [CrossRef]
43. Bai, Y.; Wang, X.; Zhao, S.; Ma, C.; Cui, J.; Zheng, Y. Sulforaphane Protects against Cardiovascular Disease via Nrf2 Activation. *Oxid. Med. Cell. Longev.* **2015**, *2015*, 407580. [CrossRef]
44. Liebman, S.E.; Le, T.H. Eat Your Broccoli: Oxidative Stress, NRF2, and Sulforaphane in Chronic Kidney Disease. *Nutrients* **2021**, *13*, 266. [CrossRef] [PubMed]
45. Santín-Márquez, R.; Alarcón-Aguilar, A.; López-Diazguerrero, N.E.; Chondrogianni, N.; Königsberg, M. Sulforaphane—Role in aging and neurodegeneration. *GeroScience* **2019**, *41*, 655–670. [CrossRef] [PubMed]
46. Schepici, G.; Bramanti, P.; Mazzon, E. Efficacy of Sulforaphane in Neurodegenerative Diseases. *Int. J. Mol. Sci.* **2020**, *21*, 8637. [CrossRef]
47. Calabrese, E.J.; Kozumbo, W.J. The phytoprotective agent sulforaphane prevents inflammatory degenerative diseases and age-related pathologies via Nrf2-mediated hormesis. *Pharmacol. Res.* **2021**, *163*, 105283. [CrossRef] [PubMed]
48. Zhang, Y.; Talalay, P.; Cho, C.G.; Posner, G.H. A major inducer of anticarcinogenic protective enzymes from broccoli: Isolation and elucidation of structure. *Proc. Natl. Acad. Sci. USA* **1992**, *89*, 2399–2403. [CrossRef] [PubMed]
49. Zhang, Y.; Kensler, T.W.; Cho, C.G.; Posner, G.H.; Talalay, P. Anticarcinogenic activities of sulforaphane and structurally related synthetic norbornyl isothiocyanates. *Proc. Natl. Acad. Sci. USA* **1994**, *91*, 3147–3150. [CrossRef] [PubMed]
50. Fimognari, C.; Hrelia, P. Sulforaphane as a promising molecule for fighting cancer. *Mutat. Res.* **2007**, *635*, 90–104. [CrossRef]
51. Juge, N.; Mithen, R.F.; Traka, M. Molecular basis for chemoprevention by sulforaphane: A comprehensive review. *Cell. Mol. Life Sci.* **2007**, *64*, 1105–1127. [CrossRef] [PubMed]
52. Zhang, Y.; Tang, L. Discovery and development of sulforaphane as a cancer chemopreventive phytochemical. *Acta Pharmacol. Sin.* **2007**, *28*, 1343–1354. [CrossRef] [PubMed]
53. Clarke, J.D.; Dashwood, R.H.; Ho, E. Multi-targeted prevention of cancer by sulforaphane. *Cancer Lett.* **2008**, *269*, 291–304. [CrossRef] [PubMed]
54. Dinkova-Kostova, A.T.; Fahey, J.W.; Kostov, R.V.; Kensler, T.W. KEAP1 and Done? Targeting the NRF2 Pathway with Sulforaphane. *Trends Food Sci. Technol.* **2017**, *69*, 257–269. [CrossRef]
55. Jiang, X.; Liu, Y.; Ma, L.; Ji, R.; Qu, Y.; Xin, Y.; Lv, G. Chemopreventive activity of sulforaphane. *Drug Des. Dev.* **2018**, *12*, 2905–2913. [CrossRef]

56. Bayat Mokhtari, R.; Baluch, N.; Homayouni, T.S.; Morgatskaya, E.; Kumar, S.; Kazemi, P.; Yeger, H. The role of Sulforaphane in cancer chemoprevention and health benefits: A mini-review. *Cell Commun. Signal.* **2018**, *12*, 91–101. [CrossRef]
57. Yagishita, Y.; Fahey, J.W.; Dinkova-Kostova, A.T.; Kensler, T.W. Broccoli or Sulforaphane: Is It the Source or Dose That Matters? *Molecules* **2019**, *24*, 3593. [CrossRef]
58. Rafiei, H.; Ashrafizadeh, M.; Ahmadi, Z. MicroRNAs as novel targets of sulforaphane in cancer therapy: The beginning of a new tale? *Phytother. Res.* **2020**, *34*, 721–728. [CrossRef]
59. Elkashty, O.A.; Tran, S.D. Sulforaphane as a Promising Natural Molecule for Cancer Prevention and Treatment. *Curr. Med. Sci.* **2021**, *41*, 250–269. [CrossRef]
60. Kuran, D.; Pogorzelska, A.; Wiktorska, K. Breast Cancer Prevention-Is there a Future for Sulforaphane and Its Analogs? *Nutrients* **2020**, *12*, 1559. [CrossRef]
61. Leone, A.; Diorio, G.; Sexton, W.; Schell, M.; Alexandrow, M.; Fahey, J.W.; Kumar, N.B. Sulforaphane for the chemoprevention of bladder cancer: Molecular mechanism targeted approach. *Oncotarget* **2017**, *8*, 35412–35424. [CrossRef] [PubMed]
62. Amjad, A.I.; Parikh, R.A.; Appleman, L.J.; Hahm, E.R.; Singh, K.; Singh, S.V. Broccoli-Derived Sulforaphane and Chemoprevention of Prostate Cancer: From Bench to Bedside. *Curr. Pharmacol. Rep.* **2015**, *1*, 382–390. [CrossRef] [PubMed]
63. Calcabrini, C.; Maffei, F.; Turrini, E.; Fimognari, C. Sulforaphane Potentiates Anticancer Effects of Doxorubicin and Cisplatin and Mitigates Their Toxic Effects. *Front. Pharmacol.* **2020**, *11*, 567. [CrossRef]
64. Kamal, M.M.; Akter, S.; Lin, C.; Nazzal, S. Sulforaphane as an anticancer molecule: Mechanisms of action, synergistic effects, enhancement of drug safety, and delivery systems. *Arch. Pharm. Res.* **2020**, *43*, 371–384. [CrossRef]
65. Wu, G.; Yan, Y.; Zhou, Y.; Duan, Y.; Zeng, S.; Wang, X.; Lin, W.; Ou, C.; Zhou, J.; Xu, Z. Sulforaphane: Expected to Become a Novel Antitumor Compound. *Oncol. Res.* **2020**, *28*, 439–446. [CrossRef]
66. Rathaur, P.; Johar, K.S.R. Metabolism and Pharmacokinetics of Phytochemicals in the Human Body. *Curr. Drug Metab.* **2019**, *20*, 1085–1102. [CrossRef]
67. Fahey, J.W.; Holtzclaw, W.D.; Wehage, S.L.; Wade, K.L.; Stephenson, K.K.; Talalay, P. Sulforaphane Bioavailability from Glucoraphanin-Rich Broccoli: Control by Active Endogenous Myrosinase. *PLoS ONE* **2015**, *10*, e0140963. [CrossRef]
68. Sivapalan, T.; Melchini, A.; Saha, S.; Needs, P.W.; Traka, M.H.; Tapp, H.; Dainty, J.R.; Mithen, R.F. Bioavailability of Glucoraphanin and Sulforaphane from High-Glucoraphanin Broccoli. *Mol. Nutr. Food Res.* **2018**, *62*, e1700911. [CrossRef] [PubMed]
69. Fahey, J.W.; Wade, K.L.; Stephenson, K.K.; Panjwani, A.A.; Liu, H.; Cornblatt, G.; Cornblatt, B.S.; Ownby, S.L.; Fuchs, E.; Holtzclaw, W.D.; et al. Bioavailability of Sulforaphane Following Ingestion of Glucoraphanin-Rich Broccoli Sprout and Seed Extracts with Active Myrosinase: A Pilot Study of the Effects of Proton Pump Inhibitor Administration. *Nutrients* **2019**, *11*, 1489. [CrossRef]
70. Petri, N.; Tannergren, C.; Holst, B.; Mellon, F.A.; Bao, Y.; Plumb, G.W.; Bacon, J.; O'Leary, K.A.; Kroon, P.A.; Knutson, L.; et al. Absorption/metabolism of sulforaphane and quercetin, and regulation of phase II enzymes, in human jejunum in vivo. *Drug Metab. Dispos.* **2003**, *31*, 805–813. [CrossRef] [PubMed]
71. Clarke, J.D.; Hsu, A.; Riedl, K.; Bella, D.; Schwartz, S.J.; Stevens, J.F.; Ho, E. Bioavailability and inter-conversion of sulforaphane and erucin in human subjects consuming broccoli sprouts or broccoli supplement in a cross-over study design. *Pharmacol. Res.* **2011**, *64*, 456–463. [CrossRef] [PubMed]
72. Mennicke, W.H.; Görler, K.; Krumbiegel, G.; Lorenz, D.; Rittmann, N. Studies on the metabolism and excretion of benzyl isothiocyanate in man. *Xenobiotica* **1988**, *18*, 441–447. [CrossRef]
73. Bricker, G.V.; Riedl, K.M.; Ralston, R.A.; Tober, K.L.; Oberyszyn, T.M.; Schwartz, S.J. Isothiocyanate metabolism, distribution, and interconversion in mice following consumption of thermally processed broccoli sprouts or purified sulforaphane. *Mol. Nutr. Food Res.* **2015**, *58*, 1991–2000. [CrossRef]
74. Hanlon, N.; Coldham, N.; Gielbert, A.; Kuhnert, N.; Sauer, M.; King, L.; Ioannides, C. Absolute bioavailability and dose-dependent pharmacokinetic behaviour of dietary doses of the chemopreventive isothiocyanate sulforaphane in rat. *Br. J. Nutr.* **2008**, *99*, 559–564. [CrossRef]
75. Zhang, Y.; Wade, K.L.; Prestera, T.; Talala, P. Quantitative determination of isothiocyanates, dithiocarbamates, carbon disulfide, and related thiocarbonyl compounds by cyclocondensation with 1,2-benzenedithiol. *Anal. Biochem.* **1996**, *239*, 160–167. [CrossRef]
76. Cornblatt, B.; Ye, L.; Dinkova-Kostova, A.; Erb, M.; Fahey, J.W.; Singh, N.K.; Chen, M.S.; Stierer, T.; Garrett-Mayer, E.; Argani, P.; et al. Preclinical and clinical evaluation of sulforaphane for chemoprevention in the breast. *Carcinogenesis* **2007**, *28*, 1485–1490. [CrossRef]
77. Oliviero, T.; Lamers, S.; Capuano, E.; Dekker, M.; Verkerk, R. Bioavailability of Isothiocyanates from Broccoli Sprouts in Protein, Lipid, and Fiber Gels. *Mol. Nutr. Food Res.* **2018**, *62*, e1700837. [CrossRef] [PubMed]
78. Ye, L.; Dinkova-Kostova, A.T.; Wade, K.L.; Zhang, Y.; Shapiro, T.A.; Talalay, P. Quantitative determination of dithiocarbamates in human plasma, serum, erythrocytes and urine: Pharmacokinetics of broccoli sprout isothiocyanates in humans. *Clin. Chim. Acta* **2002**, *316*, 43–53. [CrossRef]
79. Atwell, L.L.; Hsu, A.; Wong, C.P.; Stevens, J.F.; Bella, D.; Yu, T.W.; Pereira, C.B.; Löhr, C.V.; Christensen, J.M.; Dashwood, R.H.; et al. Absorption and chemopreventive targets of sulforaphane in humans following consumption of broccoli sprouts or a myrosinase-treated broccoli sprout extract. *Mol. Nutr. Food Res.* **2015**, *59*, 424–433. [CrossRef] [PubMed]
80. Xue, M.; Qian, Q.; Adaikalakoteswari, A.; Rabbani, N.; Babaei-Jadidi, R.; Thornalley, P.J. Activation of NF-E2-related factor-2 reverses biochemical dysfunction of endothelial cells induced by hyperglycemia linked to vascular disease. *Diabetes* **2008**, *57*, 2809–2817. [CrossRef] [PubMed]

81. Gross-Steinmeyer, K.; Stapleton, P.L.; Tracy, J.H.; Bammler, T.K.; Strom, S.C.; Eaton, D.L. Sulforaphane- and phenethyl isothiocyanate-induced inhibition of aflatoxin B1-mediated genotoxicity in human hepatocytes: Role of GSTM1 genotype and CYP3A4 gene expression. *Toxicol. Sci.* **2010**, *116*, 422–432. [CrossRef]
82. Abbaoui, B.; Riedl, K.M.; Ralston, R.A.; Thomas-Ahner, J.M.; Schwartz, S.J.; Clinton, S.K.; Mortazavi, A. Inhibition of bladder cancer by broccoli isothiocyanates sulforaphane and eruicin: Characterization, metabolism, and interconversion. *Mol. Nutr. Food Res.* **2012**, *56*, 1675–1687. [CrossRef] [PubMed]
83. Arcidiacono, P.; Ragonese, F.; Stabile, A.; Pistilli, A.; Kuligina, E.; Rende, M.; Bottoni, U.; Calvieri, S.; Crisanti, A.; Spaccapelo, R. Antitumor activity and expression profiles of genes induced by sulforaphane in human melanoma cells. *Eur. J. Nutr.* **2018**, *57*, 2547–2569. [CrossRef] [PubMed]
84. Myzak, M.C.; Tong, P.; Dashwood, W.M.; Dashwood, R.H.; Ho, E. Sulforaphane retards the growth of human PC-3 xenografts and inhibits HDAC activity in human subjects. *Exp. Biol. Med.* **2007**, *232*, 227–234.
85. Socała, K.; Nieoczym, D.; Kowalczuk-Vasilev, E.; Wyska, E.; Wlaź, P. Increased seizure susceptibility and other toxicity symptoms following acute sulforaphane treatment in mice. *Toxicol. Appl. Pharmacol.* **2017**, *326*, 43–53. [CrossRef]
86. Castro, N.P.; Rangel, M.C.; Merchant, A.S.; MacKinnon, G.; Cuttitta, F.; Salomon, D.S.; Kim, Y.S. Sulforaphane Suppresses the Growth of Triple-negative Breast Cancer Stem-like Cells In vitro and In vivo. *Cancer Prev. Res.* **2019**, *12*, 147–158. [CrossRef]
87. Alumkal, J.J.; Slottke, R.; Schwartzman, J.; Cherala, G.; Munar, M.; Graff, J.N.; Beer, T.M.; Ryan, C.W.; Koop, D.R.; Gibbs, A.; et al. A phase II study of sulforaphane-rich broccoli sprout extracts in men with recurrent prostate cancer. *Investig. New Drugs.* **2015**, *33*, 480–489. [CrossRef]
88. Shapiro, T.A.; Fahey, J.W.; Dinkova-Kostova, A.T.; Holtzclaw, W.D.; Stephenson, K.K.; Wade, K.L.; Ye, L.; Talalay, P. Safety, tolerance, and metabolism of broccoli sprout glucosinolates and isothiocyanates: A clinical phase I study. *Nutr. Cancer.* **2006**, *55*, 53–62. [CrossRef]
89. Tahata, S.; Singh, S.V.; Lin, Y.; Hahm, E.; Beumer, J.H.; Christner, S.M.; Rao, U.N.; Sander, C.; Tarhini, A.A.; Tawbi, H.; et al. Evaluation of Biodistribution of Sulforaphane after Administration of Oral Broccoli Sprout Extract in Melanoma Patient with Multiple Atypical Nevi. *Cancer Prev. Res.* **2018**, *11*, 429–438. [CrossRef]
90. Zhang, Z.; Garzotto, M.; Davis II, E.W.; Mori, M.; Stoller, W.A.; Farris, P.E.; Wong, C.P.; Beaver, L.M.; Thomas, G.V.; Williams, D.E.; et al. Sulforaphane Bioavailability and chemopreventive Activity in Men Presenting for Biopsy of the Prostate Gland: A Randomized Controlled Trial. *Nutr. Cancer* **2020**, *72*, 74–84. [CrossRef]
91. Jeffery, E.H.; Keck, A.S. Translating knowledge generated by epidemiological and in vitro studies into dietary cancer prevention. *Mol. Nutr. Food Res.* **2008**, *52*, S7–S17.
92. Liberati, A.; Altman, D.G.; Tetzlaff, J.; Mulrow, C.; Gøtzsche, P.C.; Ioannidis, J.P.; Clarke, M.; Devereaux, P.J.; Kleijnen, J.; Moher, D. The PRISMA statement for reporting systematic review and meta-analysis of studies that evaluate health care interventions: Explanation and elaboration. *PLoS Med.* **2009**, *6*, e1000100. [CrossRef]
93. Tseng, E.; Scott-Ramsay, E.A.; Morris, M.E. Dietary organic isothiocyanates are cytotoxic in human breast cancer and mammary epithelial MCF-12A cell lines. *Exp. Biol. Med.* **2004**, *229*, 835–842. [CrossRef]
94. Jackson, J.T.; Singletary, K.W. Sulforaphane inhibits human MCF-7 mammary cancer cell mitotic progression and tubulin polymerization. *J. Nutr.* **2004**, *134*, 2229–2236. [CrossRef]
95. Jackson, J.T.; Singletary, K.W. Sulforaphane: A naturally occurring mammary carcinoma mitotic inhibitor, which disrupts tubulin polymerization. *Carcinogenesis* **2004**, *25*, 219–227. [CrossRef]
96. Azarenko, O.; Okouneva, T.; Singletary, K.W.; Jordan, M.A.; Wilson, L. Suppression of microtubule dynamic instability and turnover in MCF7 breast cancer cells by sulforaphane. *Carcinogenesis* **2008**, *29*, 2360–2368. [CrossRef]
97. Ahmed, Z.; Li, X.; Li, F.; Cheaito, H.A.; Patel, K.; Mosallam, E.M.; Elbargeesy, G.; Dou, Q.P. Computational and biochemical studies of isothiocyanates as inhibitors of proteasomal cysteine deubiquitinases in human cancer cells. *J. Cell. Biochem.* **2018**, *119*, 9006–9016. [CrossRef]
98. Cao, C.; Wu, H.; Vasilatos, S.N.; Chandran, U.; Qin, Y.; Wan, Y.; Oesterreich, S.; Davidson, N.E.; Huang, Y. HDAC5-LSD1 axis regulates antineoplastic effect of natural HDAC inhibitor sulforaphane in human breast cancer cells. *Int. J. Cancer* **2018**, *143*, 1388–1401. [CrossRef]
99. Royston, K.J.; Paul, B.; Nozell, S.; Rajbhandari, R.; Tollefsbol, T. Withaferin A and sulforaphane regulate breast cancer cell cycle progression through epigenetic mechanisms. *Exp. Cell Res.* **2018**, *368*, 67–74. [CrossRef]
100. Pledgie-Tracey, A.; Sobolewski, M.; Davidson, N. Sulforaphane induces cell type-specific apoptosis in human breast cancer cell lines. *Mol. Cancer Ther.* **2007**, *6*, 1013–1021. [CrossRef]
101. Lewinska, A.; Bednarz, D.; Adamczyk-Grochala, J.; Wnuk, M. Phytochemical-induced nucleolar stress results in the inhibition of breast cancer cell proliferation. *Redox. Biol.* **2017**, *12*, 459–482. [CrossRef]
102. Lewinska, A.; Adamczyk-Grochala, J.; Deregowska, A.; Wnuk, M. Sulforaphane-induced cell cycle arrest and senescence are accompanied by DNA hypomethylation and changes in microRNA profile in breast cancer cells. *Theranostics* **2017**, *7*, 3461–3477. [CrossRef]
103. Kanematsu, S.; Uehara, N.; Miki, H.; Yoshizawa, K.; Kawanaka, A.; Yuri, T.; Tsubura, A. Autophagy inhibition enhances sulforaphane-induced apoptosis in human breast cancer cells. *Anticancer Res.* **2010**, *30*, 3381–3390.
104. Pawlik, A.; Wiczk, A.; Kaczynska, A.; Antosiewica, J.; Herman-Antosiewicz, A. Sulforaphane inhibits growth of phenotypically different breast cancer cells. *Eur. J. Nutr.* **2013**, *52*, 1949–1958. [CrossRef]

105. Yang, F.; Wang, F.; Liu, Y.; Wang, S.; Li, X.; Huang, Y.; Xia, Y.; Chunyu, C. Sulforaphane induces autophagy by inhibition of HDAC6-mediated PTEN activation in triple negative breast cancer cells. *Life Sci.* **2018**, *213*, 149–157. [CrossRef]
106. Yang, M.; Teng, W.; Qu, Y.; Wang, H.; Yuan, Q. Sulforaphane inhibits triple negative breast cancer through activating tumor suppressor Egr1. *Breast Cancer Res. Treat.* **2016**, *158*, 277–286. [CrossRef]
107. Cheng, A.; Shen, C.; Hung, C.; Hsu, Y. Sulforaphane decrease of SERTAD1 expression triggers G1/S arrest in breast cancer cells. *J. Med. Food.* **2019**, *22*, 444–450. [CrossRef]
108. Li, Y.; Buckhaults, P.; Cui, X.; Tollefsbol, T. Combinatorial epigenetic mechanisms and efficacy of early breast cancer inhibition by nutritive botanicals. *Epigenomics* **2016**, *8*, 1019–1037. [CrossRef]
109. Ramirez, M.C.; Singletary, K. Regulation of estrogen receptor alpha expression in human breast cancer cells by sulforaphane. *J. Nutr. Biochem.* **2009**, *20*, 195–201. [CrossRef]
110. Pawlik, A.; Wojewodzka, M.S.; Herman-Antosiewicz, A. Sensitization of estrogen receptor-positive breast cancer cell lines to 4-hydroxytamoxifen by isothiocyanates present in cruciferous plants. *Eur. J. Nutr.* **2016**, *55*, 1165–1180. [CrossRef]
111. Jo, E.; Kim, S.; Ahn, N.; Park, J.; Hwang, J.; Lee, Y.; Kang, K. Efficacy of sulforaphane is mediated by p38 MAP kinase and caspase-7 activations in ER-positive and COX-2-expressed human breast cancer cell. *Eur. J. Cancer Prev.* **2007**, *16*, 505–510. [CrossRef]
112. Hussain, A.; Mohsin, J.; Prabhu, S.A.; Begum, S.; Nursi, Q.E.; Harish, G.; Javed, E.; Khan, M.A.; Sharma, C. Sulforaphane inhibits growth of human breast cancer cells and augments the therapeutic index of the chemotherapeutic drug, gemcitabine. *Asian Pac. J. Cancer Prev.* **2013**, *14*, 5855–5860. [CrossRef]
113. Licznerska, B.; Szaefer, H.; Matuszak, I.; Murias, M.; Baer-Dubowska, W. Modulating potential of L-Sulforaphane in the expression of cytochrome P450 to identify potential targets for breast cancer chemoprevention and therapy using breast cell lines. *Phytother. Res.* **2015**, *29*, 93–99. [CrossRef]
114. Lubecka-Pietruszewski, K.; Kaufman-Szymczyk, A.; Stefanska, B.; Cebula-Obrzut, B.; Smolewski, P.; Fabianowska-Majewska, K. Sulforaphane alone and in combination with clofarabine epigenetically regulates the expression of DNA methylation-silenced tumour suppressor genes in human breast cancer cells. *J. Nutr. Nutrigenom.* **2015**, *8*, 91–101. [CrossRef]
115. Meeran, S.; Patel, S.; Tollefsbol, T. Sulforaphane causes epigenetic repression of hTERT expression in human breast cancer cell lines. *PLoS ONE* **2010**, *5*, e11457. [CrossRef]
116. Sarkar, R.; Mukherjee, S.; Biswas, J.; Roy, M. Sulphoraphane, a naturally occurring isothiocyanate induces apoptosis in breast cancer cells by targeting heat shock proteins. *Biochem. Biophys. Res. Commun.* **2012**, *427*, 80–85. [CrossRef]
117. Lo, R.; Matthews, J. The aryl hydrocarbon receptor and estrogen receptor alpha differentially modulate nuclear factor erythroid-2-related factor 2 transactivation in MCF-7 breast cancer cells. *Toxicol. Appl. Pharmacol.* **2013**, *270*, 139–148. [CrossRef]
118. Wang, W.; Wang, S.; Howie, F.; Beckett, G.; Mithen, R.; Bao, Y. Sulforaphane, erucin, and iberin up-regulate thioredoxin reductase 1 expression in human MCF-7 cells. *J. Agric. Food Chem.* **2005**, *53*, 1417–1421. [CrossRef]
119. Thangasamy, A.; Rogge, J.; Krishnegowda, N.; Freeman, J.; Ammanamanchi, S. Novel function of transcription factor Nrf2 as an inhibitor of RON tyrosine kinase receptor-mediated cancer cell invasion. *J. Biol. Chem.* **2011**, *286*, 32115–32122. [CrossRef]
120. Deb, M.; Sengupta, D.; Kar, S.; Rath, S.K.; Parbin, S.; Shilpi, A.; Roy, S.; Das, G.; Patra, S.K. Elucidation of caveolin 1 both as a tumor suppressor and metastasis promoter in light of epigenetic modulators. *Tumor Biol.* **2014**, *35*, 12031–12047. [CrossRef]
121. Qazi, A.; Pal, J.; Maitah, M.; Fulciniti, M.; Pelluru, D.; Nanjappa, P.; Lee, S.; Batchu, R.; Prasad, M.; Bryant, C.; et al. Anticancer activity of a broccoli derivative, sulforaphane, in barrett adenocarcinoma: Potential use in chemoprevention and as adjuvant in chemotherapy. *Transl. Oncol.* **2010**, *3*, 389–399. [CrossRef]
122. Lu, Z.; Ren, Y.; Yang, L.; Jia, A.; Hu, Y.; Zhao, Y.; Zhao, W.; Yu, B.; Zhao, W.; Zhang, J.; et al. Inhibiting autophagy enhances sulforaphane-induced apoptosis via targeting NRF2 in esophageal squamous cell carcinoma. *Acta Pharm. Sin. B* **2020**, *11*, 1246–1260. [CrossRef] [PubMed]
123. Mondal, A.; Biswas, R.; Rhee, Y.; Kim, J.; Ahn, J. Sulforaphene promotes Bax/Bcl2, MAPK-dependent human gastric cancer AGS cells apoptosis and inhibits migration via EGFR, p-ERK1/2 down regulation. *Gen. Physiol. Biophys.* **2016**, *35*, 25–34. [CrossRef] [PubMed]
124. Choi, Y.H. ROS-mediated activation of AMPK plays a critical role in sulforaphane-induced apoptosis and mitotic arrest in AGS human gastric cancer cells. *Gen. Physiol. Biophys.* **2018**, *37*, 129–140. [CrossRef]
125. Dong, Q.; Wang, Q.; Wang, L.; Jiang, Y.; Liu, M.; Hu, H.; Liu, Y.; Zhou, H.; He, H.; Zhang, T.; et al. SMYD3-associated pathway is involved in the anti-tumor effects of sulforaphane on gastric carcinoma cells. *Food Sci. Biotechnol.* **2018**, *27*, 1165–1173. [CrossRef]
126. Kiani, S.; Akhavan-Niaki, H.; Fattahi, S.; Kavoosian, S.; Jelodar, N.; Bagheri, N.; Zarrini, H. Purified sulforaphane from broccoli (*Brassica oleracea var. italica*) leads to alterations of *CDX1* and *CDX2* expression and changes in miR-9 and miR-326 levels in human gastric cancer cells. *Gene* **2018**, *678*, 115–123. [CrossRef]
127. Andělová, H.; Rudolf, E.; Červinka, M. In vitro antiproliferative effects of sulforaphane on human colon cancer cell line SW620. *Acta Med.* **2007**, *50*, 171–176. [CrossRef]
128. Rudolf, E.; Andelová, H.; Cervinka, M. Activation of several concurrent proapoptic pathways by sulforaphane in human colon cancer cells SW620. *Food Chem. Toxicol.* **2009**, *47*, 2366–2373. [CrossRef]
129. Lan, H.; Yuan, H.; Lin, C. Sulforaphane induces p53 deficient SW480 cell apoptosis via the ROS MAPK signaling pathway. *Mol. Med. Rep.* **2017**, *16*, 7796–7804. [CrossRef]

130. Gamet-Payrastre, L.; Li, P.; Lumeau, S.; Cassar, G.; Dupont, M.A.; Chevolleau, S.; Gasc, N.; Tulliez, J.; Tercé, F. Sulforaphane, a naturally occurring isothiocyanate, induces cell cycle arrest and apoptosis in HT29 human colon cancer cells. *Cancer Res.* **2000**, *60*, 1426–1433. [PubMed]
131. Pappa, G.; Lichtenberg, M.; Iori, R.; Barillari, J.; Bartsch, H.; Gerhäuser, C. Comparison of growth inhibition profiles and mechanisms of apoptosis induction in human colon cancer cell lines by isothiocyanates and indoles from Brassicaceae. *Mutat. Res.* **2006**, *599*, 76–87. [CrossRef]
132. Pappa, G.; Strathmann, J.; Löwinger, M.; Bartsch, H.; Gerhäuser, C. Quantitative combination effects between sulforaphane and 3,3′-diindolylmethane on proliferation of human colon cancer cells in vitro. *Carcinogenesis* **2007**, *28*, 1471–1477. [CrossRef]
133. Rudolf, E.; Červinka, M. Sulforaphane induces cytotoxicity and lysosome- and mitochondria-dependent cell death in colon cancer cells with deleted p53. *Toxicol. In Vitro* **2011**, *25*, 1302–1309. [CrossRef] [PubMed]
134. Byun, S.; Shin, S.H.; Park, J.; Lim, S.; Lee, E.; Lee, C.; Sung, D.; Farrand, L.; Lee, S.R.; Kim, K.H.; et al. Sulforaphene suppresses growth of colon cancer-derived tumors via induction of glutathione depletion and microtubule depolymerization. *Mol. Nutr. Food Res.* **2016**, *60*, 1068–1078. [CrossRef]
135. Shen, G.; Xu, C.; Chen, C.; Hebbar, V.; Kong, A.T. p53-independent G_1 cell cycle arrest of human colon carcinoma cells HT-29 by sulforaphane is associated with inductionof p21CIP1 and inhibition of expression of cyclin D1. *Cancer Chemother. Pharmacol.* **2006**, *57*, 317–327. [CrossRef]
136. Zeng, H.; Trujillo, O.N.; Moyer, M.P.; Botnen, J.H. Prolonged sulforaphane treatment activates survival signaling in nontumorigenic NCM460 colon cells but apoptotic signaling in tumorigenic HCT116 colon cells. *Nutr. Cancer.* **2011**, *63*, 248–255. [CrossRef]
137. Pappa, G.; Bartsch, H.; Gerhäuser, C. Biphasic modulation of cell proliferation by sulforaphane at physiologically relevant exposure times in a human colon cancer cell line. *Mol. Nutr. Food Res.* **2007**, *51*, 977–984. [CrossRef]
138. Parnaud, G.; Li, P.; Cassar, G.; Rouimi, P.; Tulliez, J.; Combaret, L.; Gamet-Payrastre, L. Mechanism of Sulforaphane-Induced Cell Cycle Arrest and Apoptosis in Human Colon Cancer Cells. *Nutr. Cancer* **2004**, *48*, 198–206. [CrossRef] [PubMed]
139. Nishikawa, T.; Tsuno, N.H.; Okaji, Y.; Shuno, Y.; Sasaki, K.; Hongo, K.; Sunami, E.; Kitayama, J.; Takahashi, K.; Nagawa, H. Inhibition of Autophagy Potentiates Sulforaphane-Induced Apoptosis in Human Colon Cancer Cells. *Ann. Surg. Oncol.* **2010**, *17*, 592–602. [CrossRef]
140. Chung, Y.K.; Or, R.C.; Lu, C.H.; Ouyang, W.T.; Yang, S.Y.; Chang, C.C. Sulforaphane down-regulates SKP2 to stabilize p27KIP1 for inducing antiproliferation in human colon adenocarcinoma cells. *J. Biosci. Bioeng.* **2015**, *119*, 35–42. [CrossRef]
141. Traka, M.; Gasper, A.V.; Smith, J.A.; Hawkey, C.J.; Bao, Y.; Mithen, R.F. Transcriptome Analysis of Human Colon Caco-2 Cells Exposed to Sulforaphane. *J. Nutr.* **2005**, *135*, 1865–1872. [CrossRef]
142. Johnson, G.S.; Li, J.; Beaver, L.M.; Dashwood, W.M.; Sun, D.; Rajendran, P.; Williams, D.E.; Ho, E.; Dashwood, R.H. A functional pseudogene, NMRAL2P, is regulated by Nrf2 and serves as a coactivator of NQO1 in sulforaphane-treated colon cancer cells. *Mol. Nutr. Food Res.* **2017**, *61*, 1600769. [CrossRef]
143. Wang, M.; Zhu, J.; Chen, S.; Qing, Y.; Wu, D.; Lin, Y.; Luo, J.Z.; Han, W.; Li, Y. Effects of co-treatment with sulforaphane and autophagy modulators on uridine 5′-diphospho-glucuronosyltransferase 1A isoforms and cytochrome P450 3A4 expression in Caco-2 human colon cancer cells. *Oncol. Lett.* **2014**, *8*, 2407–2416. [CrossRef]
144. Harris, K.E.; Jeffery, E.H. Sulforaphane and erucin increase MRP1 and MRP2 in human carcinoma cell lines. *J. Nutr. Biochem.* **2008**, *19*, 246–254. [CrossRef] [PubMed]
145. Rajendran, P.; Kidane, A.I.; Yu, T.W.; Dashwood, W.M.; Bisson, W.H.; Löhr, C.V.; Ho, E.; Williams, D.E.; Dashwood, R.H. HDAC turnover, CtIP acetylation and dysregulated DNA damage signaling in colon cancer cells treated with sulforaphane and related dietary isothiocyanates. *Epigenetics* **2013**, *8*, 612–623. [CrossRef]
146. Martin, S.L.; Kala, R.; Tollefsbol, T.O. Mechanisms for the Inhibition of Colon Cancer Cells by Sulforaphane through Epigenetic Modulation of MicroRNA-21 and Human Telomerase Reverse Transcriptase (hTERT) Down-regulation. *Curr. Cancer Drug Targets* **2018**, *18*, 97–106. [CrossRef] [PubMed]
147. Okonkwo, A.; Mitra, J.; Johnson, G.S.; Li, L.; Dashwood, W.M.; Hegde, M.L.; Yue, C.; Dashwood, R.H.; Rajendran, P. Heterocyclic Analogs of Sulforaphane Trigger DNA Damage and Impede DNA Repair in Colon Cancer Cells: Interplay of HATs and HDACs. *Mol. Nutr. Food Res.* **2018**, *62*, e1800228. [CrossRef]
148. Bessler, H.; Djaldetti, M. Broccoli and human health: Immunomodulatory effect of sulforaphane in a model of colon cancer. *Int. J. Food Sci. Nutr.* **2018**, *69*, 946–953. [CrossRef]
149. Tafakh, M.S.; Saidijam, M.; Ranjbarnejad, T.; Malih, S.; Mirzamohammadi, S.; Najafi, R. Sulforaphane, a Chemopreventive Compound, Inhibits Cyclooxygenase-2 and Microsomal Prostaglandin E Synthase-1 Expression in Human HT-29 Colon Cancer Cells. *Cells Tissues Organs* **2018**, *206*, 46–53. [CrossRef] [PubMed]
150. Jakubíková, J.; Sedlák, J.; Mithen, R.; Bao, Y. Role of PI3K/Akt and MEK/ERK signaling pathways in sulforaphane- and erucin-induced phase II enzymes and MRP2 transcription, G2/M arrest and cell death in Caco-2 cells. *Biochem. Pharmacol.* **2005**, *69*, 1543–1552. [CrossRef]
151. Kim, M.J.; Kim, S.H.; Lim, S.J. Comparison of the apoptosis-inducing capability of sulforaphane analogues in human colon cancer cells. *Anticancer Res.* **2010**, *30*, 3611–3619. [PubMed]
152. Kim, D.H.; Sung, B.; Kang, Y.J.; Hwang, S.Y.; Kim, M.J.; Yoon, J.H.; Im, E.; Kim, N.D. Sulforaphane inhibits hypoxia-induced HIF-1α and VEGF expression and migration of human colon cancer cells. *Int. J. Oncol.* **2015**, *47*, 2226–2232. [CrossRef] [PubMed]

153. Yu, R.; Lei, W.; Mandlekar, S.; Weber, M.J.; Der, C.J.; Wu, J.; Kong, A.N. Role of a mitogen-activated protein kinase pathway in the induction of phase II detoxifying enzymes by chemicals. *J. Biol. Chem.* **1999**, *274*, 27545–27552. [CrossRef]
154. Yeh, C.T.; Yen, G.C. Effect of sulforaphane on metallothionein expression and induction of apoptosis in human hepatoma HepG2 cells. *Carcinogenesis* **2005**, *26*, 2138–2148. [CrossRef]
155. Park, S.Y.; Kim, G.Y.; Bae, S.; Yoo, Y.; Choi, Y.H. Induction of apoptosis by isothiocyanate sulforaphane in human cervical carcinoma HeLa and hepatocarcinoma HepG2 cells through activation of caspase-3. *Oncol. Rep.* **2007**, *18*, 181–187. [CrossRef] [PubMed]
156. Keum, Y.S.; Yu, S.; Chang, P.P.; Yuan, X.; Kim, J.H.; Xu, C.; Han, J.; Agarwal, A.; Kong, A.N. Mechanism of action of sulforaphane: Inhibition of p38 mitogen-activated protein kinase isoforms contributing to the induction of antioxidant response element-mediated heme oxygenase-1 in human hepatoma HepG2 cells. *Cancer Res.* **2006**, *66*, 8804–8813. [CrossRef]
157. Jeon, Y.K.; Yoo, D.R.; Jang, Y.H.; Jang, S.Y.; Nam, M.J. Sulforaphane induces apoptosis in human hepatic cancer cells through inhibition of 6-phosphofructo-2-kinase/fructose-2,6-biphosphatase4, mediated by hypoxia inducible factor-1-dependent pathway. *Biochim. Biophys. Acta* **2011**, *1814*, 1340–1348. [CrossRef]
158. Liu, P.; Atkinson, S.J.; Akbareian, S.E.; Zhou, Z.; Munsterberg, A.; Robinson, S.D.; Bao, Y. Sulforaphane exerts anti-angiogenesis effects against hepatocellular carcinoma through inhibition of STAT3/HIF-1α/VEGF signaling. *Sci. Rep.* **2017**, *7*, 12651. [CrossRef]
159. Moon, D.O.; Kang, S.H.; Kim, K.C.; Kim, M.O.; Choi, Y.H.; Kim, G.Y. Sulforaphane decreases viability and telomerase activity in hepatocellular carcinoma Hep3B cells through the reactive oxygen species-dependent pathway. *Cancer Lett.* **2010**, *295*, 260–266. [CrossRef]
160. Wu, J.; Han, J.; Hou, B.; Deng, C.; Wu, H.; Shen, L. Sulforaphane inhibits TGF-β-induced epithelial-mesenchymal transition of hepatocellular carcinoma cells via the reactive oxygen species-dependent pathway. *Oncol. Rep.* **2016**, *35*, 2977–2983. [CrossRef] [PubMed]
161. Zou, X.; Qu, Z.; Fang, Y.; Shi, X.; Ji, Y. Endoplasmic reticulum stress mediates sulforaphane-induced apoptosis of HepG2 human hepatocellular carcinoma cells. *Mol. Med. Rep.* **2017**, *15*, 331–338. [CrossRef]
162. Anwar-Mohamed, A.; El-Kadi, A.O. Sulforaphane induces CYP1A1 mRNA, protein, and catalytic activity levels via an AhR-dependent pathway in murine hepatoma Hepa 1c1c7 and human HepG2 cells. *Cancer Lett.* **2009**, *275*, 93–101. [CrossRef]
163. Pham, N.A.; Jacobberger, J.W.; Schimmer, A.D.; Cao, P.; Gronda, M.; Hedley, D.W. The dietary isothiocyanate sulforaphane targets pathways of apoptosis, cell cycle arrest, and oxidative stress in human pancreatic cancer cells and inhibits tumor growth in severe combined immunodeficient mice. *Mol. Cancer Ther.* **2004**, *3*, 1239–1248. [PubMed]
164. Li, Y.; Karagöz, G.E.; Seo, Y.H.; Zhang, T.; Jiang, Y.; Yu, Y.; Duarte, A.M.; Schwartz, S.J.; Boelens, R.; Carroll, K.; et al. Sulforaphane inhibits pancreatic cancer through disrupting HSP90-p50(Cdc37) complex and direct interactions with amino acids residues of HSP90. *J. Nutr. Biochem.* **2012**, *23*, 1617–1626. [CrossRef] [PubMed]
165. Kallifatidis, G.; Rausch, V.; Baumann, B.; Apel, A.; Beckermann, B.M.; Groth, A.; Mattern, J.; Li, Z.; Kolb, A.; Moldenhauer, G.; et al. Sulforaphane targets pancreatic tumour-initiating cells by NF-kappaB-induced antiapoptotic signaling. *Gut* **2009**, *58*, 949–963. [CrossRef] [PubMed]
166. Rodova, M.; Fu, J.; Watkins, D.N.; Srivastava, R.K.; Shankar, S. Sonic hedgehogsignaling inhibition provides opportunities for targeted therapy by sulforaphane in regulating pancreatic cancer stem cell self-renewal. *PLoS ONE* **2012**, *7*, e46084. [CrossRef] [PubMed]
167. Yin, L.; Xiao, X.; Georgikou, C.; Yin, Y.; Liu, L.; Karakhanova, S.; Luo, Y.; Gladkich, J.; Fellenberg, J.; Sticht, C.; et al. MicroRNA-365a-3p inhibits c-Rel-mediated NF-κB signaling and the progression of pancreatic cancer. *Cancer Lett.* **2019**, *452*, 203–212. [CrossRef]
168. Yin, L.; Xiao, X.; Georgikou, C.; Luo, Y.; Liu, L.; Gladkich, J.; Gross, W.; Herr, I. Sulforaphane Induces miR135b-5p and Its Target Gene, RASAL2, thereby Inhibiting the Progression of Pancreatic Cancer. *Mol. Ther. Oncolytics* **2019**, *14*, 74–81. [CrossRef]
169. Chen, X.; Jiang, Z.; Zhou, C.; Chen, K.; Li, X.; Wang, Z.; Wu, Z.; Ma, J.; Ma, Q.; Duan, W. Activation of Nrf2 by Sulforaphane Inhibits High Glucose-Induced Progression of Pancreatic Cancer via AMPK Dependent Signaling. *Cell. Physiol. Biochem.* **2018**, *50*, 1201–1215. [CrossRef] [PubMed]
170. Forster, T.; Rausch, V.; Zhang, Y.; Isayev, O.; Heilmann, K.; Schoensiegel, F.; Liu, L.; Nessling, M.; Richter, K.; Labsch, S.; et al. Sulforaphane counteracts aggressiveness of pancreatic cancer driven by dysregulated Cx43-mediated gap junctional intercellular communication. *Oncotarget* **2014**, *5*, 1621–1634. [CrossRef]
171. Georgikou, C.; Yin, L.; Gladkich, J.; Xiao, X.; Sticht, C.; Torre, C.; Gretz, N.; Gross, W.; Schäfer, M.; Karakhanova, S.; et al. Inhibition of miR30a-3p by sulforaphane enhances gap junction intercellular communication in pancreatic cancer. *Cancer Lett.* **2020**, *469*, 238–245. [CrossRef] [PubMed]
172. Sharma, C.; Sadrieh, L.; Priyani, A.; Ahmed, M.; Hassan, A.H.; Hussain, A. Anti-carcinogenic effects of sulforaphane in association with its apoptosis-inducing and anti-inflammatory properties in human cervical cancer cells. *Cancer Epidemiol.* **2011**, *33*, 272–278. [CrossRef]
173. Khan, M.A.; Sundaram, M.; Hamza, A.; Quraishi, U.; Gunasekera, D.; Ramesh, L.; Goala, P.; Al Alami, U.; Ansari, M.; Rizvi, T.A.; et al. Sulforaphane Reverses the Expression of Various Tumor Suppressor Genes by Targeting DNMT3B and HDAC1 in Human Cervical Cancer Cells. *Evid. Based Complement. Alternat. Med.* **2015**, *2015*, 412149. [CrossRef]
174. Cheng, Y.; Tsai, C.; Hsu, Y. Sulforaphane, a Dietary Isothiocyanate, Induces G2/M Arrest in Cervical Cancer Cells through Cyclin B1 Downregulation and GADD45B/CDC2 Association. *Int. J. Mol. Sci.* **2016**, *17*, 1530. [CrossRef] [PubMed]

175. Rai, R.; Essel, K.G.; Benbrook, D.M.; Garland, J.; Zhao, Y.D.; Chandra, V. Preclinical efficacy and involvement of AKT, mTOR, and ERK kinases in the mechanism of sulforaphane against endometrial cancer. *Cancers* **2020**, *12*, 1273. [CrossRef] [PubMed]
176. Chaudhuri, D.; Orsulic, S.; Ashok, B.T. Antiproliferative activity of sulforaphane in Akt-overexpressing ovarian cancer cells. *Mol. Cancer Ther.* **2007**, *6*, 334–345. [CrossRef] [PubMed]
177. Chuang, L.T.; Moqattash, S.T.; Gretz, H.F.; Nezhat, F.; Rahaman, J.; Chiao, J. Sulforaphane induces growth arrest and apoptosis in human ovarian cancer cells. *Acta Obstet. Gynecol. Scand.* **2007**, *86*, 1263–1268. [CrossRef]
178. Bryant, C.S.; Kumar, S.; Chamala, S.; Shah, J.; Pal, J.; Haider, M.; Seward, S.; Qazi, A.M.; Morris, R.; Semaan, A.; et al. Sulforaphane induces cell cycle arrest by protecting RB-E2F-1 complex in epithelial ovarian cancer cells. *Mol. Cancer* **2010**, *9*, 47. [CrossRef]
179. Kim, S.C.; Choi, B.; Kwon, Y. Thiol-reducing agents prevent sulforaphane-induced growth inhibition in ovarian cancer cells. *Food Nutr. Res.* **2017**, *6*, 1–12. [CrossRef]
180. Hudecova, S.; Markova, J.; Simko, V.; Csaderova, L.; Stracina, T.; Sirova, M.; Fojtu, M.; Savastova, E.; Gronesova, P.; Pastorek, M.; et al. Sulforaphane-induced apoptosis involves the type 1 IP3 receptor. *Oncotarget* **2016**, *7*, 61403–61418. [CrossRef]
181. Chang, C.; Hung, C.; Yang, Y.; Lee, M.; Hsu, Y. Sulforaphane induced cell cycle arrest in the G2/M phase via the blockade of cyclin B1/CDC2 in human ovarian cancer cells. *J. Ovarian Res.* **2013**, *6*, 41. [CrossRef]
182. Fimognari, C.; Nusse, M.; Cesari, R.; Iori, R.; Cantelli-Forti, G.; Hrelia, P. Growth inhibition, cell-cycle arrest and apoptosis in human T-cell leukemia by the isothiocyanate sulforaphane. *Carcinogenesis* **2002**, *23*, 581–585. [CrossRef]
183. Fimognari, C.; Nusse, M.; Berti, F.; Iori, R.; Cantelli-Forti, G.; Hrelia, P. Sulforaphane Modulates Cell Cycle and Apoptosis in Transformed Non-transformed Human T Lymphocytes. *Ann. N. Y. Acad. Sci.* **2003**, *1010*, 393–398. [CrossRef]
184. Fimognari, C.; Lenzi, M.; Cantelli-forti, G.; Hrelia, P. Induction of Differentiation in Human Promyelocytic Cells by the Isothiocyanate Sulforaphane. *In Vivo* **2008**, *22*, 317–320. [PubMed]
185. Choi, W.Y.; Choi, B.T.; Lee, W.H.; Choi, Y.H. Sulforaphane generates reactive oxygen species leading to mitochondrial perturbation for apoptosis in human leukemia U937 cells. *Biomed. Pharmacother.* **2008**, *62*, 637–644. [CrossRef] [PubMed]
186. Koolivand, M.; Ansari, M.; Piroozian, F.; Moein, S.; MalekZadeh, K. Alleviating the progression of acute myeloid leukemia (AML) by sulforaphane through controlling miR-155 levels. *Mol. Biol. Rep.* **2018**, *45*, 2491–2499. [CrossRef]
187. Shang, H.; Shih, Y.; Lee, C.H.S.; Liu, J.; Liao, N.; Chen, Y.; Huang, Y.; Lu, H.; Chung, J. Sulforaphane-induced apoptosis in human leukemia HL-60 cells through extrinsic and intrinsic signal pathways and altering associated genes expression assayed by cDNA microarray. *Environ. Toxicol.* **2016**, *32*, 311–328. [CrossRef] [PubMed]
188. Wu, J.M.; Oraee, A.; Doonan, B.B.; Pinto, J.T.; Hsieh, T. Activation of NQO1 in NQO1*2 polymorphic human leukemic HL-60 cells by diet-derived sulforaphane. *Exp. Hematol. Oncol.* **2016**, *5*, 27. [CrossRef]
189. Suppipat, K.; Park, C.S.; Shen, Y.; Zhu, X.; Lacorazza, H.D. Sulforaphane Induces Cell Cycle Arrest and Apoptosis in Acute Lymphoblastic Leukemia Cells. *PLoS ONE* **2012**, *7*, e051251. [CrossRef]
190. Prata, C.; Facchini, C.; Leoncini, E.; Lenzi, M.; Maraldi, T.; Angeloni, C.; Zambonin, L.; Hrelia, S.; Fiorentini, D. Sulforaphane Modulates AQP8-Linked Redox Signalling in Leukemia Cells. *Oxid. Med. Cell. Longev.* **2018**, *2018*, 4125297. [CrossRef]
191. Misiewicz, I.; Skupinska, K.; Kasprzycka-Guttman, T. Sulforaphane and 2-oxohexyl isothiocyanate induce cell growth arrest and apoptosis in L-1210 leukemia and ME-18 melanoma cells. *Oncol. Rep.* **2003**, *10*, 2045–2050. [CrossRef] [PubMed]
192. Ishirua, Y.; Ishimaru, H.; Watanabe, T.; Fujimuro, M. Sulforaphane Exhibits Cytotoxic Effects against Primary Effusion Lymphoma Cells by suppressing p38 MAPK and AKT Phosphorylation. *Biol. Pharm. Bull.* **2019**, *42*, 2019–2112. [CrossRef]
193. Mi, L.; Chung, F.L. Binding to protein by isothiocyanates: A potential mechanism for apoptosis induction in human non small lung cancer cells. *Nutr. Cancer* **2008**, *60*, 12–20. [CrossRef]
194. Liang, H.; Lai, B.; Yuan, Q. Sulforaphane induces cell-cycle arrest and apoptosis in cultured human lung adenocarcinoma LTEP-A2 cells and retards growth of LTEP-A2 xenografts in vivo. *J. Nat. Prod.* **2008**, *71*, 1911–1914. [CrossRef]
195. Żuryń, A.; Litwiniec, A.; Safiejko-Mroczka, B.; Klimaszewska-Wiśniewska, A.; Gagat, M.; Krajewski, A.; Gackowska, L.; Grzanka, D. The effect of sulforaphane on the cell cycle, apoptosis and expression of cyclin D1 and p21 in the A549 non-small cell lung cancer cell line. *Int. J. Oncol.* **2016**, *48*, 2521–2533. [CrossRef]
196. Żuryń, A.; Krajewski, A.; Klimaszewska-Wiśniewska, A.; Grzanka, A.; Grzanka, D. Expression of cyclin B1, D1 and K in non-small cell lung cancer H1299 cells following treatment with sulforaphane. *Oncol. Rep.* **2019**, *41*, 1313–1323. [CrossRef]
197. Jiang, L.L.; Zhou, S.J.; Zhang, X.M.; Chen, H.Q.; Liu, W. Sulforaphane suppresses in vitro and in vivo lung tumorigenesis through downregulation of HDAC activity. *Biomed. Pharmacother.* **2016**, *78*, 74–80. [CrossRef]
198. Gao, L.; Cheng, D.; Yang, J.; Wu, R.; Li, W.; Kong, A.N. Sulforaphane epigenetically demethylates the CpG sites of the miR-9-3 promoter and reactivates miR-9-3 expression in human lung cancer A549 cells. *J. Nutr. Biochem.* **2018**, *56*, 109–115. [CrossRef]
199. Zhu, J.; Wang, S.; Chen, Y.; Li, X.; Jiang, Y.; Yang, X.; Li, Y.; Wang, X.; Meng, Y.; Zhu, M.; et al. miR-19 targeting of GSK3β mediates sulforaphane suppression of lung cancer stem cells. *J. Nutr. Biochem.* **2017**, *44*, 80–91. [CrossRef]
200. Wang, D.X.; Zou, Y.J.; Zhuang, X.B.; Chen, S.X.; Lin, Y.; Li, W.L.; Lin, J.J.; Lin, Z.Q. Sulforaphane suppresses EMT and metastasis in human lung cancer through miR-616-5p-mediated GSK3β/β-catenin signaling pathways. *Acta Pharmacol. Sin.* **2017**, *38*, 241–251. [CrossRef]
201. Tsai, J.Y.; Tsai, S.H.; Wu, C.C. The chemopreventive isothiocyanate sulforaphane reduces anoikis resistance and anchorage-independent growth in non-small cell human lung cancer cells. *Toxicol. Appl. Pharmacol.* **2019**, *362*, 116–124. [CrossRef]
202. Zhou, L.; Yao, Q.; Li, Y.; Huang, Y.C.; Jiang, H.; Wang, C.Q.; Fan, L. Sulforaphane-induced apoptosis in Xuanwei lung adenocarcinoma cell line XWLC-05. *Thorac. Cancer* **2017**, *8*, 16–25. [CrossRef]

203. Wang, Y.; Mandal, A.K.; Son, Y.O.; Pratheeshkumar, P.; Wise, J.T.F.; Wang, L.; Zhang, Z.; Shi, X.; Chen, Z. Roles of ROS, Nrf2, and autophagy in cadmium-carcinogenesis and its prevention by sulforaphane. *Toxicol. Appl. Pharmacol.* **2018**, *353*, 23–30. [CrossRef]
204. Chen, C.Y.; Yu, Z.Y.; Chuang, Y.S.; Huang, R.M.; Wang, T.C. Sulforaphane attenuates EGFR signaling in NSCLC cells. *J. Biomed. Sci.* **2015**, *22*, 38. [CrossRef]
205. Chen, Y.; Chen, J.Q.; Ge, M.M.; Zhang, Q.; Wang, X.Q.; Zhu, J.Y.; Xie, C.F.; Li, X.T.; Zhong, C.Y.; Han, H.Y. Sulforaphane inhibits epithelial-mesenchymal transition by activating extracellular signal-regulated kinase 5 in lung cancer cells. *J. Nutr. Biochem.* **2019**, *72*, 108219. [CrossRef]
206. Geng, Y.; Zhou, Y.; Wu, S.; Hu, Y.; Lin, K.; Wang, Y.; Zheng, Z.; Wu, W. Sulforaphane Induced Apoptosis via Promotion of Mitochondrial Fusion and ERK1/2-Mediated 26S Proteasome Degradation of Novel Pro-survival Bim and Upregulation of Bax in Human Non-Small Cell Lung Cancer Cells. *J. Cancer* **2017**, *8*, 2456–2470. [CrossRef]
207. Xie, C.; Zhu, J.; Jiang, Y.; Chen, J.; Wang, X.; Geng, S.; Wu, J.; Zhong, C.; Li, X.; Meng, Z. Sulforaphane Inhibits the Acquisition of Tobacco Smoke-Induced Lung Cancer Stem Cell-Like Properties via the IL-6/ΔNp63α/Notch Axis. *Theranostics* **2019**, *9*, 4827–4840. [CrossRef]
208. Karmakar, S.; Weinberg, M.S.; Banik, N.L.; Patel, S.J.; Ray, S.K. Activation of multiple molecular mechanisms for apoptosis in human malignant glioblastoma T98G and U87MG cells treated with sulforaphane. *Neuroscience* **2006**, *141*, 1265–1280. [CrossRef]
209. Bijangi-Vishehsaraei, K.; Reza Saadatzadeh, M.; Wang, H.; Nguyen, A.; Kamocka, M.M.; Cai, W.; Cohen-Gadol, A.A.; Halum, S.L.; Sarkaria, J.N.; Pollok, K.E.; et al. Sulforaphane suppresses the growth of glioblastoma cells, glioblastoma stem cell-like spheroids, and tumor xenografts through multiple cell signaling pathways. *J. Neurosurg.* **2017**, *127*, 1219–1230. [CrossRef]
210. Miao, Z.; Yu, F.; Ren, Y.; Yang, J. d,l-Sulforaphane Induces ROS-Dependent Apoptosis in Human Gliomablastoma Cells by Inactivating STAT3 Signaling Pathway. *Int. J. Mol. Sci.* **2017**, *18*, 72. [CrossRef]
211. Zhang, Z.; Li, C.; Shang, L.; Zhang, Y.; Zou, R.; Zhan, Y.; Bi, B. Sulforaphane induces apoptosis and inhibits invasion in U251MG glioblastoma cells. *SpringerPlus* **2016**, *5*, 235. [CrossRef]
212. Li, C.; Zhou, Y.; Peng, X.; Du, L.; Tian, H.; Yang, G.; Niu, J.; Wu, W. Sulforaphane inhibits invasion via activating ERK1/2 signaling in human glioblastoma U87MG and U373MG cells. *PLoS ONE* **2014**, *9*, e90520. [CrossRef]
213. Arcidiacono, P.; Stabile, A.M.; Ragonese, F.; Pistilli, A.; Calvieri, S.; Bottoni, U.; Crisanti, A.; Spaccapelo, R.; Rende, M. Anticarcinogenic activities of sulforaphane are influenced by Nerve Growth Factor in human melanoma A375 cells. *Food Chem. Toxicol.* **2018**, *113*, 154–161. [CrossRef]
214. Mantso, T.; Sfakianos, A.P.; Atkinson, A.; Anestopoulos, I.; Mitsiogianni, M.; Botaitis, S.; Perente, S.; Simopoulos, C.; Vasileiadis, S.; Franco, R.; et al. Development of a Novel Experimental In Vitro Model of Isothiocyanate-induced Apoptosis in Human Malignant Melanoma Cells. *Anticancer Res.* **2016**, *36*, 6303–6309. [CrossRef]
215. Fisher, M.L.; Adhikary, G.; Grun, D.; Kaetzel, D.M.; Eckert, R.L. The Ezh2 polycomb group protein drives an aggressive phenotype in melanoma cancer stem cells and is a target of diet derived sulforaphane. *Mol. Carcinog.* **2016**, *55*, 2024–2036. [CrossRef]
216. Hamsa, T.P.; Thejass, P.; Kuttan, G. Induction of apoptosis by sulforaphane in highly metastatic B16F-10 melanoma cells. *Drug Chem. Toxicol.* **2011**, *34*, 332–340. [CrossRef] [PubMed]
217. Enriquez, G.G.; Rizvi, S.A.; D'Souza, M.J.; Do, D.P. Formulation and Evaluation of drug-loaded targeted magnetic microspheres for cancer therapy. *Int. J. Nanomed.* **2013**, *8*, 1393–1402. [CrossRef]
218. Do, D.P.; Pai, S.B.; Rizvi, S.A.; D'Souza, M.J. Development of sulforaphane-encapsulated microspheres for cancer epigenetic therapy. *Int. J. Pharm.* **2010**, *386*, 114–121. [CrossRef] [PubMed]
219. Rudolf, K.; Cervinka, M.; Rudolf, E. Sulforaphane-induced apoptosis involvesp53 and p38 in melanoma cells. *Apoptosis* **2014**, *19*, 734–747. [CrossRef] [PubMed]
220. Shan, Y.; Sun, C.; Wu, K.; Cassidy, A.; Bao, Y. Effect of sulforaphane on cell growth, G0/G1 phase cell progression and apoptosis in human bladder cancer T24 cells. *Int. J. Oncol.* **2006**, *29*, 883–888. [CrossRef]
221. Shan, Y.; Wu, K.; Wang, W.; Wang, S.; Lin, N.; Zhao, R.; Cassidy, A.; Bao, Y. Sulforaphane down-regulates COX-2 expression by activating p38 and inhibiting NF-kappaB-DNA-binding activity in human bladder T24 cells. *Int. J. Oncol.* **2009**, *34*, 1129–1134. [CrossRef]
222. Shan, Y.; Wang, X.; Wang, W.; He, C.; Bao, Y. P38 MAPK plays a distinct role in sulforaphane-induced up-regulation of ARE-dependent enzymes and down-regulation of COX-2 in human bladder cancer cells. *Oncol. Rep.* **2010**, *23*, 1133–1138. [CrossRef]
223. Shan, S.; Zhang, L.; Bao, Y.; Li, B.; He, C.; Gao, M.; Feng, X.; Xu, W.; Zhang, X.; Wang, S. Epithelial-mesenchymal transition, a novel target of sulforaphane via COX-2/MMP2, 9/Snail, ZEB1 and miR-200c/ZEB1 pathways in human bladder cancer cells. *J. Nutr. Biochem.* **2013**, *24*, 1062–1069. [CrossRef]
224. Jo, G.H.; Kim, G.; Kim, W.; Park, K.; Choi, Y.H. Sulforaphane induces apoptosis in T24 human urinary bladder cancer cells through a reactive oxygen species-mediated mitochondrial pathway: The involvement of endoplasmic reticulum stress and the Nrf2 signaling pathway. *Int. J. Oncol.* **2014**, *45*, 1497–1506. [CrossRef] [PubMed]
225. Abbaoui, B.; Telu, K.H.; Lucas, C.R.; Thomas-Ahner, J.M.; Schwarts, S.J.; Clinton, S.K.; Freitas, M.A.; Mortazavi, A. The impact of cruciferous vegetable of isothiocyanate on histone acetylation and histone phosphorylation in bladder cancer. *J. Proteom.* **2017**, *156*, 94–103. [CrossRef] [PubMed]
226. Dang, T.; Huang, G.; Chen, Y.; Dang, Z.; Chen, C.; Liu, F.; Guo, Y.; Xie, X. Sulforaphane inhibits the proliferation of the BIU87 bladder cancer cell line via IGFBP-3 elevation. *Asian Pac. J. Cancer Prev.* **2014**, *15*, 1517–1520. [CrossRef] [PubMed]

227. Park, H.S.; Han, M.H.; Kim, G.; Moon, S.; Kim, W.; Hwang, H.J.; Park, K.Y.; Choi, Y.H. Sulforaphane induces reactive oxygen species-mediated mitotic arrest and subsequent apoptosis in human bladder cancer 5637 cells. *Food Chem. Toxicol.* **2014**, *64*, 157–165. [CrossRef]
228. Brooks, J.D.; Paton, V.G.; Vidanes, G. Potent induction of phase 2 enzymes in human prostate cells by sulforaphane. *Cancer Epidemiol. Biomark. Prev.* **2001**, *10*, 949–954.
229. Hahm, E.R.; Singh, S.V. Sulforaphane inhibits constitutive and interleukin-6-induced activation of signal transducer and activator of transcription 3 in prostate cancer cells. *Cancer Prev. Res.* **2010**, *3*, 484–494. [CrossRef]
230. Choi, S.; Lew, K.L.; Xiao, H.; Herman-Antosiewicz, A.; Xiao, D.; Brown, C.K.; Singh, S.V. D,L-Sulforaphane-induced cell death in human prostate cancer cells is regulated by inhibitor of apoptosis family proteins and Apaf-1. *Carcinogenesis* **2007**, *28*, 151–162. [CrossRef]
231. Carrasco-Pozo, C.; Tan, K.N.; Rodriguez, T.; Avery, V.M. The Molecular Effects of Sulforaphane and Capsaicin on Metabolism upon Androgen and Tip60 Activation of Androgen Receptor. *Int. J. Mol. Sci.* **2019**, *20*, 5384. [CrossRef]
232. Kim, S.H.; Singh, S.V. D,L-Sulforaphane causes transcriptional repression of androgen receptor in human prostate cancer cells. *Mol. Cancer Ther.* **2009**, *8*, 1946–1954. [CrossRef]
233. Herman-Antosiewicz, A.; Johnson, D.E.; Singh, S.V. Sulforaphane causes autophagy to inhibit release of cytochrome C and apoptosis in human prostate cancer cells. *Cancer Res.* **2006**, *66*, 5828–5835. [CrossRef]
234. Xiao, D.; Powolny, A.A.; Antosiewicz, J.; Hahm, E.R.; Bommareddy, A.; Zeng, Y.; Desai, D.; Amin, S.; Herman-Antosiewicz, A.; Singh, S.V. Cellular responses to cancer chemopreventive agent D,L-sulforaphane in human prostate cancer cells are initiated by mitochondrial reactive oxygen species. *Pharm. Res.* **2009**, *26*, 1729–1738. [CrossRef] [PubMed]
235. Watson, G.W.; Wickramasekara, S.; Fang, Y.; Palomera-Sanchez, Z.; Maier, C.S.; Williams, D.E.; Dashwood, R.H.; Perez, V.I.; Ho, E. Analysis of autophagic flux in response to sulforaphane in metastatic prostate cancer cells. *Mol. Nutr. Food Res.* **2015**, *59*, 1954–1961. [CrossRef] [PubMed]
236. Cho, S.D.; Li, G.; Hu, H.; Jiang, C.; Kang, K.S.; Lee, Y.S.; Kim, S.H.; Lu, J. Involvement of c-Jun N-terminal kinase in G2/M arrest and caspase-mediated apoptosis induced by sulforaphane in DU145 prostate cancer cells. *Nutr. Cancer* **2005**, *52*, 213–224. [CrossRef] [PubMed]
237. Hać, A.; Brokowska, J.; Rintz, E.; Bartkowski, M.; Węgrzyn, G.; Herman-Antosiewicz, A. Mechanism of selective anticancer activity of isothiocyanates relies on differences in DNA damage repair between cancer and healthy cells. *Eur. J. Nutr.* **2020**, *59*, 1421–1432. [CrossRef] [PubMed]
238. Lee, C.H.; Jeong, S.J.; Yun, S.M.; Kim, J.H.; Lee, H.J.; Ahn, K.S.; Won, S.H.; Kim, H.S.; Lee, H.J.; Ahn, K.S.; et al. Down-regulation of phosphoglucomutase 3 mediates sulforaphane-induced cell death in LNCaP prostate cancer cells. *Proteome Sci.* **2010**, *8*, 67. [CrossRef]
239. Singh, A.V.; Xiao, D.; Lew, K.L.; Dhir, R.; Singh, S.V. Sulforaphane induces caspase-mediated apoptosis in cultured PC-3 human prostate cancer cells and retards growth of PC-3 xenografts in vivo. *Carcinogenesis* **2004**, *25*, 83–90. [CrossRef]
240. Singh, S.V.; Srivastava, S.K.; Choi, S.; Lew, K.L.; Antosiewicz, J.; Xiao, D.; Zeng, Y.; Watkins, S.C.; Johnson, C.S.; Trump, D.L.; et al. Sulforaphane-induced cell death in human prostate cancer cells is initiated by reactive oxygen species. *J. Biol. Chem.* **2005**, *280*, 19911–19924. [CrossRef]
241. Negrette-Guzmán, M.; Huerta-Yepez, S.; Vega, M.I.; León-Contreras, J.C.; Hernández-Pando, R.; Medina-Campos, O.N.; Rodríguez, E.; Tapia, E.; Pedraza-Chaverri, J. Sulforaphane induces differential modulation of mitochondrial biogenesis and dynamics in normal cells and tumor cells. *Food Chem. Toxicol.* **2017**, *100*, 90–102. [CrossRef]
242. Beaver, L.M.; Buchanan, A.; Sokolowski, E.I.; Riscoe, A.N.; Wong, C.P.; Chang, J.H.; Löhr, C.V.; Williams, D.E.; Dashwood, R.H.; Ho, E. Transcriptome analysis reveals a dynamic and differential transcriptional response to sulforaphane in normal and prostate cancer cells and suggests a role for Sp1 in chemoprevention. *Mol. Nutr. Food Res.* **2014**, *58*, 2001–2013. [CrossRef]
243. Bhamre, S.; Sahoo, D.; Tibshirani, R.; Dill, D.; Brooks, J.D. Temporal changes in gene expression induced by sulforaphane in human prostate cancer cells. *Prostate* **2009**, *69*, 181–190. [CrossRef]
244. Gibbs, A.; Schwartzman, J.; Deng, V.; Alumkal, J. Sulforaphane destabilizes the androgen receptor in prostate cancer cells by inactivating histone deacetylase 6. *Proc. Natl. Acad. Sci. USA* **2009**, *106*, 16663–16668. [CrossRef] [PubMed]
245. Myzak, M.C.; Dashwood, W.M.; Orner, G.A.; Ho, E.; Dashwood, R.H. Sulforaphane inhibits histone deacetylase in vivo and suppresses tumorigenesis in *Apc*-min mice. *FASEB J.* **2006**, *20*, 506–508. [CrossRef] [PubMed]
246. Zhang, C.; Su, Z.Y.; Khor, T.O.; Shu, L.; Kong, A.N. Sulforaphane enhances Nrf2 expression in prostate cancer TRAMP C1 cells through epigenetic regulation. *Biochem. Pharmacol.* **2013**, *85*, 1398–1404. [CrossRef] [PubMed]
247. Beaver, L.M.; Kuintzle, R.; Buchanan, A.; Wiley, M.; Glasser, S.T.; Wong, C.P.; Johnson, G.S.; Chang, J.H.; Löhr, C.V.; Williams, D.E.; et al. Long noncoding RNAs and sulforaphane: A target for chemoprevention and suppression of prostate cancer. *J. Nutr. Biochem.* **2017**, *42*, 72–83. [CrossRef] [PubMed]
248. Hahm, E.R.; Chandra-Kuntal, K.; Desai, D.; Amin, S.; Singh, S.V. Notch activation is dispensable for D, L-sulforaphane-mediated inhibition of human prostate cancer cell migration. *PLoS ONE* **2012**, *7*, e44957. [CrossRef] [PubMed]
249. Hsu, A.; Wong, C.P.; Yu, Z.; Williams, D.E.; Dashwood, R.H.; Ho, E. Promoter de-methylation of cyclin D2 by sulforaphane in prostate cancer cells. *Clin. Epigenetics* **2011**, *3*, 3. [CrossRef] [PubMed]

250. Wong, C.P.; Hsu, A.; Buchanan, A.; Palomera-Sanchez, Z.; Beaver, L.M.; Houseman, E.A.; Williams, D.E.; Dashwood, R.H.; Ho, E. Effects of sulforaphane and 3,3′-diindolylmethane on genome-wide promoter methylation in normal prostate epithelial cells and prostate cancer cells. *PLoS ONE* **2014**, *9*, e86787. [CrossRef]
251. Vyas, A.R.; Moura, M.B.; Hahm, E.R.; Singh, K.; Singh, S.V. Sulforaphane Inhibits c-Myc-Mediated Prostate Cancer Stem-Like Traits. *J. Cell. Biochem.* **2016**, *117*, 2482–2495. [CrossRef]
252. Watson, G.W.; Wickramasekara, S.; Palomera-Sanchez, Z.; Black, C.; Maier, C.S.; Williams, D.E.; Dashwood, R.H.; Ho, E. SUV39H1/H3K9me3 attenuates sulforaphane-induced apoptotic signaling in PC3 prostate cancer cells. *Oncogenesis* **2014**, *3*, e131. [CrossRef]
253. Singh, K.B.; Hahm, E.R.; Alumkal, J.J.; Foley, L.M.; Hitchens, T.K.; Shiva, S.S.; Parikh, R.A.; Jacobs, B.L.; Singh, S.V. Reversal of the Warburg phenomenon in chemoprevention of prostate cancer by sulforaphane. *Carcinogenesis* **2019**, *40*, 1545–1556. [CrossRef]
254. Peng, X.; Zhou, Y.; Tian, H.; Yang, G.; Li, C.; Geng, Y.; Wu, S.; Wu, W. Sulforaphane inhibits invasion by phosphorylating ERK1/2 to regulate E-cadherin and CD44v6 in human prostate cancer DU145 cells. *Oncol. Rep.* **2015**, *34*, 1565–1572. [CrossRef]
255. Vyas, A.R.; Singh, S.V. Functional relevance of D,L-sulforaphane-mediated induction of vimentin and plasminogen activator inhibitor-1 in human prostate cancer cells. *Eur. J. Nutr.* **2014**, *53*, 843–852. [CrossRef]
256. Hać, A.; Domachowska, A.; Narajczyk, M.; Cyske, K.; Pawlik, A.; Herman-Antosiewicz, A. S6K1 controls autophagosome maturation in autophagy induced by sulforaphane or serum deprivation. *Eur. J. Cell. Biol.* **2015**, *94*, 470–481. [CrossRef]
257. Pei, Y.; Wu, B.; Cao, Q.; Wu, L.; Yang, G. Hydrogen sulfide mediates the anti-survival effect of sulforaphane on human prostate cancer cells. *Toxicol. Appl. Pharmacol.* **2011**, *257*, 420–428. [CrossRef]
258. Wiczk, A.; Hofman, D.; Konopa, G.; Herman-Antosiewicz, A. Sulforaphane, a cruciferous vegetable-derived isothiocyanate, inhibits protein synthesis in human prostate cancer cells. *Biochim. Biophys. Acta* **2012**, *1823*, 1295–1305. [CrossRef] [PubMed]
259. Xu, C.; Shen, G.; Chen, C.; Gélinas, C.; Kong, A.N. Suppression of NF-kappaB and NF-kappaB-regulated gene expression by sulforaphane and PEITC through IkappaBalpha, IKK pathway in human prostate cancer PC-3 cells. *Oncogene* **2005**, *24*, 4486–4495. [CrossRef] [PubMed]
260. Xu, C.; Shen, G.; Yuan, X.; Kim, J.H.; Gopalkrishnan, A.; Keum, Y.S.; Nair, S.; Kong, A.N. ERK and JNK signaling pathways are involved in the regulation of activator protein 1 and cell death elicited by three isothiocyanates in human prostate cancer PC-3 cells. *Carcinogenesis* **2006**, *27*, 437–445. [CrossRef] [PubMed]
261. Yao, H.; Wang, H.; Zhang, Z.; Jiang, B.H.; Luo, J.; Shi, X. Sulforaphane inhibited expression of hypoxia-inducible factor-1alpha in human tongue squamous cancer cells and prostate cancer cells. *Int. J. Cancer* **2008**, *123*, 1255–1261. [CrossRef]
262. Singh, K.B.; Kim, S.H.; Hahm, E.R.; Pore, S.K.; Jacobs, B.L.; Singh, S.V. Prostate cancer chemoprevention by sulforaphane in a preclinical mouse model is associated with inhibition of fatty acid metabolism. *Carcinogenesis* **2018**, *39*, 826–837. [CrossRef]
263. Herman-Antosiewicz, A.; Xiao, H.; Lew, K.L.; Singh, S.V. Induction of p21 protein protects against sulforaphane-induced mitotic arrest in LNCaP human prostate cancer cell line. *Mol. Cancer Ther.* **2007**, *6*, 1673–1681. [CrossRef]
264. Abbas, A.; Hall, J.A.; Patterson, W.L.; Ho, E.; Hsu, A.; Al-Mulla, F.; Georgel, P.T. Sulforaphane modulates telomerase activity via epigenetic regulation in prostate cancer cell lines. *Biochem. Cell Biol.* **2016**, *94*, 71–81. [CrossRef]
265. Kanematsu, S.; Yoshizawa, K.; Uehara, N.; Miki, H.; Sasaki, T.; Kuro, M.; Lai, Y.; Kimura, A.; Yuri, T.; Tsubura, A. Sulforaphane inhibits the growth of KPL-1 human breast cancer cells in vitro and suppresses the growth and metastasis of orthotopically transplanted KPL-1 cells in female athymic mice. *Oncol. Rep.* **2011**, *26*, 603–608. [CrossRef]
266. Hu, R.; Khor, T.O.; Shen, G.; Jeong, W.; Hebbar, V.; Chen, C.; Xu, C.; Reddy, B.; Chada, K.; Kong, A.T. Cancer chemoprevention of intestinal polyposis in ApcMin/+ mice by sulforaphane, a natural product derived from cruciferous vegetable. *Carcinogenesis* **2006**, *27*, 2038–2046. [CrossRef] [PubMed]
267. Shen, G.; Khor, T.; Hu, R.; Yu, S.; Nair, S.; Ho, C.; Reddy, B.; Huang, M.; Newmark, H.; Kong, A.T. Chemoprevention of familial adenomatous polyposis by natural dietary compounds sulforaphane and dibenzoylmethane alone and in combination in $Apc^{Min/+}$ mouse. *Cancer Res.* **2007**, *67*, 9937–9944. [CrossRef] [PubMed]
268. Rajendran, P.; Dashwood, W.M.; Li, L.; Kang, Y.; Kim, E.; Johnson, G.; Fischer, K.A.; Löhr, C.V.; Williams, D.E.; Ho, E.; et al. Nrf2 status affects tumor growth, HDAC3 gene promoter associations, and the response to sulforaphane in the colon. *Clin. Epigenet.* **2015**, *7*, 102. [CrossRef] [PubMed]
269. Kuroiwa, Y.; Nishikawa, A.; Kitamura, Y.; Kanki, K.; Ishii, Y.; Umemura, T.; Hirose, M. Protective effects of benzyl isothiocyanate and sulforaphane but not resveratrol against initiation of pancreatic carcinogenesis in hamsters. *Cancer Lett.* **2006**, *241*, 275–280. [CrossRef] [PubMed]
270. Li, S.H.; Fu, J.; Watkins, D.N.; Srivastava, R.K.; Shankar, S. Sulforaphane regulates self-renewal of pancreatic cancer stem cells through the modulation of Sonic hedgehog-GLI pathway. *Mol. Cell. Biochem.* **2013**, *373*, 217–227. [CrossRef] [PubMed]
271. Conaway, C.C.; Wang, C.X.; Pittman, B.; Yang, Y.M.; Schwartz, J.E.; Tian, D.; McIntee, E.J.; Hecht, S.S.; Chung, F.L. Phenethyl isothiocyanate and sulforaphane and their N-acetylcysteine conjugates inhibit malignant progression of lung adenomas induced by tobacco carcinogens in A/J mice. *Cancer Res.* **2005**, *65*, 8548–8557. [CrossRef]
272. Thejass, P.; Kuttan, G. Antimetastatic activity of Sulforaphane. *Life Sci.* **2006**, *78*, 3043–3050. [CrossRef]
273. Thejass, P.; Kuttan, G. Modulation of cell-mediated immune response in B16F-10 melanoma-induced metastatic tumor-bearing C57BL/6 mice by sulforaphane. *Immunopharmacol. Immunotoxicol.* **2007**, *29*, 173–186. [CrossRef]
274. Wang, F.; Shan, Y. Sulforaphane retards the growth of UM-UC-3 xenographs, induces apoptosis, and reduces survivin in athymic mice. *Nutr. Res.* **2012**, *32*, 374–380. [CrossRef]

275. Singh, S.V.; Warin, R.; Xiao, D.; Powolny, A.A.; Stan, S.D.; Arlotti, J.A.; Zeng, Y.; Hahm, E.R.; Marynowski, S.W.; Bommareddy, A.; et al. Sulforaphane inhibits prostate carcinogenesis and pulmonary metastasis in TRAMP mice in association with increased cytotoxicity of natural killer cells. *Cancer Res.* **2009**, *69*, 2117–2125. [CrossRef] [PubMed]
276. Traka, M.H.; Spinks, C.A.; Doleman, J.F.; Melchini, A.; Ball, R.Y.; Mills, R.D.; Mithen, R.F. The dietary isothiocyanate sulforaphane modulates gene expression and alternative gene splicing in a PTEN null preclinical murine model of prostate cancer. *Mol. Cancer* **2010**, *9*, 189. [CrossRef] [PubMed]
277. Gerhardsson de Verdier, M.; Hagman, U.; Peters, R.K.; Steineck, G.; Overvik, E. Meat, cooking methods and colorectal cancer: A case-referent study in Stockholm. *Int. J. Cancer* **1991**, *49*, 520–525. [CrossRef] [PubMed]
278. Walters, D.G.; Young, P.J.; Agus, C.; Knize, M.G.; Boobis, A.R.; Gooderham, N.J.; Lake, B.G. Cruciferous vegetable consumption alters the metabolism of the dietary carcinogen 2-amino-1-methyl-6-phenylimidazo [4,5,-b] pyridine (PhIP) in humans. *Carcinogenesis* **2004**, *25*, 1659–1669. [CrossRef] [PubMed]
279. Kensler, T.W.; Chen, J.; Egner, P.A.; Fahey, J.W.; Jacobson, L.P.; Stephenson, K.K.; Ye, L.; Coady, L.J.; Wang, J.; Wu, Y.; et al. Effects of Glucosinolate-Rich Broccoli Sprouts on Urinary Levels of Aflatoxin-DNA Adducts and Phenanthrene Tetraol in Randomized Clinical Trial in He Zuo Township, Qidong, People's Republic of China. *Cancer Epidemiol. Biomark. Prev.* **2005**, *14*, 2605–2613. [CrossRef]
280. Kensler, T.W.; Ng, D.; Carmella, S.G.; Chen, M.; Jacobson, L.P.; Muñoz, A.; Egner, P.A.; Chen, J.G.; Qian, G.S.; Chen, T.Y.; et al. Modulation of the metabolism of airborne pollutants by glucoraphanin-rich and sulforaphane-rich broccoli sprout beverages in Qidong, China. *Carcinogenesis* **2012**, *33*, 101–107. [CrossRef] [PubMed]
281. Egner, P.A.; Chen, J.G.; Zarth, A.T.; Ng, D.K.; Wang, J.B.; Kensler, K.H.; Jacobson, L.P.; Muñoz, A.; Johnson, J.L.; Groopman, J.D.; et al. Rapid and sustainable detoxication of airborne pollutants by broccoli sprout beverage: Results of a randomized clinical trial in China. *Cancer Prev. Res.* **2014**, *7*, 813–823. [CrossRef] [PubMed]
282. Riso, P.; Martini, D.; Visioli, F.; Martinetti, A.; Porrini, M. Effect of broccoli intake on markers related to oxidative stress and cancer risk in healthy smokers and nonsmokers. *Nutr. Cancer* **2009**, *61*, 232–237. [CrossRef] [PubMed]
283. Riso, P.; Martini, D.; Møller, P.; Loft, S.; Bonacina, G.; Moro, M.; Porrini, M. DNA damage and repair activity after broccoli intake in young healthy smokers. *Mutagenesis* **2010**, *25*, 595–602. [CrossRef] [PubMed]
284. Bauman, J.E.; Zang, Y.; Sen, M.; Li, C.; Wang, L.; Egner, P.A.; Fahey, J.W.; Normolle, D.P.; Grandis, J.R.; Kensler, T.W.; et al. Prevention of Carcinogen- Induced Oral Cancer by Sulforaphane. *Cancer Prev. Res.* **2016**, *9*, 547–557. [CrossRef] [PubMed]
285. Atwell, L.L.; Zhang, Z.; Mori, M.; Farris, P.; Vetto, J.T.; Naik, A.M.; Oh, K.Y.; Thuillier, P.; Ho, E.; Shannon, J. Sulforaphane bioavailability and chemopreventive activity in women scheduled for breast biopsy. *Cancer Prev. Res.* **2015**, *8*, 1184–1191. [CrossRef]
286. Zhang, Z.; Atwell, L.; Farris, P.E.; Ho, E.; Shannon, J. Associations between cruciferous vegetable intake and selected biomarkers among women schedule for breast biopsy. *Public Health Nutr.* **2015**, *19*, 1288–1295. [CrossRef] [PubMed]
287. Howell, S.J.; Campone, M.; Cortes, J.; Duhoux, F.P.; Ross, S.; Franklin, M.S. Final results of the STEM trial: SFX-01 in the treatment and evaluation of ER+ Her2- metastatic breast cancer (mBC). *Ann. Oncol.* **2019**, *30* (Suppl. 5), v122. [CrossRef]
288. Lozanovski, V.J.; Houben, P.; Hinz, U.; Hackert, T.; Herr, I.; Schemmer, P. Pilot study evaluating broccoli sprouts in advanced pancreatic cancer (POUDER trial)-study protocol for a randomized controlled trial. *Trials* **2014**, *15*, 204. [CrossRef]
289. Traka, M.; Gasper, A.V.; Melchini, A.; Bacon, J.; Needs, P.W.; Frost, V.; Chantry, A.; Jones, A.M.E.; Ortori, C.A.; Barrett, D.A.; et al. Broccoli Consumption Interacts with GSTM1 to Perturb Oncogenic Signaling Pathways in the Prostate. *PLoS ONE* **2008**, *3*, e02568. [CrossRef]
290. Cipolla, B.G.; Mandron, E.; Lefort, J.M.; Coadou, Y.; Negra, E.D.; Corbel, L.; Scodan, R.L.; Azzouzi, A.R.; Mottet, N. Effect of sulforaphane in Men with Biochemical Recurrence after Radical Prostatectomy. *Cancer Prev. Res.* **2015**, *8*, 712–719. [CrossRef]
291. Traka, M.; Melchinin, A.; Coode-Beta, J.; Al Kadhi, O.; Saha, S.; Defernez, M.; Troncoso-Rey, P.; Kibblewhite, H.M.; O'Neill, C.; Bernuzzi, F.; et al. Transcriptional changes in prostate of men on active surveillance after a 12-mo glucoraphanin-rich broccoli intervention- results from the Effect of Sulforaphane on prostate CAncer PrEvention (ESCAPE) randomized controlled trial. *Am. J. Clin. Nutr.* **2019**, *109*, 1133–1144. [CrossRef]
292. Kirkwood, J.M.; Singh, S.; Lin, Y.; Hahm, E.; Beumer, J.H.; Christner, S.M.; Rao, U.N.M.; Sander, C.; Tarhini, A.A.; Tawbi, H.A.; et al. Dose-response evaluation of broccoli sprout extract sulforaphane (BSE-SFN) in melanoma patients (Pts) with atypical/dysplastic nevi (A/DN). *J. Clin. Oncol.* **2016**, *34*, e21022. [CrossRef]
293. Pavia, M.; Pileggi, C.; Nobile, C.G.; Angelillo, I.F. Association between fruit and vegetable consumption and oral cancer: A meta-analysis of observational studies. *Am. J. Clin. Nutr.* **2006**, *83*, 1126–1134. [CrossRef] [PubMed]
294. Bravi, F.; Bosetti, C.; Filomeno, M.; Levi, F.; Garavello, W.; Galimberti, S.; Negri, E.; La Vecchia, C. Foods, nutrients and the risk of oral and pharyngeal cancer. *Br. J. Cancer* **2013**, *109*, 2904–2910. [CrossRef] [PubMed]
295. Joseph, M.A.; Moysich, K.B.; Freudenheim, J.L.; Shields, P.G.; Bowman, E.D.; Zhang, Y.; Marshall, J.R.; Ambrosone, C.B. Cruciferous vegetables, genetic polymorphisms in glutathione S-transferases M1 and T1, and prostate cancer risk. *Nutr. Cancer* **2004**, *50*, 206–213. [CrossRef] [PubMed]
296. Kirsh, V.A.; Peters, U.; Mayne, S.T.; Subar, A.F.; Chatterjee, N.; Johnson, C.C.; Hayes, R.B. Prostate, Lung, Colorectal and Ovarian Cancer Screening Trial. Prospective study of fruit and vegetable intake and risk of prostate cancer. *J. Natl. Cancer Inst.* **2007**, *99*, 1200–1209. [CrossRef]

cancers

MDPI

Review

Potential of Bioactive Food Components against Gastric Cancer: Insights into Molecular Mechanism and Therapeutic Targets

Seog Young Kang [1], Dongwon Hwang [1], Soyoung Shin [1], Jinju Park [1], Myoungchan Kim [2], MD. Hasanur Rahman [3], Md. Ataur Rahman [1,2,4], Seong-Gyu Ko [4] and Bonglee Kim [1,2,4,*]

1 College of Korean Medicine, Kyung Hee University, Hoegidong Dongdaemungu, Seoul 05253, Korea; pionasy@khu.ac.kr (S.Y.K.); d.hwang@khu.ac.kr (D.H.); red4103@khu.ac.kr (S.S.); jinjuzz98@khu.ac.kr (J.P.); rahman23@khu.ac.kr (M.A.R.)

2 Department of Pathology, College of Korean Medicine, Kyung Hee University, Hoegidong Dongdaemungu, Seoul 05253, Korea; dongoorai@khu.ac.kr

3 Department of Biotechnology and Genetic Engineering, Bangabandhu Sheikh Mujibur Rahman Science and Technology University, Gopalganj 8100, Bangladesh; hasan079@bsmrstu.edu.bd

4 Korean Medicine-Based Drug Repositioning Cancer Research Center, College of Korean Medicine, Kyung Hee University, Hoegidong Dongdaemungu, Seoul 05253, Korea; epiko@khu.ac.kr

* Correspondence: bongleekim@khu.ac.kr

Simple Summary: Recently, it has been found that cancer of the gastrointestinal tract, especially gastric cancer (GC), is the second most leading cause of cancer-related death globally. Extensive research has shown that most epidemiological investigations indicated the increased intake of naturally-occurring bioactive food components could decrease the gastric cancer risk. Several experimental studies have explained that the molecular mechanisms of action to prevent GC comprise induction of apoptosis, inhibition of cell proliferation, suppression of angiogenesis and metastasis, and regulation of autophagy. To provide an updated understanding of relationships between naturally occurring bioactive food components and gastric cancer, this study will be helpful for guiding and preventing gastric cancer by natural bioactive food products.

Abstract: Gastric cancer, also known as stomach cancer, is a cancer that develops from the lining of the stomach. Accumulated evidence and epidemiological studies have indicated that bioactive food components from natural products play an important role in gastric cancer prevention and treatment, although its mechanism of action has not yet been elucidated. Particularly, experimental studies have shown that natural bioactive food products display a protective effect against gastric cancer via numerous molecular mechanisms, such as suppression of cell metastasis, anti-angiogenesis, inhibition of cell proliferation, induction of apoptosis, and modulation of autophagy. Chemotherapy remains the standard treatment for advanced gastric cancer along with surgery, radiation therapy, hormone therapy, as well as immunotherapy, and its adverse side effects including neutropenia, stomatitis, mucositis, diarrhea, nausea, and emesis are well documented. However, administration of naturally occurring bioactive phytochemical food components could increase the efficacy of gastric chemotherapy and other chemotherapeutic resistance. Additionally, several studies have suggested that bioactive food components with structural stability, potential bioavailability, and powerful bioactivity are important to develop novel treatment strategies for gastric cancer management, which may minimize the adverse effects. Therefore, the purpose of this review is to summarize the potential therapeutic effects of natural bioactive food products on the prevention and treatment of gastric cancer with intensive molecular mechanisms of action, bioavailability, and safety efficacy.

Keywords: gastric cancer; bioactive food components; autophagy; apoptosis; angiogenesis; metastasis; chemo-resistance

Citation: Kang, S.Y.; Hwang, D.; Shin, S.; Park, J.; Kim, M.; Rahman, M.H.; Rahman, M.A.; Ko, S.-G.; Kim, B. Potential of Bioactive Food Components against Gastric Cancer: Insights into Molecular Mechanism and Therapeutic Targets. *Cancers* **2021**, *13*, 4502. https://doi.org/10.3390/cancers13184502

Academic Editor: Anupam Bishayee

Received: 26 July 2021
Accepted: 3 September 2021
Published: 7 September 2021

Publisher's Note: MDPI stays neutral with regard to jurisdictional claims in published maps and institutional affiliations.

1. Introduction

The incidence and mortality of cancer is growing worldwide, with an estimated 19.3 million new cases and 10 million cancer deaths in 2020 [1]. Gastric cancer is the fifth most common neoplasm and the fourth leading cause of cancer death, which has led to over one million new cases and an estimated 769,000 deaths in 2020 [1]. Clinically, to offer pertinent treatment, gastric carcinoma is classified as early or advanced stage [2]. Gastric carcinoma has multiple risk factors: genetics, *Helicobacter pylori* infection, gastric ulcer, gastroesophageal reflux disease (GERD), tobacco, smoking, alcohol, chemical exposure, diet, obesity, and so forth [3,4]. Surgical resection, when possible, offers the best chances of cure for early gastric cancer [5]. Adjuvant or neoadjuvant chemotherapy may be beneficial in increasing the chance of successful resection or in decreasing the rate of recurrence and/or metastasis [6–8]. For patients with unresectable advanced gastric cancer, chemotherapy is a common choice. Conventional regimens are mostly based on cytotoxic agents including antimetabolites and platinum-based anticancer drugs. However, these regimens cause severe side effects such as chemotherapy-induced peripheral neuropathy (CIPN), neutropenia, stomatitis, mucositis, diarrhea, nausea, and emesis [9,10]. Moreover, failure of first-line chemotherapy due to resistance is also an obstacle of gastric cancer treatment hampering the novel and effective therapies and imposing significant economic costs to patients [11]. Moreover, exposure to unremovable toxins (not able to be removed or non-releasable), trauma, or infection lead to mutagenic chronic inflammatory responses, which cause dysplasia [12]. Considering gastric cancer, *Helicobacter pylori* infection is a major risk factor for developing deleterious tumor microenvironments [13]. Nuclear factor kappa-B (NF-κB), c-Jun N-terminal kinase (JNK), and signal transducer activator of transcription 3 (STAT3), inflammatory cytokines, tumor necrosis factor (TNF), interleukin (IL)-1/6, tumor-derived cytokines such as fasciclin (Fas) ligand, and vascular endothelial growth factor (VEGF) are major targets of regulation for the prevention and treatment of gastric cancer [14–18]. Therefore, novel drug development against gastric cancer is strongly needed to further improve survival rates of this disease and lower the side effects of conventional therapies.

Epidemiological studies have shown that natural dietary bioactive food components decrease the risks of gastric cancer [19–22]. Extensive research was conducted to measure the value of natural products for the prevention and treatment of gastric carcinoma, leading to the discovery of major bioactive phytochemicals with anti-cancer properties, such as quercetin, silymarin, taurine, berberine, curcumin, and so forth [23–26]. However, few review articles included agents from animal or marine sources, which are also being studied with growing expectation [27,28]. The same goes for traditional medicine, despite their wide use in clinical practice to combat various illnesses including cancer [29–32]. This review explores various bioactive compounds isolated from biological resources of bioactive food components and traditional medicine in the form of single compounds that show anti-cancer properties closely targeted to gastric cancer. Moreover, the use of bioactive food components could be a promising adjuvant remedy for gastric cancer treatment as well as in developing functional food components and drugs for the treatment and prevention of gastric cancer.

2. Methods

While there have been similar reviews highlighting the anti-neoplastic efficacies of bioactive food components, few of them were written with regards to the chemical classification of each bioactive compound. This review is not only a simple compilation of previous in vitro studies testing bioactive food components on gastric cancer but goes as far as to systematically organizing previous works depending on each cancer-related pathway, namely apoptosis, autophagy, metastasis, drug-resistant capability, and more. Literature-based online databases, Google Scholar, Web of Science, PubMed, Google, and Scopus were accessed to collect information on the published articles. As there is currently no golden standard for classifying phytochemicals, we adopted a comprehensive and clear method previously demonstrated in a literature highlighting the efficacies of bioactive food components on gastrointestinal diseases. This will help researchers rule out or select appropriate candidate species of natural bioactive food products for further studies. This review only included studies published from 2014 to 2021.

3. Apoptosis-Inducing Natural Bioactive Food Components in Gastric Cancer

Apoptosis is the process of programmed cell death, characterized by distinct morphology: cell shrinking, membrane blebbing, chromatin condensation, and nuclear fragmentation [33,34]. Several bioactive compounds showing apoptosis-inducing effects on gastric cancer cells and animal models are presented in Figure 1 and Table 1. Yang et al. reported that berberine could inhibit the proliferation of SGC-7901 cells and induce apoptosis [35]. In vitro models have demonstrated that cyclovirobuxine D originated from *Buxux microphylla* Richardii. *Radix* (Buxaceae) induced apoptosis in MGC-803 and MKN-28 cells [36]. Expressions of caspase-3, cytochrome c, endonuclease G (Endo G), apoptosis inducing factor (AIF), and Smac/Diablo were upregulated in melittin-treated SGC-7901 cells. Trifolirhizin, a compound isolated from *Sophora flavescens* Aiton Radix (Fabaceae), demonstrated apoptotic activity both in vitro and in vivo [37]. Trifolirhizin induced apoptosis of MKN-45 cells in vitro via EGFR-MAPK pathways and triggered G2/M phase cell cycle arrest by impacting the CDC2/Cyclin B complex. Qian et al. discovered that ginsenoside-Rh2 originated from *Panax ginseng* C.A. Mey, Radix (Araliaceae) inhibits proliferation and induces apoptosis of SGC-7901 cells by induction of the Bcl-like protein 4 (Bax) to Bcl-2 (Bax/Bcl-2) ratio [38].

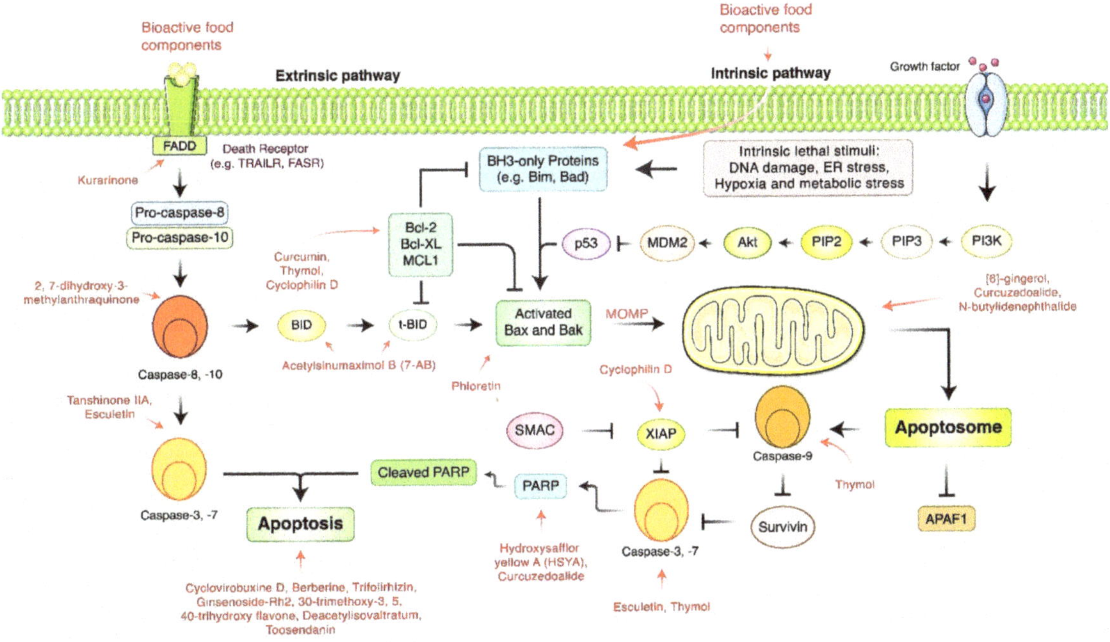

Figure 1. Schematic diagram of natural bioactive food product-mediated apoptosis signaling pathways. FADD, Fas-associated proteins with death domain; TRAILR, TNF-related apoptosis-including ligand receptor; FASR, Fas receptor; tBid, truncated Bid; PARP, poly ADP-ribose polymerase; APAF1, apoptotic protase activating factor 1; MOMP, mitochondrial outer membrane permeabilization; PIP2, phosphatidylinositol-3,4-bisphosphate; PIP3, phosphatidylinositol-3,4,5-triphosphate; PI3K, phosphoinositide 3-kinase.

Tanshinone IIA, originated from *Salviae miltiorrhiza* Bunge. *Radix* (Lamiaceae), suppressed AGS gastric tumor cells via activation of tumor necrosis factor-alpha (TNF-α), Fas, p38, JNK, p53, p21, caspase-3, and caspase-8 and inhibition of ERK [39]. [6]-gingerol treatment for 24 h to AGS cells generated ROS and decreased $\Delta\Psi$m, leading to induction of apoptosis. Perturbations of $\Delta\Psi$m were associated with deregulation of the Bax/Bcl-2 ratio at the protein level, which led to the upregulation of cytochrome c and triggered the caspase cascade. 2,7-dihydroxy-3-methylanthraquinone (DDMN), a flavone isolated from *Hedyotis diffusa* Willd. *Herba*, induced caspase-dependent apoptosis of SGC-7901 gastric cancer cells [40]. 6,7,30-trimethoxy-3,5,40-trihydroxy flavone (TTF), from *Chrysosplenium nudicaule* Ledeb. Herba, is a well-known traditional Chinese medicine for digestive diseases [41], which induced apoptosis on SGC-7901 cells. Sun et al. observed that curcumin, isolated from *Curcuma longa* L. *Rhizoma* (Zingiberaceae), induced apoptosis of SGC-7901 and BGC-823 cells by up-regulating microRNA-33b (miR-33b) expression [42]. Esculetin treatment triggered ROS formation, elevated caspase-3/9 activity, and induced poly (ADP-ribose) polymerase (PARP) cleavage [43]. Liu et al. reported that hydroxysafflor yellow A (HSYA) induces apoptosis of BGC-7901 gastric carcinoma cells via activation of the peroxisome proliferator-activated receptor gamma (PPARγ) signal through elevation of PPARγ and caspase-3 [44]. Kurarinone synergized TRAIL-induced apoptosis against gastric cancer cell line SGC-7901 [45]. Licochalcone A (LicA), a flavonoid isolated from licorice root, elucidated apoptosis by blocking the Akt signaling pathway and reducing hexokinase 2 (HK2) expression in MKN45 cells [46]. Curcuzedoalide, sesquiterpene bioactive components of *Curcuma zedoaria* Roscoe *Rhizoma* (Zingiberaceae), induced mitochondrial apoptosis induction with cleavage of PARP as well as caspase-8, caspase-9, and caspase-3 in AGS cells [47]. Thymol showed cytotoxicity on AGS cancer cells via the intrinsic mitochondrial pathway via upregulation of Bax and PARP expression, and also promoted cleavage of caspase-7, caspase-8, and caspase-9 and downregulated $\Delta\Psi$m [48].

The apoptotic ability of ophiopogonin B, the active compound isolated from *Ophiopogon japonicus Radix*, against SGC-7901 cells were suspected to be relevant with the JNK 1/2 and ERK1/2 signaling pathways through upregulation of active caspase-3 and modulation of Bax/Bcl-2 expression [49]. It has been found that phloretin, a plant-derived natural bioactive product, is an important molecule for the treatment of AGS gastric cancer via expression of Bax and was increased in dose-dependently while the expression of Bcl-2 decreased [50]. Podophyllotoxin, isolated from *Linum album* Kotschy (Linaceae), induced apoptosis and downregulated zinc finger protein 703 oncogene expression [51]. Grifolin, isolated from the mushroom *Albatrellus confluens* (Alb. and Schwein) Kotl. and Pouzar (Albatrellaceae), inhibited growth and invasion of gastric cancer cells by inducing apoptosis and suppressing the ERK1/2 pathway [52]. Tsai et al. found that 7-acetylsinumaximol B (7-AB), discovered from *Sinularia sandensis* (Alcyoniidae), showed anti-proliferative effects through apoptosis against human gastric carcinoma NCI-N87 cells via the expression of Bad, Bcl-like protein 11 (Bim), Bax, and cytochrome c, and it decreased the expression levels of phosphorylated Bad (p-Bad), myeloid cell lukemia-1 (Mcl-1), Bcl-xL, and Bcl-2 proteins. [53] Crosolic acid, isolated from *Actinidia valvata* Dunn. *Radix* (Actinidiaceae), was reported to inhibit proliferation of BGC-823 cells by downregulating the NF-κB pathway [54]. Crosolic acid inhibited phosphorylation of nuclear factor kappa B-alpha (IκBα), expression of p65, and nuclear translocation and DNA-binding activity of NF-κB. Deacetylisovaltratum, derived from *Patrinia heterophylla* Bunge, induced mitochondrial and caspase-dependent apoptosis in AGS and HGC-27 cells [55]. Li et al. demonstrated that elemene, a sesquiterpenoid mixture isolated from a traditional herbal medicine, *Curcuma zedoaria* Roscoe *Rhizoma* (Zingiberaceae), countered gastric cancer via regulation of the ERK 1/2 signaling pathway [56]. Liao et al. reported that n-butylidenephthalide (BP), a bioactive compound of *Angelica Sinensis* Diels *Radix*, activated the intrinsic apoptotic pathway of human gastric cancer cells AGS, NCI-N87, and TSGH-9201 [57]. Paeonol treatment inhibited proliferation, invasion, migration, and induced apoptosis against BGC823 cells. The protein expression of matrix metalloproteinase (MMP)-2 and MMP-9 were attenuated in a concentration-dependent manner by paeonol [58]. Pseudolaric acid B, isolated from *Pseudolarix amabilis*, commonly called golden larch, inhibited cell proliferation and induced apoptosis of the multidrug-resistant SGC-7901/ADR gastric cancer cell line [59].

Thymol is a phenolic compound isolated from *Thymus quinquecostatus* Celak. (Lamiaceae) that possesses anti-inflammatory, anticancer, antibacterial, and more biological efficacies [48]. The anticancer potencies of toosendanin (TSN), a triterpenoid found in *Melia toosendan* Sieb et Zucc *Cortex et Fructus* (Meliaceae), was discussed in two studies. Wang et al. found that SGC-7901 cells treated with toosendanin (TSN) increased early apoptosis [60]. TSN inactivated the β-catenin pathway in SGC-7901 cells and subsequently induced apoptosis following facilitation of microRNA 200a [60]. It has been reported that peptic oligosaccharide, separated from *Solanum lycopersicum* L. (Solanaceae), induced apoptosis by suppressing galectin-3 expressions [61]. Additionally, several natural bioactive products retarded tumor growth in animal models, as presented in Table 2. Wu et al. revealed that phenolic alkaloids of *Menispermum dauricum* induced apoptosis and suppressed gastric tumor growth by inducing apoptosis and inhibiting oncogenic Kirsten Rat sarcoma viral oncogene homolog (K-RAS) expression [62]. When BALB/C mice grafted with MFC mouse gastric cancer cells were treated with curcumin solution every day for 60 days, expressions of interferon gamma (IFN-γ), tumor necrosis factor-alpha (TNF-α), granzyme B, and perforin were upregulated, while differentiated embryonic chondrocyte gene 1 (DEC1), hypoxia-inducible factor-1 alpha (HIF-1α), STAT3, and VEGF expression were downregulated in the experimental group [63]. When MKN45-treated BALB/ca mice were treated with LicA, tumor growth was significantly inhibited in contrast to the vehicle group without LicA treatment [46]. Elemene retarded tumor growth in nude mice and showed better efficacy when synergized with PD98059 [56]. In a xenograft mouse model, mice treated with grifolin survived for a longer period compared to the control group [52].

Table 1. Apoptosis-inducing bioactive food components in vitro. (↑ increase, ↓ decrease).

Classification	Compound	Source	Experimental Model	Dose; Duration	Efficacy	Mechanism	References
Alkaloids	Berberine	(family: Ranunculaceae) *Coptidis japonica* Makino *Rhizoma*	SGC-7901	5, 10, 20 μM; 24, 48 h	Induction of apoptosis		[35]
Alkaloids	Cyclovirobuxine D	(family: Buxaceae) *Buxus microphylla* Richardii *Radix*	MGC-803, MKN-28	30, 60, 120 μM/L; 48 h	Induction of apoptosis	↑c-caspase-3, Bax ↓Bcl-2	[36]
Alkaloids	GFG-3a	(family: Meripilaceae) *Grifola frondose* (Diks.) Gray *Mycelia*	SGC-7901	100, 200 μg/mL; 24, 48 h	Induction of apoptosis	↑RBBP4, caspase-3, -8, p53, Bax, Bad ↓RUVBL, NPM, Bcl-2, Bcl-xL, PI3K, Akt1	[64]
Alkaloids	Melittin	(family: Apidae) *Apis cerena* Fabricius *venom*	SGC-7901	4 μg/mL; 1, 2, 4 h	Induction of apoptosis	↑caspase-3, cyt c, Endo G, AIF, Smac/Diablo, ROS ↓ΔΨm	[65]
Alkaloids, Terpenoids	Berberine, d-Limonene	(1) (family: Ranunculaceae) *Coptidis japonica* Makino *Rhizoma* (2) (family: Rutaceae) *Evodiae rutaecarpa* Bentham. *Fructus*	MGC-803	(1) 20 μM; 24, 36, 48 h (2) 80 μM; 24, 36, 48 h	Induction of apoptosis	↑ROS, caspase-3 ↑ΔΨm, Bcl-2	[66]
Flavonoids	Trifolirhizin	(family: Fabaceae) *Sophora flavescens* Aiton *Radix*	MKN-45	20, 30, 40 μg/mL; 48 h	Induction of apoptosis	↑caspase-9, -3, c-PARP, p53, p38 ↓EGFR, CDC2, cyclin B, ΔΨm	[37]
Phytosterols	Ginsenoside-Rh2	(family: Araliaceae) *Panax ginseng* C.A. Mey *Radix*	SGC-7901	5, 10, 20 μg/mL; 24, 48 h	Induction of apoptosis	↑Bax ↓Bcl-2	[38]
Phytosterols	Periplocin	(family: Apocynaceae) *Periplocae sepium* Bunge.	SGC-7901, MGC-803, BGC-823	50, 100, 200 ng/mL; 24, 48 h	Induction of apoptosis	↑Mcl-1, c-caspase-3, EGR 1 ↓pro-Bid, p-ERK 1/2	[67]

Table 1. *Cont.*

Classification	Compound	Source	Experimental Model	Dose; Duration	Efficacy	Mechanism	References
Phytosterols	Tanshinone IIA	(family: Lamiaceae) *Salviae miltiorrhiza* Bunge. *Radix*	AGS	2.0, 3.7, 5.5 µg/mL; 24, 48 h	Induction of apoptosis	↑TNF-α, Fas, p-p38, p-JNK, p53, p21, caspase-8, -3 ↓p-ERK, CDC2, cyclin A, cyclin B1	[39]
Polyphenols	[6]-Gingerol	(family: Zingiberaceae) *Zingiber officinale* Roscoe *Rhizoma*	AGS	100, 250 µM; 24 h	Induction of apoptosis	↑cyt c, Bax ↓Bcl-2	[68]
Polyphenols	2,7-dihydroxy-3-methylanthraquinone (DDMN)	(family: Rubiaceae) *Hedyotis diffusa* Wild *Herba*	SGC-7901	10, 20, 40 µM; 48 h	Inhibition of proliferation	↑Bax, Bad, caspase-3, -9, cyt c ↓Bcl-xL, Bcl-2	[40]
Polyphenols	6, 7, 30-trimethoxy-3, 5, 40 -trihydroxy flavone (TTF)	(family: Saxifragaceae) *Chrysosplenium nudicaule* Ledeb *Herba*	SGC-7901	2, 4, 8, 16, 32 µg/mL; 24, 48, 72 h	Induction of apoptosis	↑endogenous Ca2+/Mg2+ dependent endonuclease	[41]
Polyphenols	Curcumin	(family: Zingiberaceae) *Curcuma longa* L. *Rhizoma*	SGC-7901, BGC-823	5, 10, 15, 20, 40 µM/L; 24 h	Induction of apoptosis	↓XIAP ↑miR-33b	[42]
Polyphenols	Esculetin	(family: Asteraceae) *Artemesia scoparia* Waldst. et Kit, *Artemesia capillaris* Thunb.)) (family: Plumbaginaceae)	SGC-7901, MGC-803, BGC-823	12.5, 25, 50 µM; 24 h	Induction of apoptosis	↑ROS, c-caspase-9, -3, c-PARP, cyt c, Bak, Bax, CypD ↓Bcl-2, Bcl-xL, XIAP	[43]
Polyphenols	Hydroxysafflor Yellow A	(family: Asteraceae) *Carthamus tinctorius* L.	BGC-823	100 µM; 48 h	Induction of apoptosis	↑caspase-3, PPARγ	[44]
Polyphenols	Kurarinone	(family: Fabaceae) *Sophora flavescens* Aiton *Radix*	SGC-7901	5 µM; 24 h	Enhancement ofTRAIL-induced apoptosis	↓Mcl-1, c-FLIP, p-STAT3	[45]

Table 1. *Cont.*

Classification	Compound	Source	Experimental Model	Dose; Duration	Efficacy	Mechanism	References
Polyphenols	Licochalcone A	(family: Fabaceae) *Glycyrrhiza glabra* L. *Root*	MKN-45, SGC-7901	15, 30, 60 μM; 24 h	Inhibition of cell proliferation and tumor glycolysis	↑c-caspase-3, c-PARP ↓Bcl-2, Mcl-1, HK2, p-Akt, p-ERK1/2, p-S6, p-GSK3β	[46]
Polyphenols	Ophiopogonin B	(family: Asparagaceae) *Ophiopogon japonicus* Thunb *Root*	SGC-7901	5, 10, 20 μM	Induction of apoptosis	↑ROS, Bax, caspase-3 ↓p-ERK 1/2, p-JNK 1/2, ΔΨm, Bcl-2	[49]
Polyphenols	Phloretin		AGS	4, 8, 16μM; 24 h	Induction of apoptosis Inhibition of invasion	↑Bax ↓Bcl-2	[50]
Polyphenols	Podophyllotoxin	(family: Linaceae) *Linum album* Kotschy	AGS	200, 400, 600, 800, 1000 μg/mL; 24 h	Induction of apoptosis	↓ZNF703	[51]
Terpenoids	7-Acetylsinumaximol B	(family: Alcyoniidae) *Sinularia sandensis*	NCI-N87	4, 8, 16 μM; 24 h	Induction of apoptosis	↑Bad, Bim, Bax, cyt c ↓p-Bad, Mcl-1, Bcl-xL, Bcl-2	[53]
Terpenoids	Crosolic Acid	(family: Actinidiaceae) *Actinidia valvata* Dunn *Radix*	BGC-823	20, 40, 80 μg/mL; 72 h	Induction of apoptosis	↑Bax, smac, IκBα ↓Fas, Bcl-2, p65, p-IκBα, NF-κB	[54]
Terpenoids	Curcuzedoalide	(family: Zingiberaceae) *Curcuma zedoaria* Roscoe *Rhizoma*	AGS	100, 200 μM; 24 h	Induction of apoptosis	↑c-caspase-8, -9, -3, c-PARP	[47]
Terpenoids	Deacetylisovaltratum	(family: Caprifoliaceae) *Patrinia heterophylla* Bunge.	(1) AGS (2) HGC-27	(1) 4, 8, 16 μM; 24 h (2) 10, 20, 30 μM; 24 h	Induction of apoptosis	↑p21, caspase-3, c-PARP ↓p-STAT3, pro-caspase-9, ΔΨm	[55]
Terpenoids	Elemene	(family: Zingiberaceae) *Curcuma zedoaria* Roscoe *Rhizoma*	BGC-823	20, 40, 80, 160 μg/mL: 24 h	Induction of apoptosis	↑Bax, p-ERK 1/2 ↓Bcl-2	[56]

Table 1. *Cont.*

Classification	Compound	Source	Experimental Model	Dose; Duration	Efficacy	Mechanism	References
Terpenoids	Grifolin	(family: Albatrellaceae) *Albatrellus confluens* (Alb. and Schwein.) Kotl. and Pouzar	BGC-823, SGC-7901	10, 50 μM; 48 h	Induction of apoptosis	↑caspase-9, -3, CDKN2 ↓MEK1, MEKK3 MEK5	[52]
Terpenoids	N-butylidenephthalide	(family: Apiaceae) *Angelica Sinensis* Diels *Radix*	AGS	25, 50, 75 μg/mL; 24 h	Induction of apoptosis	↑REDD1 ↓mTOR	[57]
Terpenoids	Paeonol	(family: Paeoniaceae) *Paeonia suffruticosa* Andr *Root bark,* (family: Apocynaceae) *Cynanchum paniculatum* K. Schum *Radix*	BGC-823	0.1, 0.2, 0.4 mg/mL; 24, 48 h	Inhibition of proliferation, invasion, and migration Induction of apoptosis	↓MMP-2, -9	[58]
Terpenoids	Pseudolaric acid B	(family: Pinaceae) *Pseudolarix kaempferi* Gorden *Root bark*	SGC-7901/ADR	5, 10, 20 μM/L; 24 h	Induction of apoptosis	↑p53, Bax ↓P-gp, COX-2, Bcl-2, Bcl-xL	[59]
Terpenoids	Thymol	(family: Lamiaceae) *Thymus quinquecostatus* Celak *Essential oil*	AGS	100, 200, 400 μM; 6, 12, 24 h	Induction of apoptosis	↑Bax, c-PARP, caspase-8, caspase-7, caspase-9 ↓ΔΨm	[48]
Terpenoids	Toosendanin	(family: Meliaceae) *Melia toosendan* Sieb et zucc *Cortex or Fructus*	SGC-7901	0.5, 1 μM; 48 h	Inhibition of invasion, migration and EMT Induction of apoptosis	↑E-cadherin ↓β-catenin ↑miR-200a	[60]

Table 2. Apoptosis-inducing bioactive food components in vivo. (↑ increase, ↓ decrease).

Classification	Compound	Source	Experimental Model	Dose; Duration	Efficacy	Mechanism	References
Alkaloids	Phenolic alkaloids	(family: Menispermaceae) *Menispermum dauricum* DC. *Rhizoma*	Nude mice/SGC-7901	5, 10, 20 mg/kg/week; 3 weeks	Suppression of tumor growth		[62]
Flavonoids	Trifolirhizin	(family: Fabaceae) *Sophora flavescens* Aiton. *Radix*	BALB/C nude mice/MKN-45	1–3 mg/kg; 3 weeks	Retardation of tumor growth	↑c-caspase-3 ↓ΔΨm	[37]
Polyphenols	2,7-dihydroxy-3-methylanthraquinone (DDMN)	(family: Rubiaceae) *Hedyotis diffusa* Wild. *Herba*	nude mice/SGC-7901	40 mg/kg; 5, 10, 15, 20 days	Inhibition of gastric cancer cell growth	↑Bax, Bad, c-caspase-3, -9, cyt c ↓Bcl-xL, Bcl-2	[40]
Polyphenols	Curcumin	(family: Zingiberaceae) *Curcuma longa* L. *Rhizoma*	BALB/C mice/MFC	20, 40, 60 μM/L/day; 60 days	Inhibition of tumor growth Induction of apoptosis Activation of immune cells	↑IFN-γ, TNF-α, granzyme B, perforin ↓DEC1, HIF-1α, STAT3, VEGF	[63]
Polyphenols	Licochalone A	(family: Fabaceae) *Glycyrrhiza glabra* L. *Radix*	BALB/ca nude mice/MKN-45	10 mg/kg/day; 33 days	Inhibition of tumor growth		[46]
Terpenoids	Elemene	(family: Zingiberaceae) *Curcuma longa* L. *Rhizoma*	BALB/c athymic nude mice/BGC-823	200 mg/kg/day; 15 days	Retardation of tumor growth		[56]
Terpenoids	Grifolin	(family: Albatrellaceae) *Albatrellus confluens* (Alb. and Schwein.) Kotl. and Pouzar	Balb/c nude mice/BGC-823, SGC-7901	15 mg/kg; 2 days	Improvement of survival time		[52]

4. Role of Autophagy in Gastric Cancer Treatment Mediated by Natural Bioactive Food Products

Autophagy is a cellular process in which cytoplasmic contents are degraded within the lysosome/vacuole, and the resulting constituents are recycled [69,70]. Autophagy can be classified into macroautophagy, microautophagy, and chaperone-mediated autophagy (CMA) [71]. Among these, macroautophagy, which has been studied the most, is the process of forming autophagosomes that surround organelles and fuse with lysosomes, and natural products modulate autophagy [72,73]. Based on the isolation target, separate kinds of selective autophagy such as mitophagy, pexophagy, and xenophagy can be distinguished [74]. Macroautophagy consists of several sequential steps: initiation, nucleation, elongation, maturation, and fusion with the lysosome [73,75]. Phagosomes originate from omegasomes, subdomains of the ER, and associate with other organelles such as the mitochondria, golgi complex, plasma membrane, recycling endosome, etc., during its development. Four molecules, Unc-51-like kinase 1/2 (ULK1/2), autophagy-related gene 13 (ATG13), family 200-kD interacting protein (FIP200), and Atg101 form the ULK1/2 complex and initiate the process [73]. The mechanistic target of rapamycin complex 1 (mTORC1) is a major inhibitor of the ULK1/2 complex [69,76]. AMP-activated protein kinase (AMPK) inhibits mTORC1 and leads to the activation of the ULK1/2 complex [75]. The ULK1/2 complex phosphorylates the class III phosphatidylinositol-3-kinase (PI3K) vacuole protein sorting 34 (VPS34) complex consisting of VPS15, Beclin-1, and AtG14 complex, which promotes the formation of phosphatidylinositol-3-phosphate (PI3P), which is an essential lipid molecule required for the nucleation step of the phagophore [77]. Atg12 binds with Atg5 and composes a complex with Atg16L. The Atg12-5-16L1 complex lipidates LC3-I into LC3-II [78,79]. LC3-II, considered a marker of autophagy, is essential for phagosome elongation and fusion [80,81]. When the phagosome encloses and becomes a mature autophagosome, it fuses with a lysosome, and degradation and recycling processes follows. Bioactive food compounds were reported to induce autophagy along with apoptosis against gastric cancer cells, as presented in Figure 2.

It has been found that cinnamaldehyde, the bioactive ingredient in *Cinnamomum cassia*, suppressed tumor growth and the migratory and invasive abilities of gastric cancer [82]. Rottlerin, isolated from *Mallotus philipensis* Muell (Euphorbiaceae), induced autophagy and caspase-independent apoptosis against SGC-7901 and MGC-803 cells by downregulating mTOR and S-phase kinase-associated protein 2 (Skp2) [83]. Moreover, treatment of latcripin 1 protein, found in *Lentinula edodes*, activated autophagy of gastric cancer cell lines BGC-823 and SGC-7901 with autophagosome formation via the alteration of LC3-I into LC3-II expression [84]. Oxyresveratrol, found in grape, has been found to accumulate ROS production and initiated autophagic and apoptotic cell death via the FOXO-caspase-3 pathway [85,86]. Kaempferol, a natural bioactive flavonoid, induced autophagic cell death in gastric cancer via IRE1/JNK/CHOP and AMPK/ULK1 pathways [87]. It has demonstrated cytotoxic activity on AGS, MKN-45, and KATO-III human gastric cancer cells via induction of caspase activation and autophagy via the Akt/NF-κB pathway in AGS cells [22]. Pectolinarigenin, isolated from *Cirsium chanroenicum*, displayed anticancer activity through autophagy induction of human gastric cancer AGS and MKN-28 cells via the downregulation of the PI3K/Akt/mTOR pathway [88]. Perillaldehyde increased AMPK phosphorylation, leading to autophagy in human gastric cancer MFCs mouse and GC9811-P cells [89]. However, quercetin activated autophagy protection against the apoptosis in AGS and MKN-28 gastric cancer cells, which signified that autophagy might have contributed to the survival of cancer cells [90]. Therefore, autophagy induction by natural bioactive compounds might possibly be targeted as a potential therapeutic approach to control gastric cancer.

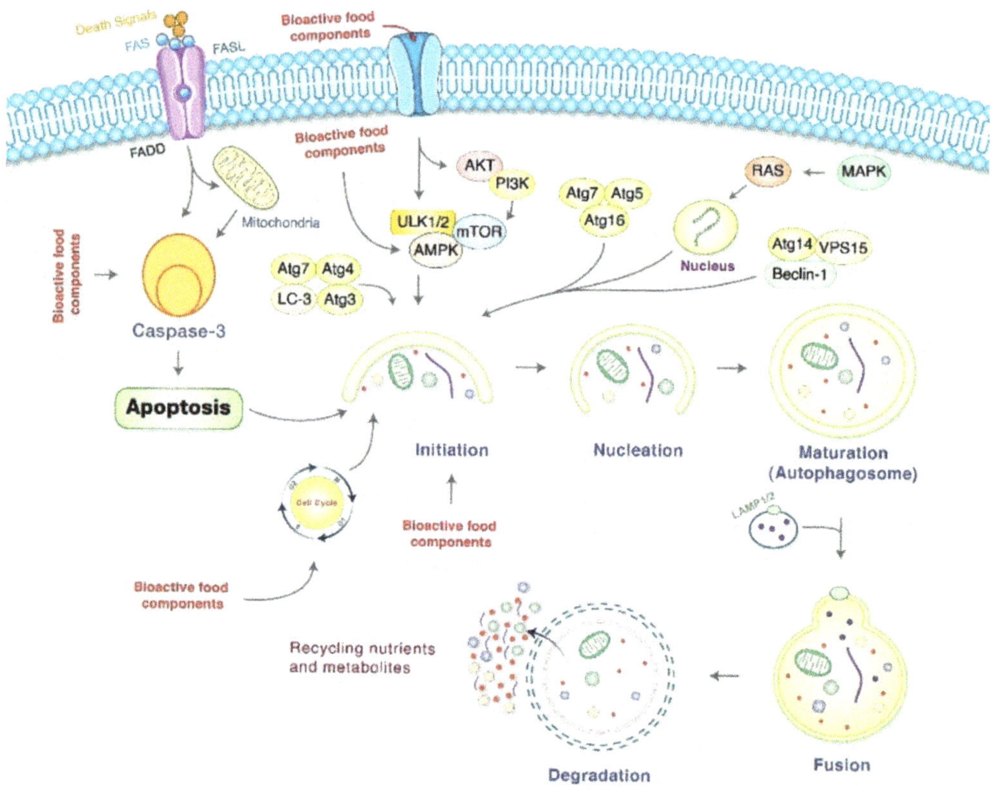

Figure 2. Bioactive compounds regulate molecular mechanisms of autophagy. Bioactive compounds initiate autophagy by the formation of a pre-autophagosomal structure via association of PI3K-AMPK, mammalian target of rapamycin (mTOR), ULK1, Vps34, and the Beclin-1 complex, which contribute to the formation of the pre-autophagosomal structure in addition to activating phagophore formation. Fusion of mature autophagosome as well as lysosome causes autolysosome formation. Lastly, elimination of molecules happens by acid hydrolases, which produce nutrients and recycle metabolites.

5. Role of Bioactive Natural Compounds to Arrest Cell Cycle in Gastric Cancer

The cell cycle is regulated through a series of control systems that in turn promote or inhibit cell division. Programmed cell death and cell cycle regulation occur together in many cancerous cells, since the tumor suppressor gene p53 and downstream proteins regulate both events [91]. A variety of natural bioactive components were described as causing cell death and inhibited cell proliferation by seizing the cell cycle according to the phase of cell cycle arrest (Table 3). Berberine, a traditional Chinese medicine normally used for gastroenteritis, inhibited proliferation of SGC-7901 gastric cancer cells in addition to inducing G1 arrest in the cell cycle phase and activated apoptosis [35]. Toosendanin, a triterpenoid, increased the proportion of cells in the G1 and S phase by activation of β-catenin signaling in gastric carcinoma [60,92]. Moreover, ginsenoside-Rh2 inhibited proliferation of SGC-7901 side population gastric cancer cells by the induction of cell cycle arrest, as well as cell apoptosis, and altered BAX/Bcl-2 protein expression [38]. Crosolic acid, isolated from *Actinidia valvata* Dunn. *Radix*, increased the sub G1 population of the cell cycle and decreased p65, bcl-2, Fas, and smac mRNA expression, and increased IκBα, bax, and survivin mRNA expression, which induced apoptosis of the human gastric cancer cell line BGC823 through down-regulation of the NF-κB pathway [54]. It has been found that rottlerin suppressed cell growth, induced autophagy as well as apoptosis, and reduced migration in addition to invasion in SGC-7901 and MGC-803 GC gastric cancer cells through mTOR and S-phase kinase-associated protein 2 downregulation [83]. Additionally, deacetylisovaltratum, a traditional Chinese herbal medicine *Patrinia heterophylla* Bunge, inhibited the cell viability of AGS and HGC-27 cells and induced G2/M cell cycle arrest via disruption of mitochondrial membrane potential as well as induction of caspase-dependent apoptosis [55].

6. Anti-Angiogenesis Effects of Natural Bioactive Products in Gastric Cancer

Angiogenesis is the most common pathway for new vessel formation in cancer [93]. Anti-angiogenic agents were studied and developed for anti-cancer therapies because angiogenesis can cause tumor growth [94]. The vascular endothelial growth factor (VEGF) signaling pathway plays an essential role in regulating tumor angiogenesis, which can be used as a therapeutic target in numerous types of human gastric cancers [95]. Inhibition of VEGF leads to anti-angiogenesis in various animal and cell line models [96]. VEGFs have an important role in forming new blood vessels, including angiogenesis and vasculogenesis (Figure 3). A dietary flavonoid, luteolin, has been found to prevent angiogenesis in gastric cancer cells of MGC-803 and Hs-746T via the suppression of Notch1)/VEGF signaling [22]. Cyperenoic acid, a sesquiterpene isolated from *Croton crassifolius*, reduced vascular endothelial growth factor A (Vegfa or VEGF-A) genes by targeting the Vegfa-Kdr and Angpt-Tie signaling pathways [97]. Moreover, zerumbone, a bioactive component of ginger, showed anti-angiogenesis activity in AGS cells by reducing VEGF expression and inhibiting NF-κB [98]. Plumbagin inhibits tumor angiogenesis of gastric carcinoma via reduction of VEGF, VEGRF2, and MVD expression in gastric carcinoma in mice by the modulating nuclear factor-kappa B pathway [99]. Moreover, nitidine chloride, *Zanthoxylum nitidum* (Roxb) DC, was found to inhibit the signal transducer as well as activator of transcription 3 (STAT3) signaling in SGC-7901 and AGS human gastric cancer cell lines, which is related to tumor angiogenesis [100]. Additionally, treatment of nitidine chloride decreased the tumor volume through angiogenesis inhibition via reduction of STAT3 and VEGF levels in a xenograft mouse model induced by SGC-7901 cells [100]. Therefore, natural bioactive compound can effectively use certain VEGF subtypes, including VEGFA156, VEGFA121, VEGFR1, and VEGFR2, for the treatment of gastric cancer.

Table 3. Cell cycle arrest by bioactive food components in gastric cancer. (↑ increase, ↓ decrease).

Phase of Cell Cycle Arrest	Classification	Compound	Source	Experimental Model	Dose; Duration	Mechanism	References
G0/G1	Alkaloids	Berberine	(family: Ranunculaceae) *Coptidis japonica* Makino *Rhizoma*	SGC-7901	5, 10, 20 μM; 24, 48 h		[35]
G0/G1	Phytosterols	Ginsenoside-Rh2	(family: Araliaceae) *Panax ginseng* C.A. Mey *Radix*	SGC-7901	5, 10, 20 μg/mL; 24, 48 h	↑Bax ↓Bcl-2	[38]
G0/G1	Terpenoids	Crosolic acid	(family: Actinidiaceae) *Actinidia valvata* Dunn *Radix*	BGC-823	20, 40, 80 μg/mL; 72 h	↑Bax, smac, IκBα ↓Fas, Bcl-2, p65, p-IκBα, NF-κB	[54]
G1	Polyphenols	Rottlerin	(family: Euphorbiaceae) *Mallotus philipensis* Muell.	SGC-7901, MGC-803	2, 4, 8 μM; 24 h	↑LC3-II ↓mTOR, Skp2	[83]
G1/S	Terpenoids	Toosendanin	(family: Meliaceae) *Melia toosendan* Sieb et Zucc *Cortex et Fructus*	(1) AGS (2) HGC-27	(1) 0.5, 1, 2 μM; 48 h (2) 0.5, 1, 2 μM; 36 h	↑c-caspase-3, -8, -9, c-PARP, Bax, p-p38 ↓Bcl-2, Bcl-xL, Mcl-1, survivin, XIAP	[92]
S	Alkaloids	Cyclovirobuxine D	(family: Buxaceae) *Buxus microphylla* Richardii *Radix*	MGC-803, MKN-28	30, 60, 120 μM/L; 48 h	↑c-caspase-3, Bax ↓Bcl-2	[36]
S	Alkaloids	GFG-3a	(family: Meripilaceae) *Grifola frondose* (Diks.) Gray *Mycelia*	SGC-7901	100, 200 μg/mL; 24, 48 h	↑RBBP4, caspase-3, -8, p53, Bax, Bad ↓RUVBL, NPM, Bcl-2, Bcl-xL, PI3K, Akt1	[64]
G2/M	Flavonoids	Trifolirhizin	(family: Fabaceae) *Sophora flavescens* Aiton. *Radix*	MKN-45	20, 30, 40 μg/mL; 48 h	↑caspase-9, -3, c-PARP, p53, p38 ↓EGFR, CDC2, cyclin B, ΔΨm	[37]
G2/M	Phytosterols	Tanshinone IIA	(family: Lamiaceae) *Salviae miltiorrhiza* Bunge. *Radix*	AGS	2.0, 3.7, 5.5 μg/mL; 24, 48 h	↑TNF-α, Fas, p-p38, p-JNK, p53, p21, caspase-8, -3 ↓p-ERK, CDC2, cyclin A, cyclin B1	[39]
G2/M	Terpenoids	Deacetylisovaltratum	(family: Caprifoliaceae) *Patrinia heterophylla* Bunge.	(1) AGS (2) HGC-27	(1) 4, 8, 16 μM; 24 h (2) 10, 20, 30 μM; 24 h	↑p21, caspase-3, c-PARP ↓p-STAT3, pro-caspase-9, ΔΨm	[55]

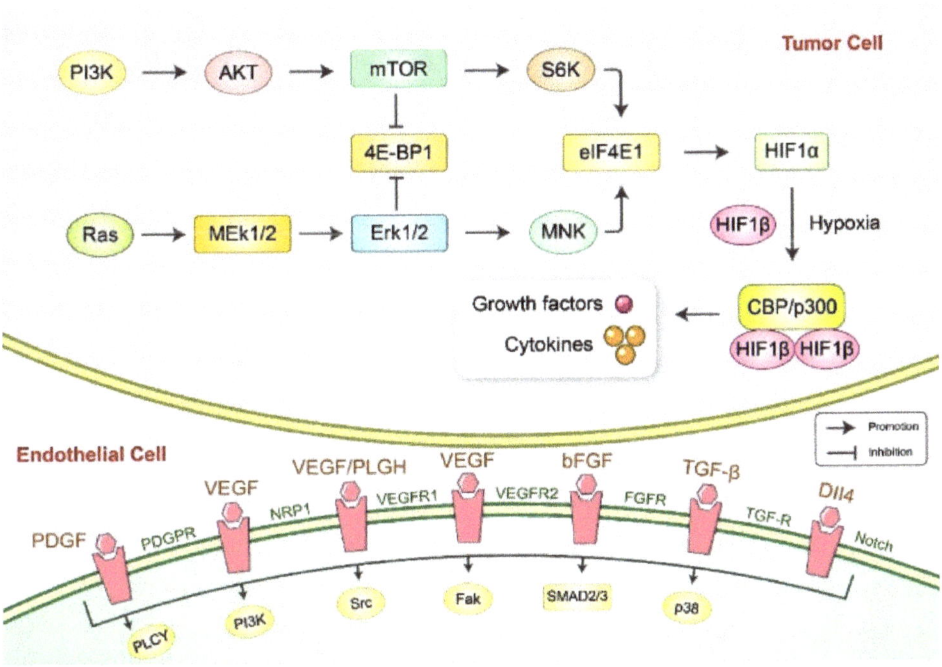

Figure 3. Schematic diagram of angiogenesis signaling pathways. PI3K, phosphoinositide 3-kinase; Akt, protein kinase B; mTOR, mammalian target of rapamycin; S6K, S6 kinase; MEK1/2, mitogen-activated protein kinase kinase 1/2; ERK1/2, extracellular signal-regulated kinase 1/2; MNK, mitogen-activated protein kinase-interacting kinase; 4E-BP1, eIF4E-binding protein 1; elF4E1, eukaryotic initiation factor 4E 1; HIF-1α, hypoxia-inducible factor-1 alpha; HIF-1β, hypoxia-inducible factor-1 beta; CBP, CREB-binding protein; p300, CBP homolog; PDGF, platelet-derived growth factor; PDGFR, platelet-derived growth factor receptor; VEGF, vascular endothelial growth factor; NRP1, neuropilin-1; PlGF, placental growth factor; VEGFR-1, vascular endothelial growth factor receptor-1; VEGFR-2, vascular endothelial growth factor receptor-2; bFGF, basic fibroblast growth factor; FGFR, fibroblast growth factor receptors; TGF-β, transforming growth factor beta; TGF-R, transforming growth factor receptor; Dll4, delta-like ligands.

7. Anti-Metastasis Effects of Bioactive Compounds in Gastric Cancer

Metastasis is a major contributor of death in cancer patients, arising from a growing tumor from which cells escape to distant organs of body [101]. Targeting metastasis is an attractive strategy in cancer treatment. Anti-metastatic ability is highlighted in diverse natural bioactive products in vitro and in vivo models. which are described below. Sulforaphane, an organosulfur compound isolated from *Brassica oleracea* var. *italica* Plenk (Brassicaceae), exerted anti-metastatic ability on AGS and MKN-45 cells [102]. Isoliquiritigenin, a phenol found in *Glycyrrhiza glabra* (Fabaceae), inhibited tumor migration and metastasis on MKN-28 cells [103]. Dehydroeffusol, a benzenoid derived from *Juncus effusus* L. *Radix et Medulla* (Juncaceae), inhibited matrix metalloproteinase 2 (MMP-2) and VE-cadherin expression, resulting in reduction of the cell-to-cell adherent junction in AGS and SGC-7901 cells [104]. Baicalein, a well-known flavone found in the roots of *Scutellaria baicalensis* Georgi *Radix* (Lamiaceae), restrains motility, migration, and invasion of AGS gastric cancer cells via downregulation of N-cadherin, vimentin, ZEB1, ZEB2, and TGF-β/Smad4 [105]. Andrographolide, a labdane diterpenoid from the herb *Andrographis paniculata* Nees *Herba* (Acanthaceae), inhibits proliferation and metastasis of gastric cancer

SGC-7901 via cell cycle arrest; upregulation of Bax, Bik, and TIMP-1/2; and downregulation of Bcl-2, CD147, MMP-2, and MMP-9 [106]. Blockages of tumor proliferation and metastasis of several bioactive compounds are presented in Table 4 and Figure 4. It has been found that evodiamine, isolated from *Evoida rutaecarpa* (Rutaceae), suppressed the epithelial–mesenchymal transition (EMT) of AGS and SGC-7901 gastric cancer cells via inhibition of the Wnt/β-catenin signaling pathway [107]. A triterpenoid found from *Melia toosendan* Sieb et Zucc (Meiliaceae), named toosendanin, has anti-metastatic capability on SGC-7901 cells through inhibition of the epithelial–mesenchymal transition of gastric cancer by upregulating miR-200a and e-cadherin and suppressing β-catenin [60]. Low-molecular-weight citrus pectin (LCP), derived from tangerines, grapefruits, lemons, and oranges, demonstrated anti-metastatic effects by treatment on AGS cells [108]. N-butylidenephthalide inhibited tumor metastasis in AGS, NCI-N87, and TSGH-9201 cells. The compound promoted e-cadherin expression while downregulating n-cadherin and vimentin slug. The activity of e-cadherin was repressed on the other hand, which inhibited EGFR kinase activity [57]. The mechanism leads to downstream regulation of multiple growth factor-related activities, which is associated with anti-metastatic activities of such natural bioactive products. In other aspects, the Bcl-2 family of proteins was also found to play a role in anti-metastatic effects of natural bioactive products [109]. Many other factors including PI3K, Akt, Rac1, and CDX1/2 play a role in anti-metastatic activity of natural bioactive compounds, some of which are also related to apoptosis of tumor cells. As it is unclear whether natural products exert anti-metastatic effects in a multi-target manner, further study is therefore required to distinguish the specific mechanism.

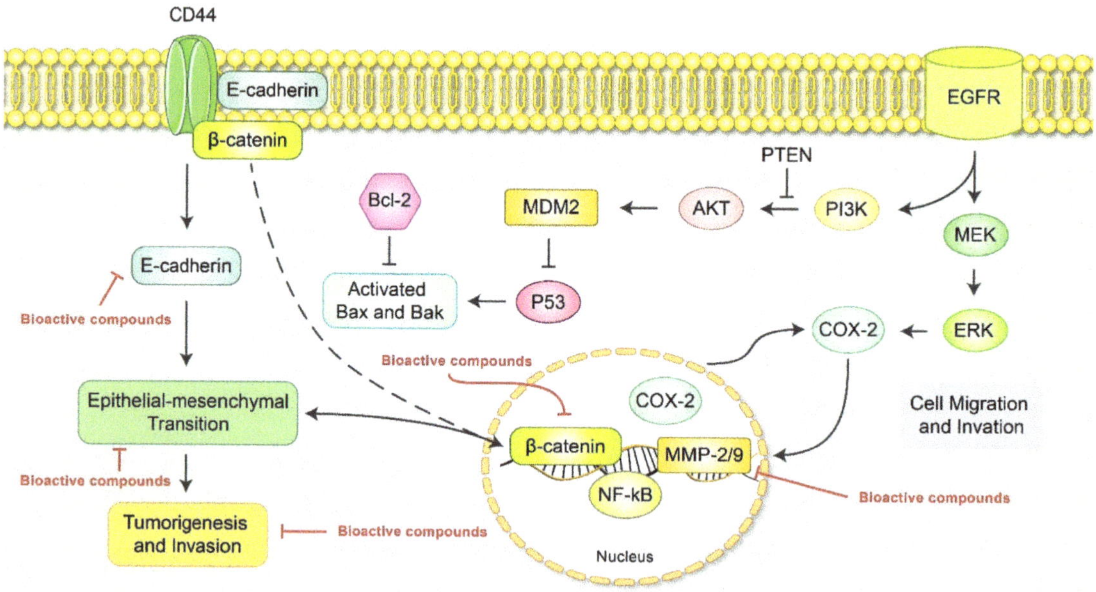

Figure 4. Schematic diagram of metastasis signaling pathways and regulation by bioactive compounds. Akt, protein kinase B; Bak, Bcl-2 antagonist/killer 1; Bax, Bcl-2-like protein 4; Bcl-2, B-cell lymphoma 2; CD44, homing cell adhesion molecule; COX-2, cyclooxygenase 2; EGFR, epidermal growth factor receptor; ERK, extracellular signal-regulated kinase; MDM2, murine double minute 2; MEK, matrix metalloproteinase-2/9; NF-κB, nuclear factor kappa-B; PI3K, phosphoinositide 3-kinase; PTEN, phosphatase and tensin homolog.

Table 4. Metastasis-inhibiting bioactive food components *in vitro* in gastric cancer. (↑ increase, ↓ decrease).

Classification	Compound	Source	Experimental Model	Doses	Efficacy	Mechanisms	Reference
Alkaloids	Evodiamine	(family: Rutaceae) *Tetradium ruticarpum*	AGS, SGC-7901	2 μM; 48 h	Inhibition of EMT	↓β-catenin, cyclin D1, c-Myc	[107]
Organosulfur compounds	Sulforaphane	(family: Brassicaceae) *Brassica oleracea* var. *italica* Plenk	AGS, MKN-45	31.25, 62.5, 125, 250 μg/mL; 48 h	Inhibition of metastasis	↑CDX1, CDX2 ↑miR-326, miR-9	[102]
Polyphenols	Isoliquiritigenin	(family: Fabaceae) *Glycyrrhiza glabra Radix*	MKN-28	20 μM; 24, 48, 72 h	Inhibition of migration, invasion, Induction of apoptosis and autophagy	↓Caspase-3, Bax, Bcl-2, PI3K, Akt, mTOR	[103]
Polyphenols	Dehydroeffusol	(family: Juncaceae) *Juncus effusus* L. *Radix et Medulla*	AGS, SGC-7901	12, 24, 48 μM; 24 h	Reduction of cell–cell adherent junction	↓VE-cadherin, MMP-2	[104]
Polyphenols	Paeonol	(family: Paeoniaceae) *Paeonia suffruticosa* Andr. *Cortex*, (family: Asclepiadaceae) *Cynanchum paniculatum* K. Schum *Radix*	BGC-823	0.1, 0.2, 0.4 mg/mL; 24, 48 h	Inhibition of proliferation, invasion, and migration, Induction of apoptosis	↓MMP-2, MMP-9	[58]
Polyphenols	Baicalein	(Lamiaceae) *Scutellaria baicalensis* Georgi *Radix*	AGS	25, 50 μM; 24 h	Inhibition of motility, migration, invasion	↓N-cadherin, vimentin, ZEB1, ZEB2, TGF-β/Smad4	[105]
Terpenoids	Andrographolide	(family: Acanthaceae) *Andrographis paniculata* Nees *Herba*	SGC-7901	5, 20, 40 μg/mL; 24, 48, 72 h	Inhibition of proliferation, invasion, metastasis	↑Bax, Bik, TIMP-1/2, ↓Bcl-2, CD147, MMP-2, MMP-9, survivin	[106]
Terpenoids	Toosendanin	(family: Meliaceae) *Melia toosendan Sieb* et Zucc *Cortex et Fructus*	SGC-7901	0.5, 1 μM; 48 h	Inhibition of invasion, migration, EMTInduction of apoptosis and cell cycle arrest	↑E-cadherin ↓β-catenin ↑miR-200a	[60]

8. Chemotherapy Resistance and Natural Bioactive Products in Gastric Cancer

Drug resistance is an important issue in cancer treatment and is known as a primary factor limiting cancer treatment [110]. Several studies have indicated that natural bioactive compounds could be used along with the primary drug to overcome drug resistance and reinforce its efficacy. In vitro drug resistance-overcoming bioactive food components in gastric cancer and their target signals are presented in Figure 5. Isorhamnetin, a flavonoid metabolite of quercetin commonly found in onions, minimized the apoptotic effects of capecitabine via inhibition of NF-κB and various NF-κB regulated gene products in tumor cells [111]. Liquiritin, isolated from *Glycyrrhiza uralensis* Fischer. *Radix* (Leguminosae/Fabaceae/Fabaceae), could circumvent the resistance of cisplatin-based chemotherapy via suppression of cell proliferation and induce apoptosis, autophagy, and G0/G1 phase cell cycle arrest against DDP-resistant gastric cancer cells [112]. Astragalus polysaccharide and apatinib co-treatment were reported to enhance apoptosis compared to apatinib monotherapy [113]. The efficacy of astragalus polysaccharide, an active component derived from *Astragalus mambranaceus* Bunge *Radix* (Leguminosae/Fabaceae/Fabaceae), arises mainly from its ability to inhibit autophagy of apatinib-resistant cells, which serves as a survival mechanism. Tanshinone IIA solution combined with doxorubicin showed anticancer effects against doxorubicin-resistant cell lines, including SNU-638, SNU-668, SNU-216, and SNU-620 [114]. Apoptosis was mainly induced by inhibition of multidrug resistance-associated protein 1 (MRP1). Although specific targets vary, most natural bioactive compounds aim to prevent drug resistance by downregulating Akt and NF-κB and following pathways (Figure 5). Mineral isorhamnetin from quercetin inhibited cell viability and prevented drug resistance by downregulating NF-κB. Liquirtin from the *Glycyrrhiza* genus promoted p53 and p21 and caspase cleavages while inhibiting cyclin activities. The compound's anti-resistant ability may be focused on apoptotic effects. Other factors such as Bax/Bcl-2 in mitochondria, and ERK1/2, MMP2, and PARP are broadly affected by many natural bioactive compounds.

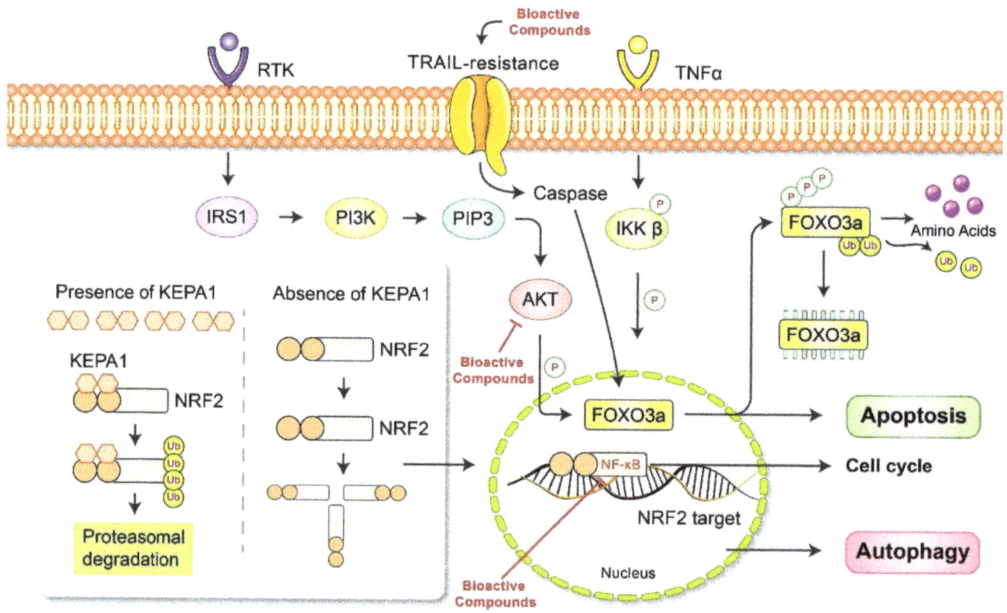

Figure 5. Schematic diagram of resistance signaling pathway. RTK, receptor tyrosine kinase; IRS1, insulin receptor substrate 1; PI3K, phosphoinositide 3-kinases; PIP3, phosphatidylinositol (3,4,5)-trisphosphate; AKT, protein kinase B (PKB); FOXO3a, forkhead box O 3; IKK-β, inhibitor of nuclear factor κB kinase subunit beta; TNF-α, tumor necrosis factor α; Ub, ubiquitin; KEAP1, Kelch-like ECH-associated protein 1; NRF2, nuclear factor erythroid 2-related factor 2.

9. Limitation and Future Perspectives of Natural Bioactive Food Products in Gastric Cancer Treatments

Gastric cancer is known to account for the fifth highest incidence and the fourth highest mortality among all cancers worldwide [1]. Chemotherapy is one of the methods typically used in advanced gastric cancer treatment, but it exerts severe side effects that limit the efficacies and decrease quality of life. Development of therapeutic remedies with less adverse effects and lower chemo-resistance is required. Natural bioactive food products are emerging as alternative resources to combat gastric carcinoma. Therefore, several natural bioactive resources obtained from dietary fruits and vegetables were discussed. Curcumin and oligosaccharide isolated from tomato, sulforaphane derived from broccoli, and citrus pectin originated from tangerine, grapefruit, lemon, and orange are good examples. These medicinal resources are still being extensively used in traditional medicine. Many natural bioactive food products were shown to exhibit multiple effects. The variety is attributed to the structural diversity and multi-target characteristic of natural compounds [115]. Additionally, clinical trials were excluded to focus on laboratory experiments highlighting specific biological pathways. Several investigations were insufficient to elucidate anti-cancer mechanisms at molecular levels in gastric cancer. They were generally focused on the cytotoxicity of the chemicals or the reporting of newly discovered compounds, which makes incisive research burdensome. By and large, more than half of the studies only carried out experiments in vitro. More in vivo studies are recommended to bridge the advance to clinical trials and therapeutic use.

Natural bioactive food products are indeed effective in the single compound to single target mechanistic perspective; however, it is worth highlighting the complex interactions between many compounds. While the importance of studying the interactions between multi-compound natural bioactive food products and other drugs was previously highlighted in many literatures, it is also important to further investigate the interactions between different natural bioactive food products, including herbal medicines, in a biochemical manner [116]. A systemic approach with a focus on structural similarities of several phytochemical compounds and human metabolites is a potential way of clearly highlighting the efficacies of multi compound drugs. Despite the value of natural bioactive food products as medicinal agents, it is important that users as well prescribers be aware of the potentially cross-reactivity and toxicity of natural bioactive food products. Indeed, it has often been stated that natural bioactive products are toxins that are taken at lower therapeutic doses. To avoid this problem, it is required to modify the natural chemical. Therefore, it is important to recognize that unmodified natural bioactive food products may have suboptimal efficacy or absorption, distribution, metabolism, excretion, as well as toxicity (ADMET) properties. Thus, for development of natural bioactive food products that lead to successful drugs, chemical modifications or combinations with other compounds are highly required. Furthermore, clinical development requires a sustainable and suitably economically viable compound supply with sufficient quantities of natural bioactive food products.

10. Conclusions

In this review, we summed up several natural bioactive food products that have anti-cancer efficacy against gastric cancer. Several epidemiological investigations have been recommended, namely that the consumption of bioactive dietary food products such as spices, vegetables, fruits, roots, bulk, and leafs are inversely related to the risk and control of gastric cancer. In vitro and in vivo studies have been exposed, namely that dietary bioactive products mainly induced cell death by apoptosis and autophagy, cell cycle arrest, inhibition of angiogenesis and metastasis, and circumvention of chemo-resistance against stomach cancer cells through various molecular mechanisms. Several compounds showed multiple efficacies, attributed to structural complexity and multiple target pathways and proteins of bioactive dietary food products. Thus, natural substances implicate possibilities of being used in nutrition or medications, which may lead to novel discoveries in alternative medicine in cancer treatment. Additionally, attention should be paid to the bioavailability and safety of dietary food product consumption and a promising approach for the management and prevention of gastric cancer. This review provides data for future research and clinical trials to develop novel drugs from natural bioactive food products for gastric cancer treatment.

Author Contributions: Methodology, S.Y.K.; validation, S.Y.K., D.H., S.S., and J.P.; investigation, S.Y.K., D.H., S.S., M.K., and J.P.; writing—original draft preparation, S.Y.K., D.H., S.S., M.K., and J.P.; writing—review and editing, S.Y.K., D.H., and B.K.; visualization, S.S., J.P., and D.H., and S.-G.K.; supervision, B.K.; project administration, B.K.; figure drawing and modification, M.H.R.; editing and reviewing, M.A.R.; funding acquisition, B.K. All authors have read and agreed to the published version of the manuscript.

Funding: This research was supported by Basic Science Research Program through the National Research Foundation of Korea (NRF) funded by the Ministry of Education (NRF-2020R1I1A2066868), the National Research Foundation of Korea (NRF) grant funded by the Korea government (MSIT) (No. 2020R1A5A2019413), a grant of the Korea Health Technology R&D Project through the Korea Health Industry Development Institute (KHIDI), funded by the Ministry of Health & Welfare, Republic of Korea (grant number: HF20C0116), and a grant from the Korea Health Technology R&D Project through the Korea Health Industry Development Institute (KHIDI), funded by the Ministry of Health & Welfare, Republic of Korea (grant number: HF20C0038).

Conflicts of Interest: The authors declare no conflict of interest.

References

1. Sung, H.; Ferlay, J.; Siegel, R.L.; Laversanne, M.; Soerjomataram, I.; Jemal, A.; Bray, F. Global Cancer Statistics 2020: GLOBOCAN Estimates of Incidence and Mortality Worldwide for 36 Cancers in 185 Countries. *CA Cancer J. Clin.* **2021**, *71*, 209–249. [CrossRef] [PubMed]
2. Hu, B.; El Hajj, N.; Sittler, S.; Lammert, N.; Barnes, R.; Meloni-Ehrig, A. Gastric cancer: Classification, histology and application of molecular pathology. *J. Gastrointest. Oncol.* **2012**, *3*, 251–261. [CrossRef] [PubMed]
3. Crew, K.D.; Neugut, A.I. Epidemiology of gastric cancer. *World J. Gastroenterol.* **2006**, *12*, 354–362. [CrossRef] [PubMed]
4. Rawla, P.; Barsouk, A. Epidemiology of gastric cancer: Global trends, risk factors and prevention. *Gastroenterol. Rev.* **2019**, *14*, 26–38. [CrossRef]
5. A Ajani, J.; D'Amico, T.A.; Almhanna, K.; Bentrem, D.J.; Chao, J.; Das, P.; Denlinger, C.S.; Fanta, P.; Farjah, F.; Fuchs, C.S.; et al. Gastric Cancer, Version 3.2016, NCCN Clinical Practice Guidelines in Oncology. *J. Natl. Compr. Cancer Netw.* **2016**, *14*, 1286–1312. [CrossRef] [PubMed]
6. Ronellenfitsch, U.; Schwarzbach, M.; Hofheinz, R.; Kienle, P.; Kieser, M.; E Slanger, T.; Jensen, K. GE adenocarcinoma meta-analysis group Perioperative chemo(radio)therapy versus primary surgery for resectable adenocarcinoma of the stomach, gastroesophageal junction, and lower esophagus. *Cochrane Database Syst. Rev.* **2013**, *2013*, 008107. [CrossRef]
7. Diaz-Nieto, R.; Orti-Rodríguez, R.; Winslet, M. Post-surgical chemotherapy versus surgery alone for resectable gastric cancer. *Cochrane Database Syst. Rev.* **2013**, *2013*, CD008415. [CrossRef]
8. Oba, K.; Paoletti, X.; Alberts, S.; Bang, Y.-J.; Benedetti, J.; Bleiberg, H.; Catalano, P.; Lordick, F.; Michiels, S.; Morita, S.; et al. Disease-Free Survival as a Surrogate for Overall Survival in Adjuvant Trials of Gastric Cancer: A Meta-Analysis. *J. Natl. Cancer Inst.* **2013**, *105*, 1600–1607. [CrossRef]
9. Gibson, R.J.; Keefe, D.M.K. Cancer chemotherapy-induced diarrhoea and constipation: Mechanisms of damage and prevention strategies. *Support. Care Cancer* **2006**, *14*, 890–900. [CrossRef] [PubMed]
10. Staff, N.P.; Grisold, A.; Grisold, W.; Windebank, A.J. Chemotherapy-induced peripheral neuropathy: A current review. *Ann. Neurol.* **2017**, *81*, 772–781. [CrossRef] [PubMed]
11. Yang, W.; Ma, J.; Zhou, W.; Cao, B.; Zhou, X.; Yang, Z.; Zhang, H.; Zhao, Q.; Fan, D.; Hong, L. Molecular mechanisms and theranostic potential of miRNAs in drug resistance of gastric cancer. *Expert Opin. Ther. Targets* **2017**, *21*, 1063–1075. [CrossRef]
12. Singh, N.; Baby, D.; Rajguru, J.P.; Patil, P.B.; Thakkannavar, S.S.; Pujari, V.B. Inflammation and cancer. *Ann. Afr. Med.* **2019**, *18*, 121–126. [CrossRef] [PubMed]
13. Lu, B.; Li, M. Helicobacter pylori eradication for preventing gastric cancer. *World J. Gastroenterol.* **2014**, *20*, 5660–5665. [CrossRef]
14. Sokolova, O.; Naumann, M. NF-kappaB Signaling in Gastric Cancer. *Toxins* **2017**, *9*, 119. [CrossRef] [PubMed]
15. Lee, H.; Jeong, A.J.; Ye, S.-K. Highlighted STAT3 as a potential drug target for cancer therapy. *BMB Rep.* **2019**, *52*, 415–423. [CrossRef] [PubMed]
16. Naylor, M.S.; Stamp, G.W.; Foulkes, W.; Eccles, D.; Balkwill, F. Tumor necrosis factor and its receptors in human ovarian cancer. Potential role in disease progression. *J. Clin. Investig.* **1993**, *91*, 2194–2206. [CrossRef] [PubMed]
17. Wang, X.; Lin, Y. Tumor necrosis factor and cancer, buddies or foes? *Acta Pharmacol. Sin.* **2008**, *29*, 1275–1288. [CrossRef]

18. Rabelo, A.C.S.; Camini, F.C.; Bittencourt, M.M.; Lacerda, K.; De Lima, W.G.; Costa, D.C. Baccharis trimera (carqueja) promotes gastroprotection on ethanol-induced acute gastric ulcer. *Adv. Tradit. Med.* **2020**, *20*, 563–570. [CrossRef]
19. Bastos, J.; Lunet, N.; Peleteiro, B.; Lopes, C.; Barros, H. Dietary patterns and gastric cancer in a Portuguese urban population. *Int. J. Cancer* **2010**, *127*, 433–441. [CrossRef]
20. Nagata, C.; Takatsuka, N.; Kawakami, N.; Shimizu, H. A prospective cohort study of soy product intake and stomach cancer death. *Br. J. Cancer* **2002**, *87*, 31–36. [CrossRef]
21. Steevens, J.; Schouten, L.J.; Goldbohm, R.A.; Brandt, P.V.D. Vegetables and fruits consumption and risk of esophageal and gastric cancer subtypes in the Netherlands Cohort Study. *Int. J. Cancer* **2011**, *129*, 2681–2693. [CrossRef] [PubMed]
22. Mao, Q.-Q.; Xu, X.-Y.; Shang, A.; Gan, R.-Y.; Wu, D.-T.; Atanasov, A.G.; Li, H.-B. Phytochemicals for the Prevention and Treatment of Gastric Cancer: Effects and Mechanisms. *Int. J. Mol. Sci.* **2020**, *21*, 570. [CrossRef] [PubMed]
23. Xu, J.; Long, Y.; Ni, L.; Yuan, X.; Yu, N.; Wu, R.; Tao, J.; Zhang, Y. Anticancer effect of berberine based on experimental animal models of various cancers: A systematic review and meta-analysis. *BMC Cancer* **2019**, *19*, 1–20. [CrossRef]
24. Hassanalilou, T.; Ghavamzadeh, S.; Khalili, L. Curcumin and Gastric Cancer: A Review on Mechanisms of Action. *J. Gastrointest. Cancer* **2019**, *50*, 185–192. [CrossRef] [PubMed]
25. Dutta, S.; Mahalanobish, S.; Saha, S.; Ghosh, S.; Sil, P.C. Natural products: An upcoming therapeutic approach to cancer. *Food Chem. Toxicol.* **2019**, *128*, 240–255. [CrossRef]
26. Kim, H.-J.; Um, J.-Y.; Kim, Y.-K. Glutathione S-transferase gene polymorphism in Korean subjects with gastric and colorectal cancer. *Orient. Pharm. Exp. Med.* **2012**, *12*, 307–312. [CrossRef]
27. Mann, J. Natural products in cancer chemotherapy: Past, present and future. *Nat. Rev. Cancer* **2002**, *2*, 143–148. [CrossRef]
28. Wang, L.; Dong, C.; Li, X.; Han, W.; Su, X. Anticancer potential of bioactive peptides from animal sources (Review). *Oncol. Rep.* **2017**, *38*, 637–651. [CrossRef]
29. Gras, M.; Vallard, A.; Brosse, C.; Beneton, A.; Sotton, S.; Guyotat, D.; Fournel, P.; Daguenet, E.; Magné, N.; Morisson, S. Use of Complementary and Alternative Medicines among Cancer Patients: A Single-Center Study. *Oncology* **2019**, *97*, 18–25. [CrossRef]
30. Li, X.; Yang, G.; Li, X.; Zhang, Y.; Yang, J.; Chang, J.; Sun, X.; Zhou, X.; Guo, Y.; Xu, Y.; et al. Traditional Chinese medicine in cancer care: A review of controlled clinical studies published in chinese. *PLoS ONE* **2013**, *8*, e60338.
31. Wode, K.; Henriksson, R.; Sharp, L.; Stoltenberg, A.; Nordberg, J.H. Cancer patients' use of complementary and alternative medicine in Sweden: A cross-sectional study. *BMC Complement. Altern. Med.* **2019**, *19*, 1–11. [CrossRef]
32. Kristoffersen, A.E.; Stub, T.; Broderstad, A.R.; Hansen, A.H. Use of traditional and complementary medicine among Norwegian cancer patients in the seventh survey of the Tromsø study. *BMC Complement. Altern. Med.* **2019**, *19*, 1–13. [CrossRef] [PubMed]
33. Elmore, S. Apoptosis: A review of programmed cell death. *Toxicol. Pathol.* **2007**, *35*, 495–516. [CrossRef] [PubMed]
34. Redza-Dutordoir, M.; Averill-Bates, D.A. Activation of apoptosis signalling pathways by reactive oxygen species. *Biochim. Biophys. Acta Bioenerg.* **2016**, *1863*, 2977–2992. [CrossRef] [PubMed]
35. Yang, Y.; Zhang, N.; Li, K.; Chen, J.; Qiu, L.; Zhang, J. Integration of microRNA-mRNA profiles and pathway analysis of plant isoquinoline alkaloid berberine in SGC-7901 gastric cancers cells. *Drug Des. Devel. Ther.* **2018**, *12*, 393–408. [CrossRef]
36. Wu, J.; Tan, Z.; Chen, J.; Dong, C. Cyclovirobuxine D Inhibits Cell Proliferation and Induces Mitochondria-Mediated Apoptosis in Human Gastric Cancer Cells. *Molecules* **2015**, *20*, 20659–20668. [CrossRef]
37. Lu, X.; Ma, J.; Qiu, H.; Yang, L.; Cao, L.; Shen, J. Anti-proliferation effects of trifolirhizin on MKN45 cells and possible mechanism. *Oncol. Rep.* **2016**, *36*, 2785–2792. [CrossRef]
38. Qian, J.; Li, J.; Jia, J.-G.; Jin, X.; Yu, D.-J.; Guo, C.-X.; Xie, B.; Qian, L.-Y. Ginsenoside-Rh2 Inhibits Proliferation and Induces Apoptosis of Human Gastric Cancer SGC-7901 Side Population Cells. *Asian Pac. J. Cancer Prev.* **2016**, *17*, 1817–1821. [CrossRef] [PubMed]
39. Su, C.-C. Tanshinone IIA inhibits gastric carcinoma AGS cells through increasing p-p38, p-JNK and p53 but reducing p-ERK, CDC2 and cyclin B1 expression. *Anticancer. Res.* **2014**, *34*, 7097–7110. [PubMed]
40. Zhu, H.; Zheng, Z.; Zhang, J.; Liu, X.; Liu, Y.; Yang, W.; Liu, Y.; Zhang, T.; Zhao, Y.; Liu, Y.; et al. Anticancer effect of 2,7-dihydroxy-3-methylanthraquinone on human gastric cancer SGC-7901 cells in vitro and in vivo. *Pharm. Biol.* **2016**, *54*, 285–292. [CrossRef]
41. Luo, Y.; Yu, H.; Yang, Y.; Tian, W.; Dong, K.; Shan, J.; Ma, X. A flavonoid compound from Chrysosplenium nudicaule inhibits growth and induces apoptosis of the human stomach cancer cell line SGC-7901. *Pharm. Biol.* **2016**, *54*, 1133–1139. [CrossRef]
42. Sun, Q.; Zhang, W.; Guo, Y.; Li, Z.; Chen, X.; Wang, Y.; Du, Y.; Zang, W.; Zhao, G. Curcumin inhibits cell growth and induces cell apoptosis through upregulation of miR-33b in gastric cancer. *Tumor Biol.* **2016**, *37*, 13177–13184. [CrossRef]
43. Pan, H.; Wang, B.-H.; Lv, W.; Jiang, Y.; He, L. Esculetin induces apoptosis in human gastric cancer cells through a cyclophilin D-mediated mitochondrial permeability transition pore associated with ROS. *Chem. Interactions* **2015**, *242*, 51–60. [CrossRef] [PubMed]
44. Liu, L.; Si, N.; Ma, Y.; Ge, D.; Yu, X.; Fan, A.; Wang, X.; Hu, J.; Wei, P.; Chen, J.; et al. Hydroxysafflor-Yellow A Induces Human Gastric Carcinoma BGC-823 Cell Apoptosis by Activating Peroxisome Proliferator-Activated Receptor Gamma (PPARgamma). *Med. Sci. Monit.* **2018**, *24*, 803–811. [CrossRef]
45. Zhou, W.; Cao, A.; Wang, L.; Wu, D. Kurarinone Synergizes TRAIL-Induced Apoptosis in Gastric Cancer Cells. *Cell Biophys.* **2015**, *72*, 241–249. [CrossRef] [PubMed]

46. Wu, J.; Zhang, X.; Wang, Y.; Sun, Q.; Chen, M.; Liu, S.; Zou, X. Licochalcone A suppresses hexokinase 2-mediated tumor glycolysis in gastric cancer via downregulation of the Akt signaling pathway. *Oncol. Rep.* **2017**, *39*, 1181–1190. [CrossRef] [PubMed]
47. Jung, E.B.; Trinh, T.A.; Lee, T.K.; Yamabe, N.; Kang, K.S.; Song, J.H.; Choi, S.; Lee, S.; Jang, T.S.; Kim, K.H.; et al. Curcuzedoalide contributes to the cytotoxicity of Curcuma zedoaria rhizomes against human gastric cancer AGS cells through induction of apoptosis. *J. Ethnopharmacol.* **2018**, *213*, 48–55. [CrossRef] [PubMed]
48. Kang, S.-H.; Kim, Y.-S.; Kim, E.-K.; Hwang, J.-W.; Jeong, J.-H.; Dong, X.; Lee, J.-W.; Moon, S.-H.; Jeon, B.-T.; Park, P.-J. Anticancer Effect of Thymol on AGS Human Gastric Carcinoma Cells. *J. Microbiol. Biotechnol.* **2016**, *26*, 28–37. [CrossRef]
49. Zhang, W.; Zhang, Q.; Jiang, Y.; Li, F.; Xin, H. Effects of ophiopogonin B on the proliferation and apoptosis of SGC-7901 human gastric cancer cells. *Mol. Med. Rep.* **2016**, *13*, 4981–4986. [CrossRef] [PubMed]
50. Xu, M.; Gu, W.; Shen, Z.; Wang, F. Anticancer Activity of Phloretin Against Human Gastric Cancer Cell Lines Involves Apoptosis, Cell Cycle Arrest, and Inhibition of Cell Invasion and JNK Signalling Pathway. *Med. Sci. Monit.* **2018**, *24*, 6551–6558. [CrossRef]
51. Asl, E.A.; Mehrabadi, J.F.; Afshar, D.; Noorbazargan, H.; Tahmasebi, H.; Rahimi, A. Apoptotic Effects of Linum album Extracts on AGS Human Gastric Adenocarcinoma Cells and ZNF703 Oncogene Expression. *Asian Pac. J. Cancer Prev.* **2018**, *19*, 2911–2916. [CrossRef]
52. Wu, Z.; Li, Y. Grifolin exhibits anti-cancer activity by inhibiting the development and invasion of gastric tumor cells. *Oncotarget* **2017**, *8*, 21454–21460. [CrossRef] [PubMed]
53. Tsai, T.C.; Lai, K.-H.; Su, J.-H.; Wu, Y.-J.; Sheu, J.-H. 7-Acetylsinumaximol B Induces Apoptosis and Autophagy in Human Gastric Carcinoma Cells through Mitochondria Dysfunction and Activation of the PERK/eIF2alpha/ATF4/CHOP Signaling Pathway. *Mar. Drugs* **2018**, *16*, 104. [CrossRef] [PubMed]
54. Cheng, Q.-L.; Li, H.-L.; Li, Y.-C.; Liu, Z.-W.; Guo, X.-H.; Cheng, Y.-J. CRA (Crosolic Acid) isolated from Actinidia valvata Dunn.Radix induces apoptosis of human gastric cancer cell line BGC823 in vitro via down-regulation of the NF-kappaB pathway. *Food Chem. Toxicol.* **2017**, *105*, 475–485. [CrossRef]
55. Zhang, D.; Zhang, B.; Zhou, L.-X.; Zhao, J.; Yan, Y.-Y.; Li, Y.-L.; Zeng, J.-M.; Wang, L.-L.; Yang, B.; Lin, N.-M. Deacetylisovaltratum disrupts microtubule dynamics and causes G2/M-phase arrest in human gastric cancer cells in vitro. *Acta Pharmacol. Sin.* **2016**, *37*, 1597–1605. [CrossRef]
56. Li, P.; Zhou, X.; Sun, W.; Sheng, W.; Tu, Y.; Yu, Y.; Dong, J.; Ye, B.; Zheng, Z.; Lu, M. Elemene Induces Apoptosis of Human Gastric Cancer Cell Line BGC-823 via Extracellular Signal-Regulated Kinase (ERK) 1/2 Signaling Pathway. *Med. Sci. Monit.* **2017**, *23*, 809–817. [CrossRef] [PubMed]
57. Liao, K.-F.; Chiu, T.-L.; Huang, S.-Y.; Hsieh, T.-F.; Chang, S.-F.; Ruan, J.-W.; Chen, S.-P.; Pang, C.-Y.; Chiu, S.-C. Anti-Cancer Effects of Radix Angelica Sinensis (Danggui) and N-Butylidenephthalide on Gastric Cancer: Implications for REDD1 Activation and mTOR Inhibition. *Cell. Physiol. Biochem.* **2018**, *48*, 2231–2246. [CrossRef] [PubMed]
58. Lyu, Z.-K.; Li, C.-L.; Jin, Y.; Liu, Y.-Z.; Zhang, X.; Zhang, F.; Ning, L.-N.; Liang, E.-S.; Ma, M.; Gao, W.; et al. Paeonol exerts potential activities to inhibit the growth, migration and invasion of human gastric cancer BGC823 cells via downregulating MMP-2 and MMP-9. *Mol. Med. Rep.* **2017**, *16*, 7513–7519. [CrossRef] [PubMed]
59. Yu, F.; Li, K.; Chen, S.; Liu, Y.; Li, Y. Pseudolaric Acid B Circumvents Multidrug Resistance Phenotype in Human Gastric Cancer SGC7901/ADR Cells by Downregulating Cox-2 and P-gp Expression. *Cell Biophys.* **2014**, *71*, 119–126. [CrossRef] [PubMed]
60. Wang, G.; Huang, Y.-X.; Zhang, R.; Hou, L.-D.; Liu, H.; Chen, X.-Y.; Zhu, J.-S.; Zhang, J. Toosendanin suppresses oncogenic phenotypes of human gastric carcinoma SGC7901 cells partly via miR200amediated downregulation of beta-catenin pathway. *Int. J. Oncol.* **2017**, *51*, 1563–1573. [CrossRef]
61. Kapoor, S.; Dharmesh, S.M. Pectic Oligosaccharide from tomato exhibiting anticancer potential on a gastric cancer cell line: Structure-function relationship. *Carbohydr. Polym.* **2017**, *160*, 52–61. [CrossRef]
62. Zhang, H.; Wu, D.; Du, J.; Zhang, Y.; Su, Y. Anti-tumor effects of phenolic alkaloids of menispermum dauricum on gastric cancer in vivo and in vitro. *J. Cancer Res. Ther.* **2018**, *14*, 505. [CrossRef] [PubMed]
63. Wang, X.-P.; Wang, Q.-X.; Lin, H.-P.; Chang, N. Anti-tumor bioactivities of curcumin on mice loaded with gastric carcinoma. *Food Funct.* **2017**, *8*, 3319–3326. [CrossRef] [PubMed]
64. Cui, F.; Zan, X.; Li, Y.; Sun, W.; Yang, Y.; Ping, L. Grifola frondosaGlycoprotein GFG-3a Arrests S phase, Alters Proteome, and Induces Apoptosis in Human Gastric Cancer Cells. *Nutr. Cancer* **2016**, *68*, 267–279. [CrossRef] [PubMed]
65. Kong, G.-M.; Tao, W.-H.; Diao, Y.-L.; Fang, P.-H.; Wang, J.-J.; Bo, P.; Qian, F. Melittin induces human gastric cancer cell apoptosis via activation of mitochondrial pathway. *World J. Gastroenterol.* **2016**, *22*, 3186–3195. [CrossRef] [PubMed]
66. Zhang, X.-Z.; Wang, L.; Liu, D.-W.; Tang, G.-Y.; Zhang, H.-Y. Synergistic Inhibitory Effect of Berberine and d-Limonene on Human Gastric Carcinoma Cell Line MGC803. *J. Med. Food* **2014**, *17*, 955–962. [CrossRef] [PubMed]
67. Li, L.; Zhao, L.-M.; Dai, S.-L.; Cui, W.-X.; Lv, H.-L.; Chen, L.; Shan, B.-E. Periplocin Extracted from Cortex Periplocae Induced Apoptosis of Gastric Cancer Cells via the ERK1/2-EGR1 Pathway. *Cell Physiol. Biochem.* **2016**, *38*, 1939–1951. [CrossRef]
68. Mansingh, D.P.; Oj, S.; Sali, V.K.; Vasanthi, H.R. [6]-Gingerol-induced cell cycle arrest, reactive oxygen species generation, and disruption of mitochondrial membrane potential are associated with apoptosis in human gastric cancer (AGS) cells. *J. Biochem. Mol. Toxicol.* **2018**, *32*, e22206. [CrossRef] [PubMed]
69. Feng, Y.; He, D.; Yao, Z.; Klionsky, D.J. The machinery of macroautophagy. *Cell Res.* **2014**, *24*, 24–41. [CrossRef] [PubMed]
70. Rahman, M.A.; Rhim, H. Therapeutic implication of autophagy in neurodegenerative diseases. *BMB Rep.* **2017**, *50*, 345–354. [CrossRef] [PubMed]

71. Kang, R.; Zeh, H.J.; Lotze, M.T.; Tang, D. The Beclin 1 network regulates autophagy and apoptosis. *Cell Death Differ.* **2011**, *18*, 571–580. [CrossRef] [PubMed]
72. Rahman, M.A.; Hannan, M.A.; Dash, R.; Rahman, M.H.; Islam, R.; Uddin, M.J.; Sohag, A.A.M.; Rahman, M.H.; Rhim, H. Phytochemicals as a Complement to Cancer Chemotherapy: Pharmacological Modulation of the Autophagy-Apoptosis Pathway. *Front. Pharmacol.* **2021**, *12*, 639628. [CrossRef]
73. Rahman, M.A.; Rahman, M.S.; Rahman, M.H.; Rasheduzzaman, M.; Mamun-Or-Rashid, A.; Uddin, M.J.; Rahman, M.R.; Hwang, H.; Pang, M.G.; Rhim, H. Modulatory Effects of Autophagy on APP Processing as a Potential Treatment Target for Alzheimer's Disease. *Biomedicines* **2021**, *9*, 5. [CrossRef]
74. Onorati, A.V.; Dyczynski, M.; Ojha, R.; Amaravadi, R.K. Targeting autophagy in cancer. *Cancer* **2018**, *124*, 3307–3318. [CrossRef] [PubMed]
75. Mandhair, H.K.; Arambasic, M.; Novak, U.; Radpour, R. Molecular modulation of autophagy: New venture to target resistant cancer stem cells. *World J. Stem Cells* **2020**, *12*, 303–322. [CrossRef] [PubMed]
76. Uddin, M.S.; Rahman, M.A.; Kabir, M.T.; Behl, T.; Mathew, B.; Perveen, A.; Barreto, G.E.; Bin-Jumah, M.N.; Abdel-Daim, M.M.; Ashraf, G.M. Multifarious roles of mTOR signaling in cognitive aging and cerebrovascular dysfunction of Alzheimer's disease. *Iubmb. Life* **2020**, *72*, 1843–1855. [CrossRef]
77. Rahman, M.A.; Cho, Y.; Nam, G.; Rhim, H. Antioxidant Compound, Oxyresveratrol, Inhibits APP Production through the AMPK/ULK1/mTOR-Mediated Autophagy Pathway in Mouse Cortical Astrocytes. *Antioxidants* **2021**, *10*, 408. [CrossRef]
78. Tanida, I.; Ueno, T.; Kominami, E. LC3 conjugation system in mammalian autophagy. *Int. J. Biochem. Cell Biol.* **2004**, *36*, 2503–2518. [CrossRef]
79. Dooley, H.C.; Razi, M.; Polson, H.E.J.; Girardin, S.E.; Wilson, M.I.; Tooze, S.A. WIPI2 Links LC3 Conjugation with PI3P, Autophagosome Formation, and Pathogen Clearance by Recruiting Atg12–5-16L1. *Mol. Cell* **2014**, *55*, 238–252. [CrossRef]
80. Rahman, M.A.; Rahman, M.H.; Hossain, M.S.; Biswas, P.; Islam, R.; Uddin, M.J.; Rahman, M.H.; Rhim, H. Molecular Insights into the Multifunctional Role of Natural Compounds: Autophagy Modulation and Cancer Prevention. *Biomedicines* **2020**, *8*, 517. [CrossRef]
81. Rahman, M.A.; Cho, Y.; Hwang, H.; Rhim, H. Pharmacological Inhibition of O-GlcNAc Transferase Promotes mTOR-Dependent Autophagy in Rat Cortical Neurons. *Brain Sci.* **2020**, *10*, 958. [CrossRef] [PubMed]
82. Pang, X.; Zhang, X.; Jiang, Y.; Su, Q.; Li, Q.; Li, Z. Autophagy: Mechanisms and Therapeutic Potential of Flavonoids in Cancer. *Biomolecules* **2021**, *11*, 135. [CrossRef]
83. Song, J.; Zhou, Y.; Gong, Y.; Liu, H.; Tang, L. Rottlerin promotes autophagy and apoptosis in gastric cancer cell lines. *Mol. Med. Rep.* **2018**, *18*, 2905–2913. [CrossRef] [PubMed]
84. Batool, S.; Joseph, T.P.; Hussain, M.; Vuai, M.S.; Khinsar, K.H.; Din, S.R.U.; Padhiar, A.A.; Zhong, M.; Ning, A.; Zhang, W.; et al. LP1 from Lentinula edodes C91-3 Induces Autophagy, Apoptosis and Reduces Metastasis in Human Gastric Cancer Cell Line SGC-7901. *Int. J. Mol. Sci.* **2018**, *19*, 2986. [CrossRef] [PubMed]
85. Kwon, Y.H.; Bishayee, K.; Rahman, A.; Hong, J.S.; Lim, S.-S.; Huh, S.-O. Morus alba Accumulates Reactive Oxygen Species to Initiate Apoptosis via FOXO-Caspase 3-Dependent Pathway in Neuroblastoma Cells. *Mol. Cells* **2015**, *38*, 630–637. [CrossRef] [PubMed]
86. Rahman, M.A.; Bishayee, K.; Sadra, A.; Huh, S.-O. Oxyresveratrol activates parallel apoptotic and autophagic cell death pathways in neuroblastoma cells. *Biochim. Biophys Acta Gen. Subj.* **2017**, *1861*, 23–36. [CrossRef] [PubMed]
87. Kim, T.W.; Lee, S.Y.; Kim, M.; Cheon, C.; Ko, S.-G. Kaempferol induces autophagic cell death via IRE1-JNK-CHOP pathway and inhibition of G9a in gastric cancer cells. *Cell Death Dis.* **2018**, *9*, 875. [CrossRef] [PubMed]
88. Lee, H.J.; Saralamma, V.V.G.; Kim, S.M.; Ha, S.E.; Raha, S.; Lee, W.S.; Kim, E.H.; Lee, S.J.; Heo, J.D.; Kim, G.S. Pectolinarigenin Induced Cell Cycle Arrest, Autophagy, and Apoptosis in Gastric Cancer Cell via PI3K/AKT/mTOR Signaling Pathway. *Nutrients* **2018**, *10*, 1043. [CrossRef] [PubMed]
89. Zhang, Y.; Liu, S.; Feng, Q.; Huang, X.; Wang, X.; Peng, Y.; Zhao, Z.; Liu, Z. Perilaldehyde activates AMP-activated protein kinase to suppress the growth of gastric cancer via induction of autophagy. *J. Cell. Biochem.* **2019**, *120*, 1716–1725. [CrossRef]
90. Wang, K.; Liu, R.; Li, J.; Mao, J.; Lei, Y.; Wu, J.; Zeng, J.; Zhang, T.; Wu, H.; Chen, L.; et al. Quercetin induces protective autophagy in gastric cancer cells: Involvement of Akt-mTOR- and hypoxia-induced factor 1alpha-mediated signaling. *Autophagy* **2011**, *7*, 966–978. [CrossRef]
91. Mrakovcic, M.; Fröhlich, L. p53-Mediated Molecular Control of Autophagy in Tumor Cells. *Biomolecules* **2018**, *8*, 14. [CrossRef]
92. Zhou, Q.; Wu, X.; Wen, C.; Wang, H.; Wang, H.; Liu, H.; Peng, J. Toosendanin induces caspase-dependent apoptosis through the p38 MAPK pathway in human gastric cancer cells. *Biochem. Biophys. Res. Commun.* **2018**, *505*, 261–266. [CrossRef]
93. Cao, Y.; Arbiser, J.; D'Amato, R.J.; D'Amore, P.A.; Ingber, D.E.; Kerbel, R.; Klagsbrun, M.; Lim, S.; Moses, M.A.; Zetter, B.; et al. Forty-Year Journey of Angiogenesis Translational Research. *Sci. Transl. Med.* **2011**, *3*, 114rv3. [CrossRef] [PubMed]
94. Wang, Z.; Dabrosin, C.; Yin, X.; Fuster, M.M.; Arreola, A.; Rathmell, W.K.; Generali, D.; Nagaraju, G.P.; El-Rayes, B.; Ribatti, D.; et al. Broad targeting of angiogenesis for cancer prevention and therapy. *Semin. Cancer Biol.* **2015**, *35*, S224–S243. [CrossRef] [PubMed]
95. Yang, J.; Wang, Q.; Qiao, C.; Lin, Z.; Li, X.; Huang, Y.; Zhou, T.; Li, Y.; Shen, B.; Lv, M.; et al. Potent anti-angiogenesis and anti-tumor activity of a novel human anti-VEGF antibody, MIL60. *Cell. Mol. Immunol.* **2014**, *11*, 285–293. [CrossRef]

96. Eklund, L.; Bry, M.; Alitalo, K. Mouse models for studying angiogenesis and lymphangiogenesis in cancer. *Mol. Oncol.* **2013**, *7*, 259–282. [CrossRef] [PubMed]
97. Huang, W.; Wang, J.; Liang, Y.; Ge, W.; Wang, G.; Li, Y.; Chung, H.Y. Potent anti-angiogenic component in Croton crassifolius and its mechanism of action. *J. Ethnopharmacol.* **2015**, *175*, 185–191. [CrossRef] [PubMed]
98. Tsuboi, K.; Matsuo, Y.; Shamoto, T.; Shibata, T.; Koide, S.; Morimoto, M.; Guha, S.; Sung, B.; Aggarwal, B.B.; Takahashi, H.; et al. Zerumbone inhibits tumor angiogenesis via NF-kappaB in gastric cancer. *Oncol. Rep.* **2014**, *31*, 57–64. [CrossRef] [PubMed]
99. Manu, K.A.; Shanmugam, M.K.; Rajendran, P.; Li, F.; Ramachandran, L.; Hay, H.S.; Kannaiyan, R.; Swamy, S.N.; Vali, S.; Kapoor, S.; et al. Plumbagin inhibits invasion and migration of breast and gastric cancer cells by downregulating the expression of chemokine receptor CXCR4. *Mol. Cancer* **2011**, *10*, 107. [CrossRef] [PubMed]
100. Chen, J.; Wang, J.; Lin, L.; He, L.; Wu, Y.; Zhang, L.; Yi, Z.; Chen, Y.; Pang, X.; Liu, M. Inhibition of STAT3 Signaling Pathway by Nitidine Chloride Suppressed the Angiogenesis and Growth of Human Gastric Cancer. *Mol. Cancer Ther.* **2012**, *11*, 277–287. [CrossRef]
101. Suhail, Y.; Cain, M.P.; Vanaja, K.; Kurywchak, P.A.; Levchenko, A.; Kalluri, R. Kshitiz Systems Biology of Cancer Metastasis. *Cell Syst.* **2019**, *9*, 109–127. [CrossRef]
102. Kiani, S.; Akhavan-Niaki, H.; Fattahi, S.; Kavoosian, S.; Jelodar, N.B.; Bagheri, N.; Zarrini, H.N. Purified sulforaphane from broccoli (Brassica oleracea var. italica) leads to alterations of CDX1 and CDX2 expression and changes in miR-9 and miR-326 levels in human gastric cancer cells. *Gene* **2018**, *678*, 115–123. [CrossRef]
103. Zhang, X.; Wang, S.; Sun, W.; Wei, C. Isoliquiritigenin inhibits proliferation and metastasis of MKN28 gastric cancer cells by suppressing the PI3K/AKT/mTOR signaling pathway. *Mol. Med. Rep.* **2018**, *18*, 3429–3436. [CrossRef]
104. Liu, W.; Meng, M.; Zhang, B.; Du, L.; Pan, Y.; Yang, P.; Gu, Z.; Zhou, Q.; Cao, Z. Dehydroeffusol effectively inhibits human gastric cancer cell-mediated vasculogenic mimicry with low toxicity. *Toxicol. Appl. Pharmacol.* **2015**, *287*, 98–110. [CrossRef]
105. Chen, F.; Zhuang, M.; Peng, J.; Wang, X.; Huang, T.; Li, S.; Lin, M.; Lin, H.; Xu, Y.; Li, J.; et al. Baicalein inhibits migration and invasion of gastric cancer cells through suppression of the TGF-beta signaling pathway. *Mol. Med. Rep.* **2014**, *10*, 1999–2003. [CrossRef]
106. Dai, L.; Wang, G.; Pan, W. Andrographolide Inhibits Proliferation and Metastasis of SGC7901 Gastric Cancer Cells. *BioMed Res. Int.* **2017**, *2017*, 1–10. [CrossRef] [PubMed]
107. Wen, Z.; Feng, S.; Wei, L.; Wang, Z.; Hong, D.; Wang, Q. Evodiamine, a novel inhibitor of the Wnt pathway, inhibits the self-renewal of gastric cancer stem cells. *Int. J. Mol. Med.* **2015**, *36*, 1657–1663. [CrossRef] [PubMed]
108. Wang, S.; Li, P.; Lu, S.-M.; Ling, Z.-Q. Chemoprevention of Low-Molecular-Weight Citrus Pectin (LCP) in Gastrointestinal Cancer Cells. *Int. J. Biol. Sci.* **2016**, *12*, 746–756. [CrossRef] [PubMed]
109. Kirkin, V.; Joos, S.; Zornig, M. The role of Bcl-2 family members in tumorigenesis. *Biochim. Biophys. Acta* **2004**, *1644*, 229–249. [CrossRef]
110. Vasan, N.; Baselga, J.; Hyman, D.M. A view on drug resistance in cancer. *Nature* **2019**, *575*, 299–309. [CrossRef] [PubMed]
111. Manu, K.A.; Shanmugam, M.K.; Ramachandran, L.; Li, F.; Siveen, K.S.; Chinnathambi, A.; Zayed, M.E.; Alharbi, S.A.; Arfuso, F.; Kumar, A.P.; et al. Isorhamnetin augments the anti-tumor effect of capecitabine through the negative regulation of NF-kappaB signaling cascade in gastric cancer. *Cancer Lett.* **2015**, *363*, 28–36. [CrossRef]
112. Wei, F.; Jiang, X.; Gao, H.-Y.; Gao, S.-H. Liquiritin induces apoptosis and autophagy in cisplatin (DDP)-resistant gastric cancer cells in vitro and xenograft nude mice in vivo. *Int. J. Oncol.* **2017**, *51*, 1383–1394. [CrossRef]
113. Wu, J.; Yu, J.; Wang, J.; Zhang, C.; Shang, K.; Yao, X.; Cao, B. Astragalus polysaccharide enhanced antitumor effects of Apatinib in gastric cancer AGS cells by inhibiting AKT signalling pathway. *Biomed. Pharmacother.* **2018**, *100*, 176–183. [CrossRef] [PubMed]
114. Xu, Z.; Chen, L.; Xiao, Z.; Zhu, Y.; Jiang, H.; Jin, Y.; Gu, C.; Wu, Y.; Wang, L.; Zhang, W.; et al. Potentiation of the anticancer effect of doxorubicinin drug-resistant gastric cancer cells by tanshinone IIA. *Phytomedicine* **2018**, *51*, 58–67. [CrossRef] [PubMed]
115. Guerra, A.R.; Duarte, M.F.; Duarte, I.F. Targeting Tumor Metabolism with Plant-Derived Natural Products: Emerging Trends in Cancer Therapy. *J. Agric. Food Chem.* **2018**, *66*, 10663–10685. [CrossRef] [PubMed]
116. Roe, A.L.; Paine, M.F.; Gurley, B.J.; Brouwer, K.R.; Jordan, S.; Griffiths, J.C. Assessing Natural Product–Drug Interactions: An End-to-End Safety Framework. *Regul. Toxicol. Pharmacol.* **2016**, *76*, 1–6. [CrossRef]

MDPI
St. Alban-Anlage 66
4052 Basel
Switzerland
Tel. +41 61 683 77 34
Fax +41 61 302 89 18
www.mdpi.com

Cancers Editorial Office
E-mail: cancers@mdpi.com
www.mdpi.com/journal/cancers

www.ingramcontent.com/pod-product-compliance
Lightning Source LLC
Chambersburg PA
CBHW061548220926
51850CB00005B/282
9783036583839